# Medical Research:
# A Midcentury Survey

*Volume II*

UNSOLVED CLINICAL PROBLEMS:
in biological perspective

*Volume I*

## AMERICAN MEDICAL RESEARCH:
### in principle and practice

*Volume II*

## UNSOLVED CLINICAL PROBLEMS:
### in biological perspective

# Medical Research:
# A Midcentury Survey

*Volume II*

UNSOLVED CLINICAL PROBLEMS:
in biological perspective

*Published for*
The American Foundation
565 Fifth Avenue, New York 17
and
Westbrook, Connecticut

*by*
Little, Brown and Company
Boston · Toronto

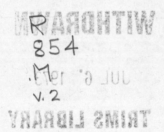
*Published simultaneously in Canada*
*by Little, Brown & Company (Canada) Limited.*
*Published in Great Britain by J. & A. Churchill Ltd., London.*

PRINTED IN THE UNITED STATES OF AMERICA BY
THE RIVERSIDE PRESS, CAMBRIDGE, MASSACHUSETTS

## THE AMERICAN FOUNDATION

# MEDICAL RESEARCH: A MIDCENTURY SURVEY

ESTHER EVERETT LAPE

*Associates*
ELEANOR M. PHILLIPS
MARGARET THOMAS EDGAR

*Secretarial staff*
HELEN C. HAHN
HAZEL BERRY
EVELYN R. HAHN

# COMMITTEE OF CONSULTANTS

The Committee of Consultants joins the American Foundation in presenting this study to the public. The American Foundation assumes the responsibility of authorship. The Committee of Consultants endorses the major intent of the report — to stress the imperative significance of basic research in solution of outstanding medical problems — and the objectivity of the American Foundation's purpose and performance.

### WALTER BAUER

*Jackson professor of clinical medicine, Harvard medical school; chief of medical services, Massachusetts General Hospital; president (1947), American Rheumatism Association*

### GEORGE H. BISHOP

*Professor emeritus of neurophysiology, Washington University school of medicine*

### AUSTIN M. BRUES

*Director, division of biological and medical research, Argonne National Laboratory; professor of medicine, University of Chicago; president (1954–1955), American Association for Cancer Research; president (1955), Radiation Research Society*

### GEORGE W. CORNER

*Director, department of embryology, Carnegie Institution of Washington; chairman, committee for research on problems of sex, National Research Council*

### RENÉ J. DUBOS

*Member, Rockefeller Institute for Medical Research*

### C. A. ELVEHJEM

*Dean, graduate school, University of Wisconsin; chairman, department of biochemistry*

### LOUIS F. FIESER

*Sheldon Emory professor of organic chemistry, Converse Memorial Laboratory, Harvard University*

### THOMAS FRANCIS, JR.

*Director, Virus Laboratory, and chairman, department of epidemiology, University of Michigan school of public health; director, Commission on Influenza, Armed Forces Epidemiological Board*

### RALPH W. GERARD

*Professor of neurophysiology, Mental Health Research Institute, University of Michigan*

### MICHAEL HEIDELBERGER

*Professor of immunochemistry, Columbia University College of Physicians and Surgeons*

### WILLIAM G. LENNOX

*Chief of Seizure Division, Neurological Institute of the Children's Medical Center; president (1945), Association for Research in Nervous and Mental Diseases*

### ESMOND R. LONG

*Retiring (1955) director, Henry Phipps Institute for the study, treatment and prevention of tuberculosis; professor emeritus of pathology, University of Pennsylvania school of medicine; chairman (1936–1939), division of medical sciences, National Research Council*

(continued)

### WILLIAM S. McCANN

*Dewey professor of medicine and head of the department, University of Rochester school of medicine and dentistry; physician in chief, Strong Memorial Hospital and Rochester Municipal Hospital*

### THOMAS PARRAN

*Dean, graduate school of public health, University of Pittsburgh; Surgeon General (1936–1948), United States Public Health Service*

### LINUS C. PAULING

*Director, Gates and Crellin laboratories of chemistry, California Institute of Technology; president (1949), American Chemical Society; Nobel laureate (1954) in chemistry*

### JOHN P. PETERS

*John Slade Ely professor of medicine, Yale school of medicine; associate physician, New Haven Hospital*

### I. S. RAVDIN

*John Rhea Barton professor of surgery and director, Harrison Department of Surgical Research, University of Pennsylvania school of medicine; chairman, board of regents, American College of Surgeons*

### FRANCIS O. SCHMITT

*Head of the department of biology, Massachusetts Institute of Technology*

### TRUMAN G. SCHNABEL

*Chairman (1949–1951), American Board of Internal Medicine; emeritus professor of medicine, University of Pennsylvania*

### W. M. STANLEY

*Director, virus laboratory, and professor of biochemistry, University of California at Berkeley; Nobel laureate (1946) in chemistry*

### DeWITT STETTEN, JR.

*Associate director in charge of research, National Institute of Arthritis and Metabolic Diseases*

### E. L. TATUM

*Professor of biology, Stanford University*

### STAFFORD L. WARREN

*Dean and professor of biophysics, school of medicine, University of California at Los Angeles Medical Center*

### PAUL A. WEISS

*Member, Rockefeller Institute for Medical Research; chairman, division of biology and agriculture, National Research Council*

### M. C. WINTERNITZ

*Chairman (1950–1953), division of medical sciences, National Research Council; dean (1920–1935), Yale school of medicine; chairman (1948–1950), committee on growth, National Research Council*

### JOHN B. YOUMANS

*Dean and professor of medicine, Vanderbilt University school of medicine*

*Both the man of science and the man of art live always at the edge of mystery, surrounded by it; both always, as the measure of their creation, have had to do with the harmonization of what is new with what is familiar, with the balance between novelty and synthesis, with the struggle to make partial order in total chaos.*

*They can, in their work and in their lives, help themselves, help one another and help all men.*

ROBERT OPPENHEIMER

*The foreword and introductory sections of Volume I have bearing also on Volume II and are therefore reprinted in this volume.*

# FOREWORD

A few words may review for those that do not already know it the general motivation of the American Foundation since its establishment by Edward Bok in 1924. I will not, in this distant year, speak directly for my father. I believe his general purposes have been reflected in the policies followed by me and my associate Esther Everett Lape, his choice and mine for the direction of our studies over the past thirty years.

In all of these studies, our objective has been to set up defenses against the lack of fact and the weight of particular propaganda that inhibit clear thinking on many important questions. We could deal with only one of these at a time. There are few public questions that would not profit from a review of all of the facts by an objective research agency that has public confidence, and from wide dissemination of the published findings.

This is the purpose that has unified the different subjects that have constituted the American Foundation's projects over the years. In all of these our dominant purpose has been the same. Our effort has been to clarify such different problems as the role, in international relations, of the judicial settlement of international disputes and the progressive codification of international law; the relations of record between the United States and the Soviet Union; the principles involved in ways of distributing and paying for medical care; and finally, in the present report, research in biology, chemistry and physics in relation to the maintenance of high standards of medical education and of medical care for the whole population.

The present survey of far-flung research that contributes to medical progress resulted from the conviction that emerged from our first medical study, that it is useless to discuss the administrative problem of distributing medical care and the economic problem of paying for it without reference to the central need of having a sufficient number of trained physicians capable of providing a type of medical care that can justify elaborate plans for distributing it and paying for it. We are convinced that the only genuine medical insurance for this country lies in making the benefits of science available to all practitioners and to all patients. It is a large order.

In the present study of medical research as the base of adequate medical care and medical education, the American Foundation acknowledges a primary debt to the investigators and to the administrators of research agencies (universities, medical schools, research institutes, industries, governmental departments and institutions) that have cooperated with us in furnishing material. We especially thank our Committee of Consultants who join us in presenting this report because they endorse its central idea and the objectivity of the Foundation's performance.

*Curtis Bok*

# CONTENTS

## Volume I

### AMERICAN MEDICAL RESEARCH:
in principle and practice

*Volume II*

UNSOLVED CLINICAL PROBLEMS:
in biological perspective

# INTRODUCTORY

*outlining why and how this study was made*

The necessity for fundamental research in biological perspective in solution of outstanding medical problems is illustrated in both volumes of the American Foundation's present report. Wherever fundamental research exists, no doubt would be expressed that medicine — meaning medical research, medical education, medical practice — is of course rooted in biology; or that the development of biological and medical research is increasingly influenced by the contributions of chemistry and physics (and atomic energy), mathematics. This truth is as yet, however, only dimly reflected in the structure of medical education or in the point of view of medical practice.

· These two volumes present a study of current trends in medical research, envisaged in the above dimensions, carried on by the American Foundation for fifteen years (it could have been many more years; the work is essentially of the kind that is never finished). The study was accomplished with the indispensable cooperation of universities and medical schools, deans, heads of departments, bureaus and divisions, individual investigators in universities, research institutes, industries, government, and with significant counsel over the years from various members of the Committee of Consultants who join the American Foundation in presenting this report.

The study of current trends in basic research that has bearing on medical progress was a natural consequence of the American Foundation's earlier study,* analyzing observations of 2,200 medical educators and practitioners on the status of medical education and medical practice. These observations resulted from an inquiry not bearing directly on either of these subjects but stimulated by the vast concentration of public interest on economic aspects of medicine. Our inquiry to medical leaders in universities and in practice was designed to establish

---

* *American Medicine: expert testimony out of court.* An analysis by medical men of current problems of medical education and medical practice; direct quotations from 2,200 leading medical scientists, educators, practitioners, investigators. Two volumes. The American Foundation, New York, 1937.

whether or not scientific men felt the need of radical change in methods of providing, distributing and paying for medical care.

Without deprecating the importance of these problems, the more profound of the replies from leaders in medical education and medical practice stressed their belief that these economic and social problems can be permanently solved only as they are related to solution of the even more challenging problem of extending and improving medical education, with consequent progressive improvement in the quality and quantity of available medical care. The vitality of both medical education and medical practice was considered to inhere in continuous contact with the currents of new knowledge, in the broadening and deepening of fundamental research directed not only toward diagnosis and treatment of specific "diseases" but also toward understanding of the total living organism.

To a public naturally enough preoccupied with the highly personal problems of getting and paying for medical care, leaders in medical science have tried to convey the truth that the only real health "insurance" consists in insuring that, as Dean Rappleye of Columbia phrased it, so far as humanly possible, physicians, dentists, nurses, public health and other health personnel are adequately trained and competent to provide modern, up-to-date health services for individual patients and the community. "The *financing* of medical service will not guarantee this. The real point that is involved must be adequate support of medical education and research."

With these views the American Foundation is in accord, and the long and arduous labors involved in the present study have been sustained by belief that the heart of the matter is the need of supporting and expanding research in medicine as a life science involving the whole field of biology and the contributions, in theory as well as in instrumentation, of chemistry, physics, mathematics.

Support of this kind of medical research is not yet the animating principle of our national policy or of prevailing public sentiment. It is true that, somewhat under the impact of the war, there has been a marked increase in a kind of abstract appreciation of the need of basic research on the part of the public. The increase has reached the extent of supporting governmental establishment of a National Science Foundation, greatly concerned with basic research (including biological and medical) but not the extent of convincing Congress of the need of appropriation adequate for the Foundation to realize its stated purposes. Every dramatic result of research is publicly acclaimed, but the need of the undramatic basic research, continuing perhaps for years without direct clinical application, is not understood. The public tends to associate the medical research of the past with control of epidemics and abolition of scourges. It tends to associate the medical research of the future with "discovery" of more and better miracle drugs. It supports drives for "conquering" cancer and preventing poliomyelitis, but still shows little realization of the many fronts along which investigative work must be pursued before there is light on the fundamental mechanisms in any disease, for instance, the nature of atypical growth in cancer. This knowledge alone can provide a fundamental *rationale* for cancer therapy, whether by beams from the betatron or by removal of the pituitary gland. This is not to say that a great amount of fundamental study has not been done before such adventurous procedures as endocrine surgery and the associated hormone replacement therapy could even be tried. In spite, however, of the degree of basic knowledge that is responsible for the very initiation of these experiments, they must, until there is further basic knowledge, remain empirical. Control and extension of an apparently successful therapy may depend upon fundamental research in areas and disciplines as yet unrelated to the field of cancer and recognizable only as "pure" research. This is true also — in spite of the amount of basic work done in devising prophylactic vaccines and in spite of a volume of work in many laboratories on chemical and immunological processes — of prophylactic mass vaccination against tuberculosis or poliomyelitis.

The most urgent of present national needs in the medical field is thus conceived to be expansion and improvement of medical education integrally related to research, and progressive improvement of medical practice, steadily lessening the empirical nature of applications of new knowledge to medicine. The medical research involved must be in biological perspective, utilizing the contributions of chemistry, physics, mathematics and the results of research on atomic energy. This is the thesis of this study; it is the point of view of the American Foundation, of its Committee of Consultants and, by every implication, of the hundreds of investigators and teachers that contributed to this work.

*Illustrative presentation of the research of the various agencies in the first volume*

While a vast amount of information furnished to the American Foundation by the above-mentioned investigators and administrators in universities, medical schools, research institutes, hospitals, industries, government departments, divisions and bureaus (reports of investigations, published and unpublished, personal communications and records) provided the essential background for both volumes, our reference to specific material is consistently only illustrative. Much of the material is not specifically mentioned; all of it was important. The necessity of highly selective procedure in any presentation of current trends in medical research in biological perspective hardly needs to be stressed; only an illustrative and selective approach would be possible where the agencies involved and the divisions of biology pertinent to medicine are so numerous.

In the discussion of the agencies of research in the third chapter of the first volume, the purpose was not to cover any one group of agencies comprehensively but rather to discuss in relative detail a few examples of each type, selected for their value in illustrating certain principles and practices. From Princeton, for instance (as a university without a medical school), are cited illustrations of the contribution of *university departments* of biology, physics, chemistry, physiology and psychology to research pertinent to medicine. Lafayette, Union and Amherst furnish illustrations of similar contributions from smaller colleges. From eight additional major university centers of biological research, material is cited illustrating contributions of university biology departments. Contributions from the *colleges of technology* to basic research in biology, chemistry and physics are illustrated by the California Institute of Technology, the Massachusetts Institute of Technology and by one program from each of two smaller technology colleges. The discussion of the contributions to medical science from *colleges of agriculture and the mechanical arts* cites only two centers (Iowa State and the University of Missouri), but the background takes into account basic research in botany, genetics, animal husbandry, agricultural biochemistry in seven other major agricultural colleges. As an outstanding illustration of work in biology relevant to medical progress, research at Stanford University is discussed apart from its medical school.

The review of fundamental research in the *medical schools* is based on material (reports and the published results of research) covering all of the medical schools; fifty-four schools (twenty-eight private; twenty-six tax supported) provided material on the organization and financing of research, and on the substance of research in every department. Research in ten private and in two tax-supported medical schools is discussed in some detail. Reference is made also to major or illustrative programs in six other tax-supported schools. In all, research in the medical school and, in many cases, biological research in the university are discussed in ten private and eight tax-supported institutions.

In the review of the *foundations* as research agencies, the Rockefeller Foundation is discussed in relative detail. Seven other major foundations, while not discussed comprehensively, furnish illustrations. In addition to these eight foundations, seventeen others provided material pertinent to medicine. In the discussion of the work of the *research institutes*, in addition to the fuller description of the Rockefeller Institute for Medical Research and the Carnegie Institution, the work and the policies of eight smaller institutes and operating foundations are cited. Approximately four hundred *hospitals* (fifty or more beds), general and special, voluntary and tax supported (a sampling of 6,000 hospitals) provided the background for discussing research in nonteaching hospitals and possibilities for research in group clinics (as illustrated by the Mayo Clinic). Research in teaching hospitals is discussed with the medical schools on which their research programs largely depend. Discussion of the contributions of *industrial organizations* to research bearing on techniques, instrumentation and materials for investigative work and on medical products is based on information from over a hundred companies, five industrial research institutes, seven industrial research foundations, a number of trade associations.

The discussions of medical research in *federal departments and bureaus* is derived from material supplied by various major departments in the federal government: by the Public Health Service, notably each of its National Institutes of Health (Department of Health, Education and

Welfare), by the Department of Defense (Army, Navy, Air Force), notably its Research and Development Board, the Atomic Energy Commission, Department of Agriculture, Department of the Interior, the National Science Foundation. The principles and practices of *eight national voluntary health societies* are used to illustrate the ways in which this group, generally, supports and promotes medical research.

The material cited above covers information at the national level. That the national pattern is followed, in principle and in practice, in substance and in financing, at the state and local levels was confirmed by results of inquiries to state and local departments (of health, hospitals, mental hygiene, education, welfare), to state colleges without medical schools, to local organizations — voluntary, charitable, social, medical.

*Illustrative presentation, in the second volume, of trends in basic research involved in solution of nine outstanding clinical problems*

The second volume develops the thesis of the report by briefly reviewing current trends in fundamental research needed for understanding mechanisms involved in nine clinical conditions. The nine "diseases" selected (there is, of course, nothing sacred or final in the number) are cancer, infertility, tuberculosis, virus infections, the rheumatic syndromes, arteriosclerosis, hypertension, alcoholism, schizophrenia. Many other diseases are actually included in the discussion of these nine: forty in the virus chapter alone, for example, at least three in the chapter on the rheumatic syndromes, a wide range of conditions in the infertility chapter. The dominant purpose in each of these chapters is the same — to present the areas of research, however vast, however remote, however little developed as yet, that seem to bear upon the metabolic mechanisms primarily involved in the given condition. This purpose is very different from an attempt to achieve an omniscient and comprehensive monograph on the particular clinical problem, and the present reviewers promptly disclaim the latter objective. The clinical name of each condition is used in the title but it is at once obvious that developing basic knowledge has already shown most clinical names to be obsolete fixations of incomplete knowledge, having little reference to the mechanisms dominantly involved.

"Outstanding" medical problems could have been selected by various criteria: those with the highest mortality and morbidity rates; those of unknown etiology; those in which, while the cause may be known, treatment remains baffling. These criteria were not operative in the selection of the nine conditions discussed in Volume II. It is true that the nine are all "outstanding" problems and that most of them figure importantly in mortality and morbidity statistics. They were selected, however, not for these reasons but because of the way in which they illustrate disturbed structure and/or function, reflecting disordered chemical processes of cellular metabolism, integration of which characterizes the normal healthy organism. Any fundamental solution of these clinical problems is seen to be referable to research in molecular biology, whether concerned with the life and activities of single cells, of specialized cells within complex organisms, or of the organism reacting as a whole through integrating and adapting mechanisms.

The newer concepts of metabolism underlying all the discussions in this report rest on work done by generations of biologists, physiologists and chemists in nurturing, developing, broadening and concretely defining Claude Bernard's concept of the steady state. "Even before the unveiling of the atomic age", Austin M. Brues pointed out, 1953, "sound interpretation of isotopic studies by Schoenheimer and his school had shown that the living organism builds itself up, and maintains itself, through a continuous process of synthesis and breakdown of chemical compounds hardly suspected by classical biochemistry. We are accordingly beginning to understand where much of the energy evolved in metabolism is used and to what purpose." The "steady state" is now seen (DeWitt Stetten, Jr., 1953) to result from "a nice balance between the rates of synthetic, in general, energy-consuming processes, and degradative, usually energy-yielding reactions". In this view, all body constituents are actually in a state of flux, are being continuously synthesized, interconverted and degraded. The rates of these processes, however, are so adjusted that the net concentration of various metabolites within or without the cell remains, as C. N. H. Long described it, "extraordinarily constant". Many of the factors involved in regulation of the rates of metabolic reactions, in the balance between release of energy and its use, and in the smooth shifts that coordinate varied metabolic reactions within the complex organism are as yet poorly understood. This survey aims to indicate converging lines of basic research that give liveliest promise of illuminating some of them.

While definite connections between altered metabolic patterns and the tissue manifestations of disease have rarely been established, concepts of metabolism have now matured sufficiently to indicate that pathological behavior of cells can be explained eventually in terms of basic normal mechanisms. Attempts to arrive at these terms recognize a new emphasis on the shapes of biological molecules and the growing possibility of relationships between detailed physical structure of molecules and the behavior of biological structures. Metabolism thus relates structure and function, becoming the chemistry and the physics of all life processes. Research in molecular biology, including all aspects of the life and activities of single cells, of specialized cells within the complex organized body, or of the organism reacting as a whole through integrating and adapting mechanisms, is thus referable to solution of clinical problems.

In this concept, it is at once obvious that each of the nine conditions used to illustrate the thesis is not to be sharply distinguished — if indeed it is to be distinguished at all — from allied disorders referable, with variations in character and in degree, to the same processes and the same mechanisms. The factors in normal and abnormal growth involved, for instance, in *cancer* are also relevant in leukemia, in Hodgkin's disease. Normal and abnormal growth as "synthetic and endothermic processes" could, as Brues put it, hardly be understood in the framework of the older, degradative biochemical methods. In studying, quantitatively and dynamically, the synthetic component in its own right, Brues suggested, lies the hope of finding the key to the nature of the inexorable process of malignant growth. While many students of cancer now look upon a tumor as a "trap" which holds on to certain substances it synthesizes and does not again release them in the normal metabolic process of exchange and turnover, it still remains to be known "what the master reaction is in this trapping process (or whether this is the right concept)".

A hallmark of *arteriosclerosis*, another of the nine illustrations, is abnormal concentration of cholesterol in the blood vessels. Abnormally high blood levels of cholesterol are found in diabetes, myxedema; excessive tissue concentration of cholesterol is exemplified in gall-stones, and in cataract, in which excess of cholesterol in the eye lens may form crystals; possible relation of abnormal metabolic products of cholesterol to cancer is under study. The "new" problems of the structure and functions of connective tissue discussed in the chapter on the *rheumatic syndromes* are involved in various other "connective tissue diseases", as periarteritis nodosa. From fundamental research oriented toward problems of the rheumatic syndromes may emerge also clarification of conditions involving degenerative, inflammatory, necrotic changes not only in the connective tissue complex but also in other tissues derived from the embryonic mesenchyme, as muscle, bone, lymphatic tissue, pertinent to study of such conditions as my-asthenia gravis, muscular dystrophy, multiple sclerosis. The mecha-nisms described in the chapter on *hyper- and hypotension* are related also to the shock syndrome, to arterial accidents, coronary or cerebral, to serious eye and ear conditions, to renal conditions (which, if they do not cause hypertension, are reflections or manifestations of it), to the toxemias of pregnancy.

The chapter on the *nature of viruses* and of nearly a half hundred *virus diseases*, in its concern with the most fundamental levels of protein and nucleoprotein metabolism, of the chemistry and activities of cells, has continuous bearing on the metabolism of the host cell under attack by any agent or from any cause. Host reactions are also stressed in the chapter on *tuberculosis*, emphasizing the host's peculiar susceptibil-ity, its power to adjust, to resist, to achieve a metabolic conquest over microorganisms or to establish symbiosis with them.

The neurophysiological and biochemical mechanisms outlined in the chapter on *schizophrenia* have bearing not only on other psychoses but also on various neurological disorders (epilepsy, cerebral palsy, various forms of paralysis). That part of the schizophrenia chapter which deals with psychological approaches is relevant to current at-tempts to assess the more general role of psychological factors, increas-ingly recognized as important manifestations or accompaniments or results or contributing causes in all diseases. Likewise the discussion of social factors in schizophrenia illustrates the universal truth that the cause, the status and the curability of any illness, mental or physical, in the individual is in some degree conditioned by his culture.

There is clearly nothing final or comprehensive either in the number of clinical conditions selected as illustrations or in the number and range of the mechanisms cited in relation to them. Additional challenging clinical conditions will immediately occur to any reader; as will also important omitted mechanisms (for instance those involved in hemorrhagic conditions). Inclusion of other diseases and other fundamental mechanisms would add to but would not change the truth that solution of all clinical problems involves fundamental biological research.

### Concepts and methods that have guided procedure in this study

In stressing work in the whole field of biology and the constantly increasing applications of chemistry and physics to biology, we may seem to have paid less than respectful attention to confusingly numerous and separate labels that are attached to investigative work — the labels of divisions of science, of academic departments, of clinical conditions or disease groups. The "splintering process" in scientific disciplines is, in a broad sense, a sign and by-product of progress; but the numerous and incoherent separate entities resulting from it are to be regarded as illogical realities of the present, perhaps expedient for pedagogic or practical purposes, but really a denial of the unity of biology and the basic sciences in medical research. There is at least a hopeful trend in universities and medical schools toward reorganizing both teaching and the planning of research by integrating work on given subjects or projects from widely diverse laboratories and departments. The integrating movement advances. Pending its consummation, our review of medical investigation in the universities, medical schools and elsewhere, while making use of the labels conventionally attached to work, recognizes that neither disciplines, departments nor diseases can accurately classify the fundamental medical research of the present. While these obsolescent and often quite misleading labels are not serviceable in accurately conveying the nature of the particular work described, they cannot distort the work and they do not greatly matter.

For limitation of the discussion of principles and practices in the first volume to the United States there is no logical justification —

other than limitations of time and space and the exhaustibility of human energy. In the second volume, although the research cited is predominantly American, the contribution of foreign workers has been included as essential to a just presentation, however illustrative, of trends in investigative work bearing on each of the outstanding medical problems discussed. We would have liked to deal with the foreign field even more fully. There are no national boundaries in scientific research. Important work here has often been stimulated from foreign laboratories, and work vaguely begun in this country has often been significantly confirmed or extended in foreign scientific centers. The only just picture of medical investigation would have no limitations of space.

The practical necessity of *time* limitation in such a study as this is immediately clear. Any presentation of "current trends" in biological and medical research must squarely face the realization that few trends, if they are lively, are "current" for very long. The betatron and synchrotron of today are likely to be the museum pieces of tomorrow. George H. Bishop commented, 1953, on the degree to which the rapid "toppling" of current theories (bearing, in this reference, on neurophysiological mechanisms) demolishes the hypotheses that have been governing an investigator's work. We have, in general, interpreted "current" as work done since 1940, and our references to *major sources* in the Appendices cite work after that year.

The major sources for Volume I in the Appendix, dealing chiefly with the agencies of research, cite comprehensively the material on organization and methods of research supplied by the various agencies but cite only illustratively the substantive material upon which the discussion of the first volume is based. The listing of major sources for the second volume adheres, selectively, to the principle of citing fundamental work, or at least work involving some fundamental approach. Certainly the major sources for the second volume are not to be looked upon as a comprehensive bibliography, in the conventional sense, covering the specific subjects of the various chapters. Such a bibliography for this volume, covering work so wide, so fractionated and on such varying levels, would have been rather a subjective record of our labors (of dubious use to the party of the second part) than an objective indication of our preoccupation with fundamental work. Selection of only one from many relevant titles over periods so long as thirty years often merely recognizes that the title included integrates the subjects covered in many preceding titles that were omitted.  Inclusion of only a few of many available titles by authors whose work is cited frequently in numerous connections and omission from the list of many authors whose work was used is due to the illustrative nature of the list. Omission of important clinical references is not to be interpreted as underestimation of the importance of clinical work; it has been used in the general background and it is often cited in the text, especially when its bearing on fundamental mechanisms is clear.

In any survey of research, it would be safer to keep to the past, but this attempt to describe fluid current trends is oriented toward the future, and is more concerned with noting the opening up of promising vistas and possibly converging lines than with recording past achievements — if indeed such a record could be honestly made.  In the historical approach, in a volatile world (even the scientific world), there is always the temptation to bridge inexplicable and disconcerting gaps by philosophy instead of by science, to chart a continuity and suggest sequences that do not in fact exist, or at least have not, as yet, been revealed.  Our mention of "discoverers" and originators in this review is, frankly, in the tradition of associating with various concepts names endorsed by time, not always by fact, some well meriting the title of discoverer, others inheriting it through associations and influences more or less fortuitous.  Even if it were possible, after the fact, justly to "attribute" work so complex and often so badly related to main investigative currents at the time the work was done, we should still view with reserve the historical technique in terms of dates and of individuals.  Both of these, in synthetic reproduction, constitute only a modified truth.  The real origins lie, as often as not, in the "barren" periods between the dates of significant discoveries and in the labors of dozens or hundreds of unknown workers who may have spent endless time barking for the right animal but up the wrong tree (or barking up the right tree but for the wrong animal), men or women who never quite succeeded in the task they set themselves but whose work, nevertheless, may have made it possible for a colleague to do so.

The true history of any discovery is rarely known in full.  Those that appreciate the labor and complexity of investigative work know that every "discovery" has a background of some kind. It would be possible to cite at quite indefinite length evidence that attempts accurately to ascribe "credit" to individuals is fraught with ancient error. Even the associations most hallowed by time and use are subject to challenge. Not long ago the American Association for the Advancement of Science published someone's observation (voicing those of others) that the degree of credit traditionally accorded to Schwann and Schleiden for the cell theory "appears to be unwarranted, because their accounts were antedated many years by the published findings of various, even superior, workers". Whatever credit Schwann and Schleiden, in spite of their much publicized "big mistakes", may deserve, it is healthy to recognize that all discovery represents, after all, a synthesis of effort.

It is enlightening, in the interest of recognition of the role of precedent fundamental research, to review the stages and the investigators that preceded an outstanding dramatic application of basic work: announcement, 1948, of the clinical effects of cortisone in rheumatoid arthritis by Hench and Kendall of the Mayo Clinic was the culmination of twenty years' work in a few laboratories, the results of which were generally regarded in medical circles as academic. From 1855, when Addison described the disease which bears his name and attributed it to insufficiency of an adrenal cortex principle, until 1930, skepticism as to the endocrine nature of the gland was profound. By 1930, extracts of the gland were obtained by physiologists, Swingle at Princeton and Hartman at Ohio State. Swingle's extract was tested in one patient at the Mayo Clinic (Rountree and Green). In the thirties metabolic effects of the adrenal cortex were studied by biochemists in animals deprived of the glands and injected with extracts: Harrop at Johns Hopkins; Britton at Virginia; Long and Lukens at Pennsylvania and Long at Yale; Ingle at the Mayo Clinic. Medical attention was still slight. Loeb at Columbia and Thorn with Emerson at Hopkins studied patients with Addison's disease and explored use of a synthetic steroid that influenced the mineral and water disturbances of the disease. Chemical studies of the extracts began in 1936 in a few laboratories: Kendall's at Mayo; Reichstein's at Basle in Switzerland; Wintersteiner's at Columbia. Of twenty-eight steroids obtained with known structures, six were shown to influence the metabolism of fat, carbohydrate and protein, and to increase resistance to stress of various kinds. Salt and water metabolism, uninfluenced by these steroids, could be restored to normal by the steroid, desoxycorticosterone, not from the gland but synthesized by Reichstein in 1938. By 1940, chemical work was renewed in efforts to synthesize the active steroids (having a structural feature unknown in other steroids), using as starting materials chemically related substances. In 1948, Compound E, later named cortisone, was synthesized from bile acids by Kendall with Sarett at the Merck research laboratories.

Thus this chemical triumph rested upon twenty years' work in organic chemistry laboratories on steroid chemistry. The trial of cortisone in rheumatoid arthritis rested upon reasoning from clinical observations by Hench, 1931 and 1938, of temporary improvement in the disease during and after attacks of jaundice, in which bile acids are involved, and during pregnancy which suggested an effect of some steroid hormone. The disciplines of chemistry, physiology, biochemistry, medicine had joined forces, 1953, to determine the physiological activity of the substance (present in extracts from which the steroids were crystallized) isolated and crystallized, 1953, almost simultaneously in Switzerland, England and the United States and named aldosterone. The powerful new steroid has the salt-regulating and life-sustaining power long ago found in the residue of extracts. Preliminary clinical reports appeared to show its efficacy in maintenance of Addisonian patients, even decreasing the pigmentation. Apparent interrelation of aldosterone with the growth hormone of the anterior pituitary (rather than with corticotropin, ACTH, which stimulates cortisone secretion) suggested new approaches to the absorbing problem of the interrelations between the adrenal cortex and the entire endocrine system presided over by the pituitary gland. The fundamental work included in this development touches upon a research area pertinent to understanding of every disease — the role of the adrenal cortex in adaptation of the organism to stress.

It takes nothing from the glory of particular names attached to the final stage, or to any stage, of an evolutionary process to realize that nevertheless names are more or less an accident *in the perspective of the whole*. Men make and pass, less as creators than as instruments. Paul plants and Apollos waters and God gives the increase — frequently to neither Paul nor Apollos. And many of the individuals that have contributed most to discovery would be first to stress the dominantly social and cooperative and cumulative character of their achievement.

Attempts to give due credit to institutions would be an undertaking even more perplexing and inaccurate than the effort to do justice to individuals. Many a university investigator has done work at three or four places; not infrequently the work published from one department or institution was actually conceived and largely done in another. An investigator trained for years in a research institute may go finally to a university where his investigative labors reach their full flowering, and from which they are published. Or he may go to a government bureau or to an industrial laboratory. A driving, curious mind may accomplish — and publish — its work in an institution which is al-most immune to the research impetus, and which "contributed" to the investigator nothing but obstacles. The research of not a few investigators is still accomplished rather in spite of than because of their environment, and with little reference to either moral support or specific funds. Even when the institution or department is inspiring, when the research impetus is a definite and continuous factor in the particular setting, it remains true that a given piece of investigative work is likely to be an indissoluble combination of influences, forces and faculties not always or easily attributable with accuracy to any given place.

There is another consideration: most human activities advance by virtue of contributions from many different types of individuals, with vastly different endowments, working at different levels. Medical investigation is no exception to this rule. Many of the current analyses of research plead for greater recognition of the "little researcher" and his contribution to the work of the seers and the pioneers. Besides the "little researcher", there are other categories to which research has often a debt — the stimulators, the gadflies, the catalysts, the plodders or the "confirming" pedestrians — and even, once in a while, the opportunists (the "apical" researchers who rush in with the capstone, flitting from one problem to another — as the climax approaches). Once oil is struck, all the neighbors busily sink wells. Some years ago, in touching upon the curious motivation of some researchers, a retiring president of the American Society of Plant Physiologists, who as a boy had lived within five hundred yards of the Ohio Canal, recalled how the neighborhood youth had fished along it, perhaps a dozen at intervals within a quarter of a mile. So soon as any one of them landed a fish larger than usual, eight or nine of the boys would run to cast their lines into the stream at that point. There were of course no more big fish in that particular spot than elsewhere; but "whenever a fellow research worker discovers an outstanding fact, literally hundreds of workers shift their investigations", hastening to cast their own lines at the lucky location. There may be a nobler aspect in this situation: as, increasingly, annual symposia and conferences indicate to research workers imminent and promising major directions and major needs, they often shift their own lines of work, but under the guidance of a scientific survey of the status of research in a given area rather than on the follow-the-leader principle. There is also, in the total research picture, an anomalous group of idea-mongers who sometimes bring grist to the mill, all unknowing what they do. They may have as little to do with the ideas of which they are the almost fortuitous carriers as the swallows perched along a telephone wire have to do with the message sent along it, but they may nevertheless form a strategic link in a circuit.

The best way to reserve "credit" for the man with the idea would really be to exalt the idea and to keep it nameless. Seifriz in the preface to his book *Protoplasm* said that he had mentioned those investigators whose work he knew best, fully realizing that another author would make another selection. "After all, names add but a human touch, always delightful in any historical account, but never important in the advancement of knowledge." Our concern in this study has been with concepts rather than persons; and while we have been driven to the use of many names, for lack of a better device, we have used them rather to identify lines of work than to attribute credit. If injustices have been done — as in some cases they inevitably must have been — it will not greatly matter in a record where the dominant interest is recognized by all of us to be not the workers but the work.

*Esther Everett Lape*

# Medical Research:
# A Midcentury Survey

*Volume II*

## UNSOLVED CLINICAL PROBLEMS:
in biological perspective

# CHAPTER I

# Current Metabolic Concepts

## *Orienting research in biology and medicine*

A progressively closer relation between biology and medicine has helped to establish the concept of the living organism in terms of continuous chemical reactions and interactions. These reactions underlie both the particular activities of highly differentiated cells (of muscle, nerve, endocrine glands, reproductive organs) and also the mechanisms of regulation and adaptation, neural and chemical, within the complex organism. By correlation of the metabolism and functions of its various parts, the organism reacts as a whole and by its adaptability to varying circumstances "the emphasis of existence may, at least for a time, be almost wholly diverted to a particular end" (C. N. H. Long, physiological chemistry, Yale, 1952). This end may be resistance against assaults from without or within and, in the profligacy of nature, the adaptive response of the organism to assaults may in itself constitute disease.

Knowledge of the interwoven patterns of metabolic processes provides the physician with a livelier appreciation of the inherent adaptability of the living organism, of its natural tendency to recover and to survive. On his knowledge of the material with which he deals as a creative workman depends his ability to cooperate with that material in which disorders are never single but always many and interrelated. A change at one point, in one molecule even, may reverberate throughout the entire system to initiate changes in seemingly unrelated organs and tissues. This concept, familiar in physics, is gaining validity in all fields of biology and medicine.

Investigative work in cancer, for example, tends increasingly toward search for a metabolic fault which changes the mechanisms of normal, controlled cell division and growth into the mechanisms of uncontrolled growth and malignancy. The lesions of arteriosclerosis increasingly suggest the need for knowledge of the structure and metabolism of the arteries in which the disease processes localize. In infectious diseases, whether caused by viruses or microorganisms, study of the multiple factors that determine infection or resistance in equally exposed individuals inevitably turns, directly or indirectly, toward metabolic cycles common to all living cells which are both the site and the armaments of the struggle between host and parasite. Research on rheumatic fever and other diseases of the connective tissue involves not only host reactions to infection but also fundamental problems of reactivity of the connective tissue complex, and (one of the oldest biological problems) the integration of chemical and mechanical phenomena in muscle. The correlation of electrical and chemical mechanisms in nervous function is fundamental to understanding the influence — old among the physician's problems and newer in medical science — of psychological and neural factors in disease and recovery. Intimately related to neural factors is balance among the hormones that influence the rates of cellular metabolism. Probably some degree of hormonal imbalance accompanies all disease. The imbalance may come about in several ways: disease, as a form of stress, may activate the pituitary-adrenal system toward increased activity; it may accelerate secretion of the adrenal cortical hormones in the effort to achieve a new equilibrium; prolonged acceleration of cortical secretion may accentuate and perpetuate a reaction of resistance into over-compensation resulting in organic disease. Certain biological concepts that have oriented medical research (in study of normal mechanisms that explain the pathological or in study of disturbed mechanisms with reference to the normal) are the substance of this chapter as they are also the framework of the chapters that follow.

## BIOLOGICAL STRUCTURE AND FUNCTION AS MOLECULAR OR METABOLIC ACTIVITY

In biology, structure and function are, like matter and energy in physics, merely two different aspects of the same thing (Ludwik Monné, University of Stockholm, 1948). Normal physiological functions are manifestations of the molecular changes that are metabolism; disease is a constellation of disturbances of finely integrated chemical mechanisms. The protean manifestations of pernicious anemia including the central nervous system pathology were traced through forty years' study to a conditioned nutritional deficiency, a metabolic failure to utilize vitamin $B_{12}$, isolated in 1948 from liver. This metabolic fault (not understood, 1954) is influenced, as are all the mysterious defects that initiate disease, by multiple factors (genetic, endocrine, neural, environmental).

For diseases that are not understood in terms of chemical mechanisms, therapy that rests upon a clear *rationale* is obviously impossible.

As yet, little is known of "the intimate chemical and physical structure of cells" and of the properties of chemical therapeutic agents on which depend their interactions with living matter (Otto Loewi, pharmacology, New York University, 1952). Understanding of health and disease becomes, therefore, a problem of molecular biology. Sickle cell anemia, which is diagnosed by microscopy at the cellular level, was described by Linus Pauling and associates (chemistry, California Institute of Technology, 1949) as a molecular disease in which abnormal hemoglobin is manufactured instead of normal hemoglobin. Some years later, other abnormal varieties of adult human hemoglobin were considered to explain other anemias not previously recognized. Further insight into the nature of disease might result, Pauling suggested, from further search for abnormal proteins in the body.

Between the microscopic and the atomic levels lie the macromolecules, huge protein complexes believed to hold the wheels and the driving power of the living machine. These giant conjugated proteins, some now visible by electron microscopy, some measurable by other physical techniques, are the chief focus of investigation in biology as the basis of medical progress. "Although an understanding of molecules is obviously not sufficient for an understanding of life, it is prerequisite to it" (Frank H. Johnson and associates, 1954). At the level of molecular and macromolecular organization, according to Francis O. Schmitt of the Massachusetts Institute of Technology, 1945, "the boundaries between morphology, physiology, and biochemistry largely disappear". Medical research is less and less concerned with symptoms and manifestations, more and more concerned with comprehension of molecular mechanisms underlying biological activities.

TOOLS AND THEORIES OF PHYSICS AND CHEMISTRY IN STUDY OF
MOLECULAR MECHANISMS UNDERLYING BIOLOGICAL ACTIVITIES

In the biological sciences, the theoretical predictions commonly used in physics and chemistry are less possible: "a biological system is a theorist's nightmare" (Kamen, 1952). After a working hypothesis has defined a biological problem, however, quantitative measurements are invoked to attack its validity or to exploit its power to permit "a peep behind the scenes of Nature's workshop" (Szent-Györgyi, 1952). The measurements use two methods, biophysical techniques with their speed and sensitivity, biochemical methods with their slower specificity. Correlation of the two is usually involved in fundamental advances.

For understanding the effects of chemicals on living matter, three types of detailed chemical knowledge were described as essential by Pauling, 1950: molecular structure of the chemical substance; molecular structure of at least some of the cell constituents acted upon; the nature of the forces involved in the intermolecular interactions. Methods of physical chemistry (X-ray and electron diffraction, microwave spectroscopy, among the newer methods) have increased the accuracy of experimental structural studies. Electron diffraction (and to a lesser extent, microwave spectroscopy), providing quantitative data on bond distances, bond angles and other information, is the basis of the theory originally proposed by Pauling that for any given molecule a small number of structures can be drawn and the properties of the molecule can be predicted. By use of this theory of bond valence, organic chemists were able, in a "remarkably short space of time", in the case of natural cortisone (a complex molecule containing twenty-one carbons, twenty-eight hydrogens, five oxygens in fused rings) to "extract it, purify it, determine its structure, manufacture it in quantity by a most complicated conversion from another substance and finally synthesize it" (E. Bright Wilson, Jr., chemistry, Harvard, 1952). Once the structure of an active compound is established, search for the unit or exact configuration essential to a given activity usually follows. Studies over many years in Pauling's laboratory have made possible prediction (with small error) of interatomic distances and the values of forces operating within molecules and between molecules. Investigators of the molecular architecture of protoplasm must deal largely with proteins which, although separable in relatively pure form from their protoplasmic *milieu*, have only recently been analyzed by methods of organic chemistry (F. Sanger, biochemistry, Cambridge, 1950) and have yet to be synthesized outside the living cell. The chemist can break them down, but their reconstruction is as impossible at present as would be the reconstruction of an airplane from its wreckage found by a skilled mechanic who had seen airplanes only momentarily in trackless flight against the sky.

## RELATION OF PROTEIN COMPOSITION AND STRUCTURE TO BIOLOGICAL ACTIVITY — LIFE

While water comprises about seventy per cent of the body's weight, proteins of muscle, connective tissue, skin represent nearly half the body's dry weight (Joseph S. Fruton, biochemistry, Yale, 1953). In every living thing, they determine form, heredity and metabolism, with its resulting activities of growth, response to stimulus and resistance. Studies of the blood proteins over thirty years in the Harvard laboratory of physical chemistry led to the conviction that almost all components of every tissue are "either protein or in a state of dynamic interaction with proteins" (Edwin J. Cohn, and associates, 1951). This assumption is supported by the recognized significance of proteins in clinical conditions, including those discussed in this volume; in growth and division of cancer cells, of the fertilized egg cell, of the bacterial cell, or virus-infected cells; in the integrity of the fibrous proteins of connective tissue; in contraction of the muscle protein complex, actomyosin, with every heartbeat; in the powerful effects of the protein hormones of the anterior pituitary gland which influence the secretion of most of the other hormones and which may, in the case of the growth hormone, influence metabolic rates directly.

The astonishingly specific proteins, built of thousands and hundred thousands of atoms in endlessly varied patterns, have molecular weights up to ten million times that of the hydrogen atom with its atomic weight of one. They are described (tentatively) as organized systems of peptide chains (chain-like groups of amino acids) alone or in combination with accessory nonprotein molecules and groupings. Some idea of the complexities of the amino acid analysis of proteins, by various microchemical and microbiological methods, is suggested by the calculation of the late Howard B. Lewis (biochemistry, Michigan), 1948, that peptides made up of twenty well-known amino acids found in the proteins of higher organisms could occur in 2,432,002,003,176,640,000 possible variations (isomers), each containing the same percentage of the same amino acids but varying slightly in their arrangement in the peptide chains. If different numbers of the various acids are included, "the number of possible combinations all but defies the imagination — many more than would seem necessary to account for the diversity of the naturally occurring substances" (Frank H. Johnson, biology, Princeton, Henry Eyring, chemistry, Utah, and Milton J. Polissar, chemistry, City College of San Francisco, 1954). Pauling estimated, 1954, that there are about 100,000 different kinds of proteins in the human body.

The globular proteins (enzymes, protein hormones, all the blood proteins except fibrinogen) are generally regarded as folded, pleated or coiled chains. The ways in which the huge protein molecules are held together, and the amino acid side chains linked to the main chain were unknown, 1953. Pauling and associates have during the past fifteen years determined the structural details (interatomic distances and bond angles) of amino acids linked together into peptide chains by the study of crystals of amino acids and simple peptides by X-ray diffraction, and have used this information to predict several reasonable configurations for polypeptide chains, which have been verified as being present in both fibrous proteins and globular proteins. That the sequence of the amino acids in the peptide chains determines the physical properties and the biological functions of individual proteins is a widely accepted hypothesis. Amino acid analysis of proteins is regarded as a necessary step toward the far-away goal of understanding protein structure.

By 1954, after more than twenty years' work in many laboratories (especially the biochemistry laboratories at Cambridge, England, at Paris, at Columbia and at Cornell in New York), complete analyses of the sequence of residues of each amino acid in the insulin molecule had been published (Sanger, 1954). As for the specificity of proteins, an example of which is the formation of specific antibodies in response to protein antigens, only beginnings have been made toward understanding "the influence of the fine structure of proteins on their immunological reactivity" (Michael Heidelberger, immunochemistry, Columbia, 1954). Something was known of the effects of molecular size and shape, but little was known of the influence of the arrangement of the constituent amino acids (to which specificity has frequently been attributed) in characteristic patterns or outcroppings on whatever functions as the surface of a protein. It has been suggested that, in the insulin molecule at least, certain groupings can be modified without loss of activity, an exception being the reduction of sulfur-to-sulfur bonds (H. L. Fraenkel-Conrat and associates, 1951). Not only the amino acid pattern of the peptide chains but also the (infinitely varied) manner of folding of the peptide chains may account for the specificity of proteins (Felix Haurowitz and Charles F. Crampton, chemistry, Indiana, 1952).

An approach to the behavior (specificity) of proteins by methods of physical chemistry (light-scattering measurements in solutions, electrophoresis, ultracentrifugation) has furnished information on the intermolecular forces (electrostatic and repulsive) that proteins exert on each other and on other molecules. It is possible (John G. Kirkwood, chemistry, Yale, 1954) that, assuming complementary surface patterns on molecules such as antigen and antibody, "relatively distant groups may influence local interactions of complementary sites on two protein molecules by serving as sources or sinks of mobile charges . . ." Electrostatic and repulsive forces were invoked by Pauling and Corey, 1951, to explain the contraction and relaxation of muscle fibers by changes in shape of the fibrous protein molecules. No more heroic task faces science than to sort out in detail the structure of proteins which will explain their specific biological activities. "Physicochemically, it is to all intents, equivalent to the problem of life itself" (W. T. Astbury, 1945).

## THE NUCLEOPROTEINS AS THE BASIS OF BIOLOGICAL ORGANIZATION, HEREDITY, ACTIVITY

Of the protein macromolecules, which consist of a protein (believed to determine the specificity of action of the molecule as a whole), attached to various nonprotein molecules (responsible for the activity), the most important are the nucleoproteins, study of which has evoked ideas reaching to the borderline between the living and the nonliving. Interpretations of the cell theory, still a theory after a century's debate, involve both of these areas. One characteristic of the cell (as the ultimate unit of living matter) is its metabolism which enables it to reproduce itself. If the viruses reproduce themselves within the cells they inhabit, are these to be regarded as subcellular, submicroscopic units of living matter? The first nucleoprotein molecule isolated as a pure rod-shaped particle was the tobacco mosaic virus which Wendell M. Stanley demonstrated, 1937, to possess the properties of the virus with ability to multiply within the cells of tobacco plant leaves. As other nucleoproteins have been studied, their replication or apparent self-duplication, although explained only by theories of building according to a model or "template" or of weaving according to a pattern, has given substance to the concept of molecular biology. Not only is the fabric of life molecular but growth itself is, in the behavior of these giant molecules, also being traced to the molecular level.

In the cell nucleus, self-duplicating genes, apparently enshrined in chain-like formation within the chromosomes, are tentatively assumed to be nucleoproteins that "grow" by producing one exact replica at cell division (mitosis). Evidence for the existence of genes as discrete units, for their duplication at cell division in the "ballet of the chromosomes" (Kurt G. Stern, chemistry, Polytechnic Institute of Brooklyn, 1952) is still almost entirely biological. The striking slightness of "the influence of chemistry on the chromosome theory of heredity" was commented upon by A. E. Mirsky (Rockefeller Institute, 1950) who had reported in 1948 the first estimate of the number of nucleic acids in one nucleus. The tobacco mosaic nucleoprotein was obtained not from the cell nucleus but from the cytoplasm (the cell substance outside the nucleus) of infected tobacco leaf cells. Proposals at a 1940 symposium that some viruses and enzymes, found in the cytoplasm, and the nuclear genes are somehow related because of their nucleoprotein nature and their ability to duplicate themselves (or be duplicated within the cell) were regarded at the time as revolutionary. By 1953, these and related ideas of the role of nucleic acids in protein synthesis, in the energy-producing mechanisms of the cell, in cellular mutation and growth had been developed into working hypotheses with many extensions into fields of genetic, virus, bacteriological, cancer research.

By newer techniques of X-ray analysis of crystals, by electron microscopic images, the framework of the giant conjugated nucleoprotein molecules "can now be seen by the mind's eye, though as in a glass darkly" (E. A. Moelwyn-Hughes, physical chemistry, Cambridge, 1950). Study of questions brought by biologists to chemists has required theoretical development of means for structural study of the protein and the nonprotein portions of these molecules and of approaches by methods of organic chemistry which depend largely upon synthesis for proof of prediction and reasoning. Proteins isolated by even the mildest physiological solvents from their biologic *milieu* have never been free from suspicion that they may be quite unlike their natural counterparts. The less-known nucleoproteins handled by the chemist may also be "unnatural". The nucleic acid portion of the molecule has been attracting increased attention as information has accumulated from research on enzymes, viruses, cancer, in microbiology and chemotherapy, and as chemical theory has provided methods of approach to their structure.

## NUCLEIC ACIDS

Nucleic acids, so named because they were discovered in the cell nucleus (by Miescher a few years after Mendel's publication of his genetic discoveries in the 1840's), were later identified as normal constituents of the cytoplasm also of all plant and animal cells and tissues. They are present inside all cells, never outside them. The types of nucleic acids are characterized by different sugar components; deoxypentosenucleic acids (formerly known as desoxyribosenucleic acids) with molecular weight of around seven millions are found only in the cell nucleus and are a constituent of chromosomes; pentosenucleic acids (formerly known as ribonucleic acids) with an approximate molecular weight of 10,000 are found in both nucleus and cytoplasm (Arthur W. Pollister, zoology, Columbia, 1952). The nucleic acids, themselves macromolecules, can be broken down into many smaller chain-like groups, the nucleotides, built in their turn of smaller nucleosides. The links that hold together the chain-like structures are phosphates or phosphoric acids. The comparison of nucleic acids with the protein molecule built of infinitely varied amino acid chains is at once obvious (A. R. Todd, organic chemistry, Cambridge University, 1950). The sequence of nucleoside residues in the nucleotide chains and finally in the nucleic acid chains provides for "a practically infinite" number of specific nucleic acids (Alexander L. Dounce, biochemistry, Rochester, 1952). From study of deoxypentosenucleic (nuclear) acids in various species Erwin Chargaff (biochemistry, Columbia) suggested, 1951, that one nuclear nucleic acid may be characteristic of each species.

The mystery of how the cells make these complex molecules that are apparently involved in what each cell is and what it does has been approached recently through theoretical structural chemistry. Early X-ray studies of nucleic acids (begun 1937) suggested a phosphoric acid axis on which the nucleotides rotate "like leaves on a long stem" (Astbury, 1945). Since 1952, electron micrographs of nucleic acids (described by S. Furberg in Sweden; Robley C. Williams, Virus Laboratory, California) have shown some resemblances to X-ray diagrams and also to helical (coiled) structures proposed by Pauling, 1953. A similar model of the structure of nuclear nucleic acids, described as two chains winding around the same axis in different directions, with specific pairing of bases between the two chains, was described (J. D. Watson and F. H. C. Crick, Cambridge University), 1953, as a possible theoretical basis for self-reproduction of the nucleic acids, a mechanism that is one of the central goals in broad fields of cancer, virus and enzyme research. Studies of enzymic mechanisms of production of energy and its use in cellular activities have emphasized the dominant role of the nucleotide, adenosinetriphosphate, in energy mechanisms.

A succession of discoveries (since 1938) showing that one of the adenine nucleotides that are found in all types of animal, plant and microbial cells is an essential means for production of energy, its transfer and use in biological processes was described as "one of the fundamental achievements of biochemistry to date" (Eugene P. Kennedy, biochemistry, Chicago, 1953). Energy from breakdown of adenosinetriphosphate was shown by C. F. Cori (biological chemistry, Washington University), 1946, to "spark" the first step in the oxidation of sugar (glucose). It seems to be able to provide the energy for contraction, *in vitro*, at least, of the complex muscle protein, actomyosin, believed to be the mechanism of contraction of the muscle cells. Because adenosinetriphosphate apparently combines with the contractile protein complex of muscle to which it conveys energy for work, Szent-Györgyi described it, 1949, as a "mortar of the living substance".

For handling energy derived from fermentation and oxidation of foodstuffs, the phosphate bonds of adenosinetriphosphate also act as storage depots and transfer systems (Fritz Lipmann, biochemistry, Massachusetts General Hospital, 1946). They operate, therefore, not only in breakdown but also in formation of such vital substances as acetylcholine which is associated with the origin and transmission of nerve impulses (David Nachmansohn, biochemistry, Columbia, 1951). The high yield of energy liberated when one phosphate bond is removed (11,500 calories of energy) is still less significant than is the stability and long life combined in this bond with high energy. This ability to conserve and transport energy (which would otherwise be dissipated as heat) amounts to one of the basic homeostatic mechanisms of living organisms (Bentley Glass, biology, Johns Hopkins, 1951).

Homeostasis describes the inherent tendency of living things to maintain equilibrium by balanced opposing reactions. In the human organism, physiological homeostasis, equilibrium, even life itself is maintained by the metabolic mechanisms of the cell which possesses certain inherent ("primitive") regulations of which the above-mentioned adenine nucleotide, adenosinetriphosphate, is one. Other nucleotides (at least five) act as coenzymes or organic molecules attached either loosely or tightly to the protein portion of enzymes. The presence of enzymes and their power to act are believed to be determined by the cellular genes containing nucleic acids. According to this concept, the controls that regulate the speed of the cell's chemical machinery are closely associated with nucleic acids. The chemical machinery itself, which produces chemical energy from foodstuffs, includes also nucleotides as parts of the complex enzyme systems of every living cell.

## THE ENZYMES

An orderly functioning of enzymes was proposed, 1948, by James B. Sumner (who in 1926 crystallized the first protein enzyme, urease) as "one way of defining life". Disease thus becomes inhibition or hyperfunction of enzymes. This idea is supported by certain recognized instances of specific changes in enzyme activity in particular disease states. In at least one form of von Gierke's disease, characterized by accumulation of glycogen in the liver and other organs, there is "an almost complete deficiency of one enzyme" (Gerty T. Cori, biological chemistry, Washington University, 1953). Prostatic cancer metastases can be detected by increased amounts in the serum of the enzyme, acid phosphatase, which occurs in the prostatic secretion (A. B. and E. B. Gutman, 1938). This enzymic alteration, however, while useful in diagnosis and in evaluation of therapy in metastasizing prostatic cancer, has little relation to theories accounting for malignant growth by loss of the biological "speedometers and brakes" that regulate the growth of normal cells.

The uncontrolled and destructive growth of cancer cells involves rapid increase in their synthesis of proteins composing, next to water, the bulk of protoplasm. This synthesis requires energy (produced by enzyme-catalyzed reactions), as suggested by evidence of requirement of this energy for making of peptide bonds which link the peptide chains of the protein molecule (Henry Borsook, California Institute of Technology, 1953). Since all enzymes that have been isolated and studied are specific, catalytic proteins (either simple or conjugated with non-protein groups), the formation of the enzymes as well as their co-ordinated activities in carrying out the smooth shifts in rates of cellular activity is one basis of normal growth. Disturbance of it is a logical suspect in cancer. Whatever type of cell (skin, liver, bone marrow, epithelium lining the stomach or uterus) and whatever physiological disasters are involved, the common mechanisms of malignant growth include some enzymic distortion.

In such rapidly acting systems, the difficulties in isolating and identifying the intermediate substances of either breakdown or synthesis are as great as those in isolating individual enzymes and their associated coenzymes that "activate" the next substance in the cycle. The minute amounts in which enzymes occur and their protein nature (which prohibits their synthesis) permit only indirect study of enzyme activity in isolated systems by measurement of the amounts of oxidation, of breakdown or synthesis of specific substances. The reactions accelerated by enzymes are chemically possible, but would not, without the enzymes, occur with sufficient speed to be effective (Sumner and Myrbäck, 1950). Although the organic chemist has never been able, for instance, to synthesize sugar, he can, by using enzymes found in living cells, synthesize cane sugar, glucose (the smaller molecules derived from the carbohydrate), plant starch and glycogen (animal starch). Biological energy, the driving power of cellular life, is produced from the "fuel" of foodstuffs under the catalytic influence of the enzymes of fermentation and oxidation, many of which, because they are proteins combined with smaller units that are nucleotides, are sometimes compared with the nucleoproteins.

## ENZYMES OF FERMENTATION AND OXIDATION

Theories postulating a relationship between the enzymes of fermentation and oxidation and genes and viruses are based largely upon chemical resemblances (a known or proposed complex protein structure) and the known or supposed power of viruses, genes and enzymes to reproduce themselves within the cell or to be reproduced by the cell. Some viruses have been shown to be nucleoproteins (a protein combined with nucleic acid); the hypothetical gene is presumed upon evidence of the chemical nature of chromosomes to be a nucleoprotein. The enzymes of oxidation and fermentation that have been isolated and analyzed have been characterized as conjugated proteins, described as a protein to which is attached a smaller organic molecule, essential to its activity. Some of the functional groups, the coenzymes, may be loosely attached to the enzyme and may shuttle back and forth between the enzymes of one class. Among the components of the known coenzymes are substances also contained in the nucleotides, *i.e.*, phosphoric acid, a purine or pyrimidine base, one of the sugars. In addition, the known coenzymes all contain one of the B vitamins (G. D. Novelli and Morris Soodak, biochemistry, Massachusetts General Hospital, 1953). In a broader sense these enzymes, as probably all others, are ultimately gene-determined, and the fact that they, as well as genes and viruses, contain nucleotides supports current concepts of the biological and metabolic significance of the nucleotide structure in all cells. Evidence has been accumulating that the coenzymes activate or prepare the (substrate) molecules for the catalyzing effect of the appropriate enzymes. It has been suggested that the activation takes place by a union of coenzyme with substrate molecule "strikingly" resembling the specific union of antigen with antibody (John Runnström, 1952).

Popular among theories explaining the specificity of enzyme action is the lock and key theory. To explain the activation of the "lock" by its "key", Pauling developed an older idea of Quastel's that the substrate molecule becomes "strained", and thus made more reactive, in order to fit perfectly the active site of the enzyme. "No lock, however, remains immune to the prying of false keys" (E. S. Guzman Barron, biochemistry, Chicago, 1949). Pauling regarded molecular architecture, rather than chemical composition, as controlling the affinity and combination of a compound with a specific cellular substance: "Even the senses of odor and taste are based upon molecular configuration rather than upon ordinary chemical properties; a molecule which has the same shape as has a camphor molecule will smell like camphor even though it may be quite unrelated to camphor chemically."

Discovery that at least five of the nucleotide groups acting as coenzymes contain B vitamin molecules has been one of the more exciting developments in biochemistry. Work on the vitamin-containing coenzymes has explained the nutritional requirements for minute amounts of nicotinamide, riboflavin, thiamine, pyridoxine and pantothenic acid. "In all cases the coenzyme form appears to be the sole bound form of the vitamin and this then becomes the only metabolically active form for these particular vitamins" (Novelli and Soodak, 1953). Pathological manifestations of acute vitamin deficiencies, as the protean generalized lesions especially of the skin, mucous membranes and nervous system in nicotinic acid deficiency or pellagra, are eloquent of the cellular disruption caused by the crippling of one oxidative enzyme system by lack of its coenzyme. On the positive side, the finding that pantothenic acid is an essential element of coenzyme A (for acetic acid or acetate) associates this vitamin with reactions that are at the very core of both energy production and the use of energy for the formation of such indispensable compounds as hemoglobin, acetylcholine and steroid hormones (Lipmann, 1948). The enzymic role of these B vitamins naturally leads to anticipation of such roles for others of the group, especially biotin, the folic acids and vitamin $B_{12}$. The necessity for study of enzymes as the core of physiological activity was implied by Green's proposal, 1946, that any substance that induces profound biological effects "does so either by participating in or by specifically affecting some enzyme system".

## CELLULAR METABOLISM

### BIOLOGICAL UNITY IN DIVERSITY

Molecular biology is largely a theoretical science comparable to physical chemistry. While physicochemical principles have long since been accepted as indispensable to practical chemistry and chemical engineering, cellular physiology has been accepted only slowly as basic in medicine. When students of pharmacology insist that the mechanisms of action of chemicals on cells is one of the most important unsolved problems of medicine, students of cell physiology reply that knowledge of what is acted upon, living protoplasm, comes first. The basic materials occurring in living matter are not different in kind from those of the nonliving world; the difference is in degree of complexity.

So far as knowledge of the behavior of living matter goes, two mechanisms resist all efforts at explanation in terms of nonliving substance: the almost incredibly delicate balance of chemical reactions within the cell; and the genic mechanisms that apparently guide, order and control these reactions (L. J. Stadler, genetics, Missouri, 1954). Increasing interest in one kind of unit, the nucleoproteins, has led to many statements (as by Monné, 1948) that nucleoproteins are intimately involved in the three basic life phenomena of building molecules, breaking them down, and irritability (expressed in growth, reproduction, development, regulation of metabolic activity). What is the significance of the nucleoproteins in the vast (but almost unimaginably minute) complex of the continuous chemical exchanges that are the life of the cell? How can we speak of the cell as a generality when it includes entities so varied as the free-living cells (the visible protozoa, the microscopic microorganisms, the blood cells) and the cells that form essential or accessory parts of complex organisms ranging from fireflies to man? How can we find unity between liver cells about 3/10,000 of an inch in diameter, the hen's egg and nerve cells, some of which with their extended fibers are three feet long? Is the growing conviction regarding the importance of nucleoproteins a will-o'-the-wisp that will vanish in the brilliant light of experimental scrutiny? The conviction appears strong that, even if application of chemical and physical concepts and techniques to study of life processes is as yet only rudimentary, tracing the threads of the nucleoproteins through the intricate pattern of the tapestry promises knowledge of those processes and ultimate application of this knowledge to understanding health and disease.

Proposals that the nucleoproteins and, with increasing emphasis, the nucleic acid portion of these giant molecules are a focal point in the biological unity of living things and also in their diversity are based on concepts as old as the theory of evolution with its doctrine of the relatedness of all natural phenomena. Since the beginning of the century, study of life has turned from dead materials, "the study of life with the life left out" (Edwin G. Conklin, 1951), toward deeper penetration to molecular levels of living cells. In the complex adult organism (onion, snail, monkey, elephant and man) structure and function approached head-on compound the diversity. On the cellular level, however, unity and simplicity are found in concrete detail, physical and chemical. The fertilized egg cell, "the narrow bottle-neck through which we have all passed, the book in which all our members were written when as yet there was none of them", (Ross G. Harrison, zoology, Yale, 1940) divides. Immediately the nucleoproteins of the two nuclei must be taken into account in seeking explanation of inheritance, of differentiation along one among many possible paths of growth.

Cell physiologists have always studied cells of plants and animals without distinction. In all of these cells, the known basic facts of "chromosomal structure and behavior, mitosis, fertilization, sex-chromosomes and cytoplastic inclusions and, of course, cell physiology are identical" (Richard B. Goldschmidt, zoology, California, 1951). In bacteria, until recently thought to lack a nucleus with localized heredity units, electron microscopic studies have demonstrated nuclei containing filamentous chromosomes and dividing by true mitosis (Stuart Mudd and associates, Pennsylvania, 1952). This type of cell division is common to all cells of the body except the egg and sperm. When these two cells unite in fertilization, equal quantities of germinal or gene substance combine and, according to the chromosome theory of heredity, the combined or double quantity is present in each cell of the body (Mirsky, 1950).

That chromosomes are or contain the nucleic acids (deoxypentose type) found only in the nucleus appears to be generally accepted. Nevertheless, Daniel Mazia (zoology, California) described, 1952, the problem of the chemistry of the cell nucleus as a series of closed doors "which we may feel we are attacking with hairpins rather than keys". More than ten years ago Muller suggested that gene nucleo-proteins could be legitimately classified as enzymes because they "effect the synthesis of specific organic compounds without being used up". More recent views tend to regard the gene theory (Morgan, 1916) developed through study of gene-enzyme interaction as a means of unifying diverse phenomena in heredity and biochemistry (N. H. Horowitz and H. K. Mitchell, biology, California Institute of Technology, 1951).

Both types of nucleic acids are found in the cell cytoplasm which behaves as a viscous liquid containing "countless chemical work-shops". Since these workshops continue to operate in good order even after the cytoplasm is thoroughly mixed up by stirring or cen-trifugation (Paul Weiss, 1949), chemical analysis of the granules or particulate bodies is possible. Various studies since 1934 in this country (R. R. Bensley at Chicago; Hoerr at Western Reserve) and in Belgium have indicated that some, perhaps all, enzymes concerned in production of energy and its use by the cell are built up and carry on their activities within the most important particles, the mito-chondria. These enzymes, acting as systems in step-wise reactions like locks in a canal, include the previously described oxidation en-zymes with their coenzymes active not only in the production of en-ergy but also in its storage, transfer and use in building cell substance.

Evidence that genes control the constitution of cellular proteins includes findings on inheritance of blood groups in man and on in-heritance of the Rh factor causing hemolytic disease of the newborn (the late Karl Landsteiner, Philip Levine, Alexander S. Wiener). Albinism, or lack of melanin pigment, is one type of gene-controlled chemical abnormality in man; another is sickle-cell anemia in which abnormal hemoglobin formation is controlled by a gene, probably through formation of an abnormal enzyme (Pauling, 1954). Evidence that enzyme action is under genic control was assembled by George W. Beadle (biology, California Institute of Technology), 1945: "whether or not a given reaction . . . can take place is gene controlled". If a particular enzyme can be blocked or altered by a gene (either normally present or mutant), not only are reactions catalyzed by the particular enzyme affected but also many other reactions are affected secondarily. The abnormality observed may be far removed from the first link in a chain reaction (Horowitz and Mitchell, 1951).

In medicine, observations are usually made in the reverse order, on the end results of chain reactions, the multiple manifestations of disease. Theories of gene-controlled enzymic changes are being integrated with theories of metabolic defects which may not be gene-controlled but which, whatever their origin, bring about widespread changes in cellular metabolism, the effects of which may first be apparent in any tissue, organ or function.

## THE DYNAMIC STATE OF CELLULAR METABOLISM

It is from study of the body's use of foodstuffs carried to the cells by the blood that newer concepts of metabolism have been developed. These concepts envisage: a constant state of dynamic equilibrium of body cells maintained through continuous breakdown and synthesis of their constituents; the wheel-like tricarboxylic acid cycle as an endlessly repeating process in which chemical energy is produced by chemical machinery; the phosphate (phosphoric acid) bond as a general pattern for parceling and transferring energy for the cell's use.

In medicine, practically every clinical condition is associated with disturbances in the smooth shifts of metabolic rates and directions of which the normal body is capable. The clinical manifestations of diabetes are referable not only to failure to use carbohydrates at normal rates but also to defects in fat synthesis, to disastrous waste of body proteins and collapse of acid-base balance. Infections involve mechanisms of synthesis of proteins: of normal proteins (the fibrous proteins that support the body's cells and tissues and form the matrix of each cell); of modified proteins (antibodies); of "abnormal" proteins (viruses). Knowledge of the machinery for making proteins, requiring channeling of energy from enzymic breakdown of foodstuffs, is fundamental to understanding of most clinical problems, as those involving muscle and connective tissue (rheumatic syndromes, cardiovascular diseases), and those involving cellular growth (cancer, infertility). Mental disorders, in the view of many workers, cannot be understood without competent knowledge of brain metabolism. In view of the finding that protein synthesis is increased in strongly stimulated neurons, Monné conjured, 1948, the possibility that synthesis of specific proteins is "the essential physical phenomenon paralleling memory, fantasy and intuition".

Cellular life cannot be considered apart from the cell's environment which is, for medicine, the community of cells with the substances they make, transform and secrete which may alter the metabolism of cells in any part of the body. Among substances made and secreted by specialized cells are the hormones which, carried by the blood to the cells they influence, "act as the traffic policemen in the crowded streets of the city" (Guzman Barron, 1949). They slow down, speed up and, in effect, channel those chemical reactions which are the life processes of cells. Study of the specific physicochemical interaction of the steroid hormones with cellular dynamic systems has been relatively neglected in favor of study of the multitude of processes, morphological and behavioral, which the hormones regulate (Thomas F. Gallagher, Memorial Cancer Center, 1954), as metabolic equilibrium, the structural and functional integrity of cells and tissues, the inscrutable biological problems of cellular growth and resistance to injurious influences from without or within.

The idea that the powerful influences of these hormones may be primarily or ultimately mediated by changes in enzymes or their activities is the basis of numerous working hypotheses, bearing on the mechanisms by which chemical agents (often in minute amounts) generally affect the body. As to the relation of drugs and enzymes in higher organisms, Loewi took a cautious position, 1952, since enzymatic effects of drugs in the living cell are difficult to separate from direct effects of drugs on excitability, contractility, etc. Others (as Welch and Bueding, Western Reserve), considered, 1946, that except in a few cases the direct action of drugs and poisons on cells appears to be through enzyme systems. Hypotheses considered include the possibility that hormones may combine at some point with enzymes or their coenzymes, or that they may act directly or indirectly in accelerating or inhibiting enzyme activities. Recent studies at the Argonne National Laboratory led to the suggestion that the action of drugs (salicylic acid, cortisone, adrenalin, aureomycin, terramycin) may depend upon the existence in the drug molecule of groupings capable of binding metals. This binding could enhance or inhibit enzyme activity, or could make available or remove the metal ion (Jack Shubert, 1954). Understanding how the body reacts in response to various pathogenic agents obviously requires knowledge of the basic biological mechanisms of the normal cell within the complex organism.

## Isotope techniques in development of this concept of cellular metabolism

The concept of the living cell as a dynamic chemical entity and of the body as in a state of chemical equilibrium in the midst of flux, first proposed by Borsook and G. L. Keighley (biochemistry, California Institute of Technology) in 1935, was elaborated by the late Rudolf Schoenheimer, David Rittenberg and others (biochemistry, Columbia), employing the isotope technique deriving from discovery of natural heavy isotopes and production of radioactive isotopes of known chemical elements. That a chemical element may be really a family of atoms, all having the same chemical characteristics but with different atomic weights and physical properties, has been known since 1912 when the different atoms of a single element were first called isotopes. Atomic structure, which accounts for differences between the naturally occurring isotopes, is usually explained in terms of the lightest of all atoms, hydrogen. The "normal" hydrogen atom is composed of one positively-charged proton in the nucleus which gives it the atomic weight of one, and one negatively-charged electron whirling through the atom's outer "shell" which gives the atom the chemical characteristics of hydrogen. The balance between the nuclear and planetary charges gives the atom its stability. Heavy hydrogen, called deuterium, a natural stable isotope, was first separated chemically in 1932 by Harold C. Urey at Columbia. Like the lighter isotope, it has one planetary electron which makes it chemically like all other hydrogen; the nucleus, still with a positive charge of one proton, contains also an uncharged neutron which increases the weight of the heavy, stable isotope to two. The atomic weight of deuterium that is incorporated into fed compounds serves to identify these compounds or their breakdown products isolated from the body tissues, blood, bones. Carbon, always present in organic chemical compounds, has two natural stable isotopes (C 12 and C 13) with nuclei twelve and thirteen times as heavy as ordinary hydrogen.

In biochemical studies, usefulness of stable isotopes is limited because analysis of their distribution in the body requires sacrifice of the animal. Artificially produced radioactive isotopes, however, can, as previously described, be followed in their course through the living body because the unstable nucleus, as it decays toward stability, emits atomic energy or radiations detectable by the Geiger counter in the living animal fed minute amounts of tagged compounds. As metabolic spies radioactive isotopes accompany groups of natural atoms through long series of chemical and biological adventures without, apparently, betraying their presence to the body cells, yet reporting all along the way to the investigator the whereabouts, size and activities of the groups into which they become incorporated. Use of tagged amino acids in confirming the assumed continual opening and closing of the peptide linkages of all the body proteins became the *modus operandi* of the dynamic equilibrium concept.

Subsequent work with the isotope technique in many laboratories extended the concept to constancy of tissue composition in the normal animal maintained by balanced synthesis and degradation of all constituents. Compounds in foodstuffs and body tissues are all broken down continually, and intermediary products are added to a common metabolic pool from which all compounds needed may be regenerated from smaller units, regardless of their origin. New formation of body tissue is not restricted to growth or repair but proceeds rapidly at all times. Deposits of fat, once regarded as static warehouses of surplus food, have been described as "more like department stores during the Christmas rush" (John E. Pfeiffer, 1953). Reactions of protoplasm to stimuli of all kinds is thus envisaged not as a turning on and off of its chemical reactions but as a maintenance of form and structure in the midst of flux.

Radioisotope experiments on protein metabolism in various species including man (the initial experiments with scarce and expensive isotopes were carried out with the rat) had, according to David Rittenberg, resulted by 1949 in a modified concept of protein metabolism in man. By this concept (falling between discarded and newer theories) the organism is partly in a dynamic and partly in an unreactive state. "The relative division depends on the particular species and upon the particular organ." Muscle protein in man, for instance, was found to require 180 days for breakdown and resynthesis; the turnover of rat muscle protein, on the other hand, required only six days. In human muscle, it was calculated, the metabolically active fraction amounts to only seven per cent of the total muscle. Rittenberg suggested that each cell may contain metabolically inert structures, whose function is to store memories of the past. On indirect evidence, some investigators consider that the deoxypentosenucleic acids, and presumably the protein complexes containing them, are built up at the time of cell division, "and are thereafter comparatively, but not completely, metabolically inert" (C. B. Brown, Memorial Cancer Center, 1954).

## ENERGY-PRODUCING CELLULAR METABOLISM

Energy needed for cellular activities is produced by oxidation-reduction reactions presided over by the complex protein enzyme systems of this class. Without these reactions, "no heart could beat, no plant could grow upward defying gravity, no amoeba could swim, no sensation could speed along a nerve, no thought could flash in the human brain" (Eugene I. Rabinowitch, botany, Illinois, 1953). So far, attempts to apply knowledge of biological energy-producing mechanisms have been directed chiefly toward investigation of known or suspected metabolic disturbances in such clinical conditions as diabetes, arteriosclerosis, radiation sickness, and of such problems as clinical reactions to drugs and hormones. DeWitt Stetten, Jr. (National Institute of Arthritis and Metabolic Diseases, 1954), found reason to suspect that the symptoms of intoxication due to dinitrophenol and other chemical agents or to excess thyroid hormone may be pin-pointed at "uncoupling" of well-known reactions in oxidative metabolism.

For energy production the chief raw materials are the carbohydrate foodstuffs. However, the amount of stored form of carbohydrate, glycogen or animal starch is only about half of one per cent of the adult's body weight (Peters and Van Slyck, 1946). On a diet completely lacking in carbohydrates, the only source of glycogen would be a wasteful conversion of amino acids, or a small conversion of fatty acids to glucose, since 1951 considered theoretically possible (Chaikoff and coworkers). It is now recognized that during a day the greater amount of carbohydrate consumed is converted to fat and then oxidized (John P. Peters, medicine, Yale, 1951). Fats, like carbohydrates, are composed solely of carbon, hydrogen and oxygen; from both are formed the same two-carbon units for oxidation to carbon dioxide and water with energy production. One explanation of the mechanism by which this energy-producing metabolism proceeds continuously, like a wheel, is furnished by the concept of the tricarboxylic or Krebs cycle according to which two-carbon units from carbohydrate, fat or amino acids serve as the common currency in energy production. The cycle was described, 1949, by Krebs (who proposed it in 1937) as a plausible means of "converting one form of energy into another — like man-made machines which require one specific form of energy". This unifying mechanism, common to animal, plant and bacterial cells, illustrates, according to Severo Ochoa (pharmacology, New York University, 1951), "the uniformity and relative simplicity of biological mechanisms".

From studies with skeletal muscle, yeast cells, blood cells and bacteria the steps in conversion of carbohydrates to the form in which they enter the oxidative cycle have been analyzed in practically complete detail and reconstructed *in vitro* with the isolated enzymes. These discoveries, with which are associated the names of investigators trained in Europe, some of whom brought their studies to America (Cori, Meyerhof, Warburg, Szent-Györgyi, Lipmann, Ochoa), approached completion around 1946. Sugar as we know it, even in contact with atmospheric oxygen, is an inert substance. Its breakdown in the body to pyruvic acid or pyruvate, one of the most reactive intermediates known, requires introduction of phosphorus.

The first step in this breakdown is activated by adenosinetriphosphate, the previously mentioned nucleotide. From sugar to pyruvate the pathway is anaerobic, that is, the reactions occur without oxygen and are known as fermentation. Cori and associates completed the isolation and identification of more than twenty enzymes active in this cycle, and of each successive phosphorylated intermediate from glucose to pyruvate. Fermentation may end, as it commonly does in yeast cells growing in plant material (grapes, grain), in formation of ethyl alcohol as an end-product; in living animal tissues it ends in formation of lactic acid which releases part of the energy stored in the carbohydrate molecule. "Anaerobic exercise is not unusual. It is required for any quick spurt of activity, for instance, a 100-yard sprint is almost entirely anaerobic exercise," (Peters, 1951). But efficiency of anaerobic breakdown of glucose is low in terms of energy release: "oxidative phosphorylation is the real mainspring of useful energy in aerobic cells, whereas glycolysis is relatively insignificant" (Albert L. Lehninger, physiological chemistry, Johns Hopkins, 1954).

Sustained use of energy, therefore, requires oxidation which begins, after the lactic acid stage of carbohydrate breakdown, with the highly reactive pyruvic acid. In his earlier studies of pyruvic acid (the cross-road at which fermentation goes on to oxidation) Lipmann discovered (1939) "accidentally" that oxidation of pyruvic acid, like the steps in fermentation leading to its formation, requires the presence of inorganic phosphate. These studies prompted the proposal of "the generalization of the phosphate bond as a versatile energy-distributing system".

From pyruvate several pathways are open, but acetic acid is the common two-carbon fragment derived from all foodstuffs. The many and continuous attempts from 1930 on to identify the fleeting, theoretically satisfying acetic acid (not in itself reactive in biological systems) succeeded only with the availability of radiocarbon in 1946. Konrad Bloch (biochemistry, Chicago, 1947) and others demonstrated that acetic acid contained most if not all of the carbon from fatty acid breakdown. As mechanisms of acetate reactions were studied by Lipmann beginning with pyruvate metabolism, by Ochoa in studies of carbon dioxide utilization in citric acid formation, by Nachmansohn in studies of chemical mechanisms of nerve function, and by others, it became obvious that an active form of acetate, possibly joined to a coenzyme, must be involved in the entrance of the common fragment into the oxidative mill. The coenzyme was identified, 1946, by Lipmann who called it coenzyme A (for acetylation) since it is apparently involved in all acetylation reactions. Shortly thereafter Nachmansohn and M. Berman identified it as the activator of acetylation of choline to form acetylcholine, and work in Lipmann's and in other laboratories extended the role of coenzyme A to other synthetic reactions, discussed later.

As study of coenzyme A developed, it became apparent that the coenzyme was involved in reactions whereby acetate was activated by adenosinetriphosphate and subsequently was transformed to a reactive product, acetyl-coenzyme A. From purely oxidative reactions, therefore, appeared a "versatile energy-distributing system" in the phosphate bond, and also a metabolic building block capable of acting as a carrier to transfer activated (energy-rich) groupings toward synthetic reactions. To describe this energy and its transfer to work performance (building of complex molecules, transfer of ions across membranes, contracting the fibrous protein complex of muscle) Eyring and associates, 1954, used the analogy of landscape levels. Low basins or valleys represent compounds, the passes over mountain ranges separating valleys or basins are activated complexes, like acetyl-coenzyme A. "The course followed by a particular activated complex from reactants to products will trace a path from the initial valleys up through one of the passes down into the final state." Stetten used an electrical analogy, envisaging adenosinetriphosphate as a storage battery, charged by breakdown processes and discharging as it "drives the motor of the biochemical ski-tow".

The possibility that coenzyme A might contain an unrecognized B vitamin was given particular attention by Lipmann's group. With the cooperation of Roger J. Williams (biochemical institute, University of Texas) the B vitamin pantothenic acid was identified in the coenzyme molecule and later, 1949, shown to be combined with a nucleotide. Work in other laboratories (University of California, National Institutes of Health) had resulted, 1952, in agreement on a structure for the coenzyme. Oddly enough, oxidative breakdown of active acetate to provide energy is preceded by its use as a building block in formation of citric acid, the six-carbon compound from which the tricarboxylic acid cycle is named (Ochoa, 1954). That a sulfhydryl group is the active group of the coenzyme was shown at Munich, 1951, by Feodor Lynen and coworkers who also isolated the compound and provided the final proof that acetyl-coenzyme A was the long-sought "active acetate" in which form the two-carbon fragment enters the tricarboxylic acid cycle. In 1951 also, Ochoa and J. R. Stern isolated the first enzyme of the Krebs cycle to be obtained in crystalline form, the condensing enzyme which, in the presence of Lynen's acetyl-sulfhydryl-CoA, catalyzes the synthesis of citric acid.

## USE OF ENERGY BY THE CELL IN SYNTHESIS

Recognition of the unifying simplicity of the energy-producing mechanisms in all living organisms has helped to open the way to understanding the use of energy derived from biological oxidation. "We do not know", Eric G. Ball (biological chemistry, Harvard) wrote, 1942, "whether all the energy released by oxidative processes is utilized by the cell or how it is utilized". A distinct gap existed between what was known ("a good deal") of production of energy and how that chemical energy is transformed into other types of energy — muscular contraction, cell division, nerve activity — and is used in all building operations of cells. By 1948 it was realized that all cells use a standard type of chemical energy, which presupposes a certain uniformity of processing (Lipmann).

Chemical energy has one source — the energy of sunlight. Plants have the power through the green pigment, chlorophyll, to store solar energy as chemical energy in molecules of carbohydrate, amino acids and fat synthesized from carbon dioxide and water, with release of oxygen. In this process between sixty-five and eighty-five per cent of the absorbed light energy is transformed by chlorophyll-bearing cells to chemical energy. Upon the products of this "giant chemical industry of the plant kingdom" the entire animal kingdom lives as "a small brood of parasites" (Rabinowitch, 1953). Indeed, the chemical and functional relationships between the green plant pigment, chlorophyll, and the red animal pigment, heme, which is the active part of the oxygen-carrying hemoglobin of the red corpuscles and also of the iron-containing oxidative enzymes, suggest an evolutionary development of mechanisms for transformation and use of energy (Sam Granick, Rockefeller Institute, 1949).

In animal cells, the packing of energy into parcels and the transfer of energy are achieved by the previously mentioned energy-rich phosphate bonds, each of which can store and distribute 15,000 calories. Lipmann, 1948, found it possible for adenosinetriphosphate, continually being regenerated, to act as the reagent for all condensations involving removal of water. These studies "foreshadowed a generality of phosphate bond generation in energy metabolism". The molecule appeared to be able to face both ways, as a part of the energy-rich phosphate pool collected from oxidation and as a contributor of energy for synthesis. Through work in many laboratories, the concept of the energy-rich phosphate pool has been extended. That "the gap between the biochemical and biological approach is narrowing down" (Lipmann, 1954) points to hope that the role of these energy transfer mechanisms in synthesis may explain formation in the body of compounds of peculiar medical interest. Progress in that direction includes identification of these mechanisms in synthesis of glutathione (a nonprotein sulfur-containing peptide) believed to have a role in brain metabolism (Bloch and associates, 1952; Heinrich Waelsch, New York State Psychiatric Institute, 1952); in the synthesis of protein, in the activation of certain enzymes, possibly as a preventive agent against radiation damage (Guzman Barron, 1952); of choline which is concerned with fat transport and deposition in the liver (Camillo Artom, biochemistry, Bowman-Gray, 1952); of the first carbohydrates in the cycle of photosynthesis in plants which, if achieved *in vitro*, might solve world-wide nutritional problems (A. A. Benson, Melvin Calvin and associates, 1952).

Study of the functions of coenzyme A has substantiated proposals of Lipmann and others that most, if not all, biochemical reactions are reversible (Ochoa, 1951). There are no blind alleys, no dead ends. If this is true, what of the carbon dioxide believed until a few years ago to be merely an end-product of metabolism in animals, a waste product of biological oxidation by way of the tricarboxylic acid cycle? Answers to this question provided with the aid of isotopes since 1941 have filled in many gaps also in the detailed picture of the tricarboxylic acid cycle (Harland G. Wood, biochemistry, Western Reserve, 1946). Observations of Wood and C. H. Werkman (bacteriology, Iowa State), 1935, and of Cornelis B. van Niel (Hopkins Marine Station, Stanford), 1941, on carbon dioxide fixation in certain bacteria that are, like man, dependent on ready-made foodstuffs, have led to investigation of the possibility that animal cells might be able to utilize carbon dioxide, in several biochemistry laboratories (at Western Reserve; Harvard; Chicago; New York University). By 1944 it had been demonstrated that by a reversal of one reaction in carbohydrate metabolism a metabolic utilization or fixation of carbon dioxide can occur in animal tissues (E. A. Evans, Jr., Chicago); by 1948 utilization of radioactive carbon, C 14, from carbon dioxide had been demonstrated in glycogen synthesis in the rat (Wood). By 1949 Ochoa with J. R. Stern had isolated and purified the enzyme for the reversible reaction by which pyruvate through carbon dioxide fixation forms citric acid and enters the oxidative cycle. Further work, according to Ochoa, 1951, has established that except for the difference in energy source, carbon dioxide fixation and photosynthesis are essentially the same; carbon dioxide can enter the cycle in animal tissues at various points and emerge as compounds to be used in synthesis.

### DYNAMIC ASPECTS OF PROTEIN SYNTHESIS

In the cell's building of its own substance, the proteins are the "master builders" (Astbury, 1945). Even in the resting cell there is continual dynamic activity. Some substances required by animal cells that lack (or have lost) ability to construct certain amino acids, fatty acids and vitamins must be supplied preformed in the diet, ultimately from plant material; of these, eight known amino acids are thus required in the human diet (W. C. Rose and associates, chemistry, University of Illinois, 1952).

Approaches to the problem of protein synthesis with isotope-labeled amino acids have yielded certain precise facts, but their interpretation and explanation are limited by theoretical development (John H. Northrop, Rockefeller Institute, 1949). Feeding labeled amino acids had demonstrated, according to Borsook, 1953, that every tissue tested, *in vivo* and *in vitro*, incorporates every known amino acid at rates varying with the amino acid and with the tissue. The incorporation of amino acids into tissue proteins involves peptide linkages, and inhibition of oxidative metabolism with consequent loss of energy inhibits the incorporation.

For protein synthesis in the above sense and for protein breakdown, many have suggested that peptide chains are the intermediaries. Hans Neurath, 1952, discussing the huge molecular size of proteolytic enzymes, suggested that the binding of the enzyme to the protein to be hydrolyzed may require the large size, and that an active center may play the dominant role. Study of fractions of physiologically active proteins has strengthened the concept of an active "core"; a fraction of the relatively pure protein adrenocorticotrophic hormone of the pituitary, corticotropin, ACTH (ten to twenty per cent molecular weight of the whole), "possessed almost all of the hormone activity" (Choh Hao Li, biochemistry, California, 1951); a relatively small fraction extracted from purified protein derivative of tuberculin was found capable of evoking a positive skin test in tuberculous individuals (Florence B. Seibert, 1950). To explain the synthesis of the vast number of specific proteins, Northrop proposed, 1949, a common protein precursor synthesized by each species or possibly by each organ, with energy derived from cellular metabolism by an autocatalytic process. From these hypothetical "proteinogens" individual proteins could, it was suggested, be formed at any time without expenditure of energy.

There are many known examples of active proteins formed from inactive precursors, as the enzyme trypsin formed from trypsinogen, pepsin formed from pepsinogen (Northrop, 1949), the blood clotting substance, thrombin, formed from prothrombin (Walter H. Seegers, physiology, Wayne, 1952). Since viruses can be grown in cultures of embryonic tissues (as the fertilized hen's egg) more easily than in adult tissues, can it be that the embryonic proteinogens are more like viruses than are adult proteinogens? From their experiments with immunological methods Haurowitz and Crampton proposed, 1952, that synthesis of specific proteins is a two-phase reaction: in the first phase each protein has species specificity (horse, rabbit serum globulin) due to the species-specific amino acid pattern of each peptide; in the second phase, folding of the peptide chains brings about specificity for use (as in formation of antibodies when serum globulin conforms in shape to an antigen). In the living animal, injection of one or more antigens (foreign substances, usually proteins) evokes production of antibodies, *i.e.*, modified serum globulins which combine specifically with the corresponding antigen but which are otherwise indistinguishable from "normal" globulin. Pauling suggested, 1940, that the normal and immune globulins might be considered isomeric forms of a native protein, differing slightly in configuration, perhaps only of terminal polypeptide chains. *In vitro* formation of antibodies from serum globulin in contact with antigen was reported in 1940 by Pauling and D. H. Campbell, and a theory of physical forces in structural conversion of these specialized proteins was developed by Pauling, 1943.

"The really fundamental concept" that embraces growth or reproduction of genes (chromosomal or cytoplasmic), of viruses, possibly of a malignant principle responsible for cancer is (Astbury, 1950) "viable growth-complexes", *i.e.*, minimum specific combinations of protein and nucleic acid which, "given an adequate physicochemical environment, can keep on turning out the same molecular pattern indefinitely". Of the various approaches (Rittenberg's involving the question whether the chromosomes are engaged in the dynamic state; Pauling's involving theoretical and structural chemistry; and others) Lipmann's approach, 1954 (in cooperation with Lynen), was based upon the mechanism of the adenosinetriphosphate-coenzyme A-acetate reaction. From these studies, models were prepared for synthesis of a peptide bond, for polypeptide synthesis, and for amino acid sequence. The model, not presented as reflecting the real mechanism, was considered useful in devising "a mechanism of genetic determination and reduplication of a specific protein" based upon amino acid sequence "as the background for specificity".

Among the factors known to influence cellular growth and division and, in molecular terms, the formation and integrity of the cellular proteins, are radiations. Study of biological effects of atomic energy requires knowledge of the mechanisms of energy production and those of energy use in synthesis. The ultimate aim of radiobiology, in which the problems are those of atomic and molecular physics and of chemistry "and not at all of nuclear physics" (Platzman, 1952), is "to follow the fate of the absorbed radiation energy through all phases, from the primary physical act to its effects on cells, tissues, and the whole organism". Dale pointed out, 1952, as have others, that our knowledge of the chemical processes within the cell is "the weakest link in the chain of events". Studies of the influence of radiations on known metabolic cycles and reactions, with use of labeled compounds, are oriented toward discovering interference with synthetic processes which ultimately induce the cell to divide (George Hevesy, chemistry, Stockholm, 1952). From studies of chromosome breakage and other disturbances of the cell nucleus induced by radiations, A. H. Sparrow and associates (biology, Brookhaven National Laboratory, 1952) concluded that there is little doubt that the change "represents an end result of radiochemical change induced either by direct ionization or by the chemical products of ionization or excitation". Breaking the structural protein or framework of the chromosomes might occur through one or more relatively small "lesions" which then "spread through the rest of the chromatid by some chain mechanism, such as enzymic hydrolysis".

Study of the mechanism of action of ionizing radiations in biological material is essentially study of cellular metabolism. Energy of radiation, insofar as physical knowledge can measure and control it, permits study of known chemical and biochemical processes in the cell that might be altered. The first requirement is a known characteristic or reaction. The next requirement is to know whether intervening effects (*i.e.*, reactions between energy transfer in the material and the end result) are relevant to that end result. Further study of these mechanisms should aid in elucidating the mechanism of action of the different types of radiations, in increasing knowledge of protection and control, in adding to "basic knowledge in many fields in physiology, pathology, and radiobiology" (A. M. Brues and G. A. Sacher, Argonne National Laboratory, 1952).

## USE OF METABOLIC ENERGY BY CELLS AND TISSUES IN COMPLEX ORGANISMS

Cells, even the "free-living" cells — sea urchins, fungi, soil bacteria — depend upon their environment whether sea water, soil or other cells in their community. Some aspects of cellular activity must be studied separately in cells in which certain activities are intensified (muscle, nerve) but activities common to all cells (division) can be studied on the basis of certain similarities. Among these the nucleotide adenosinetriphosphate and coenzyme A ("omnipresent and omnipotent") are emerging as equally important in unifying the mechanisms of cell division, of muscular contraction, of nerve cell function, thus serving to make of metabolism a continued story replacing an anthology of short stories.

While admitting a role for oxidation-reduction phenomena in cell division, L. V. Heilbrunn outlined, 1952, his colloidal theory describing cellular response to stimulation as "essentially a clotting of protoplasm", dependent primarily upon the same substances that are active in coagulation of vertebrate blood. Cell physiologists have long considered the protoplasmic property of alternation between the gel and the liquid state to be an intimate physical mechanism of cell division. Viscosity changes of the separate parts of protoplasm "are responsible for all visible mitotic movements" (Warren H. Lewis, Wistar Institute, 1951). There can be no doubt that living cells maintain closely regulated concentrations of certain inorganic ions that are in sharp contrast to concentrations of these ions in the fluid environment. A delicate balance between sodium and potassium is maintained in living cells, especially muscle and nerve cells, and its function may be related to selective binding of these elements by unknown protoplasmic constituents. In general, body fluids are poor in potassium, cells are poor in sodium. "A nice balance between falling apartness, promoted by potassium, and the structural association promoted by calcium combination of sodium complexes, could be postulated as an essential state" (H. Burr Steinbach, zoology, Minnesota, 1952).

Among methods for study of mammalian cells under controlled environmental conditions is cultivation in solutions of chemically defined nutrients of tissues or of colonies of cells derived from a single cell. Such cells can be compared with those examined immediately after removal from normal or diseased tissues, although some variations in responses naturally occur (George O. Gey and associates, Johns Hopkins, 1954). Another method is by construction of model systems: protein fibers artificially produced from globular proteins (pepsin, albumin) have been studied to throw light on chromosome structure (Mazia, 1950); proteins of the cell cytoplasm have been studied in models of proteins spread at oil-water interfaces (M. J. Kopac, biology, New York University, 1950). A model system for study of the metabolism and function of the nerve cell was prepared from single rows of electric cells of *Electrophorus electricus* (Nachmansohn,

1953). A useful model for study of muscle contraction was prepared from the isolated fibrous muscle proteins from which was obtained evidence supporting the molecular theory of muscular contraction activated by adenosinetriphosphate (Szent-Györgyi, 1951). Further study of the role of adenine nucleotide in muscle carried out in models prepared from cells (fibroblasts, liver, spleen, epithelial as well as muscle cells) led to the startling conclusion that adenosinetriphosphate "is both the agent which brings about the movements of all kinds of muscle and almost all kinds of cells and the immediate source of their working energy" (Hans H. Weber, physiology, Tubingen, Germany, 1953). Among these movements was included cell division.

Examples, to follow, of recent adventures into the molecular details of cellular activities within the body illustrate ways of integrating fundamental investigative work with broad areas of physiology which are basic to human health and disease. Several approaches to cell division and growth, which touch nearly every aspect of human health and disease, illustrate the biological unity of the lowly microbes and the highly differentiated cells of the mammalian organism. As antibiotics are increasingly used not merely empirically in chemotherapy of infectious diseases but also to promote growth of plants and of animals for the market, investigation of their mechanism of action turns to fundamental biological principles. Study of growth and attempts to inhibit growth of cancer cells by chemical agents, on the other hand begin with the complex organism although unicellular organisms are not excluded from the picture. Genetic studies on the paramecia (Sonneborn) and on the neurospora (Beadle and Tatum) have posed questions and opened new avenues in cancer research. In the nerve cell, the relations between chemical and electrical energy still puzzle neurophysiologists, but the unanswered questions here are also the unanswered questions of basic research generally. Newer concepts of muscular contraction illustrate the transformation of chemical energy into the mechanical energy used in motion, one of the simplest and most obvious manifestations of life.

## CELL GROWTH AND DIVISION ON MOLECULAR LEVELS

Chemotherapy, for all its empirical character, has been a stimulus to basic work in various fields. Problems associated with drug resistance have, for instance, heightened present interest in bacterial genetics. Observations on the effects of drugs and chemicals in cancer have been related to study of growth and division of cells in tissue culture and the direct or specific action of hormones and vitamins on certain cellular and organ sites. Study of the activities and functions of separable units (organoids) of nucleus and cytoplasm grown separately in tissue culture has increased in response to the need for knowledge of the actions of drugs and chemicals on the hereditary units to explain the effects of drugs on cell growth, on the cytoplasmic units with which enzymes are associated. Such studies have strengthened the conviction that intimate and individualized study of single cells will increase understanding of their mass behavior. Increasingly, cellular behavior in terms of movement is carried to the molecular level, as in the above-mentioned view of Weber that all cellular movement, including division, depends upon adenosinetriphosphate as a source of energy.

In cell division, one of the first visible phenomena to be recorded was a series of phases and movements within both the nucleus and cytoplasm at mitosis (by Conklin in 1902). The phases of chromosome division ending in splitting lengthwise are well known. "Growth" or division of mitochondria, the rod-shaped bodies of the cytoplasm, "the actual power plants of the cell", has been seen through stages of elongation and dividing across their length (Claude, 1950). These visible mitotic movements, for years thought to be periodic only in the act of cell division, are now regarded as part of an unceasing "endocellular traffic" (Gey and associates, 1954). These findings from newer physical techniques bring the individual cell within the universal principles of energy and motion encompassing the atoms and their nuclei, the molecules and their fragments that compose the universe from stars and planets to the epithelial cells of man. With phase optics and time-lapse photomicrography, rotation of the nucleus was recorded in epithelial cells taken from tissue cultures (C. M. Pomerat, tissue culture laboratory, Texas, 1954). In the inner sanctum of the cell, the mitochondria and other particulate bodies having different functions are continuously engaged in "free and purposeful movements" (Gey, 1954). At cell division, according to Robert Chambers (biological laboratory, Woods Hole, 1951), the nuclear membrane loses its identity and nuclear substance, except for chromosomes, mixes with cytoplasmic substance. "There are indications that the cells, during this period of nuclear and cyto-plasmic mixing, are particularly susceptible to externally applied injurious agents."

Such knowledge appears to be pertinent to studies (experimental and clinical) of inhibition of cancer growth by synthetic analogues of nucleic acid components, purines and pyrimidines (Wellcome laboratories and Memorial Cancer Center, 1954). Since at mitosis nuclear and cytoplasmic substances are mixed, formation of purines of nucleic acids which include the purine adenine (part of adenosine-triphosphate and of enzymes) theoretically could be disturbed by the presence of structurally altered purines. Such knowledge may be pertinent to the reported "indefinite" stimulation of division of cultured cells by minute amounts of a substance of small molecular weight isolated from nuclear nucleic acid (Carlos Miller, Folke Skoog, Malcolm von Saltza and F. M. Strong, botany and bio-chemistry, Wisconsin, 1955). A specific "cleavage substance" was proposed long ago by cell physiologists. Kopac suggested, 1951, that the substance may be derived from the cytoplasm, that it must be capable of energizing gelation, and that it may be adenosinetri-phosphate. Mitotic arrest was produced by terramycin, aureomycin, among other drugs, in bacteria containing a nucleus (still subject to controversy) with discrete chromosomes, following the pattern of chromosomal activity known for larger organisms (Edward D. DeLamater, microbiology, Pennsylvania, 1954).

Such fundamental findings might help to explain numerous clinical observations that antibiotics and other antimicrobial drugs that are highly effective in severe infections with rapid multiplication of the organism are slightly or not at all effective in minor infections. But present practices (use of antibiotics as "omnibiotics" in all infections, use of many separate antibiotics seriatim "one on top of the other") are undeniably not based on any clear relation between the condition treated and the efficacy of the particular antibiotic (Maxwell Finland, medicine, Harvard, 1953); in one large teaching hospital one antibiotic was prescribed solely for prophylaxis in sixty-five per cent of cases, many of which received other antibiotics at the same time. One result of improper use of antibiotics for prophylaxis or in a manner suggesting the old "shotgun" medication (whether in hospitals or in private practice without facilities for control) is development of hypersensitivity to antibiotics used in relatively small dosage. Reports of deaths attributable to hypersensitivity to penicillin have increased yearly. While penicillin is recognized to have "revolutionized" control and treatment of syphilis throughout the world (Charles R. Rein, dermatology and syphilology, New York University, 1953), it has also created serious epidemiological problems, according to a survey by the Science Fund, published by Columbia, 1954. The report pointed out that while penicillin had reduced by more than half infant mortality from congenital syphilis and also the number of neurosyphilitics admitted to mental institutions, nevertheless the methods of its use — inadequate doses for prophylaxis, dependence, in early syphilis, on single doses (which may only mask overt symptoms), complacency regarding case-finding and follow-up — were calculated to create a public health problem more serious than that of prepenicillin days.

### PROBLEMS IN CHEMOTHERAPY STIMULATING BASIC RESEARCH

Uses of antibiotics (some seventy tons per month, twenty of which were penicillin, were produced in 1953) in animal husbandry and agriculture have expanded so rapidly since 1951 that some manufacturers have established divisions of agricultural research and development. The situation has distinct bearing on human welfare. Feeding of antibiotics to increase growth and reproduction rates and to fatten animals for the market (young chicks, calves, lambs, swine) raises questions as to how far fed antibiotics are retained in animal tissues, and as to how those retained are affected by cooking. Therapeutic use of antibiotics in animals has introduced further human problems, for instance the finding that antibiotic treatment of bovine mastitis resulted in milk that inhibited the growth of cheese-making bacteria; or the finding in Food and Drug Administration laboratories, 1953, that fifty per cent of eggs laid by hens fed chlorotetra-cycline (aureomycin) failed to lose their antibiotic activity on boiling. Other problems pertinent to man are suggested by the present wide-spread interest of food manufacturers in use of antibiotics for food preservation (as adjuncts to heat and freezing, as preservatives of fresh foods in transportation, for control of contamination in fermenta-tion). General conclusions from the work reported by 1953 were that each antibiotic, each species of animal, each individual food product presents a different picture.

Therapeutic use of antibiotics in man has accomplished many "miracles" and has also raised fundamental biological questions which must be answered if antibiotics are to be safely and widely used. Destruction in body sites that are normally contaminated (oral, respiratory, intestinal, genital tracts, skin) of antibiotic-sensitive organisms is followed by persistence of nonsensitive organisms, by multiplication of those resistant originally or by mutation, or by invasion and often domination of newly implanted unsusceptibles. These changes are made more complicated by increasing use, referred to above, of multiple agents not only in all serious infections but also in "merely febrile illnesses that seem to resist treatment with individual agents" (Finland, 1953). The trend is accentuated by successive exploitation of new antibiotics (ten new antibiotics and many new combinations were reported at one 1953 conference) and by a volu-minous literature encouraging the physician to hope for an "omni-biotic" for all types of infections, thus relieving the practitioner of diagnostic responsibility.

In the not too distant future, William S. Tillett, New York Univer-sity, prophesied, the florae of the exposed areas of the human body "which have been created and presided over by universal 'anti-bioticism' will become the so-called normal florae" and will require reorientation of concepts of infection and disease. The fungus *Candida albicans* cannot successfully compete with the original florae under normal circumstances but multiplies only after the normal florae have been suppressed or killed by antimicrobial therapy and may under these circumstances give rise to such serious infections as pneumonitis. There have been reports of pneumonitis caused by bac-teria that are resistant to the usual antibiotics such as *Pseudomonas aeru-*

*ginosa* which "emerges as the dominant organism in inflammatory lesions when more susceptible bacterial species disappear and may actually cause primary pneumonia" (Paul Bunn and coworkers, medicine and bacteriology, Syracuse, 1953). Diseases caused by organisms usually considered saphrophytes or secondary invaders raise problems not only of microbiology but also of the "much neglected" host factors other than those associated with the carrier state, subclinical or latent infection, *i.e.*, physiological-biochemical disturbances that distinguish between *infection* and *disease* (Dubos, 1954). Among these, Tillett thought important "the vicious cycle of antibiosis inducing or associated with vitamin deficiency, which in turn creates local pathology, which in turn becomes vulnerable to the otherwise noninvading types of microorganisms". "There is reason to wonder whether any microorganism cannot become the cause of disease if suitable conditions are provided for it. Thus there are many circumstances, some of which are of common occurrence in human medicine, where the physical, chemical, physiological and probably psychological factors which affect the host play far more decisive parts in the causation of disease than does the presence of this or that microorganism" (Dubos, 1953).

Referable to other areas of basic research is the problem of emergence of resistant strains of organisms in infections initially susceptible to one or several or combinations of antibiotics. The staphylococcus and the tubercle bacillus illustrate this problem which has invited the interest of cell physiologists, geneticists, protein chemists and cancer investigators. In the upper respiratory tracts of the personnel of a hospital five months after introduction of a new antibiotic, erythromycin, the proportion of erythromycin-resistant staphylococci rose from zero to seventy-five per cent. "As each antibiotic is introduced, we hear first of miraculous cures, second of deleterious reactions, and third of the appearance of resistant strains . . . There are no combinations of antibiotics, so far as I know, which will prevent the emergence of resistant strains: they merely delay their appearance or diminish their numbers" (Harry F. Dowling, Illinois, 1953).

The mechanisms of drug resistance are relevant to the investigative field of biochemical genetics, which aims to discover how genes are organized at the chemical level and how they initiate and control intricate biochemical mechanisms within the cell and the organism. Controversy surrounds the question "whether resistance is acquired by individual bacteria as a result of their exposure, or whether, instead, resistance arises in a relatively small number of organisms as a spontaneous mutation, the drug acting only as a selective agent which kills off the normal sensitive organisms, and thereby promotes the survival and selective propagation of the resistant mutant" (Harry Eagle, National Microbiological Institute, 1954). The first interpretation would imply the heretical theory of inheritance of acquired characteristics, since resistance persists for many generations in the absence of the drug. The latter interpretation, widely accepted, is supported by work of M. Demerec (genetics, Carnegie Institution, 1949) and others who have demonstrated that organisms with high resistance to streptomycin and other antibiotics are derived from organisms present in the original population before exposure to the drug. That this resistance is controlled by a mutant gene was demonstrated by Rollin D. Hotchkiss (Rockefeller Institute, 1948) in studies with *E. coli*, *H. influenzae* and *Meningococci* in which resistance to penicillin, streptomycin, sulfanilamide was induced, the transforming agent always being deoxyypentosenucleic acids obtained from resistant organisms. "The strain being transformed acquires one at a time the properties previously accumulated by the donor strain as it became drug-resistant through spontaneously mutational events." The mutation is only a sign by which a genetic event is recognized.

That deoxypentosenucleic acids might act as cell-specific genic material in bacteria was demonstrated, 1944, by Oswald T. Avery, Colin MacLeod, Maclyn McCarty at the Rockefeller Institute. With a pure deoxypentosenucleic acid from virulent encapsulated Type III pneumococci, these workers transformed avirulent Type II pneumococci into the virulent Type III organism containing the specific capsular polysaccharide. The transforming agent, the specific deoxypentosenucleic acid, showed "the essential properties of the gene", and was transmitted from the parent cells to offspring indefinitely (Dubos and associates, 1952). The previously noted idea of specificity of deoxypentosenucleic acids in the nuclear genes of cells of different organisms arose from the work of Beadle, 1945, and Tatum, 1946, showing in the mold, *Neurospora crassa*, that synthesis of growth factors and amino acids is gene-controlled. "Wild" type molds do not require methionine, for example, for growth because they can make it; mutant molds (after treatment with X rays, nitrogen mustards) lose the synthetic power and require methionine in the diet as an essential amino acid. This hereditary metabolic defect consists of alteration of a specific enzyme required in the synthesis through alteration of a specific gene that controlled the enzyme. The basis of the unique specificities of deoxypentosenucleic acids from different bacteria used as transforming agents was attributed to differences in purine and pyrimidine base composition in the nucleic acids from these sources (Erwin Chargaff, chemistry, Columbia, 1951).

Progressive work on this principle in a number of laboratories made obvious the analogy between the transformed or mutant bacteria and body cells transformed into malignant or cancer cells (Rhoads, 1954). The mutant bacteria, moreover, could be selectively killed by withholding from the medium a purine required by the mutants but not by the parent normal bacteria. The hope of finding that peculiarities of composition or structure distinguish the nucleic acids of tumor cells from those of their normal counterparts had not been realized, 1954.

## CORRELATION OF ELECTRICAL AND CHEMICAL
## PHENOMENA OF NERVE FUNCTION

The discovery over a century ago that nerve activity is associated with electric manifestations appeared to open the way to understanding the functions of the nerve cells, the means of communication with the outside world and between different parts of the body. The electrical manifestations have been described, as by Nachmansohn, 1953, as merely signs that something is happening rather than as explaining the mechanism of nerve function. The electrophysiologist was described (George H. Bishop, neurophysiology, Washington University, 1952) as working in the middle "between the students of the chemical bases of metabolism which produce and modify the potential he observes, and the psychiatrists who might hope to correlate mental behavior of nervous tissue with the functioning of nerve cells in terms of the electrical activity of the cells". As with other manifestations of life activities — cell division, genetic characteristics, motion — the explanation is sought in chemical terms, in the use by the cell of energy derived from its metabolism. Heilbrunn observed, 1952, that it is a simple matter to talk in terms of magnets and electrical charges, but "much more difficult to seek interpretations in terms of the actual substances of which the cell is composed". Correlation of the rapid and precise measurements that have been developed in the recording of electrical processes in nerve tissue with the relatively slow and crude chemical measurements has proved difficult. But even without knowledge of meaning in terms of chemistry, measurements of bioelectric potentials have provided direction for research on clinical problems through the electroencephalograph and electrocardiograph.

Whether the rhythmic electrical activity of the cerebral cortex is correlated with mental function can, at present, be only assumed (Bishop, 1952). The frequency of the electric waves in all parts of the human central nervous system varies from eight to twelve a second, with other frequencies present in lower voltage. The emerging of the slower waves has now been correlated with clinical conditions including brain tumors and abscesses, various phases of epilepsy including the subclinical, other convulsive states such as insulin shock. Electroencephalography in diagnosis and in analysis of familial susceptibility as a guide to therapy of epilepsy has been studied for more than twenty years by William G. Lennox (neurology, Harvard) and associates, and in other centers, leading to search for metabolic changes underlying the electric changes. Physicochemical changes in the nerve cells cause both changes in the electroencephalographic waves and the epileptic fit (Stanley Cobb, neuropathology, Harvard, 1946).

Physicochemical changes are the basis also of the classic membrane theory of nerve impulse conduction. The membrane theory assumes that concentration of sodium ions is high outside the nerve cell membrane and low inside, the reverse being true of potassium ions. According to this theory, the membrane is electrically positive on the outside and negative on the inside; a stimulus at the surface of the membrane increases its permeability to ions. J. C. Eccles, 1949, estimated that the membrane becomes during activity about 500 times more permeable to sodium ions than it is during rest. Simultaneously the positive charge on the outside becomes negative, with generation of small currents which stimulate the adjacent regions with passage of the impulse along the fiber. These assumptions have been supported by postwar work with radioactive ions.

A. L. Hodgkin, 1951, and A. F. Huxley, 1954, at Cambridge University and investigators in Nachmansohn's laboratory have demonstrated that both sodium and potassium ions are continually moving in dynamic equilibrium across the semipermeable membrane, maintaining a positive charge on the outside and a negative charge on the inside. During passage of the impulse there is a sudden inrush of sodium and an outrush of potassium. Work of the Cambridge group suggested that the change of membrane permeability allowing the inflow of sodium changes the charge inside to positive, accounting for the rising potential. The falling phase of the potential depends upon the outflow of potassium. The membrane potential of the resting nerve was considered by Lorente de Nó (Rockefeller Institute, 1947) to be produced and maintained by the oxidative metabolism and not by ionic concentration gradients. This view was apparently supported by experiments (D. W. Bronk and associates, 1952) indicating that adenosinetriphosphate is directly involved, utilizing the mitochondrial oxidative enzyme systems, as "an essential part of the mechanism that maintains the usual ionic distribution between the inside and the outside of the cells, including axons". In other words, energy-rich phosphate is apparently generated in neural tissue by the same mechanisms as in other tissues — liver, muscle. This leaves to be answered the question as to the source or trigger mechanism of the specific change in permeability which generates the bioelectric potential for transmission of the nerve impulse along the fiber and from cell to cell. Around this point from 1937 have centered the controversial hypotheses explaining the origin of the energy that transmits the nerve impulse.

The idea of a chemical mediator acting as a direct means for communicating the nerve impulse across the synapse (between two nerve cells) and at the neuromuscular junction has been widely accepted by physiologists studying the sympathetic nervous system. First suggested by Elliott in 1904, the theory of transmission of impulses from sympathetic nerve endings to involuntary (smooth, unstriated) muscles by adrenalin (epinephrine) or adrenalin-like neurohormones was elaborated by work of Cannon and Rosenblueth at Harvard in the thirties. A similar theory of chemical transmission within the central nervous system and at the neuromuscular junction was later proposed and extended by Dale. The hypothetical chemical transmitter was acetylcholine, action of which on the cell surface was described by Loewi, 1952, as "exactly like electrical stimulation". The hypothetical mechanism was simply described by Ralph W. Gerard (neurophysiology, Illinois, 1950) as involving release of acetylcholine to produce the rising phase of the action potential and destruction of it by its enzyme as the potential falls again.

Objections to the hypothesis were many, an important one being that, since the nerve impulse is propagated along the fiber by electric currents, the basically similar propagation from nerve cell to muscle cell could not be explained by a different mechanism (John F. Fulton, physiology, Yale, 1949). Nevertheless, as one physiologist put it in the thirties, the acetylcholine-esterase system present at the neuromuscular junction could hardly have been put there by nature just to puzzle physiologists. The presence of the enzyme at the site where it is needed to break down acetylcholine cannot be taken as direct evidence, for cholinesterases have been found in high concentrations in non-neural structures such as serum and erythrocyte. Lorente de Nó, studying the effects of certain quaternary ammonium ions (acetylcholine is a quaternary amine, lipid soluble), emphasized, 1949, that these ions participate not only in maintaining the resting potential but also biochemically in the production of nerve impulses. A base of one of these ions was extracted from ox brain. He suggested that, since these ions could be used as substitutes for sodium in some fibers, the sodium mechanism is not a universal one in nerve. Ionic shifts that occur within milliseconds cannot at present be studied directly. Divergent views of permeability processes in nerve illustrate the incomplete knowledge of permeability, per se, which makes impossible definite conclusions on the events in nerve.

A degree of accommodation between electrical and chemical transmission characterized a "new conceptual scheme" (Nachmansohn) attributing the action of acetylcholine to an intracellular (not intercellular) process within the conducting membrane, increasing its ion permeability. "It forms an integral part of the elementary process by which bioelectric potentials are generated in the axon, in the nerve terminal and in the postsynaptic membrane. But the propagating agent along the axon and across the synapse is the electric currents." Study of the electric organs of fish ("the most powerful bioelectric generators which nature has created") for analysis of the generation of bioelectric potentials in general was the basis of proposals of what happens in the nerve cell. In the resting nerve cell, according to this hypothesis, acetylcholine is in a bound, inactive or storage form. Excitation of the membrane leads to breakdown of the complex, freeing acetylcholine to act upon the membrane, change its permeability and then disappear. The first reaction of breakdown of acetylcholine by its enzyme as the potential falls was demonstrated and the enzyme acetylcholinesterase isolated in high concentration from conductive tissues. The resynthesis of acetylcholine during recovery by energy from adenosinetriphosphate was demonstrated (Nachmansohn and A. L. Machado, 1943), and through work in this and other laboratories, previously noted, adenosinetriphosphate and acetyl-coenzyme A were identified in the reaction. Adenosinetriphosphate is "certainly" related to the membrane state and to discharge of currents, according to Gerard, 1952.

As in other cellular reactions, the elementary processes of generation of electric potentials within the nerve turns to study of proteins, notably of the enzyme (esterase) which breaks down acetylcholine. Study of the intermolecular forces between acetylcholine and the enzyme (Irwin B. Wilson, 1953, physical chemistry, Columbia) was motivated by the hope of obtaining clues as to the nature of the protein receptor on the cells with which acetylcholine reacts. In any case the enzyme is present in "all conductive tissues throughout the animal kingdom" in all types of nerve, all types of muscle. In the chemical and physical analysis of muscular contraction the chief focus of attention is the protein complex of the muscle cell and the role in its mechanical behavior of adenosinetriphosphate.

## CORRELATION OF CHEMICAL AND MECHANICAL MECHANISMS IN MUSCLE CONTRACTION

"From the physical point of view, muscle is an engine for the conversion of chemical energy into mechanical work, operating by means of reversible elastic strains in a solid working substance, the muscle proteins" (M. G. M. Pryor, Cambridge, 1950). Protein specificity and activities can be advantageously studied in muscle which has been the chief experimental material of physiologists for fifty years, because muscle function, motion, is easily observed and measured. Recognition of the importance of muscular function in clinical medicine has grown with realization that most diseases that incapacitate and kill involve muscle in some measure (Wallace O. Fenn, physiology, Rochester, 1941). Normal functioning of the smooth muscles underlies the health of the digestive tract, the lungs, the arteries, the inactivity of the uterus for nine months and its contraction during delivery. On the functioning of the skeletal muscles, the striated or cross-banded muscles, depend most of the movements of life, the eyes, the fingers, the limbs, the expansion of the chest in breathing. Heart muscle is a firm network of cross-connected striated muscles differing from skeletal muscle chiefly in the mechanisms of stimulation and control. In diseases such as lumbago, muscular dystrophy, heart failure, muscle dysfunction causes great suffering; and muscle failure is the immediate cause of death (Szent-Györgyi, 1949).

### REACTIONS OF MUSCLE PROTEINS IN CONTRACTION

Myosin, the contractile element of muscle, was described by Edsall and von Muralt, 1930, as the "muscle machine". Work since 1939 in biochemistry laboratories at Pennsylvania (Meyerhof), at Cambridge University (the Needhams), at Szeged, Hungary, and later at Woods Hole (Szent-Györgyi's group) and elsewhere has been concentrated upon the chemical details of muscular contraction (and relaxation, an even deeper mystery). The first problem was to take apart the molecule of the fibrous protein complex which, bound together, makes the fibers of the skeletal muscles (striated or cross-banded) and the similar heart muscles which are held together by cross-connections. The smooth muscles (blood vessels, gastrointestinal tract) are composed of spindle-shaped cells arranged in sheets or masses. But all, according to the widely accepted theory, are composed of myosin combined with a second protein, actin (isolated by Straub, 1942), into a complex, actomyosin. It is this complex protein that is believed to contract, the contraction being integrated from molecules to fibers, to cells.

In Meyerhof's laboratory at Heidelberg, generations of investigators learned through work on muscle the significance of thermodynamics for studying the sequence and cycles of intermediary metabolism. Lipmann, in his work on pyruvate metabolism, for instance, used minced pigeon breast muscle to develop the concept of the functions of the phosphate bond and acetyl-coenzyme A in energy transfer. Theories of energy sources for muscular contraction (heat generated by oxidation, surface tension) have been replaced by the previously described concepts of metabolism and function in all cells. The view that adenosinetriphosphate is the immediate provider of energy for synthesis of new compounds (as in cell growth), for osmotic work (as in shifts of ions across the nerve cell membrane resulting in generation of electric currents) and for mechanical work (as in movements of cell components in division) is the thread of the continued story which has now reached the last chapter here, the mechanism of muscular contraction. In muscle, a basic working hypothesis that the proteins contract with energy from the breakdown of adenosinetriphosphate had not been finally proved, 1953.

There is a certain agreement that the enzyme, adenosinetriphosphatase, tailored to fit perfectly the energy-carrying nucleotide and isolated from muscle (Price and Cori, 1946), is somehow associated with the actomyosin complex. This has been demonstrated in strands of the contractile protein extracted from muscle (Szent-Györgyi, 1949); it has been indicated by study of single muscle fibers (W. F. H. M. Mommaerts, biochemistry, Duke, 1952); and by studies with radiophosphate in intact muscle (E. Lundsgaard, Copenhagen, 1950). How the energy is transformed into mechanical work had not been demonstrated. Szent-Györgyi guessed, 1948, that the principle may be "regulation of energy liberated by the need of energy", the system being active only in its low-energy state and needing energy for relaxation. Dorothy Needham agreed, 1950, that relaxation is the active process; in its contracted state actomyosin becomes "enzymatically active" and splits one molecule of nucleotide per unit of actin.

Experiments with models made from living cells (fibroblasts, epithelial) when preparing for division in tissue cultures resulted (Weber, 1953) in contractions "identical" with those of muscle. Only the presence of adenosinetriphosphate was necessary; other metabolic processes could be excluded in these models. Chemical and mechanical (measuring power) studies in models, also made from smooth muscle, resulted in the same conclusion: contraction is based on the splitting of adenosinetriphosphate and relaxation is based on its binding. The contractile tissue of muscle is, like nerve, conductile and the transfer of the nerve impulse at the neuromuscular junction is electrical. Heilbrunn's general theory of stimulation and response, noted above, included all types of cells — egg, nerve, muscle — and described the response as an electrically accelerated migration of calcium ions into the interior of the cell. Weber showed in his cell models that contraction was incomplete or absent if calcium was extracted and that addition of physiological concentrations of calcium restored the response. These results seemed to him to give weight to the view "that movements of calcium connect the polarization of the membrane with the state of activity of the contractile protein". Contraction of muscle fibers was explained by "the oldest but still the most impressive fact about muscular activity — that on stimulation the structure passes over suddenly from a semi-fluid and plastic-like consistency to a state almost like that of a crystalline solid" (Astbury, 1950).

Study of muscle fibers by physical methods began (in the early thirties) with X-ray diagrams. "However valuable partial systems and models may be from the biochemical viewpoint, it is evident that, in the investigation of the structural mechanism which is characteristic of muscle, final answers will be obtained by observation of nothing less complex than the muscle fiber itself" (F. O. Schmitt, 1952). Studies of muscle by newer methods including the electron microscope reflect a growing interest in fibrous proteins, including keratin (of hair, bone, feathers), epidermin, fibrinogen and fibrin (blood-clotting proteins) and even the structural protein of certain bacterial flagella. Astbury, 1950, described the contractile mechanism of flagella as the fundamental "scheme" in all biological material, mechanism stripped to its barest essentials, "a capacity for rhythmic, energetic movement embodied in a single molecule", possibly by waves of folding or unfolding running down one side and up the other causing a waving motion.

## CONNECTIVE TISSUE AS THE FABRIC OF MULTICELLULAR ORGANISMS

A large part of the fabric of life consists of the connective tissue which, like muscle, bone and lymphatic tissues, is derived from the embryonic mesenchyme. Within this fabric or "edifice" (Sylvia H. Bensley, anatomy, Toronto, 1952) live the gel-like cells of the body which are protected and nourished by the fibrous elements and by the intercellular ground substances which store and transport compounds derived from the blood and the cells. Pathologists began more than a century ago to associate changes in the ground substance of connective tissue with disease processes (in early stages of arteriosclerosis, in scurvy).

Since 1950, study of connective tissue has been intensified by development of the concept of the rheumatic syndromes and other conditions as lupus erythematosus, scleroderma as involving connective tissue alterations. This involvement of connective tissue (which may be primary in the above-mentioned states) may occur also in other disease states, especially those in which inflammatory mechanisms are prominent. Fifteen investigators participating in the 1953 Macy conference on connective tissue had approached study of connective tissue through interest in such varied fields as infection and immunity, cardiovascular disease, ophthalmology and the nature of the vitreous humor, mechanism of action of hormones, cirrhosis of the liver, arthritis. Developing study has included functions of the ground substance in local anesthesia, in fertilization and sterility, in various aspects of the spread of cancer, in hypersensitivity, in aging.

Basic research, initially without reference to the clinical states now enveloped within an active field of research, had supplied information on the fibrous and amorphous elements of connective tissue. The proteins of connective tissue, like those of all other tissues, are partly globular and water-soluble. These globular proteins are not in great degree involved in structural elements ("you will find it rather difficult to build any mechanism out of marbles" — Szent-Györgyi, 1948). Proteins of muscle, hair, skin, and of blood fibrin account for about half the fibrous proteins of the body; the other half, by X-ray test, make up the collagenous fibers, including the white connective tissue fibers and tendons, the elastic fibers and the cartilage of joints.

Before 1930 at Leeds, Astbury set about "trying to find out by X rays something about the structure of the wool fiber for the benefit of textile technology". Those beginnings have been followed by studies, carried to the molecular level, of muscle protein, blood fibrin and bacterial flagella. Electron microscopic studies of collagen fibers (at the Massachusetts Institute of Technology, the National Institutes of Health) are aimed at knowledge of the normal as a base for investigation of disease. However, in speaking of pathological alterations of collagen (fibrous proteins of white connective tissue) in hitherto unrelated clinical states, Klemperer observed, 1950, that this immense field is "so remarkably vague and ramified that it is still a question whether we know yet what we mean by normal collagen let alone pathological collagen. . . ."

Chemical study of the ground substance got off to an earlier start with 1928 studies by F. Duran-Reynals (bacteriology and immunology, Yale) of problems of invasive infection that revealed "spreading factors", later identified with the enzymes that liquefy the mucopolysaccharides of the ground substance. These mucopolysaccharides had been isolated by Karl Meyer (biochemistry, Columbia) in 1936 during studies of vitreous humor, and later, of the ground substance of umbilical cord and other organs. These chemical revelations led to active investigative work, but as Meyer noted, 1953, there remained many unsolved problems: localization within tissues of the substances the chemist isolates from the ground substance and characterizes; specific functions of connective tissue elements in relation to growth, development, aging, calcification, salt and water metabolism, energy metabolism; interaction of connective tissue with cellular organs and with the organism as a whole. "How far does the functioning, let us say, of liver cells, or the functioning of the hair follicle, or any such structure, depend on the supporting structure? What is the interaction, or is there no interaction?" It is probably no exaggeration to say, as Meyer summarized it, that these problems include every problem of biology and medicine.

Among questions raised by therapeutic use of cortisone, hydrocortisone and the pituitary corticotropin, ACTH, in the rheumatic syndromes and numerous other diseases is the nature of the nonspecific effects of these hormones on connective tissue. There are indications that the connective tissue complex may offer a new area for study of mechanisms of action of hormones on the organism.

## CORRELATION AND ADAPTATION WITHIN THE ORGANISM AS A WHOLE

The complex organism acts as a whole in adjusting to both external and internal circumstances. "When adjustment fails completely, life ceases or, if you prefer, death takes place" (J. H. Means, medicine, Harvard, 1951). By reason of this adjustment or adaptation, the body temperature, for example, is normally held constant in spite of internal and external changes of all sorts. In normal persons the level of sugar (glucose) in the blood varies within only narrow limits between the resting metabolism of sleep, the rapid absorption of food after a meal and the high-energy expenditure of a football player carrying the ball to the goal line. Mechanisms of these and other adaptations have been sought throughout the century since Bernard described the *milieu interne*, and Cannon described homeostasis. Aside from the largely unknown adaptive mechanisms of the nervous system, the chief known regulators of cellular processes are hormones or hormone-like substances, carried by the blood stream. These are not delivered to the cells directly from the circulation (since most cells are not in direct contact with capillaries) but are diffused to the cells through the intracellular fluid or the gel-like ground substance of the connective tissue (Philip D. McMaster and Robert J. Parsons, Rockefeller Institute, 1950).

The metabolism (life) of the body cells is regulated by certain inherent ("primitive") physicochemical mechanisms governing the rates of reactions. Possibly many unicellular organisms contain only such physicochemical mechanisms to govern the rates of reactions, "and well deserve to be called 'pockets of enzymes' . . ." (Guzman

Barron, 1943). These interior regulations, however, could not completely meet the requirements of the cells within complex multicellular organisms for adjustment to environmental conditions. The
cyclic and emergency regulation of body metabolism and adjustment
to internal and external environment is therefore largely taken over
by the hormones of the endocrine glands, secreted into the blood. In
the integration mechanisms in man provided by the autonomic and
central nervous systems, hormones or hormone-like substances have
been invoked as mediators of the messages from higher centers to the
body cells that must organize for adaptation.

Two endocrine glands or organs, the adrenal medulla and the
posterior pituitary (both derived from embryonic cells that differentiate also into nervous tissue and resemble that tissue histologically)
secrete hormones that affect blood pressure, contraction of smooth
muscles and other functions controlled by the autonomic nervous
system. Epinephrine was isolated from the adrenal medulla (by
Abel at Johns Hopkins in 1902) and later crystallized and synthesized. Whether pituitrin, excreted by the posterior pituitary, contains one or more principles, whether the pressor effects and the
contraction of the uterus are exerted by a single or two separate substances had not been "settled to the satisfaction of everyone", according, 1954, to du Vigneaud who among others (Kamm at Parke Davis;
H. B. Van Dyke, pharmacology, Columbia) has studied these protein-
like fractions since the twenties. These hormones appear to be secreted in response to stimulus by the autonomic nervous system and
their action is immediate and widespread — similar to neural action.
Whether the hormones of two other glands — the parathyroid and the
pancreas which secretes the blood sugar-lowering insulin and the
blood sugar-raising glycogon, the hyperglycemic factor of the pancreas are controlled by the nervous system was unknown, 1954.
Indirect neural pathways have been traced, however, for stimulation
of other endocrine glands — thyroid, ovary, testis, adrenal cortex —
through the anterior pituitary. This tiny gland at the base of the
brain secretes at least six separate, protein-like hormones that have
been isolated and purified in varying degrees: at least two hormones
that apparently act directly upon the end-organs (prolactin on the
mammary glands, the growth hormone on body cells generally); the

trophic hormones (including ACTH) which directly stimulate the secretions of the adrenal cortex, the gonads and the thyroid.

Hormonal correlating and adapting mechanisms are best illustrated by the pituitary adrenal system. Since 1950 there has been strong support for the view that epinephrine (adrenalin, the emergency neurohormone) stimulates secretion of corticotropin by the anterior pituitary (Long, 1954). This link between neural and chemical control, at present actively investigated and debated, is basic to study of effects of the adrenal cortical hormones in certain conditions, for instance in alcoholism and schizophrenia. The growth hormone of the pituitary and the hormones of the adrenal cortex are part of the research picture on disturbances in metabolic equilibrium, on the structural and functional integrity of cells and tissues, on the inscrutable biological problem of cellular growth, and on resistance to environmental and other injurious factors.

The host's endocrine balance is in some way associated with the deep mysteries of hereditary and of acquired susceptibility and resistance to invasion and spread of infectious agents through the barriers of the connective tissue. In considering effects of corticotropin and the adrenal cortex hormones on infection and resistance, investigators have recognized the significance of accumulated knowledge concerning the effects of these hormones on metabolic rates and structural elements of the whole organism. A principle set forth, 1947, by Long appears to be generally accepted: hormones "do not initiate new patterns of cellular function; these are in the birthright of the cells themselves. All that any hormone does is either to facilitate or inhibit certain types of chemical transformation within the cells". These hormones have been found to affect the structure of lymphoid tissue (William E. Ehrich, Pennsylvania, and Joseph Seifter, Wyeth, 1953), to affect repair processes in all elements of connective tissue (Charles Ragan and associates, medicine, Columbia, 1953). These effects are not unrelated to the influence of hormones on development of antibody and hypersensitivity (Edward E. Fischel, immunochemistry, Columbia, 1953), as a basis of their clinical use in "allergies". In the rheumatic syndromes, involving the entire connective tissue complex of fibrous and gel-like substances that support and bind together cells, organs and tissues, the adrenal cortex has recently assumed a prominent place due to the temporary effects of its steroids, cortisone and hydrocortisone, on the inflammatory response of connective tissues.

In cell division and growth, the influence of the growth hormone and the adrenal hormones has been demonstrated on the level of gross and microscopically visible effects which may be explained eventually by studies gradually penetrating to the molecular level. Study of specific aspects of growth patterns is the basis of approaches to the uncontrolled cellular growth of cancer in which cell multiplication proceeds with "no function in, or integration with, any orderly cellular structure", and, in addition, "has a positive, malignant capacity to injure normal tissue" (Rhoads, 1949). Cancer cells possess a kind of autonomy in their ability to forage from the environment food for building materials and energy production needed by the normal, controlled cells of the body. But, for all that, neoplastic growth is subject to the influence of hormones, and there exists much experimental and clinical evidence that growth of certain kinds of malignant tumors can be either increased or decreased by the steroids of the gonads, of the adrenal cortex and by the growth hormone.

## Neurohormonal Mechanisms of Metabolic Equilibrium and Adaptation

Epinephrine, secreted by the adrenal medulla, is intimately associated, on the one hand, with the autonomic nervous system and, on the other, with the central nervous system through autonomic centers in the hypothalamus and brain stem. Although epinephrine is referred to as a hormone of the adrenal medulla, no syndrome referable to hypofunction of the adrenal medulla analogous to hypothyroidism has been described. The effectiveness of epinephrine as a sympathomimetic drug (in asthma), its effects on cardiovascular and respiratory function, its relation to carbohydrate metabolism and its significance in transmission of sympathetic nerve impulses have given it wide usefulness in medicine and in biological research.

Combined action of the sympathetic nervous system and the adrenal medulla in emergencies, including emotional stress, was demonstrated by the work of Cannon more than twenty years ago. One response to adrenalin secretion, acceleration of glycogen breakdown to glucose, was described as the body's chief defense against low blood sugar and its threat to the central nervous system. The theory (Cannon and Rosenblueth) of two separate "sympathins" secreted at sympathetic nerve endings and, combined with adrenalin (epinephrine), acting as mediators of sympathetic impulses to the cells and organs affected has been altered by recent work. Two transmitters, adrenalin and noradrenalin, have been described as secreted by the adrenal and by the sympathetic ganglia (U. S. von Euler, Stockholm, 1948; Z. M. Bacq, Liege, 1949; Corneille Heymans, Ghent, 1950; M. L. Tainter and associates, Sterling-Winthrop, 1947–50).

The importance of these mechanisms has been clinically recognized, for example, in theories of essential hypertension on which are based surgical removal of parts of the sympathetic nervous system and administration of drugs that lower blood pressure by so-called adrenergic blockade. The bearing which relative rates of secretion of adrenalin and noradrenalin may have on various types of mental disorder and, especially, on response of patients to electro-shock therapy was suggested by Daniel H. Funkenstein, Milton Greenblatt and Harry C. Solomon (psychiatry, Harvard), 1952. The concept that some mechanism adjusts the variable rate of secretion of the adrenal cortical hormones (and of all other hormones) to meet the varying needs of the body (Long, 1954) is fundamental to understanding correlation of metabolism and function within the organism.

A central problem concerns the mechanisms by which the pituitary is stimulated to secrete corticotropin and so activate the adrenal cortex. Integration between the anterior pituitary and its target endocrine glands has been described as a two-way phenomenon, sometimes called the axial principle: according to this concept, the trophic hormones of the pituitary are believed to stimulate secretion of the sex hormones, the thyroid hormone, and the adrenal cortical steroids, with consequent raising of the blood concentration of these substances; the amounts of each of these hormones in the blood, after reaching certain proportions, in turn decrease secretion of the corresponding trophic hormone, under normal circumstances.

## The Pituitary Adrenal System

Development of the axial principle of integration of the endocrine system through intensive investigation of the so-called pituitary adrenal axis has been described as a medical revolution.  The pituitary-adrenal relation was demonstrated by studies, in the 1930's, of Philip E. Smith (anatomy, Columbia), indicating that removal of the pituitary results in adrenal cortical atrophy; and by studies elsewhere showing that, in animals thus treated, injection of cell-free extracts of pituitary tissue stimulated the adrenal.

Isolation from the anterior pituitary and purification of the adrenocorticotrophic hormone, corticotropin, in 1943 (by Li, Evans and Simpson at California, and by Sayers, White and Long at Yale), followed by intensive work on extracts of the anterior pituitary, with newer methods of protein chemistry, provided more exact means for study of pituitary-adrenal relations.  The growth hormone, isolated in partially purified state by Li, Evans and Simpson in 1945, was later fractioned by various workers (A. E. Wilhelmi and associates, biochemistry, Georgia, 1948).  Corticotropin, soon after its preparation, was fractioned into peptide residues, collectively having the biological action of the hormone (Li, 1951; Edwin B. Astwood and associates, medicine, Tufts, 1952).  By 1953, two small fractions had been separated from what had been regarded as the relatively pure protein ACTH, one of these capable of reducing the ascorbic acid content of the gland (a measure of adrenal activity) and the other capable of maintaining and restoring the adrenals of hypophysectomized rats (cf. F. G. Young, biochemistry, Cambridge, 1953).  Of eight such fractions one (named $\beta$-corticotropin), selected for study because it was present in largest quantity, had a molecular weight of 4,566 and yielded thirty-nine residues of fifteen identified amino acids (Paul H. Bell and coworkers, American Cyanamid, 1954).

By 1955, knowledge of the adrenal cortical steroids had, by distinct stages, advanced significantly during the century since Addison in 1855 described the state of adrenal insufficiency.  By 1930, extracts of the adrenal cortex had been shown (Frank A. Hartman, physiology, Ohio State and W. W. Swingle, biology, Princeton, and their respective coworkers) to maintain life of adrenalectomized animals and relieve symptoms of Addison's disease. Later investigations provided knowledge of the relation of the cortex to sodium, potassium and chloride metabolism. Chemical studies yielded twenty-eight crystalline compounds of steroid structure and another noncrystalline (amorphous) compound, recognized by its ability to control eletrolyte metabolism. Desoxycorticosterone (DCA), a synthetic compound closely related to the steroids, but obtained only once from the adrenal cortex, had activity similar to the noncrystalline fraction which was much more powerful. The synthetic hormone was clearly not the whole answer to substitution therapy in patients with Addison's disease and could not be depended upon to restore metabolic balance and maintain life under all circumstances. Of the six steroids known to have biological activity only compound E (later, cortisone) appeared to justify attempts at large-scale production, culminating in preparation of the powerful steroid by partial synthesis from one of the bile acids and in experimental and clinical study of it. Total synthesis of cholesterol, cortisone and hydrocortisone, compound F (Robert B. Woodward and associates, chemistry, Harvard), and of cortisone (L. H. Sarett and his group at the Merck laboratories) was achieved in 1952. Current work reflects concern with chemical characterization of the amorphous fraction and with its important physiologic effects.

By 1952 the active fraction was separated and crystallized almost simultaneously (J. F. Tait, S. A. Simpson and H. M. Grundy, Middlesex Hospital, London, in cooperation with Reichstein's group at Basle; V. R. Mattox, H. L. Mason and A. Albert at the Mayo Clinic) and a dual structure was demonstrated by the English workers from which the name aldosterone was taken. By 1954, aldosterone or substances with the same characteristics and activity had been detected by various workers in adrenal venous blood of animals, in the peripheral blood of normal men and in placental tissue. It had been crystallized from the urine of a nephrotic child and tested in numerous clinical states for which the doses were minute compared with the doses of cortisone known to be clinically effective (Frederic C. Bartter, National Heart Institute, 1955). Secretion of aldosterone was stimulated by corticotropin but only slightly in comparison with secretion of cortisone; evidence suggested that secretion of aldosterone may be stimulated by the growth hormone (E. H. Venning and associates, Montreal, 1954).  Total synthesis of aldosterone was announced at the fourteenth international congress of pure and applied chemistry in July, 1955, by Albert Wettstein and coworkers (Ciba laboratories, Basle).  With the immediate prospect of abundant supplies of what may be the key adrenal hormone, investigators at the congress looked forward to possible solution of some of the mysteries of homeostasis and of disease.

Hypotheses concerning regulation of adrenal cortical secretion lead inevitably to the previously mentioned problem of regulation of secretion of corticotropin by the pituitary through which neural influences appear to operate.  Through rapid neural responses and the slower, longer-lasting chemical responses of the adrenal, at least one long-sought mechanism may be established integrating the body as a whole and the body with its environment.

According to one hypothesis (developed by George and Marion Sayers, pharmacology, Utah, 1948) in the normal state the rate of elaboration of corticotropin by the pituitary fluctuates in accordance with an inhibitory effect of adrenal cortical steroids normally present in the blood stream.  Under stress, the peripheral tissue cells use larger amounts of cortical steroids, removal of which from the blood stream abolishes the check on elaboration of corticotropin, leading to increased secretion of adrenal steroids.  This concept appears to be in accord with Ingle's suggestion, made in 1943 and recalled in 1951, that increased need for secretion of the cortical hormones in stress serves only to maintain homeostasis.  "It is certain at least that the response of the adrenal cortex during stress serves some purpose which is essential for normal resistance."  Use of the term, stress, has been broadened to include innumerable physiological insults, toxicities and changes, all of which invoke, by mechanisms not yet clarified, the response of the anterior pituitary which stimulates the adrenal cortex.  Concepts of stress in relation to pituitary adrenal stimulation raise questions of direct nervous control over the secretory functions of the anterior pituitary.

Even if, as some maintain (Sayers, 1950), a neurovascular link between the hypothalamus and anterior pituitary is not essential for discharge of corticotropin, neural factors may modify the rate of discharge of corticotropin from the pituitary. Long, 1954, thought the evidence indicated at least two mechanisms by which ACTH is released: a self-regulating humoral system, governed by the levels of adrenal cortical steroids circulating in the blood, brought slowly into action by prolonged stress; a rapid mechanism in which excitation of the sympathetic centers in the hypothalamus is followed by immediate release of corticotropin. The site of action of the increased blood level of the steroids (described as the "feed back" type) was unknown; it could be the gland itself or the adjacent hypothalamic sympathetic centers, believed, 1954, to influence the anterior pituitary, possibly through "pathways ascending the spinal cord and brain stem or from higher centers of the brain". This theory of a dual mechanism is based in part on work (Geoffrey W. Harris, physiology, Cambridge University; David M. Hume, surgery, Harvard) interpreted to show that nervous or emotional stimuli, and probably also blood levels of cortisone and adrenalin, act through the hypothalamus to stimulate secretion by the anterior pituitary (Harris, 1951). The hormonal mechanism was considered to be "only of subsidiary importance under many conditions of stress".

The relation of stress to adrenal cortical functioning belongs to both the oldest and the newest concepts of adrenal function. Inability of the adrenalectomized animal to withstand stress or to adapt to environmental changes was observed in the period when adrenal function could be studied only in reverse in the adrenalectomized animal (W. W. Swingle and associates, biology, Princeton, 1943). Clinical studies on Addison's disease showed (Robert F. Loeb, medicine, Columbia, 1941) that although Addisonian patients could be kept in good condition with adequate control of electrolytes, their lives were in jeopardy, for the crisis provoked by any stress (gastrointestinal upset, respiratory infections, physical trauma or psychic strain) was relieved only by desoxycorticosterone (the only synthetic cortical hormone then available). There appears to be general agreement that, whatever the initiating factors may be (and they are legion), activation of the pituitary adrenal cortex system is a part of the body's reaction to stress, whether as an end-result or as an intermediary mechanism.

With this concept apparently established, the objective and subjective beneficial effects of administration of cortical steroids (cortisone and hydrocortisone) or of stimulation of the cortex by administration of ACTH in a wide variety of dissimilar clinical conditions are generally interpreted as illustrating increased need for cortical hormones to enable the tissues to react favorably to stressful stimuli. In some views, reactions to stress by hormone secretion may result in injury to these tissues.

Experiments begun in 1936, showing that animals responded in a "stereotyped" manner to a variety of insults (infections, intoxications, nervous strain, temperature changes, fatigue), led to the hypothesis that the response must be a reaction to stress *per se* (Hans Selye, Institute of Experimental Medicine and Surgery, Montreal, 1950). By this hypothesis, prolonged stress and prolonged pituitary-adrenal reaction may result in a "general adaptation syndrome", in which the adaptive mechanism may be derailed and "the process of adaptation may itself become the immediate cause of diseases". As illustrations, Selye mentioned hypertension, the rheumatic syndromes, the degenerative diseases, the psychosomatic syndromes. While the mechanisms by which these hormones work are thus still an enigma, in the view, 1950, of Philip S. Hench (who carried out the first trials of cortisone in rheumatoid arthritis at the Mayo Clinic), he felt that study of hormone interrelations in disease states has nevertheless contributed to fundamental knowledge as much as study of biological effects of hormones has contributed to knowledge of disease. This relationship is illustrated by research on experimental and clinical diabetes.

## RESEARCH ON DIABETES ILLUSTRATING CORRELATION AT THE CELLULAR LEVEL AND IN THE ORGANISM AS A WHOLE

The clinical syndrome of diabetes mellitus includes a chain of metabolic phenomena, all initiated by disturbances of rates at which glucose is added to the blood and at which it is utilized in the tissues. The rate of utilization of glucose by the tissues is determined largely by the availability of insulin. Maintenance of the minimal level of blood sugar compatible with life is the "result of a complex interplay between the secretions of the anterior pituitary, the adrenal cortical hormones, and in some instances the hormone of the adrenal medulla" (Long, 1952). Aside from the hormonal aspect of carbohydrate metabolism, roles in it are also played by the gastrointestinal tract, liver, muscles and kidneys, all of which influence the blood sugar level. Diabetes represents a breakdown of the mechanisms of correlation and adaptation in which the whole organism is involved. More exact definition is not possible in the present state of knowledge: "although we have all agreed that diabetes is a world-wide problem, a disease of civilization, we cannot define precisely what we mean by the term" (Young, 1954). Elucidation of the precise disturbance (if such exists) in hormonal balance in diabetes and of the biochemical reactions that are blocked or turned aside might provide means for prevention in the genetically susceptible, perhaps even cure.

Study of diabetes has, however, revealed many of the hidden reactions of intermediary metabolism and of the interrelations of hormones in governing its rates. "The twin sisters clinical observation and laboratory experiment have walked, in the field of diabetes, very close hand in hand, to their mutual stimulation" (R. D. Lawrence, diabetes department, Kings College Hospital, London, 1954). Nevertheless the considerable work done since 1921 when Banting and Best isolated insulin from the islet cells of the pancreas and demonstrated its ability to control the blood sugar level has not, as yet, revealed the cause of the "garden variety" of diabetes in man. The factors that produce experimental diabetes in animals, while illuminating, may have nothing to do with the inciting factors in man, complicated by imponderable hereditary factors (Jerome W. Conn, metabolism and endocrinology, Michigan, 1954).

In experimental diabetes, deficiency of insulin may be complete, as in animals totally depancreatized or treated with alloxan or pituitary extracts to destroy the functioning of the pancreatic islets of Langerhans from which insulin is secreted and carried by the blood to the sites of action. Such treatments remove one or more of the regulating devices (hormones, possibly unknown compounds produced by the known hormones in reaction with body cells), thus varying the relative speeds of the processes in which a given compound, such as glucose, provides elements in the metabolic machinery, its fuel, its products. The speed and direction of the processes are then regulated by an altered pattern of hormone interrelations. Although hormonal imbalance "existing about a reaction" may be temporarily corrected by injection of one of the hormones, as insulin, "the abnormality may have been produced by a disturbance in any or all of the hormones involved" (Sol Sherry, Jewish Hospital, Cincinnati, 1953). In case the disturbance is due to an abnormal amount of one of the hormones governing the rates of intermediary metabolism, "a state of disequilibrium results which persists until a new level of adjustment is achieved"; the new level, however, leaves the organism deprived of some degree of ability to make the rapid metabolic adjustments that are essential to health or to life (Frank L. Engel, medicine and physiology, Duke, 1953). The diabetic is thus deprived of ability to increase or decrease the rate of glucose utilization according to need, and to accomplish the "smooth shifts in metabolism to meet the demands of the moment and maintain homeostasis".

The diabetic state produced in animals by injection of extracts of the anterior pituitary (Houssay, 1929–1930; by Young, 1937) involved complete destruction of the insulin-producing cells of the pancreas which apparently reacted to increased need with final exhaustion. The exhaustion was obviously nonphysiological (the anterior pituitaries of twenty-five oxen being represented in the amount given one dog) but, clinically, nonphysiological action of the pituitary might augment the diabetic syndrome (Young, 1953). The question whether the pituitary factor inducing experimental diabetes is the growth hormone or corticotropin having its effect through the adrenal cortex was considered to be answered in favor of the growth hormone (Young, 1953); or, if not the growth hormone, then another pituitary factor intimately linked with it (R. C. DeBodo and M. W. Sinkoff, pharmacology, New York University, 1953). The growth hormone in decreasing utilization of carbohydrate by the tissues may create only a relative insulin deficiency. In any case, insulin properly used can accelerate utilization of carbohydrates in the tissues and lower the blood glucose level. "It is the only hormone that does this, since all the others either do not affect the blood-glucose level or else increase it" (Long, 1952). Answers to the pivotal question in diabetes, the action of insulin in terms of individual chemical reactions, are being sought in terms of cellular metabolism many details of which have been established by tracing, by isotopic techniques, pathways in cells and tissues from diabetic animals.

In liver and muscle, at least, of the diabetic animal the immediate products of carbohydrate breakdown are formed at reduced rates and to a reduced extent. Since making of all known end-products of carbohydrate breakdown is reduced in diabetic tissues the obvious place to look for the "key" defect resulting from relative lack of insulin is in the early steps of glucose breakdown. "If traffic passing down each of several divergent roads is observed abruptly to cease, one may legitimately suspect that a road block occurs at a point prior to the divergence" (Stetten, 1955). The first requirement for glucose utilization is the penetration of glucose into the cell where it meets the enzyme systems that transform it into a metabolically reactive compound containing phosphorus, and so start it on its energy-producing way. "Obviously without transfer of glucose into the area of enzymic action, no carbohydrate metabolism could be initiated" (W. C. Stadie, research medicine, Pennsylvania, 1954). The enzyme that catalyzes this first combination with inorganic phosphorus (phosphorylation) is hexokinase.

The view that insulin may influence the permeability of cells to glucose was based on experiments with the structurally similar galactose which is not metabolized and therefore accumulates within the cell (Rachmiel Levine and associates, Michael Reese Hospital, 1950). The view that the entrance of glucose "is guided by an enzyme mechanism rather than a physical process like permeability" was based upon the observation that sorbitol, also structurally related to glucose and not used by the cell, does not enter the cell with or without insulin (A. N. Wick, D. R. Drury and E. M. MacKay, Scripps Metabolic Clinic, and physiology, University of Southern California, 1951). From another direction, the hypothesis that cellular structure is necessary for the action of insulin "and perhaps other hormones" (Stadie, 1951) is based on experiments showing that insulin combines with various tissues by an unknown mechanism, which may or may not be prerequisite to insulin action. Nevertheless, "either the combination of insulin or the action of the bound insulin is markedly affected by the diabetic state and by pituitary and adrenal factors". Further work in Stadie's laboratory led to examination of the hypothesis that "the first step in the action of insulin on intact cellular systems must be its entrance into the cell and approach within mole-◄ cule distances of the enzyme system which it affects" (Stadie, 1954).

Hope that hormonal action in the body can be traced to specific enzymic steps in known metabolic pathways has increased since the Coris' *in vitro* experiments (1946) suggesting that the first reaction involved in conversion of glucose to glycogen, the hexokinase reaction, is inhibited by anterior pituitary extracts, that the inhibition is increased by adrenal cortical extracts and that this inhibition is released by insulin. Insulin apparently acts only on glucokinase (one of the group of hexokinases) at a point in the cycle of glycogen formation before the pathways of glucose and fructose are joined (M. E. Krahl, 1951).

Progress in understanding mechanisms of energy production have shown that dietary carbohydrate is as closely related as dietary fat to fat metabolism. The idea that defects in fat metabolism (the long-debated ketosis of clinical diabetes) are related to prior defects in carbohydrate utilization was proposed by Drury, 1941, by Stadie, 1942, and developed with isotope methods by Stetten, 1944–1946, by Samuel Gurin and associates (biochemistry, Pennsylvania), 1950. Chaikoff demonstrated in diabetic rats a defect in fatty acid formation in the liver, and with radioactive carbon traced the defect to a necessary link in breakdown of glucose and a block in conversion of a two-carbon fragment to fatty acids. Contrary to earlier views, adipose tissue has been found to be active metabolically. Krahl in Cori's laboratory found, 1951, active uptake of glucose by adipose tissue *in vitro*. Stadie's studies, 1951, included adipose tissue in the demonstration that in tissues pre-treated with insulin synthesis of fat from acetate or glucose was increased.

Etching in the picture of diabetes as a syndrome involving defects in some aspect of nearly all phases of cellular metabolism and of the coordinating mechanisms of hormone interrelations is incomplete, suggesting many discrepancies. In nature there are no discrepancies and those that appear in tentative formulations therefore "represent either erroneous observation or incomplete information". We may hope that, when all the facts are in, the apparent discrepancies will be resolved (Stetten, 1955). Missing or worn out parts of a system can be replaced or repaired only if we know about them, and this knowledge, according to Szent-Györgyi, 1949, can be had only by breaking down the system, gradually step by step, always stopping to put together what has been taken apart.   Upon such analyses depend both hope of finding therapeutic substances that will relieve human suffering and hope of adding significantly to new knowledge about the fundamental "principles of life and its architecture".

# CHAPTER 2

# Cancer

*Illustrating factors that influence growth,*
*normal and abnormal*

## INTRODUCTORY

While cancer must, clinically, be considered a group of disorders rather than one specific entity, the malignant state is now regarded as involving essentially the same metabolic alteration, however diverse may be the factors influencing this change, or the cells and tissues undergoing the change. Shields Warren, 1948, observed that it would be difficult to improve upon the definition of a neoplasm given many years ago by Ewing, an uncontrolled new growth of tissue. Neoplasms occur in most vertebrates, in some insects and plants, and will probably be found eventually in all multicellular organisms. This realization, although decades in the making, was pointed to as "the largest step forward of the last few years" by Rous, 1947, who said that the investigator tackling the cancer problem "really tackles the tumor problem as a whole", all tumors being related by a common "neoplastic principle". Since, as Cowdry reminded us, 1945, cancer is a "condition that can be manifested by a wide variety of cells of the body from before birth to the point of death in more or less remote response to the action of hundreds of influences not only in man but in thousands of animal species", the understanding of malignant change must be achieved with reference to normal mechanisms which are common to all cells and to mechanisms which may be specific for each differentiated type of cell. Still, the view expressed by many over the years that we could have complete knowledge of normal growth and the factors controlling it "without having the least understanding of neoplastic growth" was considered true, 1954, by Oberling and Guérin. Search for the causes and mechanisms of malignant change envelops almost every aspect of biology, as study of clinical cancer touches all medical specialties.

The scope of the cancer problem is roughly indicated by the fact that cancer now ranks second as a cause of death in this country. The cancer toll for the country was, according to a National Cancer Institute study, 225,000 in 1953 as compared with 189,811 in 1947; statistics indicate that one half of all American homes and one in every seven persons are involved. The American people, through state and federal governments, and by public subscription, have contributed many millions for cancer control and for fundamental research which may appear to be far removed from the clinical problem, for instance, grants of more than $20,000 a year for cytochemical studies of the relation between the nucleus and cytoplasm, for the study of mutations in *Drosophila*, for the microanalysis of amino acids and proteins. But fundamental work in many different types of laboratories, widespread popular interest, vast sums of money have not as yet revealed the causes of cancer. If present knowledge and methods were universally applied, Paul Steiner estimated, 1952, the percentages of five-year cure rates could be raised from five to fifty in some types, from twenty to seventy-five in others, but in many types no improvement could be expected. Surgery and radiology can eradicate many primary cancers in man without recurrence at the original sites but, because it is nearly always impossible to remove or kill all malignant cells, cancer recurs elsewhere in the body in the form of metastatic growth. The eighty-five per cent rate of permanent or complete cure in cancer of the skin (the most accessible of all cancers), not including malignant melanoma, was compared with a one per cent cure rate in cancer of the pancreas, gall bladder, liver, and lymphatic system.

A "fundamental weakness in clinical cancer research" was faced by the Committee on Growth of the National Research Council in the first report, 1946, on the plans for its advisory work in the research program of the American Cancer Society. Admitting that both laymen and physicians look upon cancer as a "discouraging problem in terminal care", the committee designated specific clinical problems toward which facts established by experimental research have opened approaches. Since then, clinical research planned and carried out in close association with experimental programs has been aided by the Damon Runyon clinical research fellowships (recommended by the Committee on Growth); by the society's institutional research grants (begun 1948) which usually support combined clinical and experimental research; by the clinical center of the National Institutes of Health, the three cancer hospitals of the Atomic Energy Commission, and other public and private hospital research centers.

Much has been learned about the factors influencing the origin and growth of both spontaneous and induced neoplasms in experimental animals. Among tumors in experimental animals (spontaneous and induced) available for study, 1953, were carcinoma of skin, mammary gland, lung, endometrium, uterus; sarcoma of connective tissues and bone; glioma of brain; malignant tumors of liver, spleen, kidney, ovary, testis, adrenal cortex, thyroid, pituitary; lymphosarcoma and leukemias. Application to the human cancer patient of findings in experimental cancer was limited according to Homburger, 1953, to some knowledge of chemical and physical environmental factors that produce cancer (occupational cancer), to use of hormones and chemotherapeutic agents for temporary improvement in a few types of cancer. What is needed to narrow the gap is development of better methods and tools for "quantitative evaluation of biologic and biochemical phenomena in man", for there is no correlative evidence that tumors in laboratory animals are "directly comparable to human tumors" (Alfred Gellhorn, 1953).

Results of treatment are generally recognized to depend largely on early diagnosis and immediate application of available measures. Tests suitable for case finding in the general population for detection of still-localized cancer in sites not accessible to direct examination were still to be found, 1953, according to studies of the cancer control branch of the National Cancer Institute. Of chemical tests based on specific changes confined to one or another type of cancer, a few (determination of urinary steroids in functional tumors of the adrenal cortex; detection of Bence Jones protein in multiple myeloma; serum "acid phosphatase" levels in metastasizing carcinoma of the prostate) were considered by Homburger, 1953, to have had "some measure of enduring success". A method developed by Papanicolaou for the examination of free cells in the debris from body cavities has been used for the detection of cancer cells in the absence of identifiable lesions. Experience in over 40,000 cases of cervical and uterine cancer reported from a number of laboratories is regarded as promising the earlier and more effective use of surgery. E. M. Robertson discussed, 1947, the use of the cytological method of diagnosis in specimens of peritoneal exudates, pleural exudates, cyst fluid, sputum, gastric contents, feces, urine and smears from accessible lesions. J. R. McDonald and L. B. Woolner reported, 1947, the finding of carcinoma cells in either sputum or bronchial secretions in 100 cases of carcinoma of the lung. J. V. Meigs and his associates at the Massachusetts General Hospital reported, 1948, improved techniques for collecting cellular specimens by aspiration from the stomach. In forty-eight patients studied, fourteen carcinomas of the stomach were revealed at operation, twelve of which had been diagnosed correctly by cytological methods. In one case of early carcinoma, all other diagnostic procedures had been negative.

## EVIDENCES OF ORGANIZED COOPERATION

An outstanding example of organized cooperation is the research program of the American Cancer Society under the direction of the Committee on Growth of the National Research Council. The council itself, which is the operating agency of the National Academy of Sciences, represents the ninety-odd scientific societies associated with the national academy and includes on its various committees representatives of the Army, Navy, Public Health Service and other agencies of the federal government, to which it is scientific advisor. Published statements reveal a cordial relationship between the Committee on Growth and the cancer research grants branch of the National Cancer Institute. Each body responsible for the research and fellowship program has full information on applications received and on action taken by the other; undesirable duplication is avoided although grants from both bodies are sometimes made for the same projects or to the same institutions and investigators. These are considered desirable for extension of programs having several valuable aspects. Through annual campaigns, the American Cancer Society has raised from public subscription between 1938 and 1954 over 120 million dollars. The 1940 contributions amounted to a little over $210,105; in 1945, when the first wide public appeal for cancer research was made, the receipts were over $4,200,000. In that year, the society contracted with the National Research Council for advice on the expenditure of funds for fundamental cancer research and for fellowships. The council established in that year its Committee on Growth under the division of medical sciences. The Committee on Growth at the end of its sixth year, 1951, was composed of eighteen investigators representing clinical medicine and the basic sciences who were assisted by sixteen subcommittees or panels with a total membership of 108. Expenditures for grants, training fellowships and expenses of the central office, which include those for meetings and conferences, are recommended by the committee, approved by the society, and used according to the technique of coordinated research developed during the war. Between 1946 and 1952, $9,001,647 was spent for 1,226 project grants, and $1,781,397 was spent for 381 fellowships. The institutional research grants ($5,611,552 from 1947 to 1951) given by the society through its research committee to universities, medical schools, research institutes and other agencies are fluid funds for development of integrated programs of cancer research. The society is sponsor for a new bi-monthly journal, *Cancer*, reporting various phases of research, especially clinical research, and for a monthly index with classified abstracts, *Current Cancer Literature*, covering the world literature. An "electronic mind" which can organize and dispense information on chemical compounds by use of coded files of punched cards (50,000 compounds and a million and a half cards to start with) was put into operation, 1955, by the National Research Council's chemical-biological coordination center. Funds for the machines and nine years' work on developing the coding system were provided by the National Cancer Society, National Cancer Institute, the Army, Navy, Atomic Energy Commission. Data on the chemicals are available to investigators in all fields including cancer.

Coordination of experimental and clinical cancer research and teaching is illustrated in the oldest cancer research center in the country, the Memorial Center for Cancer and Allied Diseases in New York. The hospital (voluntary, independent) has long been associated as a teaching center with the Cornell medical school in which the director of the center is professor of pathology. Some years after completion of the new hospital building with research laboratories (with a grant of three millions from the General Education Board, 1937) and opening of the Sloan-Kettering Institute (built adjacent to the hospital with a gift of four millions, 1946), the institute was made a graduate division of Cornell. The James Ewing Hospital, built by the city, provided for the center affiliation with the city department of hospitals. The cancer research program, centered in the institute, was planned, 1945, to bridge the gap between established findings of experimental research and their clinical trial as part of the center's purpose of control of cancer in man. In the budget of the center (over eight millions, 1950) the twenty per cent allocated for research depends entirely upon gifts and grants. In 1950, the largest proportion of the research budget came from the American Cancer Society (institutional research grant, $250,000; funds administered by the Committee on Growth, $352,800). Grants from the federal government totaled $504,000 (about equally from the National Cancer Institute and the Atomic Energy Commission). From other sources (foundations, industry, individuals) the center received $708,000.

Gifts from *foundations* and income from cancer research endowments were, before 1940, the chief support of the research going forward in hospitals and medical schools. Present interest of the foundations in cancer research, with exception of the Childs Fund and the Anna Fuller Fund, is expressed in occasional grants apparently motivated by interest in the particular project or investigator. As illustration, the Commonwealth Fund gave, 1946–1949, a total of $90,000 for the studies of G. N. Papanicolaou on exfoliated normal and cancer cells from which the techniques of cellular diagnos's have been developed. Grants for basic research made by the division of natural sciences of the Rockefeller Foundation, over the years, particularly for basic work in metabolism, are fundamental to developing concepts now predominating in cancer research programs and may be considered as relevant to the field. Examples of such grants, 1948, are: $12,000 for research in enzyme chemistry, Massachusetts General Hospital; $15,000 for research in genetics, Jackson Memorial Laboratory; $29,600 for research on nucleic acids, Stanford University; $23,400 for research on proteolytic enzymes, Yale University. The Jane Coffin Childs Memorial Fund is the only large endowment concentrating its support upon cancer research at present. The fund, established in 1937 with a capital of approximately $4,000,000, has chosen the support of cancer research as the present purpose, with provision for transferring support to some other scientific field when progress and circumstances indicate the desirability of change. During the first years, the grants for research were given to expand programs already developing at Yale, and probably in recognition of the work of the atypical growth study unit which, without authority to supervise research programs, brings to the problems of neoplastic growth the united research interests of representatives of various university departments, *e.g.* anatomy, histology, embryology, botany, genetics, biology, chemistry, pathology and surgery. Research grants and fellowships approved by the board of managers of the fund in 1953 amounted to nearly $250,000 which was distributed to investigators in American and British laboratories.

Among the *universities*, various types of institutes, study units and coordinating committees for cancer research, in addition to the previously mentioned atypical growth study unit at Yale, have been instituted. Columbia's Institute of Cancer Research with an endowment of approximately $1,500,000 aims at integrating the activities of various medical school and university departments concerned with cancer research. Two new major cancer units at the Columbia-Presbyterian Medical Center were completed during 1949 and 1950. Additions are four new floors of research laboratories to the medical school and the Francis Delafield Hospital erected by the city. The University of Chicago announced in 1947 the establishment within the university of a committee on cancer composed of twenty-two faculty representatives of the clinical departments of medicine, surgery, pediatrics, roentgenology, obstetrics and gynecology, and the university departments of zoology, botany, chemistry, the medical school departments of bacteriology and parasitology, pathology, anatomy, physiology and biochemistry, and the institutes of radiology and biophysics, and of nuclear studies. A new $2,000,000 hospital was scheduled for completion 1950. Harvard's cancer commission administers an endowment that at the beginning of this century amounted to approximately $2,000,000. The interest of university departments in cancer research is illustrated by the distribution of research grants from the American Cancer Society in three universities between 1946 and 1952. The total of $385,463 received by Harvard was given to investigators in the departments of botany, zoology, anatomy, chemistry, biological chemistry, clinical medicine and dental science. At Pennsylvania, $322,191 was granted to investigators in departments of biophysics, chemistry, physical chemistry, surgical research and pediatrics. The $300,095 received by the University of Minnesota consisted of grants for research in departments of physics, zoology, bacteriology and immunology, physiological chemistry and cancer biology.

Among the *state universities*, Wisconsin, Texas and Missouri receive direct appropriations from state governments for cancer research. Cancer research laboratories, units, or divisions had been established in the medical schools of over fourteen public universities, 1954. The University of California inaugurated in 1948, with the aid of an appropriation from the state legislature, an interdepartmental program of cancer research, and a course in the biochemistry of cancer as a part of the regular curriculum in the biochemistry department. In addition, the laboratory of experimental oncology, a section of the National Cancer Institute, is located at the University of California medical school in San Francisco. The University of Wisconsin inaugurated in 1940 a division of oncology, housed in the McArdle Memorial Laboratory with a hospital wing (1948) for research and training cancer investigators. In 1954, New York appropriated four millions for research on lung cancer.

Outstanding among the endowed *research institutes* contributing to cancer research (in addition to the Sloan-Kettering Institute) are the Rockefeller Institute for Medical Research, the Jackson Memorial Laboratory at Bar Harbor, Maine, the Carnegie Institution laboratories at Cold Spring Harbor, the Institute for Cancer Research in Philadelphia. Studies pertinent to cancer are coordinated at the Rockefeller Institute by the appointment of a member in charge of cancer research. J. B. Murphy received from the Committee on Growth $33,000 between 1947 and 1949 for investigations in several laboratories on normal and malignant cells by electron-microscopic technique. The genetic studies of M. Demerec at the Cold Spring Harbor laboratory have been aided by grants from the Committee on Growth, 1946–1950, of $43,036. The program of experimental genetics at Bar Harbor has been supported by large gifts from the foundations, and by grants totaling, 1952, over $395,000, including $50,000 for reconstruction, from the Committee on Growth. From 1938 through 1953, grants for research on genetic and other factors in experimental cancer from the Public Health Service amounted to $402,858. The Lankenau Research Institute in Philadelphia, which has been engaged in cancer research for more than twenty-five years, has now been incorporated as the Institute for Cancer Research with a staff of 100 workers and a new building provided by a gift of $1,000,000. Institutional research grants of $450,000 have been made by the American Cancer Society to this institute, and Public Health Service research grants, $412,098, were made, 1949–1953. The Detroit Institute of Cancer Research had become, by 1949, closely affiliated with Wayne University college of medicine by joint investigations of problems by both staffs. Grants to the Detroit institute from the Committee on Growth, $412,098, and from the Public Health Service, $76,809, were received through 1953.

Direct responsibility for cancer research was assumed by the *federal government* with the passage, in 1937, of the National Cancer Act, establishing the National Cancer Institute, now one of the National

Institutes of Health under the direction of the Public Health Service. Six members of the staff of the institute serve on panels of the Committee on Growth each year. The research program of the institute has been developed on foundations laid by fifteen years of experimental cancer research carried out by the United States Public Health Service before 1937. The first appropriation under the act provided $750,000 to build the National Cancer Institute and $700,000, representing the income at that time from $20,000,000, for operating expenses. Although the research program was necessarily curtailed during the war, the annual appropriations from 1938 through 1946 averaged $464,222. During the first ten years, 286 grants-in-aid for research in other institutions, totaling $2,437,330, were made. In 1947, Congress appropriated $12,197,000 under the act for the entire cancer program of the Public Health Service and in 1948, $14,000,000 was appropriated, of which sum $9,000,000 was available for research for the year ending June 30, 1949. Grants were made to 192 different investigators in eighty-eight institutions. An additional appropriation of $8,000,000 was made for construction of cancer research facilities in medical school, hospital and other centers. The appropriations for 1950 were $18,900,000 in cash and $6,000,000 for contracts, $3,500,000 of which has been budgeted for construction. Under the auspices of the institute, the Laboratory of Experimental Cell Research was organized, 1947, at the Marine Biological Laboratory, Woods Hole, with an initial grant of $25,000; Robert Chambers, the director, received a grant for equipment and instrumentation from the Committee on Growth. Since the inception of the program, 3,950 cancer research grants representing an expenditure of $46,200,763 had been approved by September, 1953. The entire appropriations from the Public Health Service for cancer research and control, 1938, through 1950, added up to $67,851,570.

The Atomic Energy Commission, through its division of biology and medicine, established a cancer program during its first year of operation. In March, 1948, it was reported that $3,000,000 of the $5,000,000 appropriated by Congress for cancer research had been devoted to the first year's plan to explore the possible benefits of atomic energy to cancer sufferers, to assist and augment existing projects while avoiding duplication of work supported by other agencies. At that time, $450,000 was set aside for one year to supply radioisotopes to cancer investigators in the United States, free except for handling and shipping charges. The commission's committee on isotope distribution must approve the purpose of the investigations, and has set up certain restrictions governing the clinical use of isotopes. Agreements with investigators in the twenty-two foreign nations qualified to receive isotopes include reports to the commission, publication of results and permission to qualified scientists of all nations to visit and observe. Among foreign investigators who have received shipments, Lacassagne at the Pasteur Institute is using carbon 14 to synthesize benzacridines for use in cancer research. Among the thirty-four projects in biology, medicine and health physics sponsored by the commission, 1948–1949, the following investigations suggest the scope of the developing cancer program: the use of radiocobalt as a substitute for radium; the use of isotopes of carbon and nitrogen in the study of nucleic acid metabolism; the use of tagged amino acids in the study of protein metabolism in relation to cancer; radiation as a cause of cancer; and isotopes in the treatment of cancer. The commission is financing two clinical cancer research facilities: the Oak Ridge Cancer Hospital consisting of thirty-two beds in the Oak Ridge Hospital which is being operated by the deans of the southern medical schools affiliated with the Oak Ridge Institute of Nuclear Studies; the Argonne hospital, completed in 1953 at a cost of $4,180,000, operated by the University of Chicago for the use of thirty-one medical schools and universities affiliated with Argonne. It is expected that short-lived isotopes that cannot be transported far will be tested for application to human cancer in these two hospitals adjacent to the two nuclear reactors. Since 1952, radioisotopes for use in study, diagnosis and treatment of cancer have been supplied at twenty per cent of production cost, the commission finding the stimulus of free distribution no longer necessary.

Activities of *industrial organizations* in cancer research are, in general, more indirect and diffuse than those of other agencies. The work of isolation, purification and synthesis of the innumerable pure compounds that are indispensable to investigators engaged in metabolic research is one of the chief contributions of the industrial research laboratories. Among compounds tested for usefulness in chemotherapy of cancer that have been synthesized by industrial chemists and given in large amounts to outside research centers are: analogues of folic acid (Lederle); a number of purine analogues, including 6-mercaptopurine (Wellcome); cortisone (Merck). Beginning of commercial production and distribution of radioisotope-labeled compounds followed by only a few months the initiation of the Atomic Energy Commission's program, 1948, of radioisotope distribution for cancer research, diagnosis and therapy, and grants to aid these developments have been made by the commission since 1949. Since then the commission has continued its encouragement of industrial research toward development of tools, equipment and instruments, of new labeled compounds for use in research and treatment.

International, national and local research *conferences* have increased over the last decade in number and in scope of problems and approaches brought to bear on cancer. At the seventh international cancer research congress, 1947, investigators from forty nations met to revive, after the war, international cooperation and exchange. Many other later international congresses have systematized knowledge (from cytochemistry, radiobiology, protein and steroid chemistry, genetics, endocrinology) now capable of being fitted into the biological framework of the cancer problem. National conferences on cancer research held regularly since 1945 by the chemistry section of the American Association for the Advancement of Science, the American Association for Cancer Research have been held jointly with the National Cancer Institute since 1951. Periodic conferences on particular areas in the field are becoming an established means of coordination, as for example, conferences by the Committee on Growth (on nutrition), by the New York Academy of Sciences (on viruses, cellular structure, cell division, antimetabolites), by the National Cancer Institute (on gastric cancer, occupational cancer, chemotherapy).

## FOUR INTERRELATED EXPERIMENTAL APPROACHES

The urgency of the clinical problems of cancer is the impetus behind the increase in funds for cancer research during the last decade, and the resulting attraction to the field of investigators from many branches of physics, chemistry and biology bringing lines of fundamental research to bear on the central problem of the nature of malignant

change. With younger workers, often trained by the aid of cancer
fellowships or interested through increasingly numerous courses in
medical school curricula, and the body of investigators already labor-
ing in the field, cancer research programs are well staffed. From many
laboratories are reported bewilderingly numerous studies bearing on
the metabolism which is the basis of growth in all living systems.
Four major lines of approach, often interlocked, illustrate in the following discussion the breadth and sweep of the basic research from
which clinical cancer research draws its leads, its tools, its substance:
chemical carcinogens; hormones; enzymes and nucleoproteins; viruses.
Upon these four lines depend, also, the experimental testing of theories
of malignant change which, in turn, open new avenues or invite new
disciplines to aid in the attempt to find out why and how normally
functioning cells change over to the uncontrolled growth of cancer.

In the experimental production of tumors in laboratory animals,
many factors have been unraveled from the maze of controllable circumstances and analyzed for their qualitative and quantitative influence on tumor production. The first step toward bridging the gap
between experimental cancer and human cancer was made by the production of typical metastasizing carcinomas in animals by the application of chemical compounds derived from or related to tar. A new
line of research was opened with perspectives looking toward structural interrelationships between the carcinogenic hydrocarbons and a
whole series of compounds built on a sterol ring structure, including
the estrogenic hormones. At the eighth international biochemical
congress, held in Paris in October, 1948, E. C. Dodds described the
present knowledge of carcinogenic and anticarcinogenic substances
as rather depressing. "When one considers the vast amount of labour
expended during the last fifty years to gain this meager knowledge,
one wonders how much more will have to be done before the cancer
problem is solved." It seems to be undeniable that all known means
of checking or stopping neoplastic growth, once it has begun, are
indirect. It is also true, however, that more and more of the agents
known to be capable of influencing (rather than producing) the rise
and development of cancer are avoidable in proportion as they become known and understood. Standards for protection of workers
from the damaging effects of certain radiations known to induce

cancer have been slowly established, and the Atomic Energy Commission had by 1950 set standards for protection of workers with limits far below safe amounts of exposure. The commission, in stressing the need for basic research on the effects of radiation, outlined the general facts known: radiation attacks, disrupts and destroys the delicate electro-chemical balance in the atoms, molecules and protein complexes within the bodies of living things; it breaks down atoms and molecules into fragments carrying positive or negative electrical charges, which recombine in haphazard ways forming toxic substances, or causing injury in other ways. As many investigators have pointed out, the effects of ionizing radiations (these effects being qualitatively similar whether produced by radium, X ray, or neutrons and other particle radiations) are chemical alterations and their understanding depends upon knowledge of the chemistry and metabolism of living material, protoplasm. Malignant change is one outcome of exposure to radiation, as it is one outcome of exposure to carcinogenic chemicals, and investigation of mechanisms by any approach aims at the same goal, the metabolic nature of malignancy.

## CHEMICAL CARCINOGENS

The production of neoplasms in animals by the administration of organic compounds of definite and known chemical structure not only provided a powerful tool for experimental cancer research but also raised high hopes that the chemical changes leading to malignancy might thereby be discovered. The first tumors elicited by the application of chemicals appeared on the skin at the sites of application but, as time went on, investigators learned to call forth, by the action of these substances, malignant neoplasms in tissues far removed from the sites of application. The effects of these agents were not always limited to direct and local disturbances. It was hoped that if the mechanisms of malignant change could be unraveled in terms of cellular metabolism, the way might open for the development of a rational basis for chemotherapy in cancer. It was hoped, further, that a relation between chemical structure and carcinogenic activity might be discovered to provide clues pointing to carcinogens with related structure and properties which, arising in the body through abnormal metabolism, might account for the appearance of spontaneous neoplasms.  Although these hopes are still far from realization, the ideas behind them underlie lines of current research of which three illustrate major approaches: study of the action of carcinogenic chemicals on cells and tissues directly exposed; study of relations between structure and metabolism of carcinogens; study of the action of carcinogens on the cell nucleus.

Emphasis in the search for correlations between carcinogenic activity and chemical structure has shifted often during the ten or more years during which this work has been active.  It seems agreed now that these agents which are effective in producing tumors cannot be what Rous, 1943, called the "actuating" causes of the neoplasms.  They play their part and then disappear from the scene.  Even though these compounds may have no connection with any causes of human tumors, the discovery of what they do would certainly illumine the mechanisms of malignant change.  Medawar, 1947, commented upon the nonspecificity of the induction of tumors by these agents and other agents, such as radiations: "there is no specific affinity between the tumors produced by the action of one and the same carcinogen on different tissues, nor any specific difference between the tumors elicited from one and the same tissue by the action of different carcinogens." There is as yet, he observed, no definite evidence that sterols or other substances are converted by the body into a single carcinogenic principle.  Nevertheless, the possibility persists that some common structure or part of a structure, even a bond or a radical, may characterize the truly carcinogenic principle or principles which may arise in the cells through the action of these diverse agents.

Chemical carcinogenesis, beginning in 1915 when Yamagiwa and Ichikawa produced malignant tumors by painting rabbits' ears with tar, became, after 1932 when Cook and his associates at the Royal Cancer Hospital in London produced cancer in mice by the application of pure synthetic chemical substances, one of the most active lines in cancer research.  Two groups of investigators, one in England and one in Boston, brought to a close, 1941, the chemical phase, at least, of their researches on the development and synthesis of a large number of *polycyclic hydrocarbons* which had been tested as carcinogens in mice. E. L. Kennaway and his associates at the Royal Cancer Hospital published at the end of 1942 what was apparently their final paper in a series on the structure and synthesis of pure hydrocarbons. This work was summarized by Dodds, 1948: first, he said, was the demonstration that substances built of nothing but carbon and hydrogen could be carcinogenic; secondly, the identity of the active fraction of tar was established by showing that the emission spectrum was of the same type as that of the polycyclic hydrocarbons; thirdly, the first synthesis of polycyclic hydrocarbons having carcinogenic potency was reported by Cook and his coworkers in 1932. Of the hundreds of polycyclic hydrocarbons that have since been tested for carcinogenic power, only one, 3,4-benzpyrine, has been isolated from tar. The yield was minute. Hieger, of Kennaway's team, obtained in 1933 fifty grams — about the weight of eight silver quarters — from two tons of pitch. The first synthetic compound shown to be carcinogenic was 1:2:5:6-dibenzathracene and the other active substances synthesized were chiefly derivatives of anthracene, benzanthracene, benzpyrine and cholanthrene.

The American group, M. J. Shear and his associates, brought to a close their series of studies with a summary publication in 1941. These workers in the Cambridge laboratory, established by the United States Public Health Service in 1923 to initiate its cancer research, began their studies on chemical carcinogenesis in 1935. The hundreds of compounds tested in the English and American laboratories were nearly all polycyclic hydrocarbons related to 1:2-benzanthracene. The compounds tested by the English group were synthesized in their own laboratory, and the compounds tested by the Boston group were supplied by investigators led by L. F. Fieser of the Converse Memorial Laboratory at Harvard, to whom the Public Health Service gave a five-year grant of $27,550 in 1937 for this purpose. The considerable overlap in the compounds tested, the widely differing methods of synthesis, and the use of stock mice in Kennaway's laboratory and of pure strains in Shear's laboratory all enhance the significance of the essential agreement in the conclusions. The concentrated research in these and other laboratories has yielded five polycyclic hydrocarbons having well-tested carcinogenic potencies; benzpyrene, the first and generally effective carcinogen; dibenzanthracene, its close relative, a slowly acting carcinogen; methylcholanthrene, a quickly acting, powerful carcinogen; 9:10-dimethyl-1:2-benzanthracene, producing skin tumors rapidly; and the 10-methyl compound of 1:2-benzanthracene (itself inactive), more effective in producing sarcomas than skin cancers. The selection of these five compounds on the basis of their carcinogenic potencies means only that, under specific experimental conditions, they will produce cancers when brought into contact with certain tissues.

Of the substances outside the class of polycyclic hydrocarbons, those of the *azo dye group*, the most important are two: o-amino-azotoluene and 4-dimethylaminoazobenzene, which orally administered to rats produce liver cancer. While the work has been expanded by the testing of many derivatives on rats and other species, the specific power of the two original compounds to produce liver tumors has not been challenged. From the beginning of this work, many investigators have held the theory that the carcinogenic effect of the azo dye compounds must take place primarily through liver injury but this has not been proved. Tumors produced by the azo dyes are much more sensitive to dietary variations during the preliminary period than are tumors produced by other chemicals. It remains a question whether the effects of diet are primary, in that the fundamental mechanisms of malignant change are altered by diet, or secondary, in that the metabolism of the dyes is altered by diet.

By 1951, more than a thousand aromatic polycyclic hydrocarbons, azo compounds, amino compounds, nitrogen and sulfur mustards had been synthesized and, with miscellaneous organic (urethane) and inorganic compounds (arsenic, nickel, salts of beryllium, etc.) had been tested for carcinogenic power. A survey, 1951, by Hartwell, and the electronic device described above contribute to sustained investigative interest in the general problem of relation of chemical constitution and carcinogenic activity. By 1953, synthesis of three C 14-labeled carcinogenic hydrocarbons had been reported, making possible tracing the pathways of carcinogens through metabolic cycles, identification of intermediaries, determination of site or sites of interaction of active substances with the cell. Study of these interactions in terms of physical and radiation chemistry has been furthered by synthesis of two new series of carcinogens, discussed later.

Although coal tar has been associated with human cancer since the observations of Pott in 1775 on "chimney sweep's cancer" in which he related the high incidence of scrotal cancer in men of this trade to accumulation of soot on the scrotal skin, Fieser, 1945, emphasized that no evidence existed at that time that the carcinogenic hydrocarbons have any bearing on the real problem, human cancer. Benzpyrene, in recent years, has been isolated from domestic soot (Goulden and Tipler, 1949), from carbon blacks (Falk and Steiner, 1952), from atmospheric dust in cities (Waller, 1952). Atmospheric dust has been known since 1942 to be cancer-producing in animals, according to Leiter and Shear. As environmental carcinogenic chemicals are recognized (chiefly by experience) prevention of cancer through their elimination "is by all accounts superior to the best type of present-day cancer cure", in the view of W. C. Hueper (environmental cancer section, National Cancer Institute), 1953. Products obtained from mineral oils by the catalytic cracking process appear to be unusually carcinogenic in animals. A carcinogenic nitrogen-containing analogue of naphthalene, possibly formed from 2-naphthylamine which is believed to be responsible for cancer of the bladder in dye workers, produced the disease in dogs (Bonser, 1943). Study in man of environmental cancers has yielded information on susceptibility (which Hueper believed to be analogous to inherited individual susceptibility to various infectious agents) and on the complexity of carcinogenesis. There are apparently as many aspects and phases in environmental cancerous diseases as in infections.

## ACTION OF CARCINOGENIC CHEMICALS ON CELLS AND TISSUES DIRECTLY EXPOSED

Observation of the daily, even hourly, changes in living cells brought directly into contact with carcinogenic agents has the attraction of a definite problem divisible into definite parts. This is not to say that the problem is simple, for its complexities are as marked as the complexities of living protoplasm. Its solution might provide only answers to questions limited to one kind of malignant change, artificially produced and so far without any definite relation to human cancer. Its solution would certainly leave untouched the many complexities implied in Rous's statement, 1943, that the investigations of many workers "have lately made plain that the provocative carcinogens in many instances elicit tumors of a sort that the animal is more or less likely to have spontaneously". Nevertheless, some direct effect of the hydrocarbons on the exposed cells has long been thought to be probable for, as Fieser remarked, 1945, the unchanged hydrocarbon has been found in the skin from two to three months after painting and bits of unchanged hydrocarbon are sometimes found in the tumors. Cells in tissue culture, treated with 20-methylcholanthrene, were noted by Earle, 1945, to take up the chemical. He said: "We have seen some suggestions of actual droplets of fluid entering the cells. We have seen very large fragments of methylcholanthrene inside the cells. In one instance the fragment was larger than the original cell." A systematic analysis was then undertaken of changes in chemical equilibrium, in physical properties, in morphological characteristics and in functional activities of a variety of experimental material including cells and tissues exposed *in vivo* and those exposed in tissue cultures. It has also been pointed out by Spencer, 1945, that studies of free-living cells (paramecia and worms) kept in contact with chemical carcinogens can yield knowledge of biological adaptations that may be directly applicable to problems of the mechanism of action of these agents on cells of complex organisms.

For many years, malignant cells have been grown in tissue cultures and studied exhaustively to detect metabolic, cultural, cytological, and biological characteristics distinguishing malignant cells. There seems to be general agreement that Lacassagne's statement (cited by Murphy, 1942) that no specific characteristic of cancer cells has ever been established "other than a loss of subordination to the rhythm of division" remains true. It has long been hoped that, if malignant change could be chemically induced in cells growing *in vitro*, material would be available for the study of progressive changes, even changes from day to day. W. R. Earle and associates, National Cancer Institute, summarized, 1945, the data from their studies using mouse subcutaneous connective tissue fibroblasts grown in heterologous tissue cultures and exposed to 20-methylcholanthrene for periods from 116 days to 406 days. Observations without attempts at theorizing were presented. The first changes observed were morphological changes in the cell surface. The gradual changes occurred homogeneously throughout the clump as a whole rather than in isolated cells, and seemed to be permanent, no reversal being observed in more than two years after the removal of the cultures from the medium containing carcinogen. The malignancy of the treated cells was tested by injection of the cultures into strain C3H mice. The failure of some cell cultures, having all the characteristics of malignancy, to produce tumors upon injection brings up again a question which is in the minds of investigators approaching the problems of cancer from different directions: is there a stage at which cells, having undergone malignant change, may or may not grow and produce cancer? In some views, cancer prevention will eventually depend upon the environmental factors that control this phase, factors acting upon the cells that have already undergone malignant change.

Action of the polycyclic aromatic hydrocarbons is regarded by many as direct or local, tumors usually arising in cells and tissues directly exposed. In this respect, their action resembles that of radiations (Brues, 1954), whether soft X rays that induce cancer at the surface of the body or harder and more penetrating X rays producing cancer internally (in bone or hemopoietic tissues). Radioactive atoms introduced into the body produce cancer in the tissues where the chemical tends to localize, as phosphorus in bone (Brues) and iodine in the thyroid (Goldberg and Chaikoff, 1952). The hydrocarbons appear to be carcinogenic for all tissues directly exposed in contrast to the azo dyes (and a heterogeneous collection of other substances) which act "remotely" on certain specific tissues and organs (Berenblum, 1954). The explanation that appeared to cover most of the known facts (failure of such compounds to induce tumors when introduced directly into the liver, bladder or other susceptible organ) is that, since all carcinogens are metabolized in the body, the active substance in the "remotely" acting carcinogens may be an intermediary breakdown product of the compound. Or, many observations may be explained by several modifications of a two-stage theory of carcinogenesis. Berenblum considered a useful working hypothesis the concept of dormant tumor cells being induced by the primary action, and then converted into growing, fully malignant tumors by various extraneous factors. Factors known to influence tumor pathogenesis in different degrees and in different tissues are: genetic factors between species and within species; age, sex and

endocrine factors; dietary factors at varying stages of chemical carcinogenesis; solvents used for administering the carcinogens; irritation
of tissues. There may be many others. Study of regression of tar
warts in rabbits and subsequent development of progressing neoplasia
after noncarcinogenic stimuli at those sites led to a concept of "latent
neoplastic potentialities" that are irreversible but still may not be
realized (Friedewald and Rous, 1950). That a complete autonomy
of malignant cells is an extreme preceded by more responsive states is
suggested by experiments on transplantation of tumors from one
species to the anterior chamber of the eye in another species (H. N. S.
Greene, 1951). Initial dependence of malignant tumors on hormones
has been suggested by experimental interstitial cell tumors of the
testis that require estrogens for growth and persistence (W. U. Gardner, 1945); by transplantation of pituitary tumors, from thyroidectomized animals, which will grow only in other thyroidectomized
animals (Furth and Burnett, 1951). In the carcinogenic process,
studied for many years in mouse skin painted with methylcholanthrene by Cowdry with over forty collaborators, data were thought to
be consistent with the hypothesis that "the malignant transformation
is one of probably several mutations" (Cowdry, 1953). Since, however, mutations occur instantaneously, it is necessary to suppose that
the mutant cells remain "quiescent throughout the latent period".

### STRUCTURE AND METABOLISM OF CARCINOGENS

Suggestions of possible metabolic pathways of the carcinogenic
hydrocarbons in the body and of the formation of new active compounds responsible for the biological effects have come from chemical
investigation of the behavior of highly reactive groups contained in
old and new synthetic organic compounds. Pinck and his associates in
the Department of Agriculture reported, 1948, three types of Michael
condensations involved in the reactions of fluorine with dibiphenylene-
ethylene. From these reactions, compounds have been obtained
which are not carcinogenic in themselves but which, upon enzymic
dehydrogenation, yield cancer-producing compounds. As a working
hypothesis it is proposed that seven groups of organic compounds, including a cyclic aromatic hydrocarbon and an azo compound, having
electronic configurations making reactions with cell substances pos-

sible through one of the three types of Michael condensations described, are carcinogenic by virtue of their ability to initiate a series of chain reactions with cell substance. The chain of reactions once initiated would be continuous in the presence of cell substance which provides the enzymes necessary for the dehydrogenation. The author offered his theory as an explanation of the mechanisms by which minute amounts of carcinogenic chemicals initiate cancer, as a possible explanation of metastasis, and as a basis for a rational approach to chemotherapy.

Studies of the relation between electronic configuration and carcinogenesis by physical chemists in Germany (O. Schmidt 1938–1941), in France (Dandel, the Pullmans and others since 1945) and in England since the war, represent early attempts "to relate what are obviously complex biological phenomena to quantum-mechanical principles" (C. A. Coulson, 1953). Such data on molecules were included in the first survey by Hartwell, 1941, of compounds tested for carcinogenic potency, and work since then has, according to Coulson, resulted in correct predictions of potency, on purely theoretical grounds, of compounds not yet tested. If the promise of this approach should be fulfilled, problems of chemical carcinogenesis would prove to be only one facet of the whole problem of mechanism of action of chemicals on cells. Seifriz attributed, 1948, to similarity in electronic configuration the similarity in biological effects of carbon dioxide and nitrous oxide which, showing "no close chemical relationship in either composition or molecular structures", have identical effects on protoplasm.

Initial attachment of a chemical compound to the cell and its ability to act upon some enzyme within the cell are regarded by some as depending upon one specific structural region of the chemical, the "exposed bond", and by others as probably depending upon several regions. Variations of this theory applied to chemical carcinogenesis appear to include a molecule capable of diffusing into the cell, of being adsorbed or attached to an enzyme and compelling an oxidation to take place in a different region of the carcinogen. Release of energy by this oxidation, a quite conceivable mechanism (Coulson) may be parallel to the energy mechanisms of the biological effects of ionizing radiations (Anderson, 1947). Ionizing radiations produce in biological material chemical reactions that are localized in space. The most important of these from the point of view of pathology is production of short-lived free radicals or electrons which disrupt other molecules through excitation or transposition of electrons. The major effects in water (and presumably also in the water of protoplasm) are oxidative (Brues, 1954).

That the azo dye, "butter yellow", and its relatives, when fed to animals produce tumors specifically in liver has suggested that the actual carcinogen is a metabolic product of the dyes or that tumor production, in this case, requires a metabolic reaction specific to liver. Combination of these dyes with liver proteins of susceptible but not of nonsusceptible animals was found by Miller and Miller, 1952. The reaction was correlated with tumor production, also, although no protein-bound dye was found in the tumor. Studies of a highly unstable reactive form of the dye (the N-hydroxymethyl derivative) suggested that it may be the metabolite that combines with liver protein. Failure of the liver proteins of nonsusceptible animals to bind the dye could be due to absence in those species of an enzyme system required to form the reactive group. With radio-labeled carcinogenic hydrocarbons, firm binding to proteins was demonstrated in the skin of painted animals and in other tissues of intravenously injected animals (Miller, 1951; Heidelberger and Weiss, 1951). Searching ten years before these reports for possible linkages and combinations of the active hydrocarbons in body metabolism, Fieser proposed (on grounds of chemical theory) that they might combine with cell proteins by an opening of sulfur linkages.

An approach to mechanism of carcinogenic action through study of definite chemical reactions between the agents and the cell (rather than the above-mentioned specific adsorption process) was made possible by recognition of carcinogenicity in a series of biological alkylating agents. These include the sulfur and nitrogen mustards, epoxides, ethylene imines, and dimesyloxyalkanes, all of which differ widely in chemical composition and share no physical properties. They share only ability to alkylate certain groupings found in protoplasm. The nitrogen mustards, studied after the first world war as agents of chemical warfare (mustard gas), were found during the last war to be inhibitors of cell division (Jonas S. Friedenwald, 1950) and have been studied experimentally and clinically as chemotherapeutic agents in leukemia, Hodgkin's disease and allied disorders. Like ionizing radiations, the nitrogen mustards damage and kill cells (chemotherapeutic effect) and are also carcinogenic, as reported by Haddow and associates, 1948, and by many others. Similarity between the biological end results of ionizing radiations and of the alkylating compounds has led to investigations apparently supporting the concept of mechanism of carcinogenesis as a primary action on the cell nucleus. Haddow presented evidence, 1953, leading to his conclusion that a direct reaction may result in loss of genic material resulting in failure to produce an enzyme essential for growth control. These and other observations obviously call for study of reactions of these substances with proteins and nucleic acids. There was, according to Alexander, 1944, evidence that the cytotoxic alkylating agents may interfere with formation of a nucleoprotein complex (by combination of protein with nucleic acid). Certain students of electronic configuration of the hydrocarbons in relation to their carcinogenic action have suggested that several successive molecular isomerizations take place (possibly within the gene or another significant region of the cell) until the cell "mutation" becomes irreversible.

The presumably direct action of radiations on the cell nucleus with production of mutations has been a valuable tool for study of genetics in biological material ranging from unicellular organisms to higher plants and animals. In cancer research, findings suggesting that physical and chemical agents that induce mutations also have carcinogenic properties (Strong, 1947) have led to search for correlations between mechanisms of action and to theories of malignant change explained by mutations.

## ACTION OF CARCINOGENS ON THE CELL NUCLEUS: MUTATION

The use of the term mutation to describe an alteration which proves to be hereditary has led to some confusion, at least, on the part of those not trained in the exercises, disciplines and language of genetics. A question asked by Ludford some years ago points out the need for definition: "Is the malignant transformation brought about by some alteration in the genes of normal cells, or can somatic cells be constitutionally altered in some as yet unknown manner, so that specific cytological characters are transmissible independently of the gene mechanism?" Proponents of the mutation theory or theories of malignant change sometimes reason in terms of genic mutation or of somatic mutation without distinguishing clearly between these two processes. Kidd, 1946, spared no feelings when he said that if by *somatic mutation* "it is meant that one or more of the genes of a somatic cell have undergone an alteration which brings about the change to cancer and proves hereditary, then the term designates a hypothesis that must remain untestable by Mendelian methods, for the reason that cancer cells proliferate only asexually". He continued: "If the term is intended to describe the obvious fact that the profound and irreversible cancerous change is passed on from one daughter cell to the next, then it is pretentious as a descriptive term and carries a connotation that may prove false." Two approaches to these theories of carcinogenesis are through study of genetic mutations, altering susceptibility of exposed animals, and through study of mutations produced in single cells. "No final proof of gene effects in production of cancer is possible, since tissue cells are vegetative and not sexual, and since chromosome changes are not regularly demonstrable." The possibility of mutation as a mechanism of malignant change lies in the origin of cancer in localized areas, perhaps from single cells, and in the carcinogenic effects of agents that cause mutations (Rhoads, 1949).

What is meant by a gene capable of causing and transmitting susceptibility to a given tumor type? The answer is that such a gene is mutant, changed permanently so that, as it duplicates itself in each generation of cells, its progeny remain mutant. The mechanisms of gene mutation are unknown but the effects of gene mutation have been analyzed exhaustively in terms of classical Mendelian laws. Work within the past few years has resulted in two outstanding concepts: gene mutation can be analyzed not only in terms of biological characteristics such as coat color, anatomical defects and growth rates, but also now in terms of specific enzyme action; and gene mutation can be produced artificially not only by irradiation but also by the administration to animals of chemical compounds.

Beadle, 1946, outlined as reasonable and consistent the hypothesis that genes function by directing chemical (metabolic) reactions through the action of enzymes, and by controlling the specificities of enzymes and other proteins. It is assumed that genes duplicate themselves by acting as models for the synthesis of exact copies and, if this is correct, then, according to Beadle, "for every specific protein type there should exist a gene carrying this same protein". This is not a single action but, in a "multigenic" organism, a whole system of genes integrated in time and space is required. Likewise, the physiological results of a single gene mutation are so complex as to defy description. They can be compared with the results in the rat following complete deprivation of thiamine. Susceptibility in terms of genic mutation is a complex of gene-controlled biochemical or metabolic peculiarities which may or may not result in cancer.

After more than ten years' work on the inheritance of experimentally induced cancers in mice, Strong, 1947, found it possible to state "that a hereditary disease or a hereditary susceptibility to a disease, gastric cancer in mice, has been induced with chemical means". The continuous injection of methylcholanthrene into mice had resulted in the induction of "gastric adenocarcinoma as well as other types of neoplastic lesions and hyperplasias of the stomach" in the injected animals and in their untreated descendants. In addition, other biological disturbances associated with the mutation, including hereditary factors such as coat color, eye color and pigment distribution, are convincing evidence, according to the author, that "one of the effects of methylcholanthrene, or one of its metabolites, upon the organism is on the nuclear components and on the germ plasm bringing about germinal changes which are hereditarily established from their point of origin". Somatic abnormalities are regarded as probably resulting from "an unstable genetic mechanism". His experiments were considered, 1950, to confirm the findings of others that almost every physical and chemical agent that can induce mutations can also induce cancer, and *vice versa*. "The determination that some forms of cancer in experimental animals are gene controlled is not the end of the story; it is merely the beginning" (L. W. Law, 1954).

Gene mutations that result in altered susceptibility of succeeding generations are, of course, mutations within the germ cells from which the entire organism of each offspring develops. Gene mutations in body cells, as the mutations discussed above which may explain the action on body cells of carcinogenic chemicals, are transmitted only to the daughter cells formed when cells of skin, liver, bronchial epithelium divide. It is such mutations that underlie the hypotheses that explain malignant change, possibly beginning in one cell, in terms of somatic mutation. Experimental testing of such hypotheses draws upon studies of visible effects of radiations on cells in which chromosome breaks are obvious. Another approach is through study of single-cell organisms that multiply by asexual division as body cells multiply.

Tatum and Bonner reported, 1946, sex-linked genic mutations produced in *Neurospora*, the red bread mold, which is well adapted for the analysis of genic mutations in terms of enzyme action. Organisms treated with nitrogen mustard, like those treated with X rays or ultraviolet light, produce descendants which are unable to carry out one or more of the syntheses of which the parent cells were capable. It was suggested that each enzyme required is controlled by a single gene. A mutant strain of *Neurospora* was found, 1948, "to contain two apparently independent gene mutations. One controls the synthesis of p-aminobenzoic acid and the other of uridine or uridylic acid." The production of "biochemical characters" in *Neurospora* may be taken as a means by which cancer susceptibility is induced in cells by the many known carcinogenic agents. Somatic mutations affecting enzymes and hence the synthesis of cellular constituents could result in the release of a cell from the growth limitations imposed on it by neighboring cells.

Genetical studies on unicellular organisms have provided impetus for work on the action of alkylating agents in biological systems, discussed above, and for comparison of these effects with the nuclear damaging power of ionizing radiations. Reactions of these compounds with chromosomes were believed possible by Ross, 1953, on the basis of 1946 studies of the sulfur and nitrogen mustards in the laboratory of the late Max Bergmann at the Rockefeller Institute. These workers showed that the mustards can react with functional groups of proteins and of nucleic acids. Haddow's theory proposed, 1953, a primary inhibition of certain fundamental processes of genetic synthesis followed by formation of new chemically, and therefore genetically, modified nucleoprotein material. Haddow compared this action with formation of a modified serum globulin, antibody, by the presence of a foreign antigen comparable to the carcinogen. Burnet and Fenner suggested, 1947, that antibody formation results from an inherited change in mesenchymal cells affecting the pattern of synthesis of serum globulin, a change which endures long after disappearance of the antigen which brought it about originally. The change, they suggested, is brought about by formation of an adaptive enzyme, a concept with which Northrop, 1949, agreed. Advances in testing the hypothesis of combination of carcinogenic chemicals with genetic material are dependent on advances in fundamental work on the nature and structure of nucleic acids and nucleoproteins, behavior and reproduction of chromosomes at cell division, related studies of enzyme structure and synthesis.

At various points, it now appears, the work on chemical carcinogenesis, has progressed beyond the point where it must defend its value against those who view it pessimistically as an interesting laboratory exercise far removed from questions of clinical cancer. This pessimism has been evident also with regard to the immense amount of work aimed at the correlation of steroid structure with carcinogenic power to explain the action of steroid hormones.

## HORMONES

An important point in all the researches on the isomers of the carcinogenic hydrocarbons is the demonstration by Fieser, discussed retrospectively at the 1945 cancer conference, that the potency of methylcholanthrene is related to its structure as a substitution product of 1:2-benzanthracene, with a methyl group added in the 10 position, rather than to its structure as a phenanthrene nucleus to which was added a five-membered ring. This ring, called a cyclopenteno, occurs in many of the naturally occurring steroids of the body and in other biologically active substances. The proof that the cyclopenteno of methylcholanthrene is not essential to its carcinogenic power weakens but does not abolish the theory, developed since the demonstration by Cook in 1932 of the estrogenic activity of some of the carcinogenic hydrocarbons, that cancer may result from an unknown substance arising in the body from altered steroid metabolism. The structurally related substances in the body include cholic acid and desoxycholic acid from which methylcholanthrene was originally synthesized, the male hormones testosterone and androsterone, the female hormones oestrone, oestriol and progesterone, and the adrenal cortical steroids.   Other compounds having marked physiological activity, such as vitamin D derived from ergosterol, and alkaloids of digitalis, have similar structures.   Fieser's 1941 suggestion that the adrenal cortical steroids are the most likely precursors of carcinogens that might arise *in vivo* has been followed (1952) by studies of the synthesis of sterols *in vivo*, and study of intermediates of cholesterol, either normal or modified, as possible carcinogens.

Earlier experimental observations established the fact that proliferation of tissues of the vagina, uterus and breast of female mice depends to a marked degree on stimulation by the ovarian hormones. In the nonpregnant female, hormonal stimulation is cyclic and growth is controlled by the periodic ebb of ovarian secretion.   In the pregnant female a much longer period of growth overrides the cyclic fluctuations but, in the end, this growth is also controlled and retrogression follows growth.   These observations led to a question which has been approached from the biological angle in many laboratories, namely, will continued estrogenic stimulation without permitting a period for retrogression lead to atypical growth, or cancer, in the genital tissues? It has now been established that in closely inbred strains of susceptible mice, and to a lesser degree in hybrid mice, in rats, and in guinea pigs, the estrogenic hormones influence the origin and growth of tumors and cancers in the reproductive organs and in other tissues.   Clinical observations on cancer incidence have led to the same question.   Statistics of the Metropolitan Life Insurance Company, 1946, on the distribution of cancer in the general population of the United States according to the sites of the body affected show that, in women, forty per cent of cancers are located in the genital organs including the breast, and in men, fifteen per cent are located in the genital organs.   A statistical analysis, presented at the fourth international cancer research congress, of cancer incidence and mortality in New York State, where cancer has been a reportable disease since 1940, indicated that prostatic cancer in males and breast and uterine cancer in females show highest mortality.

By the use of closely inbred strains of mice having a high and predictable rate of incidence of spontaneous mammary cancer, investigators were able to reduce the mammary gland carcinoma rate to zero or almost zero by the removal of the ovaries at the time of initial sexual maturity. By progressive lengthening of the time before ovariectomy, the mammary gland cancer rate was progressively raised until the rate became the same as in unoperated mice if the operation was postponed until the tenth month of age. By the quantitative withdrawal of ovarian secretion in mice of a high-cancer strain, it was thus shown that the ovarian secretion played a definite role in the induction of this particular cancer in a strain of animals having a high hereditary susceptibility. Many investigators still speak of mammary gland carcinoma in mice as *produced by* estrogenic hormones. Biological observations over a long period led Loeb to write in 1940: "The so-called spontaneous mammary gland carcinoma is a cancer produced by the estrogen given off rhythmically in mice hereditarily predisposed to this disease."

The same conclusions were drawn from experiments conducted not by the graded removal of the estrogenic hormone but by increasing the amount of estrogenic influence over that normally present. Lacassagne (1932) produced mammary cancer by injecting castrated males, belonging to a strain in which the females have a high incidence of mammary cancer, with crystalline estrone benzoate, which had then become available. The appearance of mammary cancer in males, assumed at that time to be lacking in natural estrogenic hormones, following the administration of estrogens, established these hormones as a factor acting in conjunction with genetic susceptibility in the production of this neoplasm. These early results led to experiments in which tumors, cancers and so-called atypical growths have been reported to occur in mice and several other species after long-continued and usually massive administration of estrogenic hormones. Tumors and cancers obtained in mice by the Yale workers include cancer of the cervix uteri, mammary cancer, interstitial cell tumors of the testis, tumors of the suprarenal cortex and osteogenic tumors. Uterine fibromyomas have been reported in guinea pigs and adenomatous tumors of the pituitary in rats and mice. In addition, hypertrophy and hyperplasia of various tissues in several species have been noted. Since some hormones when appropriately applied to animals induce cancers that otherwise would not be there, "some hormones must be assumed to be carcinogenic" (Gardner, 1953). But these results occur only after prolonged exposure of tissues to these substances, most of which are normally produced cyclically so that body tissues are not exposed continuously for long periods, or at least not in the absence of some modifying hormone. Gardner and his associates, 1953, considered tenable the hypothesis "that abnormal endocrine environments may result in the expression of potentialities of the tissues, less likely to be expressed under 'normal' environment". Study of endocrine factors in experimental cancer has also strengthened the concept of the limited autonomy of certain neoplastic cells in contrast to that of complete autonomy "universally accepted for so long" (Rhoads, 1950).

Whether sex hormones play any role in etiology of cancer in man, and whether "the induction of a hormone imbalance is at all useful in the treatment of any neoplasm", were questions to which direct answers should be sought, according to Rhoads's proposal of less than ten years ago. Experimental observations by Huggins published in 1943, which showed that the activity and growth of the prostatic epithelium are stimulated by the testicular hormone, testosterone, and are inhibited by the synthetic estrogen, stilbestrol, led to the use of surgical castration, and of so-called chemical castration by means of administered estrogens, in the treatment of prostatic cancer and its metastases. In a summary of results to 1949, Huggins found that, in fifty-five per cent of treated cases, remissions were followed by relapse within two years, and that seventy-five per cent had died within five years. After eight to ten years, four of the twenty patients in the first series treated were alive and in good condition. In most cases, however, according to Huggins, the treatment provides palliation for short periods. Huggins's group was working, 1951, toward synthesis of potential antiestrogens, presumably of nonhormonal nature.

In the case of primary mammary cancer and its metastases to bone, skin, lymph nodes, lungs, pleura, liver and uterus, investigators at the Memorial Hospital found that symptomatic improvement exceeded in incidence the objectively demonstrable improvement following treatment with either estrogens or androgens. The choice of hormone depended upon the age of the patient and the sites of lesions.

The demonstration of cessation of growth of established cancers, Rous observed, "shows that even the cells of malignant growths, of cancers ordinarily fatal, are not always truly independent in their behavior". A similar observation was made by Nathanson who reported, 1947, temporary regressions, sometimes striking, in advanced cancer of the breast following estrogen therapy. The regressions in this series occurred in the primary tumor, soft tissue recurrences, lymph node and pulmonary metastases. These improvements were confined to elderly patients; in younger women, particularly in the premenopausal group, either no change or a detrimental influence was observed.

The 1951 status of hormone therapy in advanced mammary cancer, summarized by the Council on Pharmacy and Chemistry, included these evaluations of testosterone: relief of symptoms in from forty-six to ninety per cent of women; objective response in about twenty per cent; side effects of testosterone included such serious occurrences as congestive heart failure, derangements of water and electrolyte balance. Estrogens given women over sixty produced essentially the same degree of improvement in symptoms and regression of bone metastases without masculinizing effects of testosterone. Apparently direct effects of hormones on cellular growth have been reported; Pincus pointed out, 1946, that direct application of minute amounts of estrogenic substances to the vaginal epithelium resulted in marked spurt of mitosis.

Whether effects of the growth hormone of the anterior pituitary are direct or circuitous was undetermined when H. M. Evans and his co-workers announced, 1950, production of gigantism and of multiple neoplastic and hyperplastic growths in normal rats by injection of purified growth hormone; the same treatment given hypophysecto-mized rats resulted in none of these effects. Later findings, 1952, were increase in tumor growth during the first twenty-seven days followed by decrease in tumor growth. Inhibition of chemically-induced liver tumors in animals from which the anterior pituitary was removed suggested a role of both the growth hormone and ACTH in supporting tumor growth (Griffin and associates, 1953). Investigators at Memorial, at Chicago, at Harvard, at the Mayo Foundation presented at the 1951 ACTH conference their findings in human cancer treated with cortisone and ACTH: regressions for limited periods in some cases of acute leukemia, Hodgkin's disease, lymphosarcoma; profound but transitory effects in chronic lymphatic leukemia and multiple myeloma. In general, no effect on the course of any type of cancer was obtained. The converse of adrenal cortical stimulation or supplement, bilateral adrenalectomy with subsequent replacement by small doses of oral cortisone, was reported, 1952, to be followed by symptomatic improvement in prostatic cancer (Huggins) and in a variety of advanced cancers (O. H. Pearson and his group at Memorial). Huggins regarded the operation as a further tool for study of endocrine relations to neoplastic growth, obviously more complex than chemical or biological antagonism.

Proof that hormones are direct causes of cancer, in the sense of chemical carcinogenesis, "does not exist" (Gardner and associates, 1953), although the possibility of production within the body of carcinogenic substances as by-products of steroid metabolism is entertained and investigated continually. Study of steroid excretion in cancer patients and in normal controls begun at the Memorial Hospital, 1948, led Dobriner to conclude, 1952, that decreased gonadal function and an abnormal (compensative) adrenal cortical secretion "existed when cancer was present". These findings provide "one of our few indices of physiological change associated with tumor incidence". Interpretations of findings in study of hormone factors influencing the origin and growth of neoplasms are constantly being revised. Their understanding will depend upon fundamental work on synthesis and breakdown of the hormones in the body, on the action of hormones on enzymes. That hormones exert their effects on the rates of cellular metabolism by direct or indirect effects on enzyme systems, or as accelerators or inhibitors of those systems present in the cells, is an hypothesis now being investigated as fundamental to many problems, including cancer. Growth, whether normal or malignant, is the product of the chemical machinery within the cells — the organized systems of enzymes. "Protoplasm, in the last analysis, is an enzyme complex" (Seifriz, 1947).

## ENZYMES AND NUCLEOPROTEINS

The theory of cancer as a manifestation of specifically deranged metabolism centered in the energy metabolism of the malignant cells and detectable in terms of changes in enzyme patterns is not new. It springs from concepts rooted more than fifty years ago when the first steps in the development of chemical pathology were taken by a few enlightened investigators who realized that the microscopic examination of morphological changes would never answer the questions of pathological, including malignant, change. The study of the chemical composition and reactions of both normal and pathological tissues was believed by a sturdy minority to hold the clues to both normal physiology and the disturbed physiology of disease. Investigative approaches to cancer problems, discussed in previous pages, all tend to explain observed phenomena and details of unknown mechanisms in terms of chemical alterations in neoplastic cells. Theories relating the action of chemical carcinogens to enzyme mechanisms include those of the Madison group postulating that carcinogenicity of the azo dyes and polycyclic hydrocarbons is correlated with formation of protein-bound derivatives of the carcinogens and raising the question whether the protein concerned is derived from nuclear genes, cytoplasmic genes or enzymes. Proposals relating genetic mutation to malignant change lean heavily on the relation of genes to synthesis of specific proteins and enzymes (Beadle, Tatum, others). Study of possible relations of hormones to enzyme differences in neoplastic tissue has only begun.

Interest in nucleoprotein changes in malignant cells began with histological observations of striking abnormalities of the mitotic figures long before the comparatively recent beginnings of histochemical and chemical studies of nucleic acids. The importance of these substances in the "chemical anatomy" of cells and in their metabolism is beginning to be realized; progress depends on development of more refined methods for study of nucleic acids and the proteins of the complex nucleoproteins. A possible role of enzyme loss or alteration, of nucleoprotein change related to the neoplastic nature of cells, or of particular cells, would, if established, indicate a specific difference between malignant cells and their normal counterparts and suggest ways of approaching its reversal. This is the hope for rational chemotherapy of cancer which was defined by Karnofsky, 1953, as "use of a systemically administered agent which, while relatively nontoxic to the host, will interfere with, favorably modify, or destroy a neoplastic growth or alleviate its deleterious effects on the host". Such a possibility, intensively pursued at present, is thought by many to be remote. "It is almost — not quite but almost — as hard as finding some agent that will dissolve away the left ear, say, yet leave the right ear unharmed: so slight is the difference between the cancer cell and its normal ancestor" (Woglom, 1947). Nevertheless, with all the technical and experimental difficulties involved, paths are being blazed to study of specificity of enzymes and nucleoproteins in relation to cancer.

From the results of measurements of enzymatic activity in sixteen specific normal tissues of mice, Greenstein concluded, 1945, that the enzymatic pattern of each specific differentiated tissue is peculiar to that tissue and that the pattern must be correlated with its specific function. Each tissue "is metabolically (as well as morphologically) differentiated". From these studies, a concept of enzyme balance or enzyme characterization has been developed. Identification of a tissue can be made by using standard techniques of measurement applied to a suspension or extract of a tissue of unknown origin. The enzymic characterization of specific normal tissues serves as groundwork for an approach to the unanswered question whether malignant tissues have an altered metabolic balance which is capable of analysis in terms of enzyme pattern and enzyme activity. Warburg's experiments show the cellular respiration of a large variety of tumor cells to be altered in the same direction. According to du Vigneaud in his 1948 report to the Committee on Growth, the metabolic abnormality causing the high rate of glycolysis in tumor cells is yet to be discovered. Burk, 1944, set up standards of tissue slice metabolism regarded as characteristic of at least ninety-five per cent of malignant tumors. Greenstein, on the basis of his study of enzyme activity in a large variety of normal and neoplastic tissues, made some generalizations, 1950. Although there is always the possibility that further research may reveal the presence of an enzyme or enzymes in cancer tissue "unique to these tissues and absent in all normal tissues", his present results suggest that tumors have qualitatively the same kind of enzymes that normal tissues have. The quantitative patterns estimated by measurements of activity in sarcomas, carcinomas, lymphomas and adenocarcinomas arising in a variety of tissues are very nearly alike. "Metabolically, tumors resemble each other more than they do normal tissues, or than normal tissues resemble each other." A conclusion was tentatively advanced: "all tumors, no matter how or where they originate, tend toward a common tissue type." A common tissue type in terms of content of eight of the B vitamins (some if not all of which are essential parts of oxidative enzyme systems) was described for cancer tissues compared with normal tissues by Williams and his group at Texas, 1945. The tumor tissues had a higher uniformity of vitamin content than the normal tissues used, and thus resembled each other more than did the normal tissues. The tendency of tumor tissues "to converge, enzymatically, to a common type of tissue" does not appear in tumors in which enzymes peculiar to the tissue of origin have been studied.

This common enzyme pattern may have further significance if a correlation can be found between the loss of specific function (or as Greenstein called it, "metabolic de-differentiation") and loss of specific enzymic pattern. By comparisons between tumors and their normal tissues of origin, he has found that the more malignant the tumors, "the nearer they approach the kind of de-differentiated, functionless tissue presumably common to all neoplasms". This loss of function is not absolute, however, since some tumors of the endocrine glands apparently continue hormonal secretion. Needham's suggestion that cancer cells are cells that have escaped from the field of individuation may be recalled. The long-accepted dictum that cellular differentiation and growth are incompatible, but that rapidly growing embryonic tissue and neoplastic tissue have marked resemblances, has been subjected to analysis in terms of enzyme activity by Burk and by Greenstein. Enzyme activity in fetal liver and in hepatoma was reported to be nearly the same. The enzyme pattern of normal adult liver was found to be quite different. In regenerating liver, after partial hepatectomy, the enzyme activity was regarded as "fully differentiated". Since this tissue was rapidly growing, it appears that the resemblance between fetal and neoplastic tissue is not based on growth capacity alone.

While study of individual enzymes in neoplastic tissue is, as yet, a field "only superficially tilled" one practical observation was that the enzyme, acid phosphatase, known since 1935 to occur in high concentration in the prostate, also occurs in high concentration in prostatic carcinoma. High levels of acid phosphatase (presumably derived from the cancer) occur also in the serum of patients with prostatic cancer metastasizing to bone (Gutman and coworkers, 1937). Serum alkaline phosphatase was shown to be raised in patients with osteogenic sarcoma of the osteoblastic type. These observations were the first evidence that chemical characteristics of tissue may be transmitted to neoplasms arising from them. Serum enzyme levels of acid phosphatase are used for diagnosis of prostatic cancer metastasizing to bone and for evaluation of control by hormone therapy (estrogenic hormones, castration) used in prostatic cancer (Huggins, 1952).

Other examples of study of individual enzymes relate to the many-sided metabolic problem of the nature of malignancy. Fishman and his group found, 1944, that the enzyme, $\beta$-glucuronidase, widely distributed in animal tissues and catalyzing the breakdown of many glucuronic acids, occurred in high concentration in a majority of human cancers (skin, lung, breast, oesophagus, stomach, cervix, brain) compared with the concentration in neighboring, uninvolved tissues. Later, on the basis of animal experiments (Fishman, 1950) it was suggested that the enzyme facilitates conjugation of estrogens (possibly other steroid hormones) with glucuronic acid in the tissues "as a step in the utilization of the steroid glucuronide by the tissue". Although direct experimental evidence was lacking, 1953, the hypothesis was regarded as useful in suggesting experiments on the significance of the enzyme to cancer and on the mechanism of action of steroid hormones on normal and neoplastic tissue. Whether or not the enzyme hyaluronidase (which liquefies the mucopolysaccharides of the ground substance and is believed to enhance the spread of bacteria in the tissues) is associated with the invasiveness of cancer, possibly with formation of metastases, is a natural question. Simpson suggested, 1950, the working hypothesis that, since secretion of mucolytic enzymes is a property lost by adult cells of undifferentiated epithelium, epithelial cells might regain their capacity to produce the enzyme when they become malignant. However, no evidence of elevated hyaluronidase activity in tumor tissue had been found, 1953 (Fishman).

Although still far from realization, the possibility that quantitative changes in enzymes of malignant tissue account for the over-all metabolic changes suffered in certain stages of clinical cancer (and responsible for loss of appetite and weight in spite of increased caloric intake) has been suggested by many. Among findings summarized by Fenninger and Mider (National Cancer Institute), 1954, were elevated basal metabolic rates in cancer patients on low-caloric diets that produce negative basal metabolic rates in normal subjects. Even in the presence of a negative nitrogen balance, tumor growth, involving protein synthesis, has been observed in both clinical cancer patients and animals bearing transplanted neoplasms. With the isotope technique, it has been demonstrated that with inadequate protein intake nitrogen is relinquished by the host and retained by the tumor. In fact, Tannenbaum found, 1954, that evidence from fifteen years' study of nutrition in relation to cancer demonstrated that in animals undergoing a variety of nutritional deficiencies and losing fat, vitamins, minerals as well as proteins all essential cellular elements accumulate in the growing neoplasms. The next important stage of nutritional work in cancer, he thought, should deal with mechanisms underlying the many observations with promise of a better understanding of neoplastic change. Needed information on this level (Fenninger and Mider) included: the properties of malignant cells that permit them to synthesize protein at the expense of the host; the mechanisms by which a malignant cell becomes a "nitrogen trap"; the fate of nitrogen released by destroyed tumor cells.

The importance of study of nucleoproteins in neoplastic tissue is suggested by their occurrence in both the nucleus and the cytoplasm of all body cells, and by evidence that nucleoproteins are "autocatalytic" or self-reproducing, and that they are necessary for the formation of other cell proteins. Daniel Mazia reported, 1948, that desoxyribonuclease has been found to be concentrated in the nuclei of adult cells but is found in soluble form in the cytoplasm of the echinoderm embryo. The development of improved techniques for the fractionation of liver, blood and spleen proteins and for the study of nucleoprotein fractions has facilitated comparisons of the desoxyribonucleoprotein content of tissues at various stages of azo dye carcinogenesis, as reported by J. M. Luck, 1948. The idea that the nucleic acids may be specific for each type of cell derives from several lines of research. Beadle's development of the one gene — one enzyme hypothesis, 1945, led to the question whether, since the genes of cells control varying metabolic mechanisms, the genes might not contain specific nucleic acids. The demonstration by Avery and his associates, 1944, that a pure nucleic acid from one type of pneumococcus could transform the offspring of another type so that it became permanently of the first type strengthened the idea of specificity of nucleic acids. The little-studied purine and pyrimidine bases contained in nucleic acids have become of interest in cancer research in the search for chemical specificities, because rapidly growing cells must synthesize more nucleic acids. These studies are oriented toward testing synthetic antipurines and antipyrimidines as possible chemotherapeutic agents in cancer.

Although the theory of antagonism between an essential metabolite and some structurally related compound, either naturally occurring or synthesized, as a basis for a rational approach to chemotherapy is widely accepted, Green has insisted, 1946, that the explanation of this concept in terms of enzyme chemistry is essential to the development of its investigation. "Chemotherapeutic drugs may interfere either with the working of a key enzyme or with some stage in the process by which the key enzyme is synthesized. Since the synthesis of enzymes is also enzymic in nature, the primary action of chemotherapeutic drugs must still be considered as one of interference with enzymes." The results of Hertz with the retardation of tissue growth under estrogenic stimulus by the administration of a folic acid antagonist might be cited as an example of the interference of such a metabolic antagonist specifically with the growth of body cells. As B. C. J. G. Knight pointed out, 1945, the metabolic process is the essential thing, and nutrients or metabolites are essential in proportion to the need for carrying out the process. Pteroylglutamic acid (folic acid classed with the B vitamins) has, since 1943 when the first observations of folic acid deficiency were reported by W. H. Sebrell, been studied in many laboratories for its role in essential metabolic process and its inhibition by analogues acting as antagonists.

Discovery of the structure of the vitamin as pteroylglutamic acid, 1946, and its synthesis by the Lederle group in the same year led to synthesis of some 250 derivatives of the molecule, of which the 4-

amino analogues appeared to inhibit growth of some experimental tumors and to give temporary improvement in acute leukemia in children (Farber and coworkers, 1948). These early results increased confidence in the possibilities of inhibition of cancer growth by metabolic antagonists of substances essential to cellular growth in general, and also confidence in the various animal test procedures to detect compounds of potential clinical usefulness (Stock, 1954). From this point, a backward look related these studies to those of Woods and others whose work on the mechanism of action of the sulfonamides on bacteria had shown that these compounds competitively antagonize para-aminobenzoic acid which is required for synthesis by bacterial cells of the growth factor, folic acid. A forward look led to consideration of metabolism of nucleic acids of which purines and pyrimidines are components. Synthesis of these substances requires B vitamins, those of the $B_{12}$ group and either para-aminobenzoic acid or folic acid, depending upon the test organism used (Shive, 1951). Parasitic growth (bacterial, rickettsial, viral, neoplastic) is generally more rapid than that of normal body cells and presumably requires more rapid synthesis of nucleic acids. If analogues of purines and pyrimidines were found to compete with the natural constituents of nucleic acids formed in the body, then alterations in nucleic acid formation might result in selective inhibition of growth of more rapidly growing cells such as cancer cells. Of over a thousand such compounds synthesized by Hitchings's group at the Wellcome laboratories and by others the most promising was 6-mercaptopurine, a purine analogue. By 1954, efficacy of the compound to inhibit growth of embryonic and regenerating tissues, of tumors in tissue culture, of experimental tumors including mouse leukemia had been tested at Memorial Cancer Center, the National Cancer Institute and several other cancer research centers. Clinical trials, in leukemias chiefly, had been reported from twenty medical schools and hospitals in this country and from Paris, Buenos Aires, Leeds in England. Biochemical studies have indicated at least that some *in vivo* growth-inhibitory effects have been found in the case of some purines but such correlation "is based on too few examples to dignify it by calling it a conclusion" (Brown, 1954). That this inhibitory action is that of an antimetabolite was still to be established.

Although the search for metabolic antagonists capable of interfering with the growth of cancer cells has a rational basis, the empiric
approach, which has yielded brilliant results in bacterial chemotherapy, is usually an integral part of programs of cancer chemotherapy. Selection of compounds for screening, for determination
of pharmacological and toxic effects, for tests against experimental
cancers and possible clinical trials have been carried out chiefly
through coordinating centers, such as the National Research Council
Chemical-Biological Coordination Center and the National Cancer
Institute. By 1948, these two centers reported some 5,000 compounds
available for preliminary screening or already submitted to preliminary tests. Reports of trials of numerous substances for activity against
experimental and clinical cancer have shown temporary amelioration
of symptoms and cessation of cancer growth, transitory effects regarded
as limitations to chemotherapy, but by no means discouraging, by
Gellhorn and Jones of Columbia, who reviewed the status of cancer
chemotherapy, 1949. These investigators suggested, "among the
cells of a susceptible tumor there is variation in resistance to the
cytotoxic agent which may be a primary or acquired characteristic.
This would be analogous to the situation encountered in infection
when microorganisms become resistant to chemotherapeutic drugs."

Antibiotics obtained from molds and bacteria have been tested
against experimental cancer: Kidd reported, 1947, that culture filtrates (containing a substance apparently identical with gliotoxin)
of a mold isolated from the air of an animal room, and later identified as *Aspergillus fumigatus* Fresenius, inhibited growth of various
tumors *in vitro*, although no effect was observed on tumors *in vivo*.
Polysaccharide lipid complexes, isolated by Shear and his coworkers
from culture filtrates of *Serratia marcenscens*, were under study by Creech
and associates, Institute for Cancer Research. Creech reported,
1948, that these substances had been shown to destroy selectively
various tumors in mice, but that toxic and immunological properties
of the substances prevented effective clinical use. Immunological,
chemical and physical methods are being used in attempts to produce
effective, nontoxic preparations. The mechanism of action of this
polysaccharide was under study by Heilbrunn and Wilson who reported, 1950, their conclusion that initiation of "mitosis is due to a

protoplasmic clotting or gelation essentially similar to blood clotting". Heparin was found to prevent mitotic gelation and thus inhibit cell division, and further experiments showed that the bacterial polysaccharide acted like heparin in preventing cell division. The authors suggested trial of other substances which prevent blood clotting for their usefulness in preventing cell division, and possibly in cancer therapy. Green has envisaged expenditure of funds for a fundamental attack on chemotherapy, which he holds cannot be made "intelligently without a detailed knowledge of intermediary metabolism and enzyme chemistry". The impetus provided by the pioneering work on biochemical antagonisms, although still modest, was described by Woolley, 1946, as a potential current rather than "merely an eddy" in the field of pharmacology.

## VIRUSES

The early (1903) suggestion by Borrell of virus etiology for cancer was made long before the techniques now available for the study of viruses were thought of. His suggestion was based on the then prevailing theory that all disease is infectious and responsibility was attributed to virus largely because evidence against bacteria was negative. The skepticism that greeted and suppressed this idea was not due solely to lack of experimental proof, for when Rous demonstrated in 1911 that a sarcoma of the breast muscles of a hen could be transmitted by a filterable cell-free extract of the tumor, the skepticism remained. For more than thirty years evidence has been accumulating that viruses are responsible for a variety of sarcomatous growths in domestic fowl, and for tumors in cottontail rabbits and in leopard frogs. During the past ten years an agent associated with spontaneous mammary carcinoma in laboratory mice has been isolated and characterized as virus, or virus-like. In the work with papillomatous growths in cottontail rabbits, it has been found that the virus associated with these tumors can readily be obtained from the warts, but not from the cancers, although antibodies to the virus are present. It must be remembered, however, that no immune reaction could be detected at all if the virus which acts as the antigen were unknown.

These facts admit the possibility that viruses may be concerned with some tumors and cancers in man even though repeated efforts have not demonstrated the presence of a virus in human cancers. Two infectious skin diseases of man, papilloma or warts and molluscum contagiosum, have long been known to be caused by filterable agents which transmit these infections with production of growth on human, but not on animal, skin. Interest in these viruses was revived by the possibility of studying them by electron microscope and by chemical methods for analysis of nucleic acid changes in infected cells. Virus workers at Yale (Melnick, Bunting and others) described, 1952, spherical virus particles isolated from human warts or papilloma. Particles of the rabbit papilloma virus were described by Williams (California Institute of Technology), 1953, as spherical with regularly arrayed small elevations or mounds on the surface. Particles of molluscum contagiosum virus isolated from human lesions by the Yale workers were described as brick shaped, resembling the pox viruses with which it is grouped. Thin sections of cells infected with the latter virus, examined by electron microscope, provided information on effects of the virus on the infected cells: "As the virus particles are formed, they leave behind a cytoplasm which appears to be moth-eaten." Like the pox viruses, these two human viruses were described by Harvey Blank, 1952, as proliferative and destructive suggesting that the clinical skin nodules are "pseudotumors" produced by repair processes of the epithelium in response to the destructive effects of the viruses. There are investigators who consider it premature to project working hypotheses bearing on virus etiology of cancer into an area where there is so much fundamental uncertainty. Rous noted the gaps in knowledge and tended to discourage the too rapid extension of the virus hypothesis. "With so much uncertain, it is easy to suppose all tumors to be due to viruses, yet it may be easier than it is wise. When the role of bacteria in disease first reached recognition, much was referred to their action which has since turned out to be of quite other cause. Events are already taking the same course with viruses."

The investigators who recently have proposed working hypotheses of the virus etiology of cancer seem to regard the viruses as infectious agents, acquired from without the organism by transmission from one host to another, and manifesting their activities in association with tumors and cancers in ways that are compatible with the infection concept, as statements published since 1943 attest. The attributes of viruses that can explain the properties of cancer were summarized by Duran-Reynals, 1953: viruses grow only in living cells and often cause in the cells they inhabit stimulation of growth followed by cell destruction; they produce their effects after varied provocative stimuli, limited by strict species and cell specificity; their specificity can be altered by the well-known phenomenon of variation which is common to many viruses, and which enables them to infect new kinds of cells causing new lesions; they can remain latent in tissues from infancy to late in life, or may cause different lesions in young and old hosts; they can be present in the host in either a masked or overt form. Since there are some cancers certainly induced by viruses, "it is elementary logic to look for such agents when trying to find the cause of the remaining tumors of unknown etiology". In this search, Duran-Reynals thought the most important question to be why the causative viruses are overt in some cancers and masked in others.

This question and others (still unanswered) concerning the role of viruses in cancer are among problems that lie close to the center of virus research, as such: the definition of viruses as a class; their manner of reproduction within cells and the effects of viruses on the metabolism of host cells; methods of transmission from host to host and methods of spread from cell to cell. These problems also lead to questions of highest importance to research on the tumor viruses and to the whole field of virus research: relations between infection and infectious disease; relations between all the factors (genetic, hormonal, metabolic) that influence host susceptibility and resistance. What is known of the behavior of the tumor viruses cannot be reconciled completely with the barest acceptable definition of the viruses as filterable agents that are transmissible from host to host in which they cause infection and stimulate immune response. To explain discrepancies, theories have been evolved in terms of recent knowledge of submicroscopic cellular particles and constituents that can "mutate" and transmit to future generations of cells new characteristics, including abnormal growth. These theories, discussed later, range freely among the disciplines of biology and biochemistry to assemble facts of significance to one of the central problems of biology, the manner of production by cells of proteins, nucleic acids and the complex nucleoproteins that give to each type of living matter its distinctive characteristics. Our concern here is not with these theories but with the investigative work that has demonstrated in animals "a whole group of benign and malignant tumors and leukemias which are due to authentic viruses" (Oberling and Guérin, 1954). Analysis of the behavior of the known tumor viruses requires, in the view of Duran-Reynals, 1953, constant close touch with developments in the field of infection and resistance.

## Virus tumors in birds

Not long after Rous in 1911 had produced sarcoma, or cancer of connective tissue, in the breast muscle of a hen by inoculation of a cell-free filtrate of an identical naturally occurring tumor, he with Murphy and Tyler, by the inoculation of a cell-free filtrate of a sarcoma of bone in a fowl, produced in the connective tissue of another fowl a true osteosarcoma containing cells of cartilage and bone. The naturally occurring *chicken tumors* from which causative viruses have been isolated include fibromas, sarcomas, myxomas, osteomas, chondromas, lymphoid tumors, leukemia and endothelioma. According to Rous, "The chicken tumors that yield viruses are typical neoplasms in all respects, even in metabolic peculiarities, and like them they appear hither and yon in the fowl community, giving no indication of any connection with one another. The causative viruses are as various as the tumors, each engendering growths of the sort from which it was originally procured, and growths of such sort only. . . ." That these chicken tumors are directly produced by the virus agents isolated from them has been demonstrated again and again. Most of the work has been done with the virus of Rous sarcoma, or chicken tumor I, but recent studies have revealed that this virus has marked capacity for variation. When the virus varies it acquires new properties, infects new types of cells and induces new types of cancer; chickens reinfected with variant viruses develop tumors of the foreign species rather than the original chicken sarcoma.

Biological variation in the case of a pathogenic organism causing disease is often interpreted as a manifestation of the universal ability of living things for adaptation. In a broad sense infection is, as Burnet, 1941, and others have pointed out, a manifestation of adaptation on the part of the invading organism that permits it to multiply and maintain its numbers at the expense of the host. Pathogenic viruses have varying degrees of adaptability to different hosts. Some viruses attack many kinds of host while others are highly species specific. All mammals are susceptible to rabies; the virus of rabbit papilloma is specific for rabbits.

The tendency of chicken tumor I virus to adsorb upon proteins has interfered with attempts (since 1929) to isolate and purify it. "It is by no means generally agreed that the actual Rous No. 1 agent has ever been prepared" (Harris, 1953), or that its size had yet been determined (Oberling and Guérin, 1954). These workers considered that determination whether the virus ordinarily occurs in cells in the masked rather than in the particulate form touched upon a crucial point of virus-induced tumors. Of "overriding importance", according to Harris, were the fundamental problems of entrance of the virus into the cell, its effects on the cell's metabolism and the cell's response, for the tumor viruses are the only agents known to produce tumors by direct action (Rous, 1943).

Experimentally induced variations (mutations) in the chicken tumor I virus have been reported, 1945, by Duran-Reynals and his associates at Yale. These variations are considered to be demonstrated by the induction in foreign species of new histological types of tumors, including periosteal tumors and hemorrhagic blebs in the lung. The first species used in these experiments was the *duck* in which early lesions typical of the Rous tumor were produced followed by late lesions of a different sort produced by the agent which had become, according to the authors, a duck virus. On the reinjection of this virus into chickens, early lesions were typical of those produced by the duck virus, and late lesions responded perfectly to the original, now restored, chicken tumor I virus. These studies have been extended to *turkeys*, *guinea hens* and *pheasants*. Alterations or variations in the biological manifestations of the virus infection occurred in each species. Susceptibility to inoculation with the chicken virus varied in proportion to the zoological relatedness to the chicken of each species, guinea hens and pheasants being most susceptible, while pigeons were entirely resistant. Three new duck variants of the Rous sarcoma virus have now been obtained, and Duran-Reynals reported, 1947, that one strain infected pigeons of all ages and acquired an affinity for the central nervous system of chicks. From these experiments the author concluded that susceptibility, as observed, might be explained either by alteration in cellular susceptibility produced by the action of the virus, or by alteration in the virus produced by the action of the cells, "so that the agent is now virulent for that structure". Definite antigenic changes in the virus have been found to occur with the process of variation.

Fowl *lymphomatosis*, caused by a virus-like agent, is contagious in a manner similar to that of other contagious diseases. According to Burmester (Regional Poultry Research Laboratory, Lansing), 1952, at least one form of the disease complex in chickens is "truly cancerous". The virus has been cultivated *in vitro* since 1936, the most successful method being inoculation of blood or minced tissues into the embryonated fowl egg with production of leukosis in the chick embryo (Oberling and Guérin, 1954).

Work on the leukosis virus suggested early that leukemia is a form of cancer. Studies of Furth (1937) and others appeared to support this view when inoculation of the virus into suitable tissues resulted in typical metastasizing malignant tumors. This reaction has also been explained as virus variation. Studies of Burmester and Duran-Reynals, 1953, indicating that the lymphomatosis viruses are responsible for development in aging chickens of antibodies against the Rous virus, suggested that the lymphomatosis agents can cause cancer after undergoing variation.

Epidemiology of the fowl lymphomatoses has been understood only since 1917 when egg and chicken production became a large industry in the United States with development of huge incubators and rearing stations populated with pure-bred lines of fowls. The disease, apparently held in check by methods of rearing chickens in small flocks of mixed breeds, and resisting transmission by any means attempted, was regarded for forty years as a spontaneous noninfectious disease. With conditions now favorable for transmission, through the egg which produces carrier chicks as demonstrated by Waters at the Michigan station, 1945, and through aerial transmission (Waters and Bywaters, 1949), the infectious nature of a disease in every way resembling human leukemias and cancer, was established.

## VIRUS TUMORS IN ANIMALS

For some years, it has been accepted as probable that tumors of the renal epithelium occurring in *leopard frogs* found in the swamps of certain New England localities are caused by a virus. Lucké, who in 1938 obtained from these tumors an agent having the characteristics of a virus, which withstands drying and glyceration, reported that injections of tumor material, of glycerated suspensions of cellular material, and of dessicated tumor material, produced tumors in a high percentage of leopard frogs, always in the renal epithelium. Detailed study in over a thousand frogs with naturally-occurring renal tumors showed that this tumor fulfills the usually accepted criteria of a malignant neoplasm: invasion and destruction of the tissue of its origin; successful serial transplantation to other hosts; metastasis; alterations of enzymic activity in the tumor similar to those observed in mammalian cancer (Lucké, 1952). Malignancy of the tumor was regarded as further established by serial transplantation in the anterior chamber of the eye of other species of frogs and other cold-blooded animals (Lucké and Schlumberger, 1949). Although the agent had not been isolated, 1952, its characteristics in terms of behavior in cells and tissues suggested an inclusion-forming, organ-specific virus. For example, transplantation of the tumor to salamanders followed by return of the tumor to its natural host resulted in tumors of the periosteum. Rose suggested, 1952, modification or variation of the frog tumor "virus" after growth in foreign tissue (comparable variations previously noted as observed by Duran-Reynals in the Rous chicken tumor virus). He suggested that the agent may combine with certain cellular constituents of the foreign host to form a new virus with altered tissue affinity. Lucké found marked reduction in activity of catalase and phosphatase (high in normal kidney) in the renal tumor tissue, comparable to the reduction of these enzymes noted by Greenstein, 1947, in mammalian cancers.

The first definite association of a virus with neoplastic growths in mammals was reported in 1933 by Shope, who extracted a virus from papillomas found on the skin of about one in ten Western cottontail *rabbits* brought in by trappers. These warts are regarded as typical neoplasms, although they may reach such enormous size that the host succumbs. Rous described them as neoplasms on the brink of malignancy frequently progressing and developing into metastasizing squamous cell carcinomas. The malignant progression can be hastened by a number of experimental means, including trauma. These properties have suggested to investigators a relationship between the virus-induced rabbit papilloma and the virus-induced venereal warts of man, condilomas, which if neglected sometimes develop into cancers.

Early work on this virus by Shope showed that, although it is readily obtained from the papillomas of the wild rabbit, and even from dessicated fragments which had sloughed off, it could not be obtained from the papillomas produced by it in domestic rabbits, snowshoe rabbits, and swamp hares, nor from the malignant carcinomas developing from the papillomas in any rabbit. Evidence of direct progression of the papillomatous cells to the malignant state has been provided by Rous and his colleagues, Berry and his coworkers, and Kidd in this country, and by other workers abroad. Detailed study by Syverton, Berry and coworkers, published in Cancer Research, 1950, of cottontails kept under observation showed epidermoid carcinomas with metastases developing in about one fourth of the animals.

The rabbit papilloma virus under the electron microscope (Beard and associates, 1942; Knight, 1950; Kahler and Lloyd, 1952) appeared in spherical particles. Williams's electron micrographs, mentioned previously, showed in the air-dried spherical specimens "linear arrays of small elevations, or mounds on the surfaces of the particles". This first observation of a virus with regular surface structure was interpreted to reflect an internal structure showing through the dried outer layer. The virus studied by chemical and physical techniques has been obtained from the benign lesions of the wild cottontail rabbit. Although the virus cannot be obtained from other lesions, its presence has been demonstrated by the appearance of neutralizing antibodies in animals bearing them.

From studies of papillomas serially transplanted for over thirteen years, Smith, Kidd and Rous suggested, 1952, that disappearance of the virus from the malignant growths coincides with disappearance of the virus in transmissible form. The virus, they proposed, remains in the tumor in a masked form capable, however, of stimulating antibody production by the host.    Duran-Reynals, 1945, among others, favored the view that, in lesions from which the papilloma virus cannot be obtained, it is present in a masked form.    Syverton and colleagues, studying transmission of malignant tumors from the cottontail rabbit to new wild hosts, concluded, 1950, that the virus disappears completely before the malignant stage is reached.    Among various interpretations, Oberling and Guérin, 1954, favored the view that, in the rapidly developing papillomas of the domestic rabbit and in the cancers of cottontails, failure to obtain the virus is due to lack of its complete synthesis in these rapidly growing cells which may lack something for that complete synthesis.    This proposal was compared to synthesis of incomplete forms of influenza virus when inoculated in large amounts into eggs, as proposed by Henle, 1953.

Extensive work on the significance of the immune response to the papilloma virus has been carried out by Rockefeller Institute workers and by Kidd at Cornell.    Rous explained, 1942, that the tumor viruses do not kill the cells they inhabit but rather stimulate their growth so that an endless succession of virus-bearing cells results. These cells, being alive and extremely vigorous, maintain their impermeability to the antibody proteins circulating in the blood stream. "The individual cell is really the host of the tumor virus, not the organism, which becomes implicated in the disease process only secondarily . . ."    The humoral antibodies, therefore, must be of only secondary importance to the phenomenon of masking.    Their presence cannot be the only factor that neutralizes the virus, or makes its presence in extracts of the tumors undetectable.    It is possible that neutralizing antibodies may be present in the tissues.    These possibilities were brought out by Shope's experiments in which he infected the same domestic rabbit with two different strains of papilloma virus, one producing papillomas from which the virus could be extracted, and one producing papillomas from which, in that animal, the virus cannot be extracted.    The virus in one set of papillomas was masked, then, by a mechanism different from that usually attributed to antibodies.    Friedewald's experiments (1940) showed that extracts of papilloma in domestic rabbits, and extracts of liver, muscle and skin from infected rabbits neutralized the virus present in papillomas of wild rabbits.    The inhibiting effect may be due to antibodies but, if that is the case, the antibodies are present in blood-free tissues. Bernheim and associates reported, 1942, attempts to discover the nature of the antigen present in domestic rabbit warts from which no virus can be extracted. The antigen, capable of immunizing other rabbits against infection with the virus, was found to be degraded or hydrolyzed by a factor presumably an enzyme. This factor, absent in cottontail papilloma tissue, may be, according to the investigators, "a noninfectious, insoluble and possibly partially denatured degradation product of the virus". The investigators saw a possibility that the carcinomas growing from these warts may acquire such factors or enzymes in the course of malignant change. "It is an obvious possibility that such factors may prevent the recovery of a causative agent from neoplastic growths other than those associated with the papilloma virus."

Demonstration of the presence of a virus in these tumor-bearing animals by immune reactions is possible only because the associated virus has been obtained from the original papilloma in wild rabbits. Antibodies and inhibitors are the objects of a specific search with a specific antigen. Duran-Reynals mentioned Shope's observation that the experimental lesion produced by the papilloma virus "simulates the circumstance that we most often find in mammalian cancer, in that we have a tumor from which a virus cannot be isolated. If we did not know the origin of these domestic rabbit lesions, we should record them as tumors of unknown etiology."

Much has been said with respect to the tumor-producing viruses about their direct and immediate effects in actuating the tumors they produce. The carcinogenic hydrocarbons, the estrogenic hormones, and other agents such as X rays that influence the origin and growth of neoplasms are most frequently referred to as "remote" causes for various reasons but especially with regard to the time factor. The long precarcinogenic period between the application of benzpyrene to the mouse's skin and the appearance of skin cancer extends over almost two thirds of the mouse's life span. The occurrence of human cancers resulting from exposure to X rays and certain chemicals follows a similar time course. To investigators who see the possibility that all cancers may be caused by viruses, the question of the relation of the many unrelated "remote" influences to possible latent viral agents responsible for the ultimate malignant change arises in innumerable connections. One possibility is that a virus may be present but incapable of tumor-producing activity until the cells on which it can act are rendered susceptible by one or more of the "remote" causes. Experimental tests of this possibility have had to await the finding of such a viral agent, and there is now reasonable hope that such material may be available in the so-called milk influence associated with mammary carcinoma of mice.

The existence of what is now known as the *milk factor*, which affects the incidence of mammary carcinoma in *mice*, was announced in 1933 by investigators at the Jackson Memorial Laboratory. This group, Little, Bittner, Woolley, Law and others, had been engaged for a number of years in analyzing the genetic factors that influence the incidence of mammary carcinoma, a neoplasm relatively common in laboratory mice. It had become evident that individuals of a given pure strain of these animals showed a markedly uniform susceptibility to the neoplasm. In order to analyze the extent of the genetic influence, long-continued rigid inbreeding had been recognized as necessary for the stabilization of the genetic constitution in the experimental material. It was in experiments in cross breeding between high-tumor inbred strains and low-tumor inbred strains, in which the female offspring had identical chromosomal constitutions, that the extra-chromosomal influences became evident. In these crosses, the mammary tumor incidence was high in the hybrids whose female parent was taken from a high-tumor strain, and the incidence was low in the hybrids whose female parent was taken from a low-tumor strain.

The next problem was to determine where the factor was located and how it was transmitted from high-tumor mothers to their offspring. Progress on this and other questions was summarized briefly by Little, 1941: "Bittner demonstrated that the influence was commonly transferred in the milk during nursing. Woolley, Law and Little showed later that the same influence or one with similar effects could be transferred by inoculation of whole blood. Bittner showed that mammary tumor tissue or ground spleen of high-tumor strain mice could also transfer the influence but that liver could not. It was also demonstrated that the influence was stronger in the milk secreted for lactation in second and subsequent pregnancies than in that secreted for the first litter. The extent and duration of the influence in relation to age were also investigated."

Earlier opinion appeared to favor the view that the milk influence or the mammary tumor agent is not a direct cause of the cancer, as chicken tumor I virus is regarded as a direct cause of the sarcoma it produces, but rather is one factor which transmits susceptibility to mammary cancer. Bittner, who has conducted a long series of observations on many generations of hybrid mice derived from crosses between animals of high- and low-tumor strains, stated as his opinion in 1944: "hormonal stimulation, inherited susceptibility and the milk agent are of approximately equal importance in the etiology of mammary cancer in mice of known genetic constitution under normal conditions. That is, any one of the three factors of influence may be completely determining in its effects . . ." The genetic set-up provides one kind of susceptibility; the hormonal stimulation prepares the mammary gland for the activity of the milk agent or for malignant change; the tumor agent, having chemical and physical properties which indicate its virus nature, is present in the tumors. However, Dmochowski at Leeds, England, reported, 1950, some spontaneous breast cancers in low-tumor strain mice in which the milk factor was lacking. A fourth influence, an "inherited hormonal influence" which may be altered by the milk agent was proposed, 1947, by Bittner.

The announcement of the isolation and purification of the agent and the summary of its virus-like properties, published in 1946 by Bittner, were the culmination of intensive studies carried on chiefly by the group at Minnesota and by workers at the National Cancer Institute. Shimkin and Andervont noted, 1945, that the results of investigations in six or more centers in this country, in Great Britain, in Holland, France and India have shown remarkable agreement. As with the work on all viral agents, activity can be studied at present only in terms of biological effects, and it is a great drawback that tumors influenced by this agent arise only after twelve to twenty-four months following the transmission of the agent by nursing or by artificial means. Bittner reported that the active agent has the properties of a nucleoprotein, containing ribosenucleic acid, of the yeast type. Studies of the mouse virus at Columbia (Graff, Moore, Stanley, Randall and Haagensen) showed, 1947, spherical particles approximately 100 millimicrons in diameter to produce the disease in young low cancer strain females, to fulfill other criteria of virus nature, leading to the conclusion that "these particles constitute the virus responsible for mouse mammary carcinoma". Andervont reported, 1952, that wild house mice harbor in their milk a virus which has similar characteristics but which produces few tumors. Students of the milk agent appear generally to favor the idea that it is a true virus capable of long survival in a latent form and susceptible to activation by genetic, hormonal and possibly other factors (Rous, 1947; Gross, 1949; Andervont, 1949; Duran-Reynals, 1950).

Until the milk factor has been obtained in purified form with its nature established, immunological studies must be carried out with materials containing the agent. Rats and rabbits injected with extracts of the tumor produced serum antibodies which neutralized the virus *in vitro* and which conveyed passive immunity upon mice injected before receiving the agent, according to R. G. Green and Bittner. Subsequent experiments, reported, 1947, from the Minnesota laboratories, have shown that the antibodies in the immune serum combine specifically with the mammary tumor cells and that the antibodies "have an inactivating, or lethal, effect upon the cancer cell". This, according to Green, indicated that the virus had become an integral and vital part of the cancer cell which cannot survive the inactivation of the virus. It also indicated that the mouse mammary cancer cell is a species immunologically specific and distinct from the normal mammary cell. It was pointed out that the "species character modification" would of itself "remove the cell from the corporate growth control". In other words, the body exercises control over the growth of its own cells but not over "parasitic" cells of a foreign or altered species which, however, may provoke the production of antibodies specific to the foreign cell. The production of active immunity in susceptible animals had not been accomplished, 1954. The transfer of the agent by noncancerous mice suggests a latency or even an immune carrier state which is in accord with what is known of viruses in general, but which is unique among the tumor viruses. Andervont reported, 1947, observations that under certain conditions the agent becomes inactive not only in a low mammary tumor strain of mice but also in a highly susceptible strain. Further observations indicate that the agent either arises spontaneously or becomes activated in hybrid mice derived from mothers which do not develop the tumor.

Work on mammary cancer in mice has been the experimental backbone of cancer research in several lines. The evaluation of the numerous factors influencing the origin and development of this neoplasm, especially of the genetic, the hormonal and the virus influences, has resulted in data which have brought into sharp focus the crucial importance of susceptibility to cancer as the deciding influence in the action of even the most active carcinogenic agents. The chemical carcinogens and the viral agents which provoke cancer act only in susceptible animals and often only in specific susceptible tissues. This concept, according to Rous, explains in part at least how all the diverse carcinogenic agents act to "play upon the neoplastic potentialities of the cells through the disturbances they induce, with result that these become realities. The potentialities themselves may be viruses incapable of causing growths unless the local conditions happen to be right or are made right, and even then perhaps only as a result of virus variation." This and other concepts, with many elaborations and variations, underlie the newer theoretical developments supported by advances in many fields, especially cytochemistry, chemical genetics, virus and enzyme chemistry.

## THEORIES INFLUENCING CANCER RESEARCH

The newer theories are not, in the usual sense, opposing; but admitting many variations and differences they reveal a general concentration on the many-sided problem of growth, not only of cellular growth but of synthesis or growth of the complex molecules which make up the fabric of the cell and at the same time direct its metabolism. Spencer observed, 1948, that no clinical problem has created "such widespread interest among nonmedical investigators", or activated investigators in such diverse fields as has cancer research. "Malignancy", according to Berrill, 1943, "and its associated phenomena merely constitute one aspect of growth, proliferation and differentiation of cells and cell constituents. The nature of the growth controlling forces of the body, of the internal control mechanism of the cell, the relation between nuclear change and cytoplasmic and organismic expression, and determination and maintenance of cellular specializations, and the mode of reproduction of proteins, mitochondria, enzymes, genes and viruses are as little understood and equally challenging. The problem of malignancy becomes one of synthesis involving the problems of development as a whole!" These problems must draw upon findings in the fields of virus and virus diseases of plants and animals, of genetics and cytochemistry, of enzyme and protein chemistry, and especially of nucleoprotein chemistry.

The suggestion "that the key to biological reproduction must necessarily be some sort of self-reproducing protein molecule", as pointed out by Gulick, 1944, was made long ago. The nucleoprotein nature of genes is accepted on indirect evidence of various kinds, but the first substance that seemed to be a self-duplicating protein molecule to be isolated from cells was not a gene but the tobacco mosaic virus. This and several other plant viruses are nucleoproteins obtained from the cytoplasm of diseased cells. Advances in cytochemistry, meanwhile, have revealed the existence of cytoplasmic nucleoproteins in normal cells, and the enzymes which catalyze the reactions controlled by the genes are, themselves, self-duplicating proteins of various sorts. Thus it becomes evident that the thread connecting what Gulick called "chemical genetics . . . a subject capable of very broad definitions" with what investigators in the cancer field call mutations is the thread of protein chemistry. This thread is continuous in the numerous proposals and theories that attempt to describe malignant change in terms of cytoplasmic or nuclear alteration.

The concept of cancer as a *cytoplasmic* disease or aberration is not new. According to Ludford, 1941, pathologists studying, over the years, the morphological divergencies of malignant cells have reported "the mitochondria usually finer and more numerous, and the cytoplasm more granular". The present views of the nature of malignancy as a fundamentally metabolic alteration in the cytoplasm of the affected cells have developed chiefly from the growing emphasis on the possibility that malignancy is an expression of a single neoplastic principle. Kidd, 1946, observed, "it seems plain that theoretically the autonomy of cancer cells requires within them the presence of something newly activated and distinctive". The impressiveness of the current presentations lies in the essential agreement of ideas based upon experimental findings so diverse. Leo Loeb suggested, 1944, an autocatalytic substance with reference to more than thirty years' study of the influence of endocrine and genetic factors in experimental cancer. Rous suggested, 1943, the neoplastic potentiality after thirty years of work with virus tumors. Kidd proposed, 1946, a distinctive constituent of cancer cells on the basis of serological studies in tumor-bearing animals. Many proposals of cytoplasmic alteration as a basis for the hypothetical neoplastic principle call for new or different definitions of the term, virus. Some (Darlington, 1944, Haddow, 1944, Potter, 1943) distinguished between viruses as contagious, infecting agents of conventional type and viruses as altered cytoplasmic constituents (small and filterable or large and nonfilterable). The view that aggressive cellular growth can follow such cytoplasmic alterations has much in common with what is known of the effects of viruses on cells. This view proposes a spectrum from plastid to plasmagene to virus (Darlington's plant material) or from enzyme to altered enzyme, the "cancer virus" or rogue enzyme (Potter's earlier view, 1944).

In the unicellular *Paramecium*, Sonneborn, working in zoology at Indiana University, identified in one strain a cytoplasmic factor or plasmagene (among many in the cytoplasm of the organism) which is capable of killing other strains of *Paramecium*, and which is therefore designated Kappa factor. The factor is passed from generation to generation in cell division and is hereditary without, however, involving the nucleus. It resembles the gene in power of self-reproduction, but, unlike the gene, Kappa factor multiplies within the cell independently of cell division. Although virus workers, more or less committed to the concept of viruses as extraneous infective entities penetrating the cell from without, have recognized that the theories of the nature of viruses as modified cellular components deserve serious consideration, it is chiefly workers in the cancer field that are exploring these theories to explain the mystery of malignant change. Darlington sketched with bold strokes, 1944, the possible modifications in general biological concepts to be expected from study of nucleoprotein metabolism, and the new possibilities of analysis and experiment that will arise when we "have learnt the passwords to take us across" the arbitrary frontiers that exist "between the studies of heredity, development and infection".

Proponents of the theory that viruses are or may be the cause of all tumors have advanced many ideas to explain the assumed endogenous origin of tumor viruses within the tumor-bearing host. A typical proposal is that, of numerous harmless viruses residing in cells, one may respond to environmental conditions by becoming a tumor-producing variant which is adapted only to its particular environment and so is not transmitted to other animals, although the harmless nonmutant viruses may be. Investigators favoring this view in general regard all viruses as invading pathogens or nonpathogens. They have not produced evidence to account for the presence of the "silent", or masked, or latent virus from which the tumor virus may arise as a mutant. The newer theories have two chief distinctions: first, they are based on some experimental evidence that provides at least the possibility that tumor viruses may, through metabolic relationships, be formed from normal components of the cytoplasm; secondly, they include experimental evidence that such an alteration can be permanent and be transmitted at mitosis by hereditary mechanisms residing in the cytoplasm.

Virus diseases of plants were the substance of observation and experiment that led Woods and duBuy, two investigators now working at the National Institutes of Health, to develop a working hypothesis of cancer that may, according to their view, reconcile the virus and the nonvirus theories of cancer. They presented interpretations of evidence, 1945, that plant viruses arise in the course of cellular metabolism from normal mitochondria (particulate bodies in the cytoplasm) or from their derivatives, the plastids. From their studies in plants, these authors have, by analogy, proposed a theory of mammalian cancer: the plastogenes of plant cells, in their view, are comparable to the plasmagenes of animal cells; these bodies "mutate" under the influence of numerous factors known also to be associated with cancer (the mutational change occurred, in the plant cells studied, in the nucleoprotein component of the plastids).

The suggestion of R. G. Green, 1947, that the mammary tumor

agent or virus "occupies a vital position in the cancer cell" which it inhabits may be recalled in this connection. The fact that immune serum produced in rabbits by the injection of the agent has "an inactivating, or lethal, effect upon the cancer cell" indicated to the author that the cancer cell is "completely dependent upon the vital activity of the virus associated with it", and that the cancer cell is a new cell species. The description by Kidd, 1940, of a distinctive constituent of Brown-Pearce carcinoma cells, and his recent report that a specific and distinct constituent has been isolated from another transplantable rabbit cancer of unknown cause — the $N_2$ carcinoma — have led him to propose that these substances may have direct part in the proliferative activities of the tumor cells containing them. He has shown by serological methods that antibodies produced by the Brown-Pearce distinctive constituent, which is "probably a protein and perhaps a ribosenucleoprotein", suppressed the growth of the tumor cells.

Early suggestions by cytologists in Germany that the discrete particles within the cytoplasm (mitochondria, microsomes) are the sites of *enzymic* activities of the cell were confirmed (Monné, Runnström, others in Sweden; Claude, Bensley, Lazarow, Guzman Barron and others in this country) when newer techniques became available. Among findings in the active present investigations with isotopes are that ribonucleic acid, abundant in the cytoplasm, is correlated with cellular synthesis of proteins (Caspersson, 1947); that complicated complexes containing energy-rich phosphate bonds are apparently built up in the mitochondria (D. E. Green and coworkers, 1949). Spiegelman and Kamen, 1947, suggested that nucleic acids may funnel energy into the protein-synthesizing mechanism. The nucleus and cytoplasm may interact with each other largely through the nucleoproteins, the nucleus providing nucleic acids that direct the specificity of synthetic activities of the cytoplasm, and the cytoplasm possibly contributing "the more elementary steps in the synthesis" (Mazia, 1952). The possible implications of the concept of essential likeness between enzymes and viruses for cancer research were explained (Spiegelman and coworkers, 1948) in terms of carcinogenesis which may take place at the plasmagene level and "be subsequently transmitted *via* the cytoplasm from one cell generation to the next". Heston, 1948, considered it necessary to look upon the milk agent not as an entity in itself but as one of the physiologically coordinated nuclear and cytoplasmic units which comprise the cell containing it.

Suggestions of a metabolic relationship of enzymes and other nucleoproteins of the cytoplasm with viruses have been made on the basis of investigations in numerous fields. Although Claude, working in cytochemistry, has not proposed that the Rous chicken tumor agent may be derived from the nucleoprotein constituents of the cytoplasm, his findings have furnished chemical evidence that is in harmony with this suggestion. The microsomes (secretory granules) that have been found to be centers of enzymic activity have certain chemical resemblances to the active fraction of the Rous chicken tumor agent. Both are complexes of phospholipids and of nucleoproteins, containing a ribose type of nucleic acid. Haddow, who has been interested for many years in the virus theory of cancer, found, 1944, much indirect evidence to support the concept "that the changes evoked by many viruses are due to their competing for substrate with physiological elements of the cell, and thus diverting the normal metabolism . . ." Needham, on the basis of investigations in embryology, included, 1942, among related nucleoproteins that are self-duplicating, and that are concerned with growth at the molecular level, the growth-promoting factor obtained from embryonic tissue which is concerned not only with development but has been shown also to promote the growth of cells in tissue cultures and to have an acceleratory action on the healing of wounds. He suggested that the growth-promoting power of embryonic extract may reside in some nucleotide structure which may act as a "carrier for the requisite peptone bundle" or as a "bricklaying" mechanism at the site of protein synthesis. Darlington of the John Innes Horticultural Institution, England, has emphasized, 1944, the significance of the discoveries that in the cell substance there exists a molecular system depending for its permanence upon a chemical equilibrium which possesses a measure of independence but which is none the less dependent also upon the morphologically stable nucleus. This chemical equilibrium is an effective part of the biological activities of heredity, of growth, and development. Monné stated that cells deprived of the nucleus continue to display catabolism and all life phenomena that depend upon these reactions. Nevertheless, in his view, it is certain that the synthesis of cell-, organ- and species-specific proteins, and therefore the processes of "reproduction, growth and differentiation are impossible without the nucleus". These processes concern the highly specific proteins some of which are species specific, such as the reserve proteins (yolk, etc.) and defense proteins (antibodies).

The present emphasis upon the cytoplasm is not intended to rule out genetic influences and the nuclear-cytoplasmic interrelation. Thompson's concept of the dynamic interaction between all parts of a living cell, and of the corollary dynamic interaction between all parts of a complex multicellular organism, broadens the view and admits also the conception of cancer as a generalized, organismal metabolic aberration. He disregarded the separation of active and passive parts of the cell, for the "manifestations of force can only be due to the interaction of the various parts, to the transference of energy from one to another. Certain properties may be manifested, certain functions may be carried on, by the protoplasm apart from the nucleus; but the interaction of the two is necessary, that other and more important properties or functions may be manifested." From this dynamic point of view, a multicellular organism is a continuity of forces "somehow shaping the whole organism, independently of the number, magnitude and form of the individual cells, which enter like a froth into its fabric". It may be that the arguments whether transmission of malignancy in cell division takes place through the nucleus or through the cytoplasm are meaningless. Haddow pointed out that this is not susceptible to experimental proof for, in the absence of sexual reproduction in the body cells which multiply by simple division, nuclear changes cannot be distinguished from cytoplasmic changes or virus infections.

A theory of malignant change through primary action on *nuclear* material and secondary change in the cytoplasm was developed by Haddow, 1953, on the basis of previously mentioned study of mechanism of action of the nitrogen mustards and other chemicals the action of which on cells resembles that of X rays. He cited work indicating that, in cells so exposed, chromosome fragments "are characteristically ejected into the cytoplasm". If such a fragment were of molecular dimensions, "it might then be capable of reproducing itself in the cytoplasm indefinitely". Much may be expected, he thought, from future studies of the effects of certain carcinogens that combine with nuclear material, and of the effects induced in the cell as a whole (genetic and cytological). Studies are in progress in numerous laboratories to test the mutagenic properties of known carcinogens; Strong raised the question, 1949, whether every carcinogenic agent is not also mutagenic, and *vice versa*. There have been suggestions, as by Bjorksten, 1951, that the unusual sensitivity to radiations and nitrogen mustards of cells that are active in the synthesis of protein and desoxyribonucleic acids is related to cross-linking between the proteins. This cross-linking appears to be identical with that taking place in aging proteins, aging rubber and similar substances. Aging tissues, then, may be characterized by cross-linking of proteins (with consequent reduction of ability to retain water, loss of elasticity and acquired brittleness). Such a view disposes of the necessity for specific carcinogens and provides for action of the known cancer-producing agents as expediting changes in genetic protein, which would in any case occur with age.

### PERTINENCE OF THESE CONCEPTS TO HUMAN CANCER

An affirmative answer to the natural question whether these fundamental concepts have any relevance to the prevention and control of human disease can be given only if the kind of "control" contemplated is based on knowledge of mechanisms and causes. Kidd, who regarded the theoretical developments as the most reasonable explanation of the experimental facts established for the Brown-Pearce carcinoma, held that "understanding of the factors and principles involved in the continuing causation of malignancy is important as providing the basis for an intelligent approach to the problems of cancer prevention and cancer cure". The more fundamental approach to the problem of the nature of malignancy and of malignant change in terms of molecular alteration, or metabolism, was specified as the only rational approach by the Surgeon General's committee reviewing the status of cancer research in 1938. Murphy, analyzing the committee's conclusions, said "that substantial advancement in the methods of treatment will come only with a fuller knowledge of the formal genesis or the mechanism by which the growth capacity of cancer is maintained". Stanley's vision of the possibility of eliminating "the disease-producing viruses by supplanting them with innocuous viruses produced in the laboratory by chemical means from pathogenic viruses" may be realized for cancer when the neoplastic principle or principles can be determined.

Other possibilities of potential clinical usefulness have been suggested by investigators who have explored the stages of cancer development. H. N. S. Greene's experiments, mentioned previously, on transplantation of tumors to the anterior chamber of the eye as an inoculation site have resulted in a description of cancer development as not "a sudden transition of normal cells", but rather "a progressive developmental process during the course of which the primary neoplastic focus passes through successive stages of anaplastic cellular change, local tissue invasion, foreign tissue invasion and eventually metastasis". One of the most practical (although seemingly academic) results of all the work on endocrines in relation to cancer is the proof that malignant growth is dependent upon the "endocrine environment". Rhoads, 1954, looked toward the day when it will be possible by analyzing this environment to arrive at means for cancer prevention.

In both the neoplastic and the virus field there is wide skepticism concerning attempts to alter the internal composition or metabolism of cells that have either been infected by viruses or have become neoplastic, without at the same time injuring or killing the unaffected cells of the host. Search for compounds that will do this, still in its initial phases, rests upon the general concept that virus growth and multiplication and malignant change, especially in the latent or early stages, are metabolic processes probably involving nucleoprotein elements in the affected cells. If these processes could be precisely defined (even though they may be different for each virus infection and for each different neoplasm) there would be hope of interrupting processes that lead to destruction of cells by viruses and to uncontrolled growth of neoplastic cells. Horsfall subscribed to such a hope in describing, 1952, to the Harvey Society his experiments looking toward hope of chemotherapy of virus infections.

As contrasted with study of chemotherapeutic agents that inhibit the growth of specific body cells and, therefore, of neoplastic cells derived from them (the sex hormones, for example, in breast and prostatic cancer), and with study of chemotherapeutic substances that appear to inhibit the growth of cells that are actively dividing (the antifolic acid compounds in leukemia, for example) the search appears to be opening for compounds that may specifically inhibit nucleo-protein alterations that take place in the earliest stages of neoplastic change. The immense amount of work on chemical and metabolic differences between original (wild) and mutant strains of bacteria suggests an analogy with normal and possibly mutant mammalian cells with neoplastic properties (Rhoads, 1954). The number of highly differentiated cells with specific metabolic functions in the normal body makes expectable a high degree of difference among neoplastic cells derived from them. Yet the variations in microorganisms and in the diseases they produce did not impede the search for chemo-therapeutic compounds for infections when success had once been demonstrated. Selective inhibition of the growth of cancer cells would be much more difficult, but not sufficiently more difficult to justify pessimism, according to Rhoads, who pointed out that cancer deaths generally are due to only a few types of cancer.

For goals so distant and targets so invisible the best present hope may be "guided missiles", aimed by logical theoretical reasoning supported by closely interpreted experimental findings. Study of regulating mechanisms that channel the multiple enzymic reactions toward different pathways will, Guzman Barron pointed out, 1949, clarify the role of enzymes in growth processes and help us in under-standing the change from normal, controlled growth to the uncon-trolled growth of cancer. If some, at least, of the known carcinogens act by elimination of gene or enzyme mechanisms that control syn-theses essential for cell division and growth, Haddow envisaged possibilities "which may feasibly lead, in due time, to the chemical or enzymatic means of its reversal or control". The adventurous in-vestigator is content with such a basis for his hypotheses.

CHAPTER 3

# Infertility

*Resulting from defects in the female
and/or male reproductive tract*

## INTRODUCTORY

Selection of infertility as an outstanding medical problem might, at first blush, seem curious at a time when the nation's birth rate has reached an all-time high and the nation's infant mortality rate an all-time low. The urgency of the problem is sufficiently defined, however, by the wide range of diseases and accidents involved in infertility and not less significantly by the psychological hazards to marriage which infertility presents. As used in this discussion of investigative

135

work, infertility covers not only barriers to conception but also anything that prevents production of a normal child capable of continued
growth and development, including spontaneous abortion, premature
birth, stillbirth, neonatal death, congenital abnormality. It is doubtful whether a Mongolian idiot or an infant doomed at birth to die
before it is one year old or to be institutionalized sooner or later for
motor disorders or mental defect would be regarded by an infertile
couple as an improvement on the barren state. That the male as well
as the female may be responsible for infertility has been recognized
medically within the past two decades, in line with the view advanced
by biologists more than fifty years ago that fertility represents the reproductive capacity of *pairs* of male and female organisms.

There are no dependable statistics defining the extent of the medical
problem of infertility. The National Research Council's committee
on human reproduction noted, 1950, that the best available figures
suggest that approximately ten per cent of all marriages in the United
States are involuntarily sterile. Nicholson J. Eastman estimated,
1950, that ten per cent of all pregnancies terminate in spontaneous
abortion and that, in spite of significant reduction, half the maternal
mortality that occurs each year in the United States as a result of child
bearing is still preventable. The total infant loss (stillbirths, deaths
attributed to premature birth or congenital defect) represented more
than ten per cent of deaths from all causes reported in 1948 by the
National Office of Vital Statistics. "Maternal, infant and fetal deaths
add up to the third leading cause of all deaths", according to the
Children's Bureau, 1950.

Obstacles in attempts to determine the causes of infertility are: the
fact that failure to conceive comes to the physician's attention only on
the initiative of the childless couple; that infertility is not a dramatic
hospitalizable illness; that dependable diagnostic methods are lacking
for determining capacity to produce normal ova and spermatozoa;
that there is not available a sufficient body of normal material to make
it possible to define deviations; that it is not possible to externalize
hidden reproductive processes; that length and complexity of the human fertility cycle make it impossible to recognize how frequently and
how far infertility goes back to faulty maturation in earlier periods.
Failure in spermatogenesis or in ovulation discovered only in adoles-

cence may have originated in developmental events that go back to childhood, even to the developing embryo: adult cryptorchidism, for instance, results from failure of the testes to descend in the last month of fetal life from the abdomen to their normal location, the scrotum. Investigators, whether biologists or animal husbandry workers, endeavoring to explain parts of the long and complex cycle, are repeatedly driven back to antecedent events: Carl G. Hartman, in his study of the primate embryo, found he needed to know the prefertilized ovum and was so launched on a fifteen-year study of ovulation in monkeys; George B. Wislocki and Edward W. Dempsey, in the course of their study of the pregnant uterus, found it necessary, 1945, "to become acquainted with the *antecedent* preimplantation endometrium". Clinicians unable to find specific therapies for the later aspects of infertility have been forced to recognize the significance of earlier physiological changes: Cary, 1944, considered that at least thirty-three per cent of his cases of adult infertility could be traced to abnormal conditions in puberty; Charny, 1950, described adult infertility as "almost too late for treatment", urging "more attention to the study of testicular development in the growing boy" in order to understand deviations from fertility in the man. With Conston and Meranze, he made a beginning in this direction, 1952.

While animal experimentation over the past thirty years certainly charted the course for investigation of human infertility, literal application of the results of animal research to correction of human infertility has been thus far disappointing. Not useful to human medicine, for instance, is the biologists' procedure in producing complete sterility in mouse, rat, rabbit, monkey by removing various organs or tissues. Medical men are less interested in complete sterility than in depressed fertility, hopefully regarded as amenable to medical aid by stimulation. Equally inapplicable to the human problem are many of the procedures of animal husbandry, the chief objective of which (until recent years) has been less to correct infertility (since sterile animals may be killed for meat and replaced by more fertile strains) than to increase fertility beyond normal limits: to stimulate the bull that normally fathers sixty calves to sire five hundred; to induce cows and sheep, by hormonal stimulation, to shed more ova and produce twins and triplets; to induce animals to breed outside the normal breeding season and so make it possible to send "spring" lamb to market at any season. The unbiologic nature of such stimulation is recognized in S. A. Asdell's reference to increased yield of milk induced in cows under the heightened metabolic rate resulting from thyroxine stimulation: "One wonders whether the cow will be able to stand up to the strain of an increased rate of living." Commenting on facile transfer to humans of hormonal stimulation of ovarian function in animals, one anatomist observed, "a woman is not a cow". Many biologists have pointed out that up to the present the mammalian species explored have been too few to justify generalizations that would place human fertility in biological perspective. Over-simplified hypotheses of menstrual bleeding constructed on the basis of twenty years' research on the rhesus monkey (whose menstrual cycle resembles woman's) were challenged by the later finding that in other species of monkeys there is no external sign of bleeding.

## MAJOR SOURCES OF INVESTIGATIVE WORK IN INFERTILITY

Only cursory reference is possible to the many divisions of biology and medicine now contributing to knowledge fundamental to solution of human infertility. Research on human infertility, moreover, ranges far beyond the fields of biology and medicine to include anthropological, social, psychological observations, studies of population problems. The basic biologic lines from which present investigative work developed were laid in the first thirty years of the present century by zoologists, anatomists, embryologists, physiologists, gynecologists (and some obstetricians) and, during the past twenty years, also by biochemists, geneticists, animal husbandrymen. Many of the workers that led in opening the whole field to investigation in the twenties and earlier have continued to be major contributors to basic work. Their work may, it is true, have moved to events antecedent or subsequent to the stage originally studied, may have passed from morphological to chemical, biochemical, cytochemical emphasis. Frederick L. Hisaw's work in Wisconsin's zoology department, 1928, on the corpus luteum of menstruation had moved on at Harvard, 1952, to the corpus luteum of pregnancy. Herbert M. Evans's work, 1952, in California's laboratory of experimental biology, on the chemical nature and physiological effects of pituitary gonadotrophins goes back to his classic study, 1922, with J. A. Long, of estrus in the rat. Philip E. Smith's work on spermatogenesis in monkeys (Columbia's anatomy department) may be traced to his Stanford work, 1928, demonstrating the gonadotrophic role of the anterior pituitary in the rat. Histochemical studies of the placenta, conducted since 1943 in Harvard's anatomy department by Wislocki and his associates, followed twenty years of comparative work on evolution of the placenta. George W. Corner began in Mall's laboratory at Johns Hopkins the work on the corpus luteum that led, 1929, in Rochester's anatomy department, to isolation with Willard M. Allen of crude progesterone and, 1944, to histochemical evidence of the origin of the cells of the corpus luteum. These are part of the program of the Carnegie Institution's laboratory of embryology (now directed by Corner) which includes research on other stages of the reproductive cycle, implantation (Elizabeth M. Ramsey), pregnancy and parturition (Samuel R. M. Reynolds), fetal growth and nutrition (Louis B. Flexner). Frank R. Lillie's research on the chemistry of fertilization during the first two decades of the present century led to the program on the biology of sex, now in its thirtieth year in Chicago's zoology department, with especial interest in the work of Carl R. Moore on the biology of the testes. A complementary program on ovarian physiology with especial reference to menstruation in primates has been conducted by George W. Bartelmez in the anatomy department.

The past ten years have seen marked advances in application to biology and medicine of such contributions from animal husbandry as the programs developed a decade ago on the biochemistry of spermatozoa (H. A. Lardy and his associates in Wisconsin's department of agricultural biochemistry), on the physiology of sperm (S. A. Asdell and his associates in Cornell's agricultural school), on structure and function of the male accessory organs (Fred F. McKenzie and his associates in the Missouri Agricultural College), on chorionic gonadotrophins in the mare (George H. Hart and H. H. Cole, in California's agricultural college). In England, studies on reproduction in university biology, physiology, biochemistry departments, work in medical school departments of obstetrics and gynecology, in agricultural colleges and institutes, supported by the government's Agricultural Research Council and its Medical Research Council, have been brought together by consultative arrangements between the two councils and by grants from both for common biological problems. As a result, recent research on the biology of spermatozoa has been conducted not only by the staff of the Agricultural Research Council (studies of T. Mann at the Molteno Institute) but also in the biochemistry department of the University of Cambridge, with grants from the council, and in the National Institute of Medical Research (investigations of A. S. Parkes also engaged for over twenty years in research on the nature and function of steroid hormones in sex and reproduction). The work of the generation oriented by F. H. A. Marshall's synthesis of existing knowledge in his *Physiology of Reproduction*, published, 1910, from the physiology department of the University of Cambridge, appears in the 1952 edition, in contributions from staff members of the Agricultural Research Council (Joseph Barcroft on fetal physiology, J. Hammond on gestation and parturition in the rabbit), the Medical Research Council, university, agricultural, medical school investigators.

The declared aims of investigative committees formed at different times by the National Research Council during the past thirty years reflect changing emphasis and objectives in infertility research. The work demonstrating the physiological role of the gonadotrophic and gonadal hormones in the sex cycle of mammals (estrous cycle of animals, menstrual cycle of primates), stimulated and coordinated in some twenty biology, anatomy, zoology, biochemistry departments, by the council's committee for research on problems on sex (established 1921, still functioning with diminished funds), has now shifted to the more difficult problem of discovering the place of origin of these hormones, the mechanisms of their synthesis, utilization, breakdown, excretion. In 1952, the council's division of biology established a committee on development "to stimulate better correlation of knowledge coming from the various tributaries of the field, to detect major gaps in knowledge, to organize group meetings to point up research needs". Efforts to reduce the stillbirth and neonatal death rate reflect the growth of developmental physiology during the last ten years. The committee on human reproduction formed, 1947,

through contract with the National Research Council, by representatives of biology, obstetrics, gynecology, psychology, sociology, public
health to plan long-term research designed to clarify the mechanism of
conception, the possibility of correcting infertility, the causes of prematurity, abortion, the nature and mechanism of factors that influence
development of the embryo, was dissolved, 1951, for lack of funds.

In view of the amount of work still to be done before physiological
hypotheses of reproduction and embryonic development advanced
during the past twenty years can be proved, it is perhaps not surprising
that a comprehensive program on the scale that proved effective for
the program on sex has not yet emerged in human reproduction.
Biologic research is only now moving from investigations of the sex
cycle to the more complex problems of the pregnancy cycle. In their
fundamental approach biologists often owe a degree of guidance to
clinical suggestion. Observations during surgery from a group of
Viennese gynecologists at the close of the last century on cytological
changes of the uterus oriented biological investigation and contributed to the concept of the ovary as a secretory organ at least
twenty years before the ovarian hormones were isolated. From a
gynecologist also came Bernard Zondek's demonstration, 1926, of the
gonadotrophic role of the anterior pituitary in the rat, the isolation,
1927, of estrogenic substances from human pregnancy urine, facilitating analysis and, later, synthesis by organic chemists. Combined
training in gynecology and embryology enabled John Rock and Arthur
T. Hertig to add new chapters to the life of the early human embryo
through their collection of fertilized ova at various early stages. In
some medical schools (Vanderbilt, Yale, Johns Hopkins, Columbia,
Harvard) anatomists pursuing physiological problems in monkeys
have worked with obstetricians to throw light on problems of human
reproduction. The combined efforts of a urologist and an anatomist,
Robert S. Hotchkiss and John MacLeod, led to studies of human infertility in the male that have been productive on both the clinical and
the fundamental level. A coordinated study of the physiology of
human fertility and conception begun, 1950, in the Sloane institute
for research in human reproduction by members of Columbia's
departments of anatomy, biochemistry, pediatrics, medicine, urology,
psychology, under Howard C. Taylor, Jr., chairman of the gynecology

and obstetrics department, aimed at focusing "public . . . and foundation interest on the fundamental character of the medical problems
incidental to the reproductive process and on the necessity of expanding research in this field".

Research on fertility mechanisms has opened up spectacular approaches to medical problems considered more catastrophic than
infertility, and support for research on these problems has outdistanced
support for research on infertility.   Research on the sex hormones has
been "diverted" from their role in reproduction (in the study of
which they were discovered) to their role in hemopoiesis, normal protein anabolism and growth, cancer.   While this associated research
will ultimately aid in clarifying the role of the hormones in fertility,
the "diversion" does emphasize lack of a comprehensive, intensive and
unified attack on infertility.   Nothing of the extensive work done on
animals can be counted as wasted in the attack on human infertility:
as Rock observed (at a 1949 conference on human reproduction), "all
research on the physiology of reproduction, whether in virus or chimpanzee, may eventually help the human individual at will to achieve
or to suppress his reproduction"; the present investigative picture,
however, discloses many undeveloped areas, many still unanswered
questions.   The committee on human reproduction pointed, 1950,
to fundamental research as the best hope for preventing tragic loss
from premature labor, toxemias of pregnancy, habitual abortion
"since in over half of the fatalities associated with pregnancy, the
fundamental biology of the reproductive process is at fault".   The
"fundamental research" includes work that will explain ovulation, the
chemistry of sperm and of ovum, the mechanism of their transport, the
factors responsible for poor quality of either or both.

## CAUSES OF INFERTILITY

### Physiological Variables Affecting Fertility in Both Sexes

The causes of infertility (for certain of which there may be neither
overt pathology nor clear evidence of functional failure) are multiple
and may be referable to factors and functions outside the reproductive
system.   The primitive concept of reproduction as an isolated func-

tion, fostered by the fact that the gonads may be removed from animals and man without endangering life (as would removal of the heart), has given way to modern biological concepts recognizing the chemical web that links "system" with "system" in a dynamic metabolic exchange.

While among factors that appear to have a bearing on infertility (inability to conceive, stillbirth, birth of defective infants) stress has been laid upon *age*, "very little is known", according to Taylor, 1949, about the relation of age to the curve of declining fertility in normal women. To questions raised at a 1949 conference on human reproduction by population experts regarding frequency of conception at different ages, incidence of tubal closure and of sperm inadequacy (frequently cited causes of infertility) with advancing age, medical men replied that available statistics are not adequate to furnish replies. The menstruation known to occur without ovulation for several cycles in early puberty as well as at the beginning of the menopause (not to be confused with pathological anovulatory menstruation during adult reproductive life) represents a kind of "physiologic infertility" associated with reproductive as distinguished from chronological age. That a parallel type of infertility may be associated with immaturity and senility in the male was suggested, 1939, by Jacob Yerushalmy's finding stillbirths more numerous when fathers were very young or very old, without regard to the age of the mother. Maternal age, however, influences the stillbirth rate: in Scotland, 1950, women over forty accounted for twice as many stillbirths as women under twenty. "Advancing maternal age" was cited (Penrose, 1954) as the most striking single feature associated with Mongolian idiocy, "one of the most baffling problems in medicine".

Deficiency of particular *nutritional elements*, vitamins, proteins, minerals, experimentally demonstrated to have a specific role in infertility in mice, rats, horses, bulls, cows, chickens, has not been shown to cause human infertility. Gertrude van Wagenen observed, 1946, as have others, "while the necessity for adequate protein nutrition in pregnancy scarcely admits of doubt, actual establishment of standards awaits rigorous experimentation". W. J. Darby, R. G. Cannon and M. M. Kaser pointed out, 1948, that biochemical measurements are available for few of the forty or more nutritional essentials. Their study, by the most objective quantitative methods available, of the nutritional status of 1,700 pregnant women at a Vanderbilt University clinic led them to regard biochemical assessment of nutritional level during pregnancy as still a subject for investigation. Landrum B. Shettles, at a 1942 conference on the biology of sperm, described the relation between diet and spermatogenesis as "a virgin field for study". Since Evans and Bishop found, 1922, that vitamin E deficiency resulted in testicular atrophy in male rats (but not in several farm animals subsequently studied by others) and, in females, in absorption or abortion of the fetuses before term, vitamin E has been used increasingly to promote spermatogenesis in men, to prevent abortion in women. Opinions as to its clinical value have ranged from Shute's 1944 report of prompt and striking effect upon spermatogenesis to Edmond J. Farris's conclusion, 1949, from tests in man, "vitamin E does not stimulate spermatogenesis". One suggestion offered by investigators in the anatomy, pharmacology and pathology departments at Columbia (Hans Kaunitz and C. A. Slanetz with others), 1949, is that vitamin E deficiency "is deeply involved in the processes which accompany aging", as are various other deficiency states, symptoms of which include changes in the reproductive cycle and infertility.

That nutrition may influence the part played by hormones in reproductive capacity has been suggested by numerous experiments with laboratory and barnyard animals within twenty years past. John Hammond, Jr., observed, 1945, that use of gonadotrophins to induce ovulation in domestic animals is ineffective in poorly nourished animals. Huseby and Ball in the same year reported that cutting by one third caloric intake of young mice resulted in persistence of juvenile ovaries, castration effects in the uterus and other evidences of a low level of gonadotrophins. Work on less extreme deficiencies and on specific nutritional factors has been less conclusive. Karl E. Mason, 1944, summarized various reports indicating that gonadal-hypophyseal dysfunctions found in the vitamin E-deficient rat are more likely to be "the result of, rather than the cause of, the reproductive disturbances characteristic of the deficiency state". Illustrating claims that various hormones will correct atrophic changes in reproductive tissues attributed to deficiencies of vitamin B factors, Roy

Hertz (National Cancer Institute's endocrine section) told the American Society for the Study of Sterility, 1947, that folic acid deficiency impaired the biological effects of even maximal doses of estrogens in both birds and monkeys. Studying the role of the liver in the inactivation of estrogens and androgens (in rats) since 1939, M. S. Biskind concluded that in vitamin B deficiency the liver loses its ability to inactivate estrogens but continues to inactivate androgens, causing an imbalance, excessive estrogens, leading to infertility in the male. In 1943 he reported, with Falk, that vitamin B treatment of thirteen infertile men resulted in "apparent restoration of fertility in eight". Although experimental evidence for the breakdown of estrogens in the liver is widely accepted (current work is directed toward identification of the specific enzymes involved) and although the finding that several B vitamins function as coenzymes has added weight to the suggestion that thiamin and riboflavin play a part in estrogen metabolism (R. D. H. Heard and J. C. Saffran, 1949), developing research has revealed paths other than the liver for metabolism of sex steroids. Fundamental students of metabolism of the sex steroids regard it, therefore, as premature to assign to the liver an exclusive etiological role in disturbed steroid metabolism associated with infertility.

Recognition of infertility accompanying states of extreme endocrine deficiency and general preoccupation with the influence of *hormones* in the biology of reproduction have led to wide empirical use of hormones in attempts to deal with clinical infertility. Outstanding in reports of such clinical trials is the lack of controls, if controls in the strict scientific sense could be set up in the absence of means for exact determinations of hormone activity. Newer methods of study of endocrine function (to replace what has been called the "shoot and see" principle) have made possible the beginnings of a new cytochemical anatomy, a new approach to study of the metabolic activities of the hormones affecting the specific target organs and affecting the rates and directions of intermediary metabolism. Among the newer methods in use for tracing biological activities of hormones at the molecular level are: tracer studies with radioactive carbon and other substances; modification of endocrine function by chemical means (rather than by experimental ablation) such as use of hormone antagonists; histochemical, cytochemical, microdissection methods for study of sites of origin of hormones; tissue culture techniques; methods of enzyme chemistry for study of mechanisms of action on target cells, mechanisms of inactivation of the hormones. Among insistent questions underlying the possibility of using hormones to nullify certain suspected causes of infertility are: How do the hormones reach the cells of their end organs? How do the hormones of the anterior pituitary act upon their end organs, the individual endocrine glands? To what degree is secretion of the trophic hormones of the pituitary controlled by the influence of other endocrine glands, by the nervous system? What governs the competence of the particular tissue to respond to particular hormones? "The truly impressive progress" resulting from the "enormous volume" of work on identification, isolation, purification and even synthesis of hormones was contrasted, 1953, by Paul Weiss, with the "wholly inadequate" attention spent on efforts to discover how a hormonal target organ can respond selectively to its proper hormone. These unanswered questions emphasize the impossibility, in the present state of knowledge, of conducting clinical trials of hormones in infertility according to the accepted (if imperfect) standards for clinical trials of drugs; they emphasize the inconclusive nature of published results of use of thyroid, gonadotrophic, sex hormones in treatment of infertility.

Although a clinical role for the thyroid has been recognized for many years (because of heightened activity noted in many individuals during periods of changing sexual function, as adolescence, pregnancy, menopause), there has been less work on the thyroid than on the pituitary gonadotrophins and the sex steroids. Hamblen, who noted hypothyroidism in from twenty to twenty-five per cent of childless women seen in his clinic, attributed, 1945, ten per cent of pregnancies achieved to thyroid therapy; other clinical reports have mentioned higher percentages. The mechanism by which the thyroid influences human gonadal function is unknown, not only, as Edward T. Tyler pointed out, 1949, because "controlled studies of infertile patients who have been successfully treated with thyroid are few" but also because it is difficult to evaluate the effect of thyroid combined, as it commonly is, with other measures. Development of more dependable tests of thyroid function, introduction of thyroid antagonists (as thiouracil) providing a cheaper and more convenient tool than gland ablation in animals have contributed to revival of investigative activity on the role of the thyroid. Experimental studies include a report on the role of the thyroid in the menstrual cycle of monkeys (Earl T. Engle, 1944), in testicular function of rats (James H. Leathem), a report (William C. Young and his associates, 1952) on a long-term study of the role of the thyroid in fertility. Administration of generous amounts of thyroid early in pregnancy to prevent abortion, offered as suggestive by John P. Peters and his associates at Yale, 1951, was based upon several years' determination of serum iodine; a rise in iodine occurred during normal (but not in disturbed) pregnancy. Results of measurement of precipitable serum iodine before and during pregnancy were discussed in relation to the controversial question whether moderate thyroid hyperplasia recognized in from sixty to ninety per cent of normal pregnancies is associated with actual hyperfunction. Other unanswered questions in thyroid physiology, discussed by J. H. Means, 1949, relate to the mechanism of thyroid hormone synthesis, its storage, delivery, transport; to mechanisms controlling these activities; to its action on specific cells of the body and to the fate of the hormone after it has exerted its action. Answers to such questions (applicable to all endocrines) will perhaps throw light on the influence of subtotal hormonal failures in infertility.

The fundamental questions raised concerning the thyroid are also raised concerning the adrenal cortex: whether it exerts a specific, direct effect on the gonads, whether its effect is mediated through the anterior pituitary, whether its effect on fertility is a part of what Dwight J. Ingle called, 1951, a "permissive" action, the hormones of the adrenal cortex being necessary, but not responsible, for a particular response. Although a clinical role for this gland has also been suggested by the sterility seen in severe adrenal cortical disease, the significance of depressed adrenal function for fertility remains to be established, in spite of the volume of experimental research over the last twenty years on the relation of the gonads to the adrenals.

Fundamental research of the past quarter century demonstrating that the anterior pituitary stimulated the gonads in representative animals in all of the vertebrate classes so far back in the phylogenetic series as certain primitive insects stimulated hope of achieving a hormonal specific for depressed human fertility. Cushing had observed that pituitary tumors ultimately result in sterility in males and other clinical observation had associated sterility with pituitary failure in Simmonds's disease. Since 1930 when several groups (Zondek and Aschheim; Hisaw, Fevold and Leonard) postulated two gonadotrophic factors in the anterior pituitary, two components have been separated from anterior pituitary extracts: a follicle-stimulating hormone (FSH) which in the female animal stimulates growth of the follicle, and in the male, spermatogenesis; a luteinizing hormone (LH) which in the female, when added to FSH, stimulates ovulation and transformation of the follicle to the corpus luteum and which, in the male, mediates the secretion of androgen. Although increasing purification has established them as distinct chemical entities, each with its own physiological effects (varying, however, with the experimental animal, its physiological state and the relative amounts of each extract), the belief entertained by some chemists that the anterior pituitary secretes into the blood two separate gonadotrophic hormones is not shared by a number of biologists (Smith, Engle, Cole) chiefly because effects obtained with the separate fractions may be secured with undivided extracts; and because certain results (notably ovulation) secured by combining the two factors cannot be secured in some species by either factor alone. Evans, in whose laboratory FSH was prepared in pure form by C. H. Li, 1949, observed, 1950, "It is by no means certain that the pituitary secretes two gonadotrophic hormones." A third pituitary factor, luteotrophin, has been suggested by several investigators as necessary for initiating secretory activity in the corpus luteum and for maintaining it in a functional state, but it has not been demonstrated whether this third factor is identical with the lactogenic hormone or whether it is a fourth, separate factor, as suggested by Edwin B. Astwood, 1941.

The number, nature, cell of origin and physiological effects of the various pituitary gonadotrophins are not the only problems in assessing their role in fertility. Why the gonads begin to respond to gonadotrophins when they do is not known since it is now recognized that gonadotrophins are secreted, if at a low level, before puberty, and the administration of gonadotrophins to young boys for undescended testes has shown that the gonads possess the capacity to respond before puberty. Engle suggested that the gonads can respond to gonadotrophins only after they have experienced a certain amount of ripening which may be independent of the pituitary. Up to 1947, no anterior pituitary extracts suitable for routine medical trial in infertility had been accepted by the Council on Pharmacy and Chemistry and the trials of those available had not proved encouraging. Tyler, 1949, summarized the use of follicle-stimulating pituitary substances for seminal deficiency in infertile men as even more discouraging than the use of such substances to stimulate ovulation in infertile women. Since FSH and LH as foreign proteins (derived from sheep and hog pituitary) involve danger of shock, therapeutic trial has been made of gonadotrophins from nonpituitary sources, e.g., chorionic gonadotrophins (isolated, 1927, by Aschheim and Zondek from the urine of pregnant women) and equine gonadotrophins (discovered by Cole and Hart, 1928, in the blood of pregnant mares). The enthusiasm stirred in the early thirties by trials of human chorionic gonadotrophins for human infertility has been succeeded by frank disappointment at their failure to stimulate spermatogenesis or ovulation. One explanation suggested by recent studies is the luteinizing nature of their major component. For the use of such substances for ovarian disturbances, *New and Nonofficial Remedies* found, 1950, no scientific rationale. Of equine gonadotrophins, shown to possess both follicle-stimulating and luteinizing properties, the council, 1950, reported that "no preparation of this material" had been accepted. Biologists and medical men (P. E. Smith, 1938; Jailer and Leathem, 1940; Leathem and Abarbanel, 1943) have also reported formation, following the use of pituitary extracts (equine) in mice, monkeys, humans, of antihormones which, by antagonizing the patient's available supply, add a further barrier to his fertility.

The disappointment that followed clinical trial of gonadotrophins in various hypogonadal states in both sexes followed also loss of the early hope that androgens and estrogens would prove a specific remedy for various causes of infertility. The former belief that the gonads are an exclusive source of sex-specific steroids was shaken by the discovery that males and females alike produce both androgens and estrogens; that tissues other than the gonads (adrenal, placenta, perhaps others) are also a source of such substances; that these hormones are not sex specific but organ specific, exerting their characteristic effects on parallel tissues in both sexes (accessory sex organs, genital tract, skin, skeleton). Perhaps the greatest barrier to their rational use is realization that differences in response to hormones are governed not by dosage alone, by the character of the numerous synthetic substitutes now available, but also by the target organ's competence to respond. A further barrier to their use as substitutes for presumptive deficiencies has been absence of dependable ways of measuring estrogen and progesterone produced in the body. It should be recognized that the use of hormonal stimulants although disappointing to date and premature because not based on the needed degree of fundamental knowledge has nevertheless aided in carrying hormonal research to a deeper level. It has focused attention on the intermediary metabolic mechanisms that will explain function, and confirm or disprove such hypotheses as that hormones exert their effects as accelerators of enzyme systems.

Contradictory as the concept "inherited sterility" may seem, it is known that such *genetic factors* as inherited structural defects in reproductive organs are responsible for infertility in domestic animals, chiefly cattle and sheep, but also some species of cats, canaries, mice. Inherited sterility in plants and mice, resulting from irradiation, became more than a laboratory curiosity with initiation of studies in Nagasaki and Hiroshima by the joint commission for the investigation of the effects of the atomic bomb, in association with experimental work in biology laboratories in this country with grants from the National Academy of Sciences under contract with the Atomic Energy Commission. Among immediate reversible effects, the commission noted, 1949, that ionizing radiations from the bombs caused reduction in spermatozoa and, in those closest to the center of explosion, profound destructive changes in the testes, evident so early as the fourth day with "almost complete loss of the germinal epithelium". The ovaries appeared more resistant; the number of abortions, however, appeared to be directly related to proximity to the center of explosion. Citing, 1950, experimental work on inherited effects of radiation upon fertility, George D. Snell (referring to semisterility resulting from irradiation in six strains of mice bred since 1933, and Paula Hertwig's work in Germany since 1935) noted that mice irradiated with 800 roentgen-units showed cessation of spermatogenesis and were sterile for the next nineteen weeks. Although sperm already mature appeared normal and motile, genetic damage was evident in offspring of irradiated males mated to normal females, the litters being smaller and about half the offspring semisterile. Since H. J. Muller showed, in 1927, that exposing fruit flies to X radiation increased the rate of chromosome mutations among offspring, this tool has widened the field of genetic research. While there is general agreement that penetrating radiation, demonstrated to increase the mutation rate in animals and plants, affects the mutation rate in man also, the quantitative rate has not been established. This point, which the commission's studies aim to clarify by data accumulated on three generations on the Japanese islands, illustrates the deeper biological levels to which research touching reproduction extends.

In addition to the above-mentioned physiological variables (age, nutritional elements, hormones, genetic factors as yet little explored), considered to influence fertility in men and women more or less indirectly, more specific causes of infertility, also applicable to both sexes, include: barriers (caused by congenital defects, by infections, whether localized in the genital tract or systemic) to transport of sex cells to the site of fertilization; inadequate development of the gonads (perhaps congenital, perhaps related to some failure in adolescent assumption of function) or of the accessory organs (hypoplasia of the uterus). These obvious physiological and developmental phenomena are naturally more often discussed in the clinical literature than are more remote biological problems fundamentally affecting fertility, as origin of the primary sex cells; factors (genetic, embryonic) responsible for differentiating the potentially bisexual embryo into male or female with its appropriate genital tract; physiological factors involved in production and maturation of sex cells; the finer structure, the chemistry and metabolism of sex cells in relation to their maturation, their transport to the site of fertilization and their role in it.

While fundamental logic would dictate discussion of these problems without sex division, the partial and limited nature of investigative approaches accounts for the expedient of dealing fractionally with processes that are biologically indivisible.

## BIOLOGICAL ASPECTS OF MALE INFERTILITY

One reason why study of male reproductive physiology has lagged behind study of female may be, Hartman suggested, 1952, because barren marriages were so long attributed only to female sterility. So lately as 1949 Rock described the physiology of the male tract as "lamentably obscure". Assessment of male fertility is based largely on analysis of semen with emphasis on the number, morphology, motility of spermatozoa, according to prevalent arbitrary standards of the normal. While Moench, 1944, emphasized the proportion of morphologically abnormal forms found in a sample of semen and Farris emphasized the significance of the total number of actively motile sperm, others (R. S. Hotchkiss, J. MacLeod, A. I. Weisman, L. Michelson) considered the composite picture the best available guide until controlled investigations provide, for assessing the significance of each factor, a more dependable basis than clinical observations from veterinary and human medicine. Dissatisfaction with present standards has been variously referred to facile transfer of criteria from animals to man, to insufficient studies of infertile men and of the normal range (MacLeod, 1949) as seen in men of known fertility.

As to number: although sixty million sperm per cc is widely accepted as a requisite minimum, M. H. Jackson and Clare Harvey, 1948, reported fertility with less than twenty million; L. and R. P. Michelson, 1951, noted at least five pregnancies resulting from sperm under one million and two resulting from less than a half million; MacLeod, finding among a thousand fertile men numerous cases of low sperm that produced pregnancies, suggested considering thirty million sperm per cc the low limit of the normal. More significant than number, according to M. C. Chang, 1946, is concentration of sperm. Testing equal numbers of rabbit sperm in three degrees of dilution, he found that the least diluted produced approximately ten times as many pregnancies as the others, a finding confirmed, 1948, by C. W. Emmons and G. I. M. Swyer.

After Williams and Savage, 1925, correlated decreased fertility in domestic animals with number of morphologically abnormal sperm, Moench made similar correlations in man, beginning with his 1931 report that when abnormal sperm heads exceed eighteen to twenty-five per cent of the total normal fertility is impaired, and that at twenty-five per cent clinical sterility appears. MacLeod's 1950 comparison of 1,000 fertile with 800 infertile men revealed, however, that thirty-nine per cent of 874 of the fertile group exhibited more than twenty per cent abnormal forms, three per cent over fifty per cent abnormal forms. On the basis of rabbit tests, Chang concluded, 1946, that morphologically normal sperm may be physiologically abnormal. Opinion has been divided as to whether abnormal forms are a result of defective spermatogenesis, imperfect maturation, or whether they are degenerated forms of normal, mature sperm. In cytological studies of human testes, Engle traced the origin of abnormal cells to aberrant cell divisions in the primary and secondary spermatocytes. The functional significance of some parts of the sperm cell is not fully understood and the metabolic events associated with the well-known stepwise cell divisions that transform the primary spermatocyte to a mature spermatozoon are unknown. Both problems are under investigation. The difficulty in getting clear photographs of head and body because of the opacity of human sperm has as yet made it impossible to determine whether or not certain details (reported in various studies, 1941–1952) are artefacts, whether they serve any purpose in fertilization. First reports of electron-microscopic studies of mature ram spermatozoa (J. T. Randall and M. G. Friedlander, 1950) indicated "complexity . . . much greater than has often been supposed"; these studies of ram sperm aim at eventual correlation of structure and metabolism. Reports were offered, 1952, on the headcap and acrosome of spermatids (rodent, ram, bull, man) and on changes occurring with maturation by Yves Clermont on the basis of histochemical staining reactions. Commenting on lack of knowledge of reasons for abnormal patterns of germinal epithelium sometimes observed in apparently healthy men, Hotchkiss, 1949, considered it increasingly "evident that the quality of spermatozoa is determined in the germinal epithelium". He suggested studies of prepuberal and adolescent testes; increased attention to indirect factors influencing testicular function, among them intermediary metabolism of steroid hormones (especially in the liver), subclinical testicular inflammation, the "formidable problem" of the relation of the glands of internal secretion to the testis.

Farris, 1949, considered sperm motility the best index of fertility in man; Moench considered it no criterion; MacLeod, while considering motility alone no criterion, found poor motility associated with low count in 800 infertile men compared with the 1,000 fertile men of his study. Chang found motility decreased with fertilizing capacity in rabbit suspensions containing lower sperm concentration. Animal experiments do not support assumptions that motility is synonymous with fertilizing capacity, that spermatozoa motile in the semen remain so up to their arrival at the site of fertilization in the upper female tract (points that cannot be tested in man since the only test of fertilizing capacity is demonstrated pregnancy): S. A. Asdell and G. W. Salisbury, 1941, found that in the rabbit fertilizing capacity lasted from eight to ten days while motility lasted from fourteen to thirty-eight days; they and others (Walton, Chang) reported that immotile sperm (rabbit) could retain capacity to fertilize ova while some motile sperm lacked capacity to do so.

Search for sources of energy for sperm motility and the metabolic mechanisms that release it has led animal husbandry workers to attempt correlations of number, motility, fertilizing capacity with sperm metabolism and so to use swifter chemical methods (glycolysis, fructolysis) for assessing fertilizing capacity of animal semen. While these recent advances result from extensive studies of the last decade aimed at developing media to preserve the fertilizing capacity of stored sperm for artificial insemination of cattle, they were made possible by fundamental investigations over the preceding twenty years on metabolism of spermatozoa of lower forms and within the last decade of humans. Following a succession of earlier investigators (Walton, Hammond and Asdell, 1928; Baker, 1930; Ivanov, 1931; Redenz, 1933, among others) who attempted to determine the relative role of respiration and glycolysis in motility of sperm, (of rabbit, dog, bull, boar), MacLeod in this country began, 1939, a study of the metabolism of human spermatozoa. He concluded for isolated human sperm, as the earlier workers had for those of lower species, that most of the energy for motility is obtained from anaerobic glycolysis or fermentative breakdown of some seminal sugar. This "reducing sugar of semen" at identification of which research has been aimed since 1928 was shown, 1945, to be fructose by Mann, who isolated it from the semen of many mammals, including man, and crystallized it. This occurrence of "a high concentration of a fermentable sugar which can be, and is, utilized by human spermatozoa for the purpose of obtaining energy for motility" was characterized by MacLeod, 1952, as "the first obvious functional relationship of a chemical substance in semen". Mann reported that this sugar was metabolized by sperm both aerobically and anaerobically. By 1951 fructose had been identified in the semen of the ram, bull, rabbit, boar, stallion, goat, guinea pig, rat, mouse, hamster, opossum and man, chiefly in seminal vesicles but also, in some species, in the prostate gland; at the site of origin (testis, epididymis) where sperm are immotile, fructose is absent; motility is at its height when sperm come in contact with accessory organs containing fructose. In poor semen fructolysis is low. While, according to Mann, "information as to how male accessory glands generate this rather unusual sugar" is still lacking, available evidence "points strongly" to a metabolic mechanism whereby blood glucose is converted into seminal fructose with glycogen and phosphohexoses functioning as intermediary compounds. He considered fructose a measure of the functional ability of the accessory glands.

A functional role has been sought by a few investigators for an increasing number of chemical substances (amino acids, carbohydrates, various enzymes, ascorbic acid) which have been identified, since 1933, in seminal fluid from various animals and man. MacLeod, 1952, pointed out that human seminal fluid is chemically far too complex to be merely a medium for transport of spermatozoa from the male genital tract to the female, the only function that can be assigned to it on the basis of present evidence. More extensive research on the chemistry of seminal fluid has been repeatedly described as requisite for understanding not only the metabolism of spermatozoa in whole semen but also the role of the accessory organs (epididymis, vas deferens, seminal vesicle, prostate) about the structure and function of which much remains to be learned.

The longevity of sperm in the epididymis when both ends of this organ are tied off, demonstrated in various species (rabbit, Asdell, 1941; rat, Shettles, 1940; horse, Phillips, 1941), confirmed the belief that it functions as a storage place but apart from this function the participation of the epididymis in the nutrition and metabolism of spermatozoa is "far from clear" (Mann, 1949). Several workers have shown that epididymal sperm although not showing active motility have produced conception. The demonstration that spermatozoa from the end of this organ have higher fertilizing capacity than those from the beginning led to the suggestion by Charles A. Zittle and G. Henle, 1942, that part of the ripening process spermatozoa are believed to undergo in the epididymis may involve a change in function of their enzyme systems, an hypothesis explored by other workers also: John F. Lasley and Ralph Bogart, 1944, attributed changes in viability of sperm as they proceed along the epididymis and other parts of the male tract to changes within spermatozoa rather than to changes in their chemical environment; Lardy, Hansen and Phillips, 1945, considered increases in endogenous respiration of epididymal sperm after storage an aspect of their maturation; Lardy and certain of his associates have published further reports (1946–1952) in a long-term study comparing ejaculated with epididymal bull sperm. Present knowledge of the epididymis was described by MacLeod, 1952, as "rudimentary" although its role in the transport and maturation of spermatozoa bears "singular significance to problems of infertility".

The function of the prostate, according to Hotchkiss, 1944, "other than that of affording a vehicle for spermatozoa", is not known. Its "only certainly known function", according to Charles B. Huggins, 1945 (after twelve years' work on the chemistry of prostatic secretions), is "thinning and increase in the volume of semen".

These and other developing studies, including his own, led Chang to observe, "any disturbance of the accessory glands may affect the fertility of a male though clinical data on this point are still scarce"; M. Edward Davis and W. W. McCune considered, 1950, that the high incidence of accessory organ disease in man has had little attention in attempts to determine causes of clinical infertility.

While artificial insemination with either husband's or donor's semen (1941 estimates suggested that 9,000 live children had been thus produced in the United States up to 1940) has been represented as lessening the urgency of fundamental research on sperm, the problems (medical, genetic, legal, psychological, religious) associated with artificial insemination and the obvious logic of dealing more physiologically with infertility have inclined medical men to join biologists in urging more research on the biology of spermatozoa, and the individual chemical components of semen. Work in this direction was, 1951, not only limited but also often confusing, because of failure to distinguish sperm enzymes from enzymes of accessory organ secretions. The developing research of the last decade on accessory organ secretions has suggested not only possible new factors influencing male infertility but also a possible link between the little studied generative and the more actively studied secretory functions of the testes. By 1937 medical trials had demonstrated that androgens temporarily depressed spermatogenesis with resulting testicular damage, including atrophy of germinal elements, but, after a few months, functional recovery occurs in the germinal epithelium and spermatogenesis is resumed. Recent reports (Heller, Nelson, Maddock and associates, 1950, 1952; Heckel and associates, 1951, 1952) indicate that in some cases the "rebound" is associated with a higher sperm count than at the pretreatment level. A central problem appears to involve the testicular regulator of pituitary gonadotrophins. The testis, like most endocrine glands, depends for its functional integrity upon the trophic hormones but it is not clear whether the level of pituitary gonadotrophins is regulated by testosterone or some other testicular secretion. An inhibiting role has been sought for estrogen, isolation of which (estradiol) from human testes was reported, 1951, by Goldzieher and Roberts; whether the source of the estrogen is the Sertoli cells (Scott, 1949), the Leydig cells (Nelson, 1952) or the seminiferous tubules (McCullagh and Schaffenburg, 1952) is not settled. A nonsteroidal water-soluble substance, "inhibin" (originating in the seminiferous tubules), has been proposed as inhibitor of gonadotrophin levels. Another hypothesis proposes for an inhibiting hormone at most only a supplemental role in regulating the pituitary and considers the levels of gonadotrophic hormones in the body fluids dependent upon whether or not the testes utilize the gonadotrophic hormones (Nelson, 1952).

Since Charles W. Hooker, 1944, characterized the evidence for the interstitial cells of Leydig as the site of androgen production "after forty years of study" as "for the most part unsatisfactory", further indirect evidence for this view has accumulated on additional species: Wislocki, 1949, using histochemical methods, concluded from studies of deer testes at the two extremes of the yearly breeding season, "steroid hormones are formed in the interstitial tissues"; S. Kumaran and C. W. Turner, 1949, concluded from a polarized light study that the site of hormone secretion in the white Plymouth Rock is the interstitial tissue.   Hooker, 1948, on the basis of observations of tubular and interstitial tissue as androgen levels rose (in the bull) from early to adult life, could see no changes in the tubules; the greatest rise in androgens occurred on vacuolation (regarded as evidence of secretion in some species) of the Leydig cells.   Nelson and Heller, however, consider vacuolation of Leydig cells in man indicative of degenerative rather than secretory activity.   James B. Hamilton and William Montagna, from histological studies of human testes, concluded, 1951, "the problem of the origin of testicular hormones is not settled"; in their view histological criteria used for demonstrating testicular hormones in other animals are not applicable to the human testes; "if they are, then the presumptive sites of hormones should include . . . the seminiferous epithelium as well as the cells of Leydig".   Sniffen considered, 1952, that "interstitial cells appear to hold the key position in testicular function for the tubules are never normal if the Leydig cells are abnormal or absent".   Simpson, Li and Evans reported, however, 1951, that homogeneous preparations of FSH injected into hypophysectomized rats resulted in spermatogenesis without appearance of Leydig cells.

## FEMALE INFERTILITY — ILLUSTRATIVE BIOLOGICAL PROBLEMS

Detailed comparative studies in the present century establishing the common pattern of mammalian ovarian function in the estrous cycle of lower animals and the menstrual cycle of primates have radically altered concepts of the human ovarian cycle, inducing a marked physiological (as opposed to dominantly surgical) trend in obstetric and gynecologic practice.   Much of this work, however, has been focused on the hormones of the ovary.

Referring to the greater attention during the preceding thirty years to secretory than to generative functions of the ovary, Edgar Allen dryly observed, 1942, "however, the production of eggs is still the primary function of the ovaries".   In spite of almost a century of research, biological opinion is still divided as to how eggs are first formed in the embryonic ovary and as to whether the adult ovary is capable of continuing to form ova as testes continue to form sperm after puberty, or whether the ripened ova discharged once a month during woman's reproductive span are drawn from the thousands of ova known to be present at birth.  Whether during embryonic development primordial germ cells originating in the segmenting egg remain unmodified and migrate into the developing gonad (theory of the continuity of germ plasm) or whether they arise locally (and from which tissues and at which stage) remain controversial questions. Newton B. Everett, 1945, found "as great diversity of opinion regarding the postnatal formation of germ cells as exists regarding their embryonic formation".  Other aspects of ovarian embryology, of adult intraovarian structure (vascular, neural) and function remain to be clarified.  Hisaw emphasized, 1947, the need of going behind the results of the last thirty years' research on the response of the Graafian follicle to pituitary gonadotrophins in order to discover how the follicle becomes able to respond to them; he outlined as a working hypothesis derived from his own and other work since 1941 four stages of follicular development each with its possibly characteristic organizing force. Although maturation division of the ovum has been correlated with secretion of liquor folliculi in many mammals, M. C. Chang and Gregory Pincus, 1951, found "not easy to answer" the question whether the maturation of ova is induced directly by the pituitary hormone, as claimed by some investigators, or indirectly by growth of follicle and by changes in the liquor folliculi.  The actual dynamics of follicle rupture (directly visualized in the anesthetized rabbit by Hammond so long ago as 1927, subsequently in other species) are still to be conclusively determined in woman.  Although present opinion appears to favor the view that follicular rupture is caused by accumulation of follicular fluid, the origin of the fluid, as the mechanism of rupture, is still to be explained.  J. H. Burr and J. I. Davies, 1951, suggested, in a study of ovulation (rabbit), that the fluid is in part formed by capillary wreaths and in part forced into follicles as a result of ovarian swelling (following increased permeability of capillaries and veins, in which lymphatics play a part).  This is one of a few developing studies (illustrated by the long-term programs of Bartelmez, 1943–51; Reynolds, 1946–51) which after two decades of concentration on the uterine vasculature have recently directed investi-

gative attention to vascular events in the ovary. Reynolds's redis-
covery (1947–50) of the spiral arteries of the ovary (rabbit, woman)
led to a comparison of blood vessels in human ovaries taken from different reproductive stages suggesting that the ovary's main blood
vessels may be undeveloped before and after adult reproductive life
but that as cyclic ovarian function is established at adolescence the
intrinsic blood supply grows in response to increasing amounts of
estrogens; primary or abortive ovarian failure during adolescence,
he suggested, might plausibly be explained as "failure of ovarian
vasculature to grow". Questions concerning the origin of the ovarian
steroids include which follicular tissue elaborates the ovarian steroids,
the theca interna, as the majority believe, or the granulosa cells; the
question whether the lutein cells come from the theca interna (Dempsey and Bassett, 1943; McKay and Robinson, 1947), whether they
result from proliferation of the granulosa (a widely held view), or
whether they are derived from both (Corner, Evans). Other evidences of increasing interest in the effect of intraovarian estrogens
on ovarian structure and function (rather than on such target tissues
as the vagina, cervix, uterus, tubes) include: Hisaw's suggestion that
estrogen might serve, in the second stage of follicular development,
as the intrinsic organizer sensitizing the follicle to pituitary gonadotrophins; S. H. Sturgis's monkey study (completed 1949) indicating
that the whole process of follicular atresia (the rate of which had been
unknown) takes five weeks and may augment production of estrogen
at a time when the hormone is necessary for ovulation and for lutein-
ization of the one follicle that is destined to rupture. However, "the
mechanism of selection of the particular ovum or ova destined to be
shed is still", according to J. D. Boyd and W. J. Hamilton, 1952, "a
matter for speculation". Slowly increasing investigative interest in
intraovarian structures reflects medical dissatisfaction with present
indirect methods of assessing ovarian function in infertile women.
Taylor, who began, 1949, a long-term study of the quantitative interrelation of various morphological elements of the ovary, observed,
1950, "the morphologic basis of ovarian dysfunction is, with the exception of extreme degrees of atrophy, not understood, and scarcely
explored".

In clinical infertility, the first requisite is to determine whether a functioning ovary is producing ova; the second to determine when ovulation occurs, for the limited life of spermatozoa and ovum make conception impossible if fertilization does not occur within from twelve to twenty-four hours after ovulation. For biologists, the time of ovulation is important not only for dating and correlating events at various levels of the female reproductive tract with ovarian changes but also for reckoning the earliest stages of embryonic development and correlating initial changes (cytological, cytochemical, vascular, hormonal) in the pregnancy cycle. For the breeder of domestic animals who in estrus has some indication of ovulation, the time of ovulation of domestic animals (now known for most species) is of great economic importance, since, as in the infertile woman, it determines the time for normal mating or artificial insemination.

The conclusion of Allen and his associates, 1928, from recovery of ova in the fallopian tubes, that ovulation occurs *approximately* on the fourteenth day of a twenty-eight-day cycle has been confirmed in monkeys and women by a number of indirect methods and by a limited number of inspections of ovaries during surgery. Unfortunately, expanding experimental and clinical attempts to refine all tests of ovulation and so to correlate several of them as to narrow the range of difference have only emphasized individual variation in the length of the ovarian cycle among normal women, in the time within the cycle when normal women may ovulate. Hartman, 1944, found no answer to the question whether the individual monkey or woman tends to ovulate on about the same day of the cycle in successive cycles. There exists as yet no specific method of determining the exact time of ovulation and it is now recognized that many tests widely employed throughout the last fifteen years and the present indicate not the release of a ripe ovum but physiological changes associated with ovulation. Endometrial biopsy, determination of pregnanediol (metabolite of progesterone), demonstration of urinary gonadotrophins, of changes in cervical mucus are employed in diagnosing infertility as circumstantial evidence that the follicle converted to a corpus luteum has actually released a live ovum. But "there are as yet no criteria for recognizing a healthy, viable egg — one that may be fertilized and develop normally", even in experimental studies that have been made on a few mammalian species (R. J. Blandau, 1954).

Although the vaginal smear proved immensely useful in the hands of anatomists during the twenties as a tool for establishing time of ovulation and length of the ovarian cycle for a number of animals, it has not proved adaptable to routine clinical use in infertility attributed to ovarian dysfunction. It proved useful in G. N. Papanicolaou's studies of women, and in Inés L. C. de Allende's detailed studies, 1941–50, of vaginal cytology of monkeys and women in connection with ovarian function and pathology. Much, however, remains to be learned concerning the cytology, the embryology (controversial), and the metabolism of the vagina. The vaginal acidity that is known to be unfavorable to sperm motility is attributed to lactic acid from the breakdown of glycogen of unknown origin present in vaginal epithelium throughout all stages of the menstrual cycle.

The midcycle changes in quantity and quality of cervical mucus, first noted in 1855, correlated with ovulation (1933) by Sequy and Simmonet (by direct inspection of ovaries during surgery), confirmed in monkeys and in women (Shettles, Lamar, Delfs, 1940, 1943), have stimulated investigations of the chemical and physical properties of cervical mucus, and have been interpreted as a sign of ovulation. In studies, between 1942 and 1952, of the chemistry of cervical mucus, Pommerenke and his associates (Breckenridge, Viergiver, Pederson) reported that carbohydrates (glucose, maltose, glycogen) capable of being used by sperm are present in cervical mucus in all phases of the menstrual cycle, as is also an enzyme, diastase, capable of breaking down glycogen to the more readily utilizable glucose and maltose. Up to 1951, however, "the source of glycogen in cervical mucus remained a question". Other identified substances of unknown function included seventeen amino acids, which were found (Pommerenke, 1950) to decrease at midcycle, and lipids. A complex neutral mucopolysaccharide associated with the viscosity that makes mucus less penetrable to sperm was found to decline at ovulation when the mucus becomes more fluid. In a 1945 report to the Royal Society of Medicine on his studies of the physical properties of human cervical mucus, A. F. Clift suggested, on the theory that human cervical mucus is not a truly viscous fluid, the possibility of improving results of artificial insemination by adding to the semen a substance (as egg-white) having rheological properties resembling those of midcycle cervical secretions. Shettles, working on the chemistry of cervical mucus, observed, 1949, of infertility in which no defect could be established in either partner, "an incompatibility between the semen and cervical mucus in some of these couples can be proved". While some physicians attribute to cervical infections up to seventy per cent of the infertility in their practice, controlled studies of cervical infections are few. Basic studies of the cervix include a few comparative studies (Blandau, 1939–1945; Belonoschkin in Stockholm, 1946) of the cervix of various animals in relation to the physiology of insemination, and chemical, physical, bacteriological, histological, cytochemical studies, most of them initiated since 1943, emphasizing Corner's reference, 1949, to the significance of the cervix uteri through which sperm cells must travel inward for conception and through which the infant must pass outward at birth.

Corner's reference, however, was not to the cervix uteri alone but to the whole uterine lining, the endometrium, subject, during the past twenty-five years, of extensive cytological research; much of this has concerned endometrial changes in response to withdrawal and administration of ovarian steroids, and use of these changes to follow the cyclic changes of the hidden ovary in lower animals (estrous cycle) and in primates including woman (menstrual cycle). As a result of these studies, endometrial biopsy became a major diagnostic dependence in assessing female infertility, the progestational (secretory) changes in the endometrium characteristic of its response to the luteal hormone (progesterone) being considered circumstantial evidence that a functioning corpus luteum has developed from a follicle which has released a viable ovum. While endometrial biopsy remains a major diagnostic aid, it is now recognized that cytological changes occurring in the part of the endometrium from which the specimen is taken may not extend to the whole endometrium; that follicles that have lost their ova may nevertheless produce progesterone; and that there is no way, unless pregnancy results, of knowing whether an ovum is viable at the time of follicular discharge. Urinary levels of pregnanediol are not, as numerous students have pointed out, a dependable "test" of ovulation since abnormal urinary levels may signify dysfunction not specific to the ovary but possibly referable to any one of the four organs (ovary, endometrium, liver, kidney) concerned in secretion, metabolic utilization, destruction, excretion of progesterone.  Study of the metabolism of progesterone has, since 1945, been accelerated by new tools permitting investigation in the living animal, as development of an apparently specific method for determining blood levels of progesterone (C. W. Hooker and T. R. Forbes, 1947), use of radioprogesterone in mice and rats (Byron Riegel, W. L. Hartop, Jr., G. W. Kittinger, 1950).

Although the changes occurring in the endometrium under the influence of ovarian hormones released with follicular maturation and ovulation have for some time been believed to represent preparation for implantation and for nourishing the fertilized ovum, this has not been directly demonstrated.  A functional role in this connection has been sought for only a few substances identified in the endometrial lining; and little has been done, until recent years, with earlier suggestive findings concerning enzymes identified in the endometrium in association with the rise of estrogens.  Recent studies, 1944–1952, on hormone-induced changes in alkaline phosphatase content of the uterus, cervix, vagina, of the rat, mouse, recent comparisons of the concentration and distribution of this enzyme in women during different stages of the reproductive cycle represent the beginnings of the more intensive search for the intermediary metabolic processes by which hormones exert their effects, particularly the mechanisms involved in synthesis and breakdown of glycogen.  Glycogen deposition has been known to increase in the epithelial lining of the uterus, and also in the cervix and vagina under the influence of estrogen.  Zondek, who, in 1940, noted the increased concentrations of glycogen after ovulation, in 1947 reported (with Hestrin) higher concentrations of the enzyme phosphorylase which has been associated with increased deposition of glycogen.  Increased concentrations of diastase, E. C. Hughes suggested, 1945, may be concerned in breakdown of glycogen to simpler sugars more readily utilized by the fertilized ovum.  The biochemical significance of the high concentration of alkaline phosphatase reported in the endometrium and correlated with the presence of estrogen in rat and mouse experiments (W. B. Atkinson, 1950, Bing, 1950) at the time when glycogen concentrations also increase remains "as yet undetermined" (Pommerenke and Breckenridge, 1952).  Evidence from other tissues (chiefly liver) has led some investigators to suggest that alkaline phosphatase may be predominantly responsible for degradation (hydrolysis of various phosphate esters) rather than synthesis. On resolution of this point, not yet achieved, depends the validity of other hypotheses concerning the relevance of alkaline phosphatase to normal reproductive functions. Meanwhile clinical correlations suggest a higher incidence of spontaneous abortion and sterility when glycogen is absent in the luteal phase, or when it is present in other phases of the cycle (Zondek, 1942; Hughes, 1945). Comparing biopsy specimens from the endometria of sixty-eight normal women and of 324 women with a history of infertility, E. C. Hughes, W. A. Van Ness and C. W. Lloyd, 1950, found evidence of abnormal glycogenesis (glycogen and alkaline phosphatase in smaller amounts, in unusual distribution) in fifty-eight per cent of the abnormal group.

In spite of continued attempts to refine and correlate methods for detecting ovulation, it is recognized (McLane, 1949; Palmer, 1949) that vaginal smears, endometrial biopsies, hormone assays do not consistently agree and patients that may give evidence of ovulation by one or more of these "tests" may still not become pregnant. Probably, according to Rock, 1949, because of the number of independent biological factors involved in the whole process of ovulation, "no sign of the exact moment of ovular release will ever be recognizable".

In similarly implied criticism of the unbiologic nature of many of the hypotheses invoked during the past twenty years to explain menstruation, Bartelmez described, 1951, the rhythm in female primates as "not a rhythm of gears and levers, but that of a living pulsating organism attuned to various influences, both internal and external". He noted that in the human species as in the rhesus the normal range of the menstrual cycle is from three to five weeks rather than the generally assumed twenty-eight days; that cycles of the same length may differ radically; that variability is inevitable in a cycle controlled by a system of balanced endocrine forces, fluctuation in any one of which may change the whole configuration; that the target organs and different areas of the same organ may vary greatly in susceptibility. In a report on 197 selected specimens from rhesus monkeys, Bartelmez emphasized the notable lack of comparable normal human material.

The relation of menstruation to ovulation and the significance of menstrual disorders in infertility are not yet clear in spite of thirty years of cytological and endocrine research. Although regression of the endometrium on withdrawal of the ovarian hormones is found in all mammals in which the ovarian cycle has been studied, menstrual bleeding occurs only in some, notably the rhesus and woman. Just why the sudden drop in concentration of ovarian hormones in the blood at the end of the ovarian cycle causes the blood vessels in one particular organ, the uterus, to break down with ensuing hemorrhage remains "one of the outstanding mysteries of human biology" (Corner, 1949). Opinion remains divided as to whether hemorrhage can be explained as a purely local, vascular, mechanical event related to changes in the coiled arteries that invest the superficial layer of the endometrium, a conclusion suggested by J. E. Markee's direct investigation in the living monkey and histological study of human material. With regard to the role ascribed to these changes as with regard to the question whether withdrawal of estrogen or of progesterone causes menstruation, Hisaw reported to the 1952 meeting of the American Association of Anatomists experiments in which daily administration of estradiol or progesterone or both to castrated monkeys for periods ranging from a hundred days to a year had resulted in morphological uterine changes varying widely but demonstrating that all the animals were capable of menstruation. His conclusion was that menstruation is a stromal phenomenon (that is, occurring in the connective tissues of the uterus and not merely in its epithelial layer) which occurs on withdrawal of a supporting stimulus (estrogen or progesterone) and which will take place regardless of presence or absence of uterine glands, surface epithelium, coiled arterioles. More investigative attention to neural factors that may trigger anterior pituitary gonadotrophins in menstruation has been urged by various biologists (among them Asdell, Hisaw, Zuckerman). Investigations of such neural factors (focused on the hypothalamus) have been reported by G. W. Harris, 1948–1952, from Britain, by D. M. Hume, 1950, from Harvard; others. So recently as 1950, Asdell observed of research on menstruation, "we are back to our position of ignorance". That menstruation can occur without ovulation is, finally, well established in women. Hypotheses advanced to explain anovulatory menstruation include the suggestion that gonadotrophic function of the anterior pituitary may be depressed to levels not sufficient to induce actual release of the ovum from the follicle but sufficient to stimulate secretion of the hormones necessary to build up the endometrium which, on hormonal withdrawal, undergoes the characteristic breakdown and hemorrhage.

The mechanisms (physical, metabolic, hormonal, neural) by which the released ovum gains access to the fallopian tubes are not yet clear. From his experiments revealing transport of the ovum through an abdominal "window" in the living rabbit (later in monkeys) and from roentgenographic study of one human subject, A. Westman of the Stockholm women's clinic suggested, 1950, that, while movements of both ovary and the mouth of the tube play a part in drawing closer together at ovulation, increased motility of the tubal musculature plays a dominant part in sucking in the ovum. That tubal function is under neural as well as hormonal control was also suggested by his observations (rabbits, women) after transection of presacral nerves. Deviations from the ideally wide, flaring end (ampulla) of the tube were described by Rock, 1949, as possibly "very significant to fertility". Occlusion of the hair-thin lumen of the tube is a commonly mentioned barrier to the meeting of spermatozoa and ovum at the site of fertilization in the upper tube. Little is known, however, concerning the histology and histochemistry of the tubal lining. C. L. Buxton, 1950, commenting on the question (raised by a patient who possessed functioning ovaries but no tubes) whether ova are fertilizable if not subjected to the chemical environment of the tubes, observed that the whole physiology of the tubes is as important in producing pregnancy as their patency. Referring to as yet unpublished studies suggesting that tubal fluid in the rabbit favorably conditions the spermatozoa for activation of eggs, Rock, 1949, recommended analyses in a number of species and in women to determine the role of tubal fluids in fertilization. Studies (D. W. Bishop, 1953) of the hydrogen-ion concentration in tubes were designed to check a suggestion that this is responsible for dispersion of cumulus cells surrounding the ovum.

Although the time required for spermatozoa to move through the female tract to the site of fertilization in the upper tube has been estimated for a number of species, human findings in this regard are few: R. L. Brown, 1944, estimated twenty-seven minutes to traverse the human uterus, forty-two minutes to traverse the tubes; to M. Edward Davis was attributed, 1950, an estimate of three hours for the whole journey. The degree to which sperm motility, and/or structural, functional, metabolic factors of the female reproductive tract influence the time of sperm transport is not known. "In general, the mechanism of sperm transportation is still not clear", according to Chang and Pincus, 1951. Little is known, in their view, of the fertilizing power of spermatozoa recovered from different parts of the female tract, although observations have been made concerning the motility and longevity of sperm found at different levels of the tract or subjected to *in vitro* incubation in vaginal fluids (the poorest medium for motility), in cervical, tubal, uterine, follicular, peritoneal extracts. Boris B. Rubenstein and his associates, 1951, found that sperm introduced in fifty-one women about to undergo surgery migrated through the cervix, fundus, fallopian tubes within thirty minutes after introduction into the vagina at any time during the menstrual cycle and retained motility in any part of the female tract for at least fifty hours. In view of reports of longer sperm survival, they recommended further study.

Delay in fertilization resulting in aging of either sperm or ova may affect fertility at later stages in the reproductive cycle. Witschi's 1952 report that the aging ova of the frog resisted penetration by sperm or, if penetrated, resulted in developmental defects in offspring, confirmed earlier studies. Blandau considered it conclusively demonstrated, 1954, that, in both rat and guinea pig, aging of spermatozoa in the female reproductive tract may affect ability to penetrate the egg, but whether this applies to other animals is "still to be determined". Aging eggs of these species resisted penetration by sperm and even when greatly overripe rat eggs could be penetrated "various abnormalities of development may result which are not compatible with continued growth". Whether only moderate overripeness of mammalian eggs also leads to developmental defects in the fetal and postnatal period is "as yet unexplored".

## BIOLOGICAL AND BIOCHEMICAL FACTORS IN FERTILIZATION

Referring to the finding that in a number of species (rat, rabbit, ferret, pig, sheep, cow) sperm reach the site of fertilization from five to thirty hours before the ova are liberated, Chang and Pincus suggested, 1951, that to insure fertilization this interval may be needed to effect some physiological change in sperm or to permit accumulation of a large number. How many spermatozoa arrive at the site of fertilization in woman is not known and the function served by all but the one that accomplishes fertilization of the ovum is not fully understood in mammals. An early theory was that the large number of sperm might be required to provide a sufficient amount of some "cumulus-dissolving factor" (presumably an enzyme) to facilitate sperm entry into the ovum by dissolving the follicular mass surrounding ova as they enter the tubes. The *in vitro* demonstration that the proteolytic enzyme, hyaluronidase, liquefies the mucus clot containing cumulus cells surrounding the ova of rats (D. McLean and I. W. Rowlands, 1942) and of mice (E. A. Fekete and F. Duran-Reynals, 1943) led to the suggestion that this is the function of hyaluronidase in fertilization, a theory supported by subsequent demonstration of the enzyme in the testes and sperm of several species (mouse, rat, rabbit, boar, bull, man) but not in species (birds, reptiles) having ova without follicular cell cumuli. The report (I. W. Rowlands, 1944) that addition of hyaluronidase to sperm suspensions greatly decreased the number of spermatozoa required for conception after artificial insemination of rabbits stimulated trial of the enzyme (now commercially available from bulls) in human infertility attributed to low sperm count. Favorable early reports were not, however, confirmed. Chang's report, 1947, that purified hyaluronidase showed no significant effect on the *in vivo* fertilizing capacity of rabbit spermatozoa (he attributed the favorable effects reported by Rowlands to the seminal plasma employed as the source of hyaluronidase) has cast doubt on the specific function envisaged for hyaluronidase, denudation of the egg, attributed by Chang to some tubal factor. Subsequent reports that ova are penetrated by sperm before complete denudation in the rat (S. L. Leonard and his associates, 1946) and rabbit (Austin, 1948) cast further doubt on the necessity of denudation in all species and on the exclusive role of hyaluronidase in this step in fertilization. A role in human infertility is implied in the 1950 autopsy findings (W. H. Perloff and J. H. Nodine) that factors that depressed spermatogenesis in their series (age, anemia, cardiac failure, fever, severe weight loss) depress concentration of this enzyme in spermatogonia and their derivative cells in all stages of maturation. A powerful inhibitor of hyaluronidase, which possessed no ordinary spermicidal action in the amounts used, was reported (A. S. Parkes, 1953) to prevent fertilization when added to rabbit semen before insemination. An antifertility effect of phosphorylated hesperidins orally administered to rats and mice (G. J. Martin and J. M. Beiler, 1947–1952) was also attributed to its inhibitory action on hyaluronidase; the "startling claims of clinical effectiveness" (preliminary report, B. F. Sieve, 1952) of phosphorylated hesperidin given orally to 300 couples over thirty months (in continuous ten-day doses to insure blood saturation), with restoration of fertility by omission of the drug for a forty-eight-hour period, cannot, according to Parkes, be accepted without confirmation.

Concerning the generally unknown mechanism of penetration of sperm into the mammalian ova, Chang and Pincus, 1951, suggested that tubal contraction and ciliary activity may play a part, the former by guiding the angle at which the spermatozoa enter the ovum. Referring to Barker's report, 1948, that the specific glycoprotein of the zona pellucida (the exposed layer of the ovum after denudation) may change under the influence of luteal hormone, Pincus and Chang observed, "the biochemical changes occurring in the zona pellucida before and after denudation of the ova, and after the penetration of spermatozoa, require further study", as do also biochemical reactions of sperm in relation to fertilization. Lardy, 1950, raised the question whether biochemical reactions involved in sperm motility may not also play a part in sperm penetration of the egg, activation of the egg to divide and develop, possibly even in the genetic contribution made by the male.

The development of a coherent theory of fertilization has been, for forty years past, the objective of biologists' experiments on the sperm and ova of marine animals. The earlier view that sperm aggression (suggested by motility) is responsible for penetration of the egg yielded, as a result of experiments with sea urchin gametes during the first decade of the present century, to the concept that sperm are attracted or attached to the egg through an agglutinating substance on or within the egg. Lillie furnished support for this hypothesis in his theory (set forth in *Problems of Fertilization*, 1919) that a protein substance on or within sea urchin eggs, fertilizin, reacts with a sperm receptor. The eggs became infertilizable when fertilizin was washed out, and fertilizable when it was returned. Developing chemical knowledge (especially of enzymes) and methods have made possible amplification and modification of this hypothesis which has continued to stimulate chemical work on fertilization in sea urchins (by John Rünnstrom in Stockholm, in this country by Albert Tyler). Rünnstrom's experiments led to his theory that a polysaccharide in the mature, unfertilized egg serves as a natural inhibitor to further development, a view supported by a 1950 report (Monné and Slautterback) of cytochemical evidence of polysaccharides in the egg cortex and the inhibiting effect (L. V. Heilbrunn and others) of polysaccharides (heparin) on fertilization of invertebrate eggs.

Since little is known of the mechanism underlying mammalian fertilization, adaptation of these chemical and physical theories to mammals would at present, according to Chang and Pincus, 1951, be speculative. In summarizing the accumulated knowledge (chiefly cytological) of the last twenty years on the physiology of fertilization in laboratory animals (mouse, rat, rabbit, guinea pig, cat, ferret, dog), in farm animals, in monkey and in man, Chang and Pincus pointed out that investigative work on the physiology of fertilization in mammals has not yet reached the stage of biochemical study. They emphasized the need of investigating physiology of the fallopian tubes where fertilization occurs, physiology of sperm in the female tract, interrelation between spermatozoa and ova in the tubes, histochemistry of ova before and after penetration of spermatozoa, in short the need of research that will throw light on the degree to which the chemical constitution of sperm and ova, the chemical fluids to which they are subjected under the influence of gonadal and other hormones, condition the ultimate metabolic role of both in fertilization.

## BIOLOGICAL PROBLEMS IN PREGNANCY

Since in most animals thus far studied (mouse, rabbit, guinea pig, pig, cow, monkey) passage of the fertilized ovum through the oviducts to the uterus has required from three to four and a half days, it has been assumed that in woman passage requires between three and four days. Some investigators (Corner, Reynolds) have suggested that the slower rate of migration in the lower part of the tube may be needed to allow time for progesterone to prepare the uterus for implantation and nourishment of the arriving ovum or for tubal fluids to exercise some needed function, acting perhaps not merely as a transport medium but also, as suggested by Hertig, 1950 (on finding a two-cell fertilized ovum in human tubes), "somewhat in the manner of an incubator". On the other hand, the absence of tubal fluid did not appear to interfere with development of fertilized mouse ova removed from the tube and transplanted to the anterior chamber of the eye where they continued to grow, as demonstrated, 1947, by Runner, also by Wislocki, Fawcet and Waldo.

These studies are part of renewed experimental attempts to resolve a long-standing controversy as to whether the activity of the embryo or of the maternal uterine mucosa is dominantly responsible for implantation. One school of thought has attributed implantation to elaboration by the embryo of some specific cytolytic chemical (an enzyme?) and considered the part of the uterus passive; another school has considered the part of the embryo passive, attributing implantation to endometrial sensitivity (induced by progesterone) in response to mechanical forces (trauma) due to growth of the ovum. Wislocki, Fawcet, Waldo, 1947, while attributing the initial hemorrhage accompanying invasion of the endometrium by the ovum to a chemical substance (possibly a cytolytic enzyme) released by the ovum to secure food in this hemorrhagic fluid until connection with the maternal circulation is established by the placenta, concluded that sensitization of the endometrium is also important. Neither is chiefly responsible for implantation: "ovum and uterine mucosa no doubt have mutually supporting roles". Blandau, 1949, in experiments employing inert glass beads of the size and specific gravity of ova to determine whether they induce decidual reactions in the endometrium and implant, and culturing fertilized ova on protein substrates to determine whether they produce a proteolytic enzyme, found a species difference: the endometrial response to trauma occurred in the rat but not the guinea pig; guinea pig ova when cultured elaborated a "proteolytic ferment" but rat ova did not.

Detailed studies of the vascular pattern of the endometrium in this country (Doris H. Phelps, 1946; I. H. Kaiser, 1949; Elizabeth

Ramsey, 1949–50) and in Copenhagen (E. Hasner) have led to the suggestion that the coiled arterioles of the endometrium are important not in menstrual bleeding but in implantation, representing adaptation enabling the endometrium to supply blood rapidly to the placental villi of the invading ovum when it begins to implant. Rock and Hertig deduced from a series of normal human ova, ranging in developmental age from 7.5 to 16.5 days, that implantation in the human occurs during the late sixth or early seventh day of its development. Their finding that all of these normal ova implanted on the posterior wall of the uterus, while four abnormal ova implanted on the anterior wall, raised the questions whether there is a "normal" site of implantation, whether the pathologic ova are attributable to abnormality of ovum or of uterine metabolism. Although a preferred site of implantation has been attributed by some to heavier concentrations of glycogen, adequate evidence for this view has never been offered. Streeter, on the basis of twenty years' work with early embryos of monkeys, suggested that while the site of attachment seemed to be definitely regulated the regulating influences are not known. Failure of the fertilized ovum to implant in its normal site within the body of the uterus may lead to spontaneous loss of the ovum, to surgical termination of the extrauterine pregnancy if it is recognized, to maternal death if it is not. Little agreement exists concerning the factors that influence the fertilized ovum to implant in such abnormal sites as ovary, abdomen, tubes. The fact that the blastocyst normally implants on the endometrium has stimulated controversy as to whether errant endometrial tissue may be a factor in attracting the fertilized ovum to an abnormal site.

Discussion of all possible interruptions of pregnancy goes beyond the limits of this review. Any disease, pathological growth, infection, physiological, or metabolic disorder that afflicts a nonpregnant woman may afflict a pregnant woman, and any one of them may be a direct factor (acting on the reproductive mechanism) or an indirect factor (acting *via* the maternal system) in loss of the products of conception or in termination of pregnancy to save the life of the mother. In a recent ten-year analysis, only 7.2 per cent of forty-four indications for interrupting 280 pregnancies (Kuder and Finn, New York Hospital) were peculiarly obstetric or gynecologic conditions. On the influence of intercurrent disease on pregnancy, investigations since 1947 in this country and England have shown that so long as twenty years before the onset of recognized diabetes fetal mortality and fetal gigantism may occur. The possible relation to infertility of diabetic endocrine imbalance attributed to insulin is suggested by the rise in fertility rate from the two per cent cited (Eastman, 1949) for the preinsulin period (when pregnancy in the diabetic was a "medical curiosity", and when twenty-five per cent of the mothers and fifty per cent of the infants died) to the current 28.6 per cent. Observation that statural as well as genital development is frequently retarded in juvenile diabetics (Priscilla White, 1942), that the offspring of diabetic mothers are often unusually large (adding another hazard to labor) carried an implication that the growth factor of the anterior pituitary may be involved in diabetic infertility. Experimental investigations of diabetes (by B. A. Houssay, C. N. H. Long) and of infertility (by H. H. F. Barns and M. E. Morgans, M. E. Davis and N. W. Fugo) have included recent reports on the possible involvement of the anterior pituitary hormones in premature delivery, abortion, fetal resorption, stillbirth, fetal gigantism in the diabetic dog, rat, rabbit. Referring to the "significantly low" fetal survival rate generally recognized to prevail in diabetic pregnancies, White observed, "the controversial points include an explanation of the mechanism, particularly which of the endocrine glands is primarily at fault, the placenta, the pituitary, the adrenal or all three". Management of diabetic pregnancy was still (1951) controversial.

Fifty years of clinical research on the symptom complex known as toxemias of pregnancy, for which an "ominous" number of explanations have been offered, have resulted in little agreement with regard to the etiological role of maternal systemic factors (circulatory, renal, neural, nutritional) exacerbated by the physiological adjustments incident to pregnancy, of factors peculiar to pregnancy (placental hormones, ischemia, pressor substances, "toxins"), or of fetal factors. To the toxemias, once described by Peters as neither "toxic" nor peculiar to pregnancy, were attributed (1951, United States, Britain) between one third and one fourth of maternal deaths associated with pregnancy.

"The fairly large group of women in whom conception may occur with relative frequency only to terminate in spontaneous abortion may", according to Tyler, 1949, "for practical purposes be considered infertile." About ten per cent of all pregnancies terminate in abortion (Eastman), about 4.1 per cent of these resulting from recurrent factors; three or more spontaneous abortions are described as habitual abortion. Opinions differ as to therapies for habitual abortion and even as to desirability of treatment in view of the spontaneous cure rate. Malpas calculated, 1938 (on the basis of a study of 6,000 pregnancies including analysis of 115 abortion and stillbirth sequences), that after one abortion seventy-eight per cent would not abort; after two abortions, sixty-two per cent would have a normal pregnancy; after three, twenty-seven per cent would go to term normally; and after four only six per cent would have a chance of favorable outcome. Opinion is divided also as to whether abortion is caused by defective germ plasm resulting in a pathological fertilized ovum or by some failure in uterine environment. From fifty to eighty per cent of abortuses are pathological, lacking an embryo. Hertig, 1953, comparing the fertilized ova with the maternal environment in a series of 185 potentially pregnant women whose uteri and fertilized ova were directly examined after hysterectomy (prior to the first missed menstrual period), considered that the defective ova suggested about a twelve per cent clinical incidence of spontaneous abortion. In some views, abortion late in pregnancy is probably attributable to failures in maternal environment, abortion early in pregnancy to germ plasm defects, genetic (lethal genes) or physiological factors (as, delayed arrival of sperm at the site of fertilization allowing the ova to "age").

Outstanding among therapeutic approaches to spontaneous abortion has been the use of various hormones (as progesterone from the corpus luteum; steroid hormones presumed to come from the placenta) suggested by research during the last fifty years as possibly necessary to maintain gestation. At least a decade before progesterone was isolated, aqueous solutions of the corpus luteum were being tried, 1918, in threatened abortion on accumulated experimental evidence of the preceding decade that the corpus luteum played a part in maintaining gestation. Although subsequent investigations demonstrated that removal of the corpus luteum after implantation does not terminate pregnancy in women and monkeys, in a number of species abortion results unless progesterone is substituted. The factors (pituitary, estrogenic) that extend the life of the corpus luteum of menstruation into early pregnancy, as those responsible for regression of the corpus luteum during pregnancy (decline of pituitary gonadotrophins, production of chorionic gonadotrophins by the developing embryo) are subjects of current investigation.

So also are the questions whether the placenta takes over production of progesterone after regression of the corpus luteum, whether placental gonadotrophins (possibly placental estrogens) are necessary in this transfer of secretory function from the corpus luteum to the placenta. George Van S. Smith and Olive Smith have employed estrogens alone to prevent abortion (associated with diabetes, toxemia, premature delivery) on the theory (based on hormone estimations, 1936–52, in pregnant women) that estrogens stimulate placental secretion of both estrogens and progesterone which influence vascular supply to reproductive tissues; they emphasized a reciprocal relation between vascular supply to the uterus and to the placenta, and considered that adequate vascularity is as essential for normal production of steroid hormones by the placenta as is adequate hormonal support from the placenta for increased vascularity of the pregnant uterus. A. E. Rakoff and N. W. Vaux, however, employed estrogens and progesterone because they believed that the rough parallel which they found between levels of the two indicated that deficiency of one is probably accompanied by deficiency of the other, and because their studies (and those of others) failed to reveal a stimulating effect (claimed by the Smiths) by estrogens on production of progesterone. Their observation that such treatment did not result in normal serum estrogen levels prompted the question whether the defect might be not in production but "in some abnormality of estrogen-progesterone metabolism". The interrelation of these two steroids, puzzling with regard both to mechanisms of menstruation and to maintenance of gestation, will, it is hoped, be clarified by developing research concerned with discovering their paths (separate?) of conversion, utilization, metabolism, excretion in a sufficient number of mammalian species to give biological significance to the findings. That rational use of hormones to prevent abortion is not imminent follows from the fact stated by Hooker, 1946, that "the role of the various hormones during pregnancy remains obscure, perhaps to a large extent because the identity and the time and degree of fluctuations in levels of these hormones are not yet known with certainty". The role of hormones remains obscure also because of lack of agreement concerning hormones produced by the placenta. While G. O. Gey, M. K. Gey and G. E. S. Jones, 1943, demonstrated gonadotrophins in human placental tissue maintained in tissue culture, and Wislocki and his associates confirmed this finding by histochemical studies of the placenta of a number of species, including the human, these two groups (and others that have attempted to confirm their findings) are not agreed that steroid hormones are also produced by the placenta. Earlier workers, having correlated the appearance of chorionic gonadotrophins with formation of the chorion, consider that spontaneous abortion is especially likely to occur in this formation period. Among several suggestions as to the functional role of such chorionic gonadotrophins in maintaining gestation is that of Hisaw, 1944: having calculated from experiments with monkeys that the ovum, when fertilized, becomes embedded before disappearance of the corpus luteum of menstruation, he suggested that the gonadotrophin produced by the fetal chorion passes into the maternal blood stream to maintain the corpus luteum for fifteen to sixteen days, into early pregnancy; and that the corpus luteum during pregnancy may secrete an estrogen, perhaps even after it has ceased to produce progesterone. Those who believe that the placenta is responsible for production of progesterone after regression of the corpus luteum (a view based on demonstration of this hormone after removal of the corpus luteum in pregnancy and on histochemical evidence offered by Wislocki and his associates) have suggested that spontaneous abortion is an especial hazard at the time of transfer of secretory function from the corpus luteum to the placenta. W. H. Newton's statement that the mechanism involved in the maintenance of pregnancy "is evidently dependent on some or all of the hormones secreted by the placenta which seems capable of superseding to a varying degree both ovaries and pituitary" summarizes the basic framework orienting present investigative attempts to discover the mechanisms and establish the details that will prove this.

Concern with placental hormones in normal and disturbed pregnancy represents part of the attempt since 1905 to determine whether the fetus or placenta exerts a controlling influence on mechanisms responsible for maintenance of gestation. Newton's experiments with mice and rats, 1935–40, repeated by Gertrude van Wagenen with monkeys, 1943, demonstrated that removal of the fetus with retention of the placenta does not interfere with continued differentiation and survival of the placenta and delivery of it at the time when parturition would normally occur. Although development under these conditions of major physiological changes associated with normal pregnancy offers confirmation of the role of the placenta in maintaining gestation, the study of placental physiology is, according to Hammond and Huggett, 1952, still "in its infancy". Finding functional significance in the impressive body of comparative morphological data accumulated in the last eighty years in studies of evolution of the placenta is complicated by great species variation in placental structure and by its complexity (its numerous layers, not separable in woman; changes in number and structure of layers as pregnancy progresses). "It is doubtful", E. C. Amoroso observed, 1952, "if any anatomical structure has given rise to keener or more prolonged controversy."

In noting that "practically every known constituent substance for which search has been made in the placenta has been found there", Joseph Needham, 1942, added, "yet we are still a long way from having a complete account even for the placenta of one single species as to how its chemical constitution varies with the development of the fetus". The functional significance of a wide range of substances, carbohydrates, fats, proteins, pigments, vitamins, enzymes isolated from the placenta is still undetermined. Hammond and Huggett observed, 1952, that Claude Bernard's "attractive hypothesis of almost a century ago" that the placenta acts as the fetal liver "is somewhat negatived" by the finding that placental glycogen remains unchanged while fetal blood sugar fluctuates (as in diabetes, maternal asphyxia) with that of the mother. They suggested that placental glycogen appears to be "an endogenous metabolic product associated with the structure and growth of the placenta as a transfusion agent". Wislocki and Dempsey similarly distinguished between "passage" iron in the placenta, en route from mother to fetus, and intracellular iron related to the metabolic activity of the placenta; in their histo-chemical studies of steroid secretion they interpreted the presence of ribonucleic acid, of fat globules, as evidence not merely of the presence of hormones but also of intracellular metabolic activity connected with placental secretory function. Developing studies of this type have replaced the concept of the placenta as a passive filter for transfer of substances between mother and fetus by the concept of it as a "robust structure" with "an order of metabolism comparable to the most active organs of the adult body".

This concept distinguishes placental substances involved in the metabolic activity of the placenta (as a secretory, excretory, trans-fusing, storage organ) from substances passing between mother and fetus. In support of the concept that the placenta in early preg-nancy functions primarily as a storage depot, for nutrition of the fetus, in which energy is expended in anabolic processes, Wislocki and Dempsey cited the cytoplasmic basophilia attributed to ribo-nucleoprotein, found high in the placenta (cat, rodent, human) early in pregnancy; as pregnancy progresses, ribonucleoprotein falls and alkaline phosphatase rises, a phenomenon interpreted by these workers as evidence that the placenta's energy production lessens as it becomes primarily a diffusing organ for exchange of substances between mother and fetus. This inverse relationship between cytoplasmic basophilia attributable to ribonucleoprotein and alkaline phosphatase which Wislocki and Dempsey considered characteristic of the normally aging placenta was found prematurely (at five months) in human placental tissue from toxemic patients, but whether the aging was a cause or a result of toxemia these workers did not suggest. The "placental aging" frequently invoked as a pos-sible cause of toxemias, premature labor, spontaneous abortion has been related more often to "degeneration products" released as the placenta ages than to metabolic activity connected with its precise function in maintenance of gestation.

In spite of the voluminous literature that has grown up on sub-stances (toxins and antitoxins, metabolites, hormones, chemothera-peutic agents, anesthetics, bacteria, spirochetes, viruses, agglutinins, other antibodies) that do or do not pass the placenta, much remains to be learned concerning the placenta as a transfusing organ. Since

Needham, 1942, described as "a wide field for future study" the whole correlation of progressive changes in placental permeability with progressive development of the fetus, British and American investigators have made a beginning. The conclusion that permeability is not progressive to term, that it is not a generalized process uniformly affecting all layers of the placenta was reached in the studies of Louis B. Flexner and Alfred Gellhorn (rabbits, 1942; women, 1947). They found that although placental permeability rises progressively throughout pregnancy, it decreases toward term (in rabbits from the beginning of the last trimester to the end of gestation); and that, while radioactive sodium passed the placenta (rabbits; women) in progressively increased amounts as pregnancy progressed, the greatest increase occurred only when the chorion disappeared, suggesting that this layer had actually functioned as a barrier throughout pregnancy. Flexner and his associates concluded from these and other studies of the rate of transfer of physiological substances (as heavy water, 1941, radioactive sodium, 1942, 1947) that the rate of transfer roughly parallels increase in fetal weight, the larger the fetus the greater the turnover of water.

Joseph Barcroft's studies, 1936–46, also emphasize the relationship between placental function and fetal nutrition. In his 1947 monograph, *Researches on Prenatal Life*, reporting fetal respiration and circulation in the living fetus (sheep) still attached to its mother, he described how the fetal need for oxygen throughout the course of pregnancy is met by placental adjustments between maternal and fetal circulations. The orienting concept in these studies, that mechanisms involved in placental transfer are governed by a reciprocal relation between the morphology of the placenta and the nutritive requirements of the fetus, derived from morphological studies of placental circulation (Mossman in the rabbit, 1925; Spanner in woman, 1935; Barcroft and Barron in sheep, 1942) and the comparative work on placental structure that preceded it. On developing research on placental permeability depend answers to many urgent clinical questions, for instance why poliomyelitis virus fails to pass the placenta while rubella virus passes it to cause serious congenital defects in the fetus; or why Rh-positive agglutinogens pass from fetus to an Rh-negative mother to induce specific maternal antibodies which then return across the placenta to react with fetal agglutinogens to destroy fetal erythrocytes, causing hemolytic damage ranging from mild forms of hemolytic disorder, jaundice and anemia in the newborn, to mental deficiency and death from erythroblastosis fetalis. This mechanism, according to Hammond and Huggett, 1952, is "quite clearly extendable to other naturally occurring proteins". Whether by reason of its secretory, nutritional, transfusing, or other functioning, the significance of the placenta in the successful outcome of pregnancy cannot be denied on the basis of such findings as Hertig's, whose analysis of the pathology of a thousand abortions revealed anomalies in placental development in 9.6 per cent.

Prematurity, a leading cause of neonatal death, was, 1948, eighth among causes of death in persons of all ages listed by the National Office of Vital Statistics. In spite of a measurable salvage of premature infants, no major clinic, according to Clement A. Smith, 1948, appeared to have effected a progressive decrease in the rate of premature births. To causes previously mentioned as possibly explaining premature initiation of labor (premature aging of the placenta, deficiencies or imbalances of placental hormones presumed to be important in the maintenance of gestation) have been added interrelated effects of the posterior pituitary oxytocic factor. The trend, however, is to replace the search for a specific precipitant of labor by attempts to balance withdrawal of factors (chiefly hormonal) believed to be responsible both for maintenance of gestation and inhibition of uterine contraction against the gradual rise of positive influences (perhaps of the posterior pituitary) increasing uterine motility. Reynolds stressed the significance of the whole uterine environment in maintenance of gestation, initiation of parturition. In integration of "the triad of basic functions" — uterine growth, motility, vascularity (operating through four interacting mechanisms, neural, hormonal, metabolic, vascular) — lay, in his view, hope of a unified concept of uterine function, "nidation, uterine accommodation of the products of conception, parturition". Only approach to these as interrelated functions, he pointed out, 1951, can provide a fundamental base for solution of outstanding problems of infertility. His investigations support theories developed in the thirties by Hammond's studies of uterine accommodation of the products of conception (rabbit) from which Hammond concluded that enlargement of the uterus in pregnancy is more than mere dilation, representing active growth effects on the part of the muscular tissue (myometrium) in response to two influences: control by internal secretions "the origin of which is not known but believed to be the placenta" (Hammond and Huggett, 1952), and the mechanical distention (increased by progesterone) resulting from contact between embryo and uterus. The increase in the growth rate of the uterus which Hammond showed in the seventh month was subsequently confirmed by Scammon's measurements of the human uterus. Reynolds, whose recent investigations in animals and, with Johns Hopkins obstetricians, in women (extending Hammond's work), have been directed to the relation between changing rate of growth and changing shape of the fetus, the resulting tension on the uterine wall and its effect on uterine blood flow, concluded, 1949, that with respect to space in the uterus and conditions of uterine blood circulation, the seventh month may be an especially hazardous period with reference to premature birth.

Of extensive attempts over the past twenty years to measure the duration and propulsive forces of contraction in the various stages of labor, or from various segments of the uterus, Davis, 1950, observed that, since uterine contractions involve humoral, endocrine, chemical enzymatic, mechanical, neural factors, the problem "obviously goes beyond simply recording uterine activity in labor". Besides Reynolds's studies of the interrelations of hormonal, vascular, physical factors, a beginning has also been made, since 1945, on some of the enzymatic and other chemical elements that may be involved in uterine contractions in studies reported 1947–51 and later. A. I. Csapo, oriented by Szent-Györgyi's theories of muscular contraction (especially inability of the contractile element of muscle, actomyosin, to contract without adenosinetriphosphate), has since 1947 reported findings on isolated muscle strips taken at various stages of pregnancy from several species, including woman. He found actomyosin concentrated most heavily and in its most active form in human uterine muscle toward term, less concentrated in the nonpregnant uterus, least concentrated and poorest in contractile quality in women who had been sterilized by X ray. The slight amount and poor contractile quality of actomyosin in menopausal women, disappearance of actomyosin on removal of ovaries and return of it under estrogen administration implied (1950–51) hormonal regulation. This also was the implication of histochemical correlations made by Elftman and Atkinson, 1946, between the presence of estrogen and the presence and distribution in uterine muscle (rodent) of adenosinetriphosphatase, a finding which Csapo confirmed in isolated human uterine muscle. Reynolds, 1951, emphasized the significance of these findings when they shall have been extended from test tube demonstrations on isolated muscle to the living subject.

## CAUSES OF FETAL AND NEONATAL DEATH

Death occurs approximately twice as often among prematures alive at birth as among full-term infants. Pathological study of neonatal death attributable to *prematurity* discloses sometimes "uncompleted" structure, more often "uncompleted" function. A 1953 conference, focused on prematurity and other major causes of the million neonatal deaths that occur annually, considered the metabolic significance of imperfect development in prematures of enzymes responsible for different steps involved in utilization of carbohydrates (upon which the brain is especially dependent) and also the significance of immaturity of the endocrine system. The anemia of prematures, more serious than anemia in full-term babies, was attributed to deficient synthesis of fetal hemoglobin that would have been adequate had the baby lived out its normal span of uterine life (I. Schulman, 1953). Health department records used to discover common factors in the history of cerebral palsy cases indicated an "almost constant" association with prematurity (A. M. Lilienfeld, 1953).

Since 1940 when H. W. Mossman described physiology of the fetus as "even yet almost a virgin field" for study, further investigation has been made of various fetal functions (respiratory, renal, vascular) and of changes in function that occur in transfer from intrauterine to extrauterine life. The modern discipline, "developmental physiology", includes contributions from many fields: physiologists hope in embryological development to throw light on adult function; biochemists concerned with the metabolic basis of function seek to correlate histochemical changes in fetal organs and tissues with assumption of active function; chemical and experimental embryologists seek clarification of chemical stimuli, metabolic exchanges that will explain differentiation and development at the very beginnings of life. Selected for mention here from far-ranging investigations are only a few bearing on the more frequently cited causes of fetal and neonatal death, or on serious disabilities in children attributable to processes before and during birth.

Of the 300 stillbirths and neonatal deaths out of every 10,000 births (Clement A. Smith, 1951), about seventy are primarily due to *anoxia*. It was considered the final cause of death in the vast majority of cases of fetal and neonatal loss by the international conference on anoxia of the newborn arranged by the World Health Organization in 1953; prenatal and postnatal anoxia were described as inseparable. Proximate causes of anoxia may lie in mother, fetus, placenta. Toxemias and qualitative changes in maternal blood associated with anemia or cardiac decompensation are considered to disturb pressure gradients of oxygen and carbon dioxide between mother and fetus, resulting in anoxia before birth. A premature infant with "immature" or otherwise defective lungs, circulation, brain (controlling higher respiratory centers) may be unable to make the transfer from placental oxygenation to extrauterine pulmonary respiration. Eric Denhof and R. H. Holden reported, 1951, that of 100 children with cerebral palsy thirty-seven per cent had required oxygen (and/or transfusions) at birth. Among known causes of anoxia are cord abnormalities interfering with circulation between placenta and fetus, partial or complete detachment of the placenta during pregnancy or on initiation of labor (because of abnormal implantation over the cervix), birth trauma (cerebral hemorrhage and consequent depression of higher respiratory centers), narcotization of the fetus during birth from prolonged or poorly administered analgesics and anesthetics. One clinician's 1951 comment, "until we know why most babies breathe when they emerge from the uterus we shall scarcely be sure why some babies do not", touches on a critical question in investigative work, when respiration begins.

The trend appears to be away from the earlier belief that pulmonary respiration initiates a new form of activity and toward the view that it is a continuation of respiratory movements begun early in fetal life. Such movements have been observed in several species including the human, and their basis in the progressive nervous development of respiratory movement has been described in extended observations on the living fetus still attached to the anesthetized sheep by Joseph Barcroft and Donald H. Barron, 1942, 1947, who also correlated anoxic breathing with inadequate involvement of the higher nervous centers required for normal respiration. By sectioning the central nervous system at each of four stages in the development of respiratory movements, Barcroft concluded that nervous control of respiratory movement developed from below upwards. Under such circumstances, he reasoned, it should be possible to initiate respiration either by depressing the upper inhibitory centers (that come into operation last) to release the lower centers, or by excessive stimulation of the lower centers to overcome inhibitory influence of the higher. Respiration was produced in the fetal sheep by both methods but when the higher centers associated with rhythmic respiration were depressed the result was the gasp characteristic of the earlier development of discontinuous respiratory movements under the lower centers. Similar gasps were observed by Barcroft in cyanotic infants seen in the course of nine consecutive human deliveries. On the basis of his experimental work Barcroft characterized the difference between normal respiration and anoxia in terms of the nervous centers involved. Although noting that two chemical events occur when the umbilical cord is tied or the placental circulation fails, i.e., oxygen is cut off, and carbon dioxide accumulates, Barcroft did not enter the long-standing controversy concerning the primarily chemical theory that stimulation of the respiratory center and initiation of respiration occur by reason of increased amounts of carbon dioxide in the circulating blood.

Long-standing disputes concerning the morphological changes that occur at birth in the lungs seem more or less resolved by recent work suggesting that this pattern is also established well before birth. A considerable literature has grown up on how the air spaces (alveoli) in the lungs, formed by the terminal dilatations of the bronchioles, change from structures lined by a continuous layer of epithelium in early life to structures in which the walls are largely composed of capillaries. Some maintain that the epithelial cells originally covering the capillaries are cast off at or before birth so that the capillaries lie in direct contact with the air spaces, others that the epithelial covering cells remain intact but flatten out as alveoli expand and remain as permanent but invisible platelike structures covering the capillaries. Potter's studies of fetal lungs (in 1946 with Davis, in 1951 with Loosli) supported neither view but indicated that long before fetal maturity "the uncovered capillaries lie in direct contact with the air spaces and the pattern that exists in the lung after birth is established"; the epithelial cells are not shed but squeezed up and separated by capillaries so that they appear smaller; by the time of birth the alveoli are composed largely of naked capillaries in direct contact with the pulmonary lumen.

Congenital defects rank high as a cause of fetal and neonatal death. The disability (physical, mental, psychological) they account for in the living is not similarly measurable both because minor defects are not reported and because figures on serious defects are based chiefly on proportions found in institutions for the feebleminded. Congenital defects cause death more frequently before than after birth; D. P. Murphy, 1947, found congenital defects five and a half times more frequent in stillborn than in infants alive at term. The implication (voiced by some pathologists, obstetricians, pediatricians, investigators of developmental physiology) that nature tends to dispose of babies not structurally prepared for life and growth has stimulated a certain amount of doubt concerning present efforts to salvage smaller and smaller premature infants. Smaller size has been especially emphasized in incidence of retrolental fibroplasia, an ocular condition developing after birth, recognized, 1942, by T. L. Terry, and since found to include vascular changes in the eye, later changes that may lead to retinal detachment, gross changes ranging from impaired vision to total blindness. Terry's finding (Massachusetts Eye and Ear Infirmary) that ninety-two out of a hundred children with this condition had been born prematurely has been widely confirmed. Search for less obvious ocular defects in children known to have been born prematurely has resulted in finding exophthalmos, strabismus from muscular imbalance, delay in attainment of full central vision.

Of the many attempts made to find the cause of retrolental fibroplasia, in 1953 first among causes of blindness in children in the United States, the most profitable line of research appeared, 1953, to lie in study of oxygen concentration maintained in incubators: several reports (as Campbell, 1951) have indicated a considerably higher incidence in prematures maintained at higher concentrations of oxygen than at lower; other reports have noted a significant reduction (Crosse and Evans, 1952) in incidence when oxygen has not been routinely used for all prematures.   Holt, 1953, and others have stressed the need of transferring a degree of the available investigative interest from postnatal to prenatal conditions. Although prenatal conditions have been hypothetically suggested as causative factors by several, none had been conclusively demonstrated, 1953. Among causes suggested but not proved have been various nutritional deficiencies (iron, vitamins A and E) suggested by studies (animal and human) over the last thirty years to be significant in fetal nutrition, sometimes in the mother, sometimes in the infant. In the case of the blind offspring of pigs fed during pregnancy on a diet deficient in vitamin A, it has been difficult to determine whether the blindness resulted from specific vitamin A deficiency or was merely one manifestation of a generalized assault upon development.  Josef Warkany and his associates in a series of investigations (1940–50) on the role of nutrition in blindness and other congenital defects noted in the offspring of rats on a vitamin A deficient diet during pregnancy cleft palates, eye defects, malformations of the extremities and of the genitourinary tract, ectopic kidneys, cardiovascular defects, undescended testes, vaginal aplasia.   Finding, 1947, "no way at present of estimating how frequently maternal dietary deficiency is actually a factor in the etiology of mammalian monsters", he stressed the apparent certainty that improved nutrition after the period of early development cannot in animals repair damage already done and may indeed (by enabling the mother to carry to term) result in a higher incidence of congenital malformation in living offspring.

The role of diet in the production of congenital defects is part of the larger question of fetal nutrition (in both early and late pregnancy) now under reinvestigation as the result of new biological concepts, and new tools (as radioactive substances).  Extension of studies of fetal nutrition generally may throw light on the statistical evidence that diet (particularly vitamins and proteins) affects not only the course of pregnancy but also the normality of the offspring.   The "theory of partition of nutrients", the hypothesis that tissues with higher metabolic rate have a prior call on blood stream nutrients over those with lower metabolic rate, was first advanced by C. M. Child in 1920 with reference to the single organism. Applying this to the placenta, fetus and uterus, Hammond, 1952, suggested that the young cells of the fetus and fetal placenta, having a higher metabolic rate than old cells of maternal tissue, account for a growth gradient by which the fetus will grow even if maternal tissues may lose weight. The truth of the general hypothesis was demonstrated by Wallace, 1944–48; the nervous system (with the highest metabolic rate) of fetuses in sheep fed a diet on a high and on a low plane was shown to be least affected, the flesh most affected. Differential effects observed in other organs and tissues were also correlated with metabolic rates. "The final birth weight was dependent upon the plane of nutrition in the last part of pregnancy; little effect resulted from diet in early pregnancy."

The effect on the fetus of maternal infection during early pregnancy has received considerable attention since the 1941 report of the Australian ophthalmologist, N. M. Gregg, tracing unusual incidence of congenital cataract in infants of the same age group to rubella in their mothers. Investigators elsewhere added to ocular defects (cataract, atrophy of the iris, etc.) cardiac defects, deaf mutism, dental anomalies, physical and mental retardation. In contrast to the higher rate suggested by some, H. C. Miller, of the committee on congenital malformation of the American Academy of Pediatrics, estimated, 1950, on the basis of 32,000 cases, that only forty per cent or less of the infants born to mothers that had contracted rubella in the first trimester of pregnancy would have congenital defects. Charles Swan, however, concluded from statistical analysis of various reports, including his own studies since 1942 in Australia and in England (for the British Medical Research Council), that the mother with rubella in the first four months of pregnancy will in three cases out of four bear a congenitally defective infant; with A. L. Tostevin, 1946, he recommended therapeutic abortion for every woman that contracts the infection during this period. More than thirty years ago biologists pointed out that specific congenital defects are governed rather by the developmental stage of the fetus than by the particular character of the agent, an observation induced by the early finding that a number of chemical and physical agents (salts of lithium, magnesium, cold, heat) produced the same defects at a given developmental stage of lower animals. Attention has been called to the need of investigating generally in higher species the possible effect upon the offspring of a wide range of influences in early pregnancy including all types of viruses, bacterial and other infecting organisms, nutritional substances, as well as other chemical and physical agents.

Many factors besides diet and infection have been studied in the search over centuries for an explanation of human "monsters" and of lesser defects on which obstetricians and pediatricians are now uniting in a nation-wide attempt to decrease the death rate associated with them.

While advancing maternal age has consistently, as previously noted, been statistically associated with incidence of Mongolism, knowledge is still lacking, as Worcester pointed out, 1953, as to "which of the many variables that may be associated with the aging process" is responsible. Ingalls thought, 1954, that age "is hardly to be considered among direct causes but is rather an index of intrinsic anatomical and physiological factors". His experiments with mice at Harvard supported the hypothesis that Mongolism may be a "stage-specific defect of about the eighth week of fetal life, induced in a potentially normal embryo" which has weathered a period of critical, almost lethal stress and survives "but with a permanent arrest of tissues differentiating during the period of stress". Among physiological variables influenced by age, Benda has suggested (on the basis of pregnancy history of the mothers of Mongoloid children) a "borderline" hormonal status in women approaching the menopause. Penrose, however, expressed, 1954, the view that "if an endocrine disturbance is to be held responsible for *all* cases, it must be of a kind not yet known to clinical medicine". Hanhart, 1944, suggested the genetic background of Mongolism to be a single dominant gene. Penrose, 1953, on the basis of his own studies over twenty years, preferred the hypothesis of a single recessive gene. Ingalls considered a simple Mendelian explanation unlikely. The trend appears to be away from attributing Mongolism and other congenital anomalies and defects exclusively to genetic or exclusively to maternal influences;

as Hogben put it, "whatever gene differences are involved . . . appear to require a special prenatal environment to make them recognizable". Ingalls observed, 1952, "it is man's environment that is susceptible to manipulation, not his genes and chromosomes". In 1954, he thought that the possibility of even beginning a program of control measures was dependent on giving to epidemiological considerations "as much weight" as is now accorded "to clinical diagnosis and custodial care of these blighted beings". Penrose, 1954, stressing how little is known of the outcome of very late pregnancies in wild animal populations as opposed to laboratory stocks, suggested that wider biological study might facilitate study of the human problem.

Murphy's 1929 report, based on replies from gynecologists and radiologists to his inquiry on the status of infants born to mothers subjected during pregnancy to therapeutic doses of pelvic irradiation, that of seventy-six full-term children twenty-five showed defective development (seventeen of those with microcephaly being mentally defective), has experimental support in a wide variety of skeletal, ocular, cranial anomalies in the offspring of irradiated animals. The previously mentioned joint commission's long-term study in Japan (associated with experimental work in this country) aims to follow through several generations the effects of irradiation on the offspring of pregnant women exposed to the Nagasaki and Hiroshima bombs.

A genetic basis for some human defects is suggested by the Mendelian pattern of transmission traced in some families for certain defects, as brachydactylism, polydactylism, albinism, hemophilia, more recently hydrocephalus (Bickers and Adams, 1949), cataract (Saebb, 1949). Curt Stern outlined, 1950, the possibility of making a "genetic prognosis" for some defects on the basis of accumulating knowledge from studies of human pedigrees, twins and from experimental work: in brachydactylism, for instance, two possibilities exist since it is caused by a dominant gene; an abnormal gene from the affected parent may join a normal gene from the normal parent resulting in a child with this abnormality; a normal gene from the affected parent (only half of whose genes are abnormal) may join with a normal gene resulting in a normal child. Albinism, on the other hand, being a recessive gene, requires for transmission an abnormal gene from both parents, both of whom may have normal appearance.

Geneticists now recognize that defects known to be genetic in origin may be copied by defects produced by nongenetic influences. Shortly after L. C. Dunn and Walter Landauer of the University of Connecticut reported that "rumplessness" in fowl also on occasion occurred spontaneously as a nonhereditary character, C. H. Danforth (1932) produced the same character by manipulation of (incubator) temperature. Later, 1945, E. Zwilling induced it by incising the backs of young embryos and Landauer reported, 1945, that injection of insulin would induce the same defect in genetically normal chicks. Landauer, 1948, suggested that the various abnormalities produced result from interference with carbohydrate metabolism which Needham, 1942, had suggested as the source of energy for growth and differentiation of the chick embryo in these early stages. Commenting on the variety of ways by which rumplessness may be induced, Danforth, 1946, found it "increasingly apparent that this trait, like some others involving developmental failure, may be induced by either dominant or recessive genes and likewise by a diversity of extragenic disturbances occurring before some as yet undetermined period of embryonic life has been reached". Recent reports on twins offer a certain support for a view that some of the defects known to be genetic can apparently be induced by interaction of genetic and environmental factors. Referring to recent (1948–51) reports on clubfoot, hypertrophic pyloric stenosis and Mongolism, in which while one twin showed the given defect the other was spared, F. C. Fraser and T. D. Fainstat observed, 1951, that while excess of concordant cases in the genetically identical group suggested genetic origin, the fact that some genetically identical pairs are unlike with respect to the given defect indicated that nongenetic factors must also be involved.

This broadened biologic picture appears as yet to have percolated only to a limited degree to medical practitioners who, on the whole, appear to favor genetic rather than environmental causes of congenital defect. Murphy concluded from study of the families of 800 defective children "gross, human, congenital malformations arise solely from influences which affect the germ cells prior to fertilization . . . hence are hereditary in origin". The statistical bases for this view included: the finding that families with one malformed child are twenty-four times more likely than families in the general population to have further malformed children; that one child's malformation frequently appeared among its brothers and sisters, and in thirty-nine cases was found in forty-one per cent of distant relatives; that rare defects were duplicated in two children born to the same mother; that the same defect appeared in children having different mothers but the same father. Corner, noting (Ourselves Unborn, 1944) that the genetic basis of some congenital defects seems to be affirmed by experimental evidence accumulated in the last thirty years, added, "it will be a very long time before enough is known about human heredity to make possible prediction of unfavorable human crosses, except in a few obvious cases". Among potential causes of congenital abnormalities he noted defects of ovum and sperm (which may be genetic, or the result of nongenetic constitutional influences), of fertilization, of maternal environment ranging from faulty transportation of the fertilized ovum, failure of implantation, hormonal failure in pregnancy, mechanical disorders, to infections of the reproductive tract or of the embryo, toxic factors, nutritional defects. Geneticists have pointed out that as gaps in knowledge of reproductive physiology are filled, it will become easier to assess purely genetic factors in congenital defect.

The association of congenital defect not only with spontaneous abortion, fetal and neonatal death and prematurity but also with periods of sterility has raised the question whether common factors may not operate in all of these. In noting, 1947, that of 501 mothers of defective children, 226 (forty-five per cent) bore no further offspring in the five-year period studied, that periods of relative sterility were four times more common preceding the appearance of congenital defect than preceding the birth of normal offspring in the same family, that in the 430 pregnancies that subsequently occurred in fifty-five per cent of his series, 100 terminated in abortion, premature births, stillbirths, or a repetition of malformation, Murphy considered these facts to favor a common cause.

CHAPTER 4

# Arteriosclerosis

*With especial reference to the metabolic
basis of arterial changes*

## INTRODUCTORY

A United States government survey showed that almost half of the 1950 deaths from cardiovascular disease (consistently shown by vital statistics to be the major killer in this country) were attributed to arteriosclerosis, thirty per cent to arteriosclerosis combined with hypertension.

The term, arteriosclerosis, is greatly in need of definition. Even a brief review of current investigative work in this field needs to take into account certain important distinctions, not all of which are even now susceptible to precise definition but some of which havle certainly been progressively clarified by scientific advances. Among the ancient errors that have obscured precise values in the pubic mind is the widespread view that the "hardening of the arteries" supposed to describe arteriosclerosis is simply one manifestation of senility, inevitable in all mammals (if they live long enough) and irreversible. The idea that vascular change inevitably accompanies the aging process has been modified by evidence that arterial "aging" is not necessarily identified with chronological age. Albert I. Lansing (anatomy department, Washington University) found, 1951, marked calcification in the elastic fibers of the media (middle coat of the arteries) in some persons of twenty; arteriosclerosis was found at autopsy in soldiers during the first world war in over thirty per cent at twenty years of age, in over forty-five per cent at twenty-five (cited by Louis N. Katz and D. V. Dauber, Michael Reese Hospital, 1945). On the other hand, M. A. Goldzieher found, 1951, in a group of nonagenarians arteries which he thought most middle-aged people would have been glad to own.

The popular misconception that arteriosclerosis is an inevitable concomitant and sign of aging is not the only fallacy that has confused the arteriosclerosis picture. In medical as well as in popular discussions, the generic term, arteriosclerosis, has been roughly and inclusively used to cover all arterial pathology, all forms of sclerosis, Mönckeberg's sclerosis, hyperplastic arteriosclerosis, atherosclerosis. While all the conditions included are characterized by some thickening of the artery wall, they vary greatly in severity, in location and character of lesions. Mönckeberg's sclerosis, involving degeneration and calcification of the two outer arterial coats (adventitia consisting of loose and elastic connective tissue, media consisting of smooth muscle fibers and noncellular connective tissue elements), affects chiefly the extremities and is comparatively benign. Atherosclerosis, on the other hand, involving especially the intima or innermost lining of the arteries (although the elastic layer may also be affected) may, especially in coronary or cerebral arteries, progress to a fatal issue in coronary occlusion or in cerebral hemorrhage. While in the present rapidly changing state of knowledge a definitive description of all of the arterioscleroses could hardly be justified, it is at least clear that the term arteriosclerosis is applied to entities that are diverse. "Awareness of this fact" was described, 1952, by Katz as "absolutely essential for progress in this field". He pointed out that the attention of investigators is "correctly focused today" on atherosclerosis "since this is the lesion among the arterioscleroses which is overwhelmingly responsible for morbidity and mortality in man". In the present brief review of current trends in investigative work in this field attention is also focused on atherosclerosis, but with due recognition of certain facts and factors: first, that some outstanding investigators still tend to use atherosclerosis and arteriosclerosis almost interchangeably; secondly, that the criteria that distinguish the various entities among the arterioscleroses are still in process of evolution and not yet subject to precise summary; thirdly, that arteriosclerosis and atherosclerosis may conceivably both be present. Since the character of the intimal lesions in atherosclerosis can be proved only by pathological examination of sections, clinical distinction remains difficult. In short, the assumption that atherosclerosis is a distinct entity in the sense that it has a uniform etiology and pathogenesis is, in the present state of knowledge, untenable. These considerations will explain the use of both arteriosclerosis and atherosclerosis in the following discussion, the latter term being reserved for reference to the condition in which intimal atheromatous lesions are stressed.

## Major Investigative Approaches

Current research on arteriosclerosis includes: studies of long-neglected problems of structure, function and metabolism of arterial tissues in departments and laboratories of anatomy, pathology, cytology, zoology, physiology, medicine, gerontology; studies of metabolic and biochemical aspects of the disorder in departments of medicine, nutrition, biochemistry, physiology, pathology, medical physics and biophysics, cardiovascular divisions and departments in various universities, hospitals, research institutes. Progressively more discernible is the trend toward accumulation of accurate chemical and physical data which will facilitate formulation of arteriosclerosis problems in terms of metabolism. Structure and function of the arterial walls are regarded by many as essential base lines for study of etiology. In the past, studies of human arteries were largely confined to autopsy material, a situation reminiscent of the state of cancer research before 1915 when the first experimental cancers produced by chemical carcinogens opened the way to study of cellular and metabolic changes that precede malignant transformation. Among pathological studies of arterial tissues directed specifically toward changes preceding development of atherosclerosis in both animals and men are those reported, 1938, by workers in the Yale pathology department under M. C. Winternitz who expressed hope that new directions in study would lift the problem of arterial structure and function "out of the limbo of 'degenerations'" and into the area of metabolism. The inseparability of structure and function was stressed at a 1951 conference on connective tissue by D. Murray Angevine (pathology, Wisconsin): "They are the same. There is no anatomy and chemistry; chemistry is anatomy at the atomic level."

Since Anitschkow's time (1911) there has been marked concentration of interest in the relation of lipid metabolism to atherosclerosis. A favorite hypothesis has been that the cholesterol deposition that characterizes the intimal atheromatous lesions of human atherosclerosis results from hypercholesterolemia. One gap (pointed out by I. L. Chaikoff, physiology, California, 1953) in the evidence offered for this hypothesis is lack of study of possible passage of serum cholesterol, under physiological conditions, through the vessel wall. John P. Peters (internal medicine, Yale, 1952), reviewing what he considered to be certain fallacies in earlier investigative preoccupation with an hypothesis that derives from experimental production of atherosclerosis in rabbits by feeding cholesterol, stressed the possibility that the rabbit may be (as he believes) unique; he also emphasized the danger of losing sight of the concept, repeatedly suggested over the years, that antecedent injury to arterial tissues is a condition precedent to atheromatous deposition.

Dead ends in various avenues of investigative work and challenging questions arising from inapplicability of experimental work to human atherosclerosis have raised the broad question whether the most direct approach may lie not through investigation of disease at all (in animals or men) but rather through fundamental investigation of the processes of normal metabolism. Forrest E. Kendall (biochemistry, Columbia) suggested, 1951, that the lipid complexes now under active investigation may be part of the normal mechanism of lipid transport, that high serum concentrations may only reflect cellular defects in utilization of fats. Discussion of the relative expediency of approach from the pathological to the normal or *vice versa* at the 1951 Macy conference seemed to end in agreement that at the structural and the cellular levels it is probably better to start with the pathological, but at the molecular level with the normal (or usual or average).

## WORK ON THE STRUCTURE, FUNCTION, METABOLISM OF ARTERIAL TISSUES

Exploratory physical studies of the fine structure of tissues composing the arterial walls include electron-microscopic observations: of collagen fibrils of connective tissue (R. W. G. Wyckoff, National Institute of Arthritis and Metabolic Research, 1952); of reticulin (A. H. T. Robb-Smith, pathology, Radcliffe Infirmary, Oxford, 1952); of elastin extracted from elastic tissues (Jerome Gross, Massachusetts Institute of Technology, 1950; C. M. Franchi and E. de

Robertis, Institute of General Anatomy and Embryology, Buenos Aires, 1951). Chemical studies of elastin, not yet isolated in pure form but generally considered to be the insoluble portion of elastic tissues remaining after treatment with acid or alkali, were undertaken by A. I. Lansing and associates. Their analyses of human aortic elastic fibers showed, 1951, differences between young and old elastin in mineral content (young elastin being mineral-free while older elastin showed increasing phosphorus and calcium) and in amino acid content (increase with age in aspartic and glutamic acids). From the age of thirty, fraying and fragmentation of elastic lamellae (discs or plates) are progressive, the mineralization and aggregation of which account for Mönckeberg's sclerosis in the extremities. These changes affect the media alone and occur whether or not atherosclerosis is present in the intima. Elastic fibers in the media dissolved by elastinase (prepared from crude pancreatin by the Hungarian workers, Balo and Banga, 1950) yielded what appeared to Lansing and his coworkers to be a lipid component. Studies thus far have not revealed changes with age in the lipid content of the media comparable to those in the intima.

Need for further knowledge of the cytochemistry of arterial tissues, for deeper penetration into the early stages and mechanisms of arterial changes has motivated such histological and pathological studies of human coronary arteries as those reported, 1951, by James F. Rinehart, H. D. Moon and Louis D. Greenberg (pathology, California). In these studies, early lesions of atherosclerosis were characterized by accumulation of a mucoid substance in the intima, increase in connective tissue cells, deposits of collagen and elastic tissues; advanced lesions were characterized by lipid deposition. Late manifestations frequently described include aneurysms, surface ulceration, deep necrosis. Especially in the coronaries, scars or arterial injuries have been attributed to arteritis produced by hypersensitivity, and to other types of intimal hyperplasia resulting from infection, bacterial intoxication, increased arterial tension (Otto Saphir and Ira Gore, Michael Reese Hospital and Armed Forces Institute of Pathology, 1950). In general, morphological and histological analysis of lesions lags behind biochemical approaches, in the view, 1950, of Rudolf Altschul (anatomy, University of Saskatchewan); interested morphologists, comparatively few, "will have to add new zest to their endeavors". Study of early spontaneous lesions in dogs by Chaikoff and associates (Stuart Lindsay and J. W. Gilmore), 1952, revealed in the older dogs signs of arterial injury in fraying, splitting or fragmentation of the internal elastic tissue. The earliest change in the intima was "fibroblastic proliferation associated with deposition of mucoid ground substance". Lipid deposition was a late development; small amounts of finely divided lipid material (not cholesterol) appeared in the cytoplasm of the fibroblastic cells of the thickened intima (in nine of fourteen dogs). "It is clear that lipids are not involved in the early aortic disease of the dogs", some of the lesions of which "bear a remarkable resemblance to coronary arteriosclerosis of the human being".

Revival of interest in the theory that development of atherosclerotic lesions varies inversely with the blood supply to the arterial walls goes back to previously mentioned studies of the biology of arteriosclerosis by the Yale pathology group (Winternitz and associates) published in 1938. Their examination, in various animal species, of fresh specimens of blood vessels supplying the walls of coronary, cerebral arteries, aorta, veins, etc. (vasa vasorum) resulted in the conclusion that distribution and extent of arterial vascularity are related to both age and disease. Morbid processes in mural vascular channels were described as: occlusion by thrombus; stasis of blood and subsequent lith formation; obstruction and closure by overgrowth of surrounding connective tissue; degeneration and necrosis in association with similar involvement of the tissues of the vessel wall. Although presence of vasa vasorum in the outer coats of the normal artery (adventitia and the outer half of the media) is generally accepted, this is not true as to the normal inner media and the intima; in the latter, however, the Yale studies showed vascularity which reacts to injurious agents, as do other tissues, by exudation and proliferation. Hemorrhage, common in the arterial wall and regarded as an exaggerated form of exudation, was found in the elective sites of atheroma and the sites of origin of vasa in the normal arteries of man and many animals. "With no further evidence, some relation between the three factors — vascularity, hemorrhage, sclerosis — would seem likely." Some evidence for the idea that hemorrhage and exudations from the vasa into the vascular wall might be one source of materials deposited within atheroma was offered by Katz and Dauber, who, in 1943, described a correlation between cholesterol-induced lesions in chickens and number of vasa in the arterial walls. Repeated emphasis on mechanisms of cholesterol transport rather than on serum cholesterol concentrations makes important the suggestion that the vasa vasorum may be at least one mechanism by which cholesterol may reach the intimal endothelium (Winternitz and associates). The theory that arterial lesions are caused by pathology in the vasa vasorum in the outer layers or by hemorrhage from intimal networks was described by Altschul, 1950, as merely shifting the problem of etiology to the smaller vessels. He considered the theory invalidated by the gradual "foamy transformation" of the intimal endothelium together with lack of changes in the media. Comparison of aortic vascularization of several species in health and disease (J. Schlichter and R. Harris, Michael Reese Hospital, 1949) led to a general hypothesis that arterial lesions may result from conditions (hypertension or physiological growth of vessels) increasing the demand of the arterial wall for blood, especially oxygen, without proportional increase in the supply, or reducing the blood supply by destroying the vasa vasorum or by producing prolonged anoxemia. Experiments have indicated, first, the necessity of adequate circulation in the vasa vasorum (in dogs, J. F. O'Neill, surgery, Bowman Gray, 1947), and, secondly, correlation between vascularity of the aorta and varying susceptibility to experimental or spontaneous atherosclerosis in different species (studies of the aorta in dog, man, chicken, rabbit, Schlichter, 1948; comparative studies of the vasa in dog and human aortas, Charles A. Woerner, anatomy, University of Louisville, 1951).

One process described, 1951, by Melvin H. Knisely (anatomy, formerly Chicago, later South Carolina) as of regular occurrence (on the basis of observing it in five thousand patients with sixty different conditions) was formation of blood sludges or masses of agglutinated red cells. Knisely suggested that these sludges apparently associated with disease (on the basis of comparative studies, including those of investigators in Denmark, Finland, Tennessee, conducted over a twenty-year period, of the circulation in thousands of living animals of many species and of presumably normal persons), might have a possible role in thrombosis and in forcibly decreasing rates of blood flow through the small vasa vasorum, participating in the initial pathologic histological changes of human atherosclerosis. At a 1951 conference on aging, Lewis V. Heilbrunn (zoology, University of Pennsylvania) emphasized the constant equilibrium *in vivo* between clotting and anticlotting factors and, since sludges occur near injured tissues which liberate thromboplastic substance, an apparent relation between the two phenomena. Nitrogenous lipid constituents of tissues that are active in blood coagulation and formation of clots within the blood vessels were reported under microchemical study, 1950, by Erwin Chargaff (biochemistry, Columbia). In 1946 in England J. B. Duguid (pathology, University of Durham) revived a view advanced a century ago by Rokitansky (but not endorsed by Virchow) that the fibrous thickening of atherosclerotic arteries, described by most modern investigators as fatty degeneration with fibrous overgrowth of the intima, is in reality a blood product. This theory suggests that fibrinous deposits may partially occlude the vessels, become covered with endothelium and appear to be part of the intima; multiple mural deposits in the same location might explain the progressive nature of atherosclerotic lesions. Occurrence of atheroma in arteries but not in veins (N. G. B. McLetchie, pathology, Dalhousie University, Halifax, 1952) may be referable to the greater stress in arteries. Potentially significant also would be demonstration of deficiency of fibrinolysin in the blood of arteriosclerotic patients which Hans Selye (Institute of Experimental Medicine and Surgery, University of Montreal, 1950) thought might indicate a deficiency of the enzyme that breaks down fibrin, resulting in abnormal deposits of fibrinoid material on artery walls. To test the hypothesis that organized mural thrombi may result in primary pulmonary arteriosclerosis in man, C. V. Harrison (morbid anatomy, Postgraduate Medical School, London, 1948) produced small emboli in the pulmonary arteries of rabbits by intravenous injection of finely fragmented fibrin clot; the resulting lesions were said to be "morphologically indistinguishable from spontaneous arteriosclerosis". In 1951, Knisely was attempting to produce in monkeys multiple minute obstructions in the cerebral arteries and to correlate changes in the brain and in cerebral vessels with psychological and physical changes in the animals.

Duguid admitted that the thrombosis hypothesis leaves unsolved the problem of fatty changes in atherosclerosis, but suggested that the lipid substances, appearing also in the fibrinous vegetations in endocarditis, are blood products forming mural thrombi; other lipid substances causing the superficial fatty streaking in the human aorta, and cholesterol-induced fatty deposits in the rabbit aorta he attributed to generalized metabolic disturbances. The view that "changes in the chemical composition of arterial tissue are, in large part, a reflection of its plasma environment" was challenged by M. D. Siperstein, I. L. Chaikoff and Sidney S. Chernick, 1951, who showed that slices of aortic tissue (rabbit, chicken) synthesized cholesterol from isotope-marked acetate. In any case, demonstration of the metabolic capabilities of arterial tissue, indicated by the presence of enzymes known to be active in synthesis or breakdown of specific metabolites, argues against the assumption that all cholesterol, calcium, protein compounds found in arterial lesions are carried preformed to these sites by the blood stream. Reactions known to result from activities of a large number of competing and cooperating enzyme systems (formation of fatty acids and phospholipids) were demonstrated in rat aorta *in vitro* by Chaikoff and associates, 1949. Presumptive evidence of utilization of carbohydrate by rat arterial tissue was obtained by use of enzyme inhibitors. Phosphatases, enzymes involved in phosphorus and calcium metabolism, demonstrated in human aorta by J. E. Kirk and coworkers (gerontology, Washington University, 1950), "will have to be considered in future discussions on arterial calcification". Studies of normal and atherosclerotic human aortic tissues with reference to mineral metabolism (R. C. Buck and R. J. Rossiter, University of Western Ontario, 1951) indicated a ratio of calcium to phosphorus similar to the ratio in bone and only slight mineral increase in atherosclerotic portions of the aorta compared with the total increase associated with aging.

While other vessels, as the splenic artery, show extensive atherosclerotic changes, sclerosis of coronary, cerebral and renal arteries has become an especially important focus in investigative work because of the vital character of the circulation in heart, brain, kidney. "The

peculiar susceptibility [to atherosclerosis] of a few tenths of a gram, or
at most a few grams, of coronary intima", which appears to explain
the chief cause of death of American men during their period of
highest earning capacity, led William Dock (Long Island College of
Medicine) to test the theory that one factor in this susceptibility is a
peculiar thickness of the intimal layer in male coronaries; his observations, 1946, indicated in new-born males an intima three times
thicker than in new-born females.   In line with the possibility that
local mechanical factors might determine the first sites of atheroma
formation in the coronaries, Dock, 1950, was "tempted to think of
vibrating collagen fibers as churns which form visible aggregates from
cholesterol in solution or suspension in the interstitial fluid".   An experimental approach to the influence of pre-existing injury (local
injury of coronaries of dogs followed by intravenous injections of egg
yolk emulsions) was described as indicating accumulation of cholesterol in extensive lesions in the injured areas, which, however, showed
measurable recovery after cholesterol injections were stopped (Levin
L. Waters, pathology, Yale, 1953).

Susceptibility of cerebral arteries to atherosclerosis was referred by
Stanley Cobb and Daniel Blain (neuropathology, Harvard, 1933) to
cerebral circulatory factors, to the metabolism and oxygen requirements of the brain.   The small cerebral arteries differ from arteries
of the same size elsewhere in that the adventitia is very thin, and in
the thicker media there is, as pointed out by A. E. Cohn over a decade
ago, less elastic tissue and muscle, with collagen appearing earlier
and in larger amounts.   The question why, since atherosclerotic
lesions may occur in arteries anywhere, certain areas of the brain
should manifest distinctive "local vulnerability" and greater susceptibility to ischemia or massive apoplectic hemorrhage was raised,
1951, by Karl Stern (psychiatry, McGill, later Ottawa).   The answer
suggested was that the patterns of arteries entering the brain determine the points that will suffer most from pulsation and from thrombi.
The consequences include not only the hazard of death by hemorrhage
but also of deterioration resulting from anoxia due to decreased blood
flow.   Seymour S. Kety and associates (pharmacology, Pennsylvania)
recalled, 1951, their finding in earlier experiments with normal young
men that reduction of cerebral venous oxygen content for even so

short a period as thirty minutes resulted in "definite mental changes". In later studies also, of ten cases of senile psychosis (six of them attributed to cerebral arteriosclerosis), the Kety group thought that the degree of anoxia of brain tissue which they found "could in itself be responsible for most of the mental deterioration in these patients". They considered, however, that "unequivocal demonstration that psychosis depends upon the reported circulatory and metabolic changes" would depend upon repeating the studies in a comparable series of elderly individuals without psychosis. The importance of the possible connection is suggested by figures (National Institute of Mental Health) indicating that in 1951 for sixteen per cent of first admissions of psychotic patients in all public and private hospitals the diagnosis was psychosis associated with arteriosclerosis.

Whether sclerotic lesions in the renal arteries induce hypertension by initiating a chain of events involving a renal pressor mechanism, or whether generalized atherosclerosis is a morphological change in arteries subjected to the stress and strain of hypertension is an unresolved controversy. Amplifying the former theory, that atherosclerotic lesions in the major renal arteries antedate hypertension, Jonas S. Friedenwald (Wilmer Ophthalmological Institute, Johns Hopkins) observed, 1947: "When such a lesion is sufficient to mimic a Goldblatt clamp, a humoral and renal phase of the hypertensive disease will be superimposed on the previous atherosclerotic phase." To test the latter theory that atherosclerosis results from hypertension, a few experimental approaches have been devised: Katz, with Jeremiah Stamler, 1950 and 1951, found that salt-induced hypertension without a cholesterol supplement had no effect on the incidence, extent and severity of atherosclerosis in the chick. In rabbits, dogs, sheep and goats on diets without cholesterol supplement, hypertension alone did not induce atherosclerosis. Hypertension induced in chicks and rabbits with hypercholesterolemia apparently, however, accelerated formation of atheromata. Certain pathological evidence (Dock, 1953) has indicated correlation of atherosclerosis with the levels of arterial pressure. Locally, the occurrence of atheromata in the aorta may be "massive" at its forked division into two branches when in the arch only a few small plaques are seen. Clinical observations have noted five times more frequent occurrence of myocardial infarction between the ages of twenty and sixty in a hypertensive than in a normotensive population (Kendall, 1950).

## STUDIES OF METABOLISM OF LIPIDS GENERALLY IN RELATION TO ATHEROSCLEROSIS

Investigative interest in atherosclerosis over many years has been concerned largely with the metabolism of lipids. Much speculation has been directed toward attempts to define the role, in the characteristic changes of atherosclerosis, of simple lipids as neutral fats, compound lipids as phospholipids, cholesterol. Concentration of interest upon cholesterol especially has been due to various factors, several of which were briefly mentioned previously: the fact that cholesterol has been a consistent finding, over the years, in atheromatous deposits; experiments showing that excessive dietary cholesterol produces a high serum cholesterol concentration and atherosclerosis in rabbits and chicks; observations in some (but not all) recent studies that average concentrations of serum cholesterol are higher in persons with coronary occlusion than in normal subjects of the same age groups. From these unrelated findings and from deductions (often criticized as unwarranted) developed the hypothesis that dietary cholesterol produces hypercholesterolemia in man as it does in rabbits, and that there is a cause and effect relation between excess of cholesterol in the blood and deposition of cholesterol in human arteries. Many workers still look toward unraveling the mysteries of cholesterol metabolism as the liveliest hope of discovering the cause of atherosclerosis and possibly its prevention and cure.

On the other hand, there are those who feel that preoccupation with cholesterol has greatly and harmfully narrowed the investigative picture; that instead of centering attention upon cholesterolemia it is necessary to consider not only the concentrations but also the proportions of lipids in the serum, in which the free lipids (i.e., neutral fat and other lipids not bound by or combined with protein) may be quite as significant as cholesterol; that cholesterol synthesized by body tissues, including arterial tissue, may be of greater importance in the pathogenesis of spontaneous arteriosclerosis than has hitherto been supposed (Chaikoff and associates, 1951); that investigation of the significance of cholesterol must be brought within "the framework of the chemistry and physiology of lipids" generally (Peters, 1952). There are also the questions and reservations inevitably involved in all applications of experimental work to human conditions: with reference, for instance, to the "decisive significance" (Anitschkow) of hypercholesterolemia, resulting, in rabbits, from dietary cholesterol, it was pointed out by C. B. Taylor and R. Gordon Gould (biochemistry, Illinois, 1950) that rabbits respond to dietary cholesterol, as do other animals, by a decrease in synthesis of cholesterol from labeled acetate, but they differ in having normally a much slower rate of synthesis (and therefore of disposal) of cholesterol, "and this may be of significance in explaining their remarkable sensitivity to dietary cholesterol". Arterial deposits of cholesterol in the rabbit are only a part of a general lipoidosis in which many tissues, including the liver, appear to be involved. The normal rabbit, as Peters put it, reacts to cholesterol "as other animals do only when they are hypothyroid". In man, fatty diets may increase the fat stores of the body but they do not produce hyperlipemia (Peters and Man, 1953). Ancel Keys (physiological hygiene, Minnesota) and associates, however, reported, 1952, that changes in fat intake, either vegetable or animal, "have a profound effect" on cholesterol concentrations "even if caloric and cholesterol intake are constant". On the other hand, there appears to be agreement that, in man, excess dietary cholesterol is without effect on blood cholesterol concentrations (Peters and Man, 1953; Keys and associates, 1952; Gertler and associates, 1950); Keys added, however, "if calorie and fat intake are constant". Thus the simple narrative of excess dietary cholesterol, then excess cholesterol in the blood, then deposition in the intima of the arteries becomes measurably complicated. More must be known of the physiology and metabolism of lipids generally. And beyond this are apparently other still unknown factors that determine arterial susceptibility to lipid deposition. Peters, in summary, observed: "The available evidence suggests that cholesterol accumulates in the walls of the arteries when these are affected by degenerative processes or suffer local injury. The nature of the noxious influences which pave the way for the deposition of cholesterol remains to be discovered."

Evidence supporting the local injury hypothesis includes such observations as that of Lansing and associates (1950) that intimal fibrosis (hyperplasia) occurs frequently without deposition of either cholesterol or calcium in the intima; that of Waters (1950) showing that, in the dog, injected lipids, or under some conditions the body's own fat, accumulate selectively at sites of injury in the coronary arteries.

So long as the mechanisms of the "noxious influences" that injure arterial tissues and make them susceptible to lipid deposition remain unknown, the problem of atherosclerosis cannot be completely solved. Meanwhile work reported in connection with both of the approaches outlined above marks stages in developing knowledge. And the two approaches should be viewed perhaps not as antithetic but as counter and corrective hypotheses that lead to progressively sounder perspective.

## Work Illustrating Dominant Investigative Interest in Cholesterol

What is known of the nature of the sterol, cholesterol, and its metabolism is pertinent in all attempts to define its relation to atherosclerosis. It has been related to fats because it resembles them in solubility, because it combines with fatty acids to form cholesterol esters, and because its concentration in the serum of normal persons varies with that of phospholipids which are connected with the metabolism of fat. While the functions of many of the compound and derived lipids, of which cholesterol is one, are "quite obscure" (Peters, 1952), some information concerning their formation and fate has been gained by labeling them with isotopes or peculiar fatty acids. While free cholesterol is found in all tissues, cholesterol esters (combinations of cholesterol with fatty acids) occur only in the circulating plasma (where they exceed free cholesterol), the intestinal mucosa and the tissues in which steroids are synthesized (liver, adrenal cortex, sex glands). "The esterification of cholesterol, therefore, seems to be connected with the metabolic activities of cholesterol itself." Esters are not found in most cells. The inference is (Peters, 1952) that, if esters gain access to the cells of arterial walls in which they are not normally found, "the antecedent integrity and vitality of the cells must be questioned". In arterial cells already injured, deposition of foreign matter (as esterified cholesterol) would be exaggerated by increased concentration of foreign matter in the serum. In point here are Chaikoff's previously mentioned studies of atheromatous lesions in dogs (which are subject to spontaneous atherosclerosis but peculiarly resistant to hypercholesterolemia); lipids were found in the older lesions but in early lesions there was evidence only of degeneration, cell necrosis and scar tissue.

Those that look toward cholesterol as the most likely clue to solution of the problems of atherosclerosis naturally attach investigative significance to measurements of serum cholesterol often regarded as a symbol of serum lipids in general. Since 1940, however, it has been clear that cholesterol concentrations alone are inadequate indications of blood lipids and that relative concentrations of cholesterol, phospholipids, serum proteins are more revealing (Hirsch and Weinhouse, 1940). For this reason and because concentrations of lipid components vary extremely in the serum of normal individuals, any single determination of cholesterol is to be interpreted "only with the greatest reserve" (Peters, 1952). Practically in point also is the fact that accurate measurement of serum lipids is a difficult and time-consuming procedure, beyond the capacity of the ordinary clinical laboratory. The newer methods (ultracentrifuge, tagged isotopes) are progressively clarifying the character and relations of blood lipids and colloidal complexes.

Among recent studies reporting that average concentrations of serum cholesterol are higher in persons with arteriosclerosis than in normal subjects of the same age is the Harvard coronary research project (Menard M. Gertler, Stanley M. Garn, Paul D. White, Jacob Lerman, others). Findings in this project, comparing ninety-seven men who had had coronary heart disease before forty with 146 healthy men in all of whom factors that might influence serum cholesterol concentrations were matched, indicated in the coronary disease group higher values of serum cholesterol (total, free and, especially, esterified), of serum phospholipids and markedly higher cholesterol-lipid phospholipid ratios. The final concentration of serum cholesterol was considered to result from several interdependent factors — utilization, synthesis and availability of the substance for metabolic needs. Maximum concentrations were found by Keys and associates (1950) in presumably normal men at about fifty-five years, the age at which, in males, severe or fatal coronary atherosclerosis occurs most frequently. Other studies (W. B. Kountz and associates, gerontology division, Washington University, 1945) have suggested lack of correlation between blood cholesterol and arteriosclerosis: elderly female patients had higher blood cholesterol concentrations although onset of arteriosclerosis was earlier in the males; in patients (both sexes) with low serum cholesterol concentrations peripheral arteriosclerosis was more common. These more or less confusing results of attempts to establish correlations in human atherosclerosis could be in part referable to wide natural variation in cholesterol values in the population. Eskimos in the East Canadian Arctic suggested to R. G. Sinclair and associates (biochemistry and medicine, Queens University, 1949) that part of the population, both young and middle-aged, have (like rabbits) high and unstable cholesterol values, sensitive to added cholesterol or to diets rich in fats and calories; others (like dogs) maintain concentrations under 200 mgm. on rich diets; in an intermediate group high calorie, high fat and cholesterol diets seemed to provide "the straw to break the camel's back".

Always recurrent is the question as to just what experimental cholesterol-induced atherosclerosis has to offer by way of throwing light on human atherosclerosis. Without doubt experimentally induced atherosclerosis has raised a great many questions, has answered some of them in ways helpful to investigative work on human atherosclerosis, and has left others unanswered. Among the latter is, for instance, the question whether the rabbit lacks a metabolic mechanism for handling a substance foreign to the diet. The rabbit, however, synthesizes cholesterol from the same small molecular units from which other mammals synthesize it. Comments on the significance of the rabbit findings include the view that because rabbits resemble other mammals qualitatively in their metabolic processes, it cannot be inferred that they do not differ quantitatively. Data on susceptibility to cholesterol-induced atherosclerosis in different species increases, with almost yearly changes in the list of susceptibles and nonsusceptibles: the 1952 list of susceptible species, in addition to rabbit, chicken and dog, included guinea pig, golden hamster, prairie gopher, goose; the nonsusceptible list included rat, mouse, cat, goat, fox, pigeon, parrot, monkey. Repeated failure of cholesterol feeding to induce atherosclerosis in young rhesus monkeys (Hueper, 1946) was considered by Rinehart and Greenberg "a potent argument against the cholesterol theory as a major influence in the pathogenesis of atherosclerosis" in man, although these investigators described, 1949, production in these monkeys, by dietary means (prolonged pyridoxine deficiency), of lesions resembling human atherosclerosis. In the New World cebus monkey, used by a group of investigators in nutrition and pathology at Harvard (G. V. Mann, S. B. Andrus, Ann McNally, F. J. Stare) primarily interested in development of a dependable experimental animal for atherosclerosis research, aortic lesions were reported, 1953, following diets high in cholesterol and deficient in sulfur amino acids. Continuing work on chicken and dog has pointed to distribution of lesions very similar to that in man. In rabbits following cholesterol feeding, cholesterol deposits appear in the reticuloendothelial system and viscera before arterial lesions develop. While certain workers had reported no change in cerebral vessels in the experimental disease, careful examination of rabbits fed dried and heated egg yolk as a source of cholesterol revealed foam cell formation in the lining and around the wall of cerebral vessels (Altschul, 1946); the degree of change was less than that in human cerebral vessels, however, and the morphology was not identical.

The contention that man is the only mammal in which spontaneous atherosclerosis occurs in significant degree (absence of lesions having been reported in large numbers of domesticated, laboratory, zoological garden animals living out their full lifespan) has been partly invalidated by finding of spontaneous atherosclerosis in birds, especially chickens (usually asymptomatic and not lethal) and in dogs (including coronary artery and heart disease in older dogs). Comparative studies (Chaikoff and associates, 1950) of spontaneous coronary lesions in birds and lesions induced by diethylstilbestrol injection and cholesterol feeding showed marked differences: spontaneous lesions consisted of intimal plaques entirely free of lipid; lesions induced by stilbestrol, confined to the media, consisted of lipids; lesions induced by cholesterol feeding appeared to be intimal and medial and contained lipids. Spontaneous atherosclerosis was found (Katz and associates, 1948, and the California workers) in chickens on diets practically devoid of cholesterol although with dietary cholesterol the lesions developed more rapidly. Lesions produced in dogs by feeding thiouracil and cholesterol (Alfred Steiner with Kendall and others, 1949) were regarded as identical with cholesterol-induced lesions in other species and "but a part of a widespread deposition of cholesterol in many tissues" (Chaikoff and associates, 1952); on the contrary, in spontaneous lesions in the dog, even older lesions, minimal lipid infiltration was "not related to cholesterol deposition".

### STUDY OF FACTORS THAT MAY INFLUENCE CHOLESTEROL METABOLISM OR OCCURRENCE OF ARTERIOSCLEROSIS

Factors, in addition to species differences, to which work on chicken and dog has pointed as possibly influencing cholesterol metabolism or arterial pathology include: diet and obesity; hormone influences; lipotropic substances; the diabetic state. While Keys's 1952 studies at Minnesota, Oxford and Naples produced no definite evidence of correlation of obesity with high cholesterol levels, Keys, in 1949, had found in a group of five hundred apparently normal men that fatter men tended to have higher cholesterol values even at the same age and with substantially the same basal metabolism. Precise chemical studies seem to indicate that obesity is not directly correlated with hyperlipemia (Peters, 1952): that high calorie diets, while they may increase the fat stores in the body, do not produce hyperlipemia (Steiner, 1948; Wilkinson and associates, 1950); that administration of cholesterol does not disturb normal lipid interrelations (Entenman and Chaikoff, 1940; Keys and associates, 1950). It is generally admitted that definite undernutrition lowers serum cholesterol (but this is a pathological dietary state).

Opinions concerning a relation of obesity to incidence of arteriosclerosis are sharply divided. Experimental evidence was interpreted in favor of obesity as a factor by J. B. Firstbrook (Banting Best

Institute, Toronto, 1950), in whose cholesterol-fed rabbits low initial body weight or loss of body weight inhibited development of atherosclerosis. In the cholesterol-fed chick, however, restriction of the rest of the diet to two-thirds of normal failed to prevent development of atheromatosis (Rodbard, Bolenc, Katz, 1951). In a study of 1,300 autopsies at Bellevue Hospital, Sigmund L. Wilens (pathology, New York University, 1947) found advanced arteriosclerosis ten times as common in the obese of each age group, while twice as many of the poorly nourished had little or no arteriosclerosis. Among reports of correlation between incidence of arteriosclerosis and wartime or otherwise limited diets was Steiner's 1951 finding that of a hundred autopsied cases in all age groups among the poor of Okinawa (who live virtually without animal food products) only seven showed arteriosclerosis (minimal) of the aorta and no coronary disease. In the other direction, various reports correlate rising incidence of atherosclerosis in postwar Norway, Sweden, Finland with increased consumption of cholesterol, fat and calories. The difficulty of restricting dietary cholesterol in man, except by rigid exclusion of all dairy and animal products, was pointed out, 1950, by Keys who found that at least two hundred mg. of cholesterol are consumed daily in diets containing only ordinary amounts of lean meat and skimmed milk. The previously mentioned coronary research project at Harvard and the Massachusetts General Hospital adds to clinical evidence challenging the hypothesis that dietary cholesterol and fats are causally related to coronary heart disease and atherosclerosis; serum cholesterol concentrations were considered to result not from ingested cholesterol but from interplay of availability of building materials and rate of synthesis, on the one hand, and of rate or means of utilization on the other, that is, on metabolic variants. Variants influencing cholesterol metabolism in animals include: deficiency of pantothenic acid reported to decrease in rats the high liver and serum cholesterol following addition of one per cent to the diet (R. R. Guehring, L. S. Hurley and A. F. Morgan, biochemistry, California, 1953); deficiency of certain amino acids resulting in cholesterol-induced atherosclerosis in the nonsusceptible cebus monkey (Stare and coworkers, 1953); complete failure of absorption of cholesterol from the intestinal tract in the absence of bile, and prevention of rise in serum cholesterol and of atheromata in chickens by feeding ferric chloride, known to precipitate bile *in vitro* (Chaikoff and associates, 1953).

Evidence associating several hormones with cholesterol metabolism and atherosclerosis in various species is largely of the older type of metabolic experiment and observation (measurements of blood levels, examination of tissues to determine rates and sites of deposition, study of effects of hormone administration on development of gross lesions.) The thyroid is believed by many to decrease hypercholesterolemia by aiding deposition in various tissues or by suppressing shifts from tissue depots to the blood stream. Administration of thiouracil to depress thyroid activity in dogs simultaneously with cholesterol feeding was found (Steiner and Kendall, 1949) to produce more marked hypercholesterolemia and earlier lesions than "unphysiological" cholesterol feeding alone which required a year for production of gross lesions. Desiccated thyroid was found (Katz and associates, 1950) to reduce atherosclerosis induced in chicks by repeated implantations of diethylstilbestrol, although it had no sustained effect on concentration of plasma and tissue lipids. It was suggested that relations between ovary and thyroid were probably mediated by the pituitary. Two years after complete removal of thyroid and pituitary, twenty-one dogs (Lindsay, Chaikoff with others, 1952) showed high plasma lipid concentrations; early aortic and coronary lesions "identical with" those described previously in normal dogs; lesions in the coronaries with primary lipid deposition; small amounts of cholesterol, not found in the spontaneous lesions. Broader metabolic implications as to hormonal influences are suggested by a 1949 report from Chaikoff's laboratory that thyroid increased tissue respiration of the excised rat aorta and thiouracil decreased it; by observations with radioactive tracers (DeWitt Stetten, Jr., Public Health Research Institute, New York, 1949) that hyperthyroidism may lead to disproportionate increase in hepatic degradation of fat. Rapid increases in concentration of the blood lipids in dogs after thyroidectomy was shown by Entenman, Chaikoff and Reichert (1942) to depend upon adequate caloric intake. While the nutritional state was not the sole factor, it, rather than the thyroidectomy, was considered to be essential in production of hyperlipemia. Studying, in a small group of patients, the hypercholesterolemia that followed thyroidectomy performed to alleviate angina pectoris and congestive heart failure, Herrman L. Blumgart and associates (medicine, Harvard, 1952) concluded that the hypothyroid state with its hypercholesterolemia does not necessarily produce coronary atherosclerosis. It has been emphasized (Chaikoff, 1953) that findings in estrogen-induced atherosclerosis in birds (peculiar in the ovarian control of lipid metabolism) are not applicable to man. All of these observations are in keeping with the established finding that the hormones do not initiate metabolic processes but merely alter the rates of the reactions, acute hypothyroidism, for instance, lowering the rate of utilization of dietary lipids. Understanding hormonal control of mechanisms of lipid synthesis ("almost completely unknown") requires (Samuel Gurin and Roscoe O. Brady, physiological chemistry, Pennsylvania, 1953) study of individual metabolic steps, just beginning.

A belief on the part of some workers that lipotropic substances (derived from the pancreas; choline, or its precursors, methionine and betaine), known to inhibit development of fatty livers in a number of species, might prevent lipid deposition in the arteries has led to their clinical use. An early observation (in Macleod's laboratory at Toronto, 1924) that fatty livers in depancreatized dogs treated with insulin over several years could be prevented by adding raw pancreas to the diet was related (Charles H. Best and C. C. Lucas, Banting and Best Research Institute, 1943) to factors other than insulin in the pancreas. Continuing work at Toronto and at Michigan (H. C. Eckstein, biological chemistry) established that dietary choline (active constituent of the phospholipid, lecithin), methionine and casein had similar lipotropic activity; choline prevented deposition of neutral fat and also of cholesterol in the liver and accelerated removal of both from it. Demonstration that the effects of feeding pancreas fractions to depancreatized dogs could not be accounted for by their choline or methionine content pointed (Chaikoff and Entenman, 1948) to another type of antifatty liver factor in the pancreas. Reports of tests of the efficacy of choline in inhibiting induction of experimental atherosclerosis by cholesterol continue to be contradictory (Steiner, 1948; Davidson, Meyer, and Kendall, 1951). Liver lipids and serum lipids are not directly correlated; on the contrary, the dietary fatty liver is usually accompanied by hypolipemia, not hyperlipemia. For this reason, Peters commented, 1953, attempts to prove the beneficent effect of lipotropic factors are "not altogether logical". A Michael Reese Hospital group expressed in 1950 a view that "neither on theoretic, nor experimental, nor clinical grounds is there today a firm scientific basis for the widespread clinical use of costly lipotropic preparations in the prophylaxis and/or therapy of human atherosclerosis".

Diabetics, it has been observed, develop atherosclerosis earlier and in greater severity than nondiabetics. Cardiovascular-renal disease (atherosclerosis predominantly) rose as the proximate cause of death in diabetics from 17.5 per cent, 1897–1914, to 70.1 per cent, 1944–1949 (E. P. Joslin, New England Deaconess Hospital, 1950). Whether the two conditions are conceivably "two branches of the same tree" (Henry T. Ricketts, Mayo Clinic, 1947) is not established. Recent evidence, however, points definitely to an effect of insulin on the rates of formation of fat from two-carbon compounds (Gurin and Brady, 1953). The disturbance of serum lipids in diabetes appears to be referable not to the disease itself but to the numerous disorders which accompany it. The lipids vary greatly in diabetes according to the state of the patient, defying gross statistical analysis (Peters and associates, 1953). The assumption that diabetic retinitis is a localized form of atherosclerosis was repudiated, 1947, by Friedenwald, who attributed the retinitis to generalized capillary fragility related in some unknown way to the metabolic disturbances of diabetes. Clinical studies of diabetics have indicated correlation of hyperlipemia and phospholipid-cholesterol ratios with severity of atherosclerosis but not with the state of the diabetic condition (Julius Pomeranze, New York Medical College, and H. G. Kunkel, Hospital of the Rockefeller Institute, 1950; L. T. DeWind, G. D. Michaels and L. W. Kinsell, Highland Alameda County Hospital, California, 1952). Findings of comparable hypercholesterolemia in cholesterol-fed normal and diabetic rabbits but less severe aortic atherosclerosis in the latter (G. Lyman Duff and associates, pathology, McGill, 1948) have been attributed to loss of body weight in the diabetic animals (Firstbrook, 1951), to tearing down of body tissues, including atherosclerotic lesions during starvation (Chaikoff, 1953). Chaikoff and Hotta suggested, 1952, that evaluation of factors influencing early development of arteriosclerosis in the diabetic should include study of possible increased rate of cholesterol synthesis by the liver. While Brady and Gurin had concluded, 1950, that the ability of the diabetic liver to synthesize cholesterol is unimpaired, Chaikoff's group reported "definite increase in cholesterol formation" by livers from untreated diabetic rats, while livers from insulin-treated rats showed a definite reduction.

## RECENT APPROACHES TO SYNTHESIS AND BREAKDOWN OF CHOLESTEROL

Clearly, elucidation of the assumed role of cholesterol in arterial disease processes depends (Konrad Bloch, biochemistry, Chicago, 1950) upon prior solution of basic problems of intermediary lipid metabolism generally. Whether or not deposition of cholesterol in arterial lesions is related to increased synthesis of cholesterol or to faulty disposal of cholesterol cannot be proved without knowledge, still lacking, of the metabolic steps by which cholesterol is broken down and built up by body cells. According to Bloch, 1952, "information on the biological role of cholesterol has only recently begun to accumulate and we are still in the process of establishing the molecular details by which the steroids are synthesized and broken down in the animal cells". In 1951, confirmation of the structure of cholesterol by its total synthesis in the laboratory was announced by Robert B. Woodward and associates (Converse Memorial Laboratory, Harvard). Since 1937, there has been evidence that many small molecules are used in cholesterol synthesis *in vivo*. Between 1942 and 1946, study of cholesterol synthesis in animals with the aid of isotopic markers (Bloch, Schoenheimer and Rittenberg in the Columbia biochemistry department) had produced abundant indirect evidence that the carbon incorporated into the steroid nucleus of cholesterol (its claim to relationship with the steroids) is derived from acetic acid or closely related two-carbon units. This knowledge, relating cholesterol to the common currency of metabolic interchange (two-carbon fragments attached as an acetyl group to coenzyme A, as shown by Fritz Lipmann and associates, 1947–1951) emphasized that cholesterol synthesis is not dependent upon dietary fat. Rather, the two-carbon fragments are derived from carbohydrate, most amino acids, acetaldehyde and other sources, and enter the metabolic pool upon which cells draw for their synthetic activities and for energy to carry them on. Bloch, 1952, considered carbohydrate to be the most important source of building materials for cholesterol and also probably a source of energy for its synthesis. Fatty acids (in which the two-carbon fragments are also used) were synthesized in surviving liver tissue from glucose in 1950 experiments in Chaikoff's laboratory. The two-carbon fragments may not be incorporated directly into the cholesterol molecule but may be used first in synthesis of intermediates, as yet unknown. Lack of knowledge of these intermediary compounds, believed to be built up rapidly and as rapidly transformed, has created an *impasse* in all attempts to trace the steps leading to synthesis and involved in breakdown of cholesterol *in vivo*.

Renewed attempts to identify intermediates are naturally concerned with the sites of these activities. The hypothesis that end products of cholesterol identified in bile and in intestinal contents may not arise from breakdown in the intestines but may be formed by metabolic conversion in the liver was under study (Page and Menschick, 1952; Meyer Friedman and coworkers, Mt. Zion Hospital, San Francisco, 1950–1953; Harry J. Deuel, Jr., biochemistry, University of Southern California, 1948). Another approach attempts to increase reduction of cholesterol in the intestines to the unabsorbable coprosterol (Robert B. Gordon, S. C. Kraft and Richard J. Jones, medicine and surgery, Chicago, 1953). Efforts to determine sites of cholesterol synthesis (the liver, although an important is not the sole site) look toward eventual study of these reactions in cell-free preparations at the molecular level. In rats and mice, synthesis from C 14–labeled acetate was reported, 1950, to occur in intestinal mucosa, liver, skin and other tissues (C. B. Taylor and R. G. Gould, Presbyterian Hospital, Chicago); synthesis in arterial tissue was reported, 1951, from Chaikoff's laboratory. Although steroid synthesis has been observed only in systems containing intact cells, preparation from pigeon liver of a cell-free system capable of incorporating C 14–labeled acetate into long-chain fatty acids was reported, 1951 (Brady and Gurin); cholesterol was synthesized from such precursors only in intact tissues *in vitro*. The site of cholesterol esterification and synthesis in the cell and the effect of cholesterol feeding on these cell functions were under study, 1953, by Deuel and associates.

Whether or not rates of cholesterol synthesis are related to development of atherosclerosis, knowledge of the mechanisms by which the rates are normally maintained is essential to study of possible disturbance of the rates. That endogenous synthesis of cholesterol continues at rates far in excess of that required for synthesis of steroid hormones and bile acids, of which cholesterol is an intermediary (Bloch, 1950), was considered certain by Kellner, who estimated, 1952, that so much as 1,500 to 2,000 mg. is synthesized daily by normal man. Evidence for the existence of a homeostatic mechanism in the liver, "the most likely site for the synthesis of plasma cholesterol" (Chaikoff), for regulation of cholesterol synthesis was found in depression of synthesis by dietary cholesterol (Taylor and Gould, 1950; Chaikoff and associates, 1953; Langdon and Bloch, 1953), raising again the question of the advantage of dietary restriction (Chaikoff). Search for compounds involved as intermediates in cholesterol synthesis, for mechanisms of regulation of synthesis and metabolism of cholesterol, for means of inducing a reduction in cholesterol synthesis without feeding cholesterol, was active, 1953, in a number of other biochemistry laboratories (Harland G. Wood, Western Reserve; David M. Greenberg, California; Harry J. Deuel, Jr., Southern California). Endogenous cholesterol synthesized from labeled acetate was found (Gould, 1950) widely distributed in the body, and changes in distribution after the first four hours during which synthesis was active "must be due to transport or to metabolic conversion".

## MECHANISMS OF LIPID TRANSPORT AND STABILIZATION IN THE BLOOD STREAM IN RELATION TO ATHEROSCLEROSIS

Rapid advances in knowledge of chemistry and metabolism of the lipids have revealed that these substances, many of which were formerly considered inert (depot fat) or metabolically inactive (cholesterol), are intimately involved in the continuous exchange of metabolic cycles. One of the questions that have particularly baffled chemists and biologists is how water-insoluble lipids — cholesterol, cholesterol esters, phospholipids, neutral fat — are carried by the blood plasma. The possible mechanisms of lipid transport have recently come under review in connection with atherosclerosis research. Quite aside from the question whether or not the lipids, especially cholesterol, in arterial lesions are deposited there by the blood, these mechanisms would have a certain background interest and significance. More than forty years ago, pathological study in atheromatous lesions of large globular phagocytic cells filled with lipids ("foam cells") led to theories (based upon Virchow's concept) that these cells had become loaded with cholesterol (an inert, "foreign" substance) in the fixed reticuloendothelial cells of the liver, spleen and other tissues, and had carried their load *via* the blood stream directly to the subendothelial layer of the intima. By another view, the cholesterol was taken up initially by the arterial endothelial cells themselves from the plasma that bathes their surface and then either passed on to the subendothelial layer or carried into it by migration of the endothelial cells which then appear as foam cells. Objections to these theoretical concepts have been supported by studies with newer methods: Gofman's studies, 1951, with ionium-labeled colloids (which are ordinarily taken up by the fixed cells of liver, spleen, bone marrow) indicating no evidence of such migratory transport in development of rabbit lesions; Duff's studies, 1950–1951, using a wetting or surface-active agent (Tween 80) to facilitate accumulation of lipids in the fixed cells, indicating abundant foam cells in the blood stream but only minimal arterial lesions and no plugging of vasa vasorum with foam cells. Duff, 1951, concluded, as had others previously (Hirsch and Weinhouse, 1940; W. C. Hueper, 1945) that, in the genesis of experimental cholesterol atherosclerosis, the relation of serum cholesterol to other serum lipids, especially phospholipids, and to the serum proteins is even more important than the concentration of cholesterol itself.

Ratios between cholesterol and phospholipids in the serum, long regarded as important in lipid transport (W. R. Bloor, biochemistry, Rochester, 1943), have more recently been studied in relation to arteriosclerosis, and other disease states, as infectious hepatitis and obstructive jaundice (Peters and associates, 1950). The latter investigators demonstrated a close relationship of the serum phospholipids to the free cholesterol, even when the ratio of free to total cholesterol was markedly distorted. Attempts have been made to test experimentally and clinically the concept that disparity in this ratio might be correlated with development of atherosclerosis: by Kellner and associates at Cornell, 1951; by Pomeranze and Kunkel, 1950; by Ahrens and Kunkel, 1953. Whatever the significance of turbid serum to atherosclerosis may be, there is obvious need of greater knowledge of the mechanisms governing the stability of the serum lipids. In studies since 1947, aimed at discovering the stabilizing mechanisms, H. S. Simms and associates (pathology, Columbia) followed in tissue cultures of chicken and human arteries two agents obtained from serum and named lipfanogens and antilipfanogens. Lipfanogens were described as substances taken up from the plasma by living cells and converted into visible fat; segments of arteries incubated in medium containing lipfanogen were reported to develop lipid deposits similar to early lesions *in vivo*. Antilipfanogens were described as substances in the albumin fraction of serum capable of preventing fat deposition. Studying the ratios of the two agents in human serum, these workers reported, 1951, higher proportionate values for lipfanogen in males, and in patients with diabetes, coronary disease, nephrotic syndrome. Continuing study aims at determining factors that influence the normal inactivation of lipfanogen by combination with antilipfanogens to form an inactive complex.

Combination of serum lipids with serum proteins has long been suggested and the combined macromolecules are referred to as lipoproteins. Such a complex had been described by K. O. Pedersen in Sweden, 1945, as the "x-protein", a labile compound the constituent parts of which could be dissociated by physical manipulations. In connection with the continuous program of studies on serum proteins in the department of biochemistry at Harvard, E. J. Cohn and his group developed quantitative methods for separating the protein components of human plasma. Findings with respect to lipoproteins, discussed before the Faraday Society in 1949 by Cohn with F. R. N. Gurd, John L. Oncley, John T. Edsall, included separation from human plasma of two lipoproteins identified electrophoretically as alpha and beta globulins which, between them, carry almost all the plasma lipids. The beta lipoprotein, isolated in pure form, has been found to be water-soluble although it contains seventy-five per cent lipid. Oncley, Gurd, and M. J. Melin, 1950, described the alpha lipoprotein as composed of fifty per cent protein and fifty per cent lipid, the latter containing cholesterol and phospholipid in equal molecular proportions; the beta lipoprotein contains two molecules of cholesterol to one of phospholipid. As a result of ultracentrifugal study of serum lipoproteins and of the patterns in individual sera of the molecules of different flotation and migration values, J. W. Gofman and his group (medical physics, Berkeley, clinical medicine, San Francisco, University of California) concluded that in human sera one portion of the spectrum of these molecules, the class with relatively low flotation and migration values, ten to twenty, appeared to be correlated with the presence of arteriosclerosis; in rabbits a similar correlation of migration and flotation values of the serum lipoproteins (ten to thirty) appeared to be correlated with presence of atherosclerosis. Although tests of sera from large groups of patients with coronary artery disease and with other diseases thought to predispose to arteriosclerosis were reported to show higher proportion of macromolecules of the ten to twenty class, sera from a large number of presumably normal persons also showed high proportions. The proposal that proportionate levels of these giant molecules may be used to diagnose or predict arteriosclerosis has been received with reservations. Keys thought it "unjustifiable", 1951, to assume that these measurements have greater virtue than simple serum cholesterol measurements. Kellner, 1951, described as "impressive" the association between serum concentration of these lipoprotein molecules and severe atherosclerosis but warned of the pitfalls in diagnosis (clinical or post mortem) of a "practically universal" disease. That increase in proportion of low density complexes (*i.e.*, low in the column of ultracentrifugate) may be explained by "increased proportion of fat in lipoprotein-fat complexes" was proposed, 1952, by Roy H. Turner and associates (medicine, biochemistry and biophysics, Tulane), who have studied since 1948 a system of lipoproteins containing phospholipid and fat but no free cholesterol and little or no esterified cholesterol. Patterns of distribution (proportions of phospholipids) in the system without free cholesterol, and concentration of the system as a whole showed "a tendency toward constancy" in health, under control of a highly efficient regulatory mechanism. Its function of lipid transport "may be of major importance in energy metabolism". Distortion of the patterns at levels where significant concentration of free cholesterol occurs was marked in sera from patients with miscellaneous diseases. The authors proposed study of deviations from normal "under dietary stress or because of disease" as possibly contributing "to a better understanding of normal and pathological physiology of lipids". The view that increased amounts of lipoproteins of various descriptions now under study indicate aberrations in lipid transport suggests that a person with a high level of lipoproteins of the ten to twenty migration and flotation class may not be transporting abnormal amounts of lipid but may be suffering from a piling up of fractions not utilized by cells with faulty metabolism.

The new approaches by physical techniques may supplement the indispensable chemical analyses in breaching the wall that still bounds a large uncharted area in this field. Aside from the practical values for atherosclerosis which may emerge from studies of the tissues of the circulatory system, of the intermediary metabolism of steroids and other lipids, of the physical state of blood lipids, all of these types of study are progressively developing a new biological knowledge which is valuable in itself, and which is capable of constantly stimulating the imagination, strengthening the persistence and mitigating the frustrations of those committed to investigating the unknown.

CHAPTER 5

# Hypertension

*Illustrating developing knowledge of mechanisms
involved in normal and deranged blood pressure*

## INTRODUCTORY

Estimates of the incidence of hypertension in the population fail to
furnish a dependable total because they are arrived at on such varying
principles.   Some of the generally high estimates are based on single

sources (military, industrial, insurance or hospital records); some of them are based on casual or single blood pressure readings, failing to take into account temporary rises from temporary causes; in general, they are based on varying diagnostic criteria which may, for instance, include among hypertensives individuals with elevated systolic but normal diastolic pressure. Work governed by more uniform and more selective principles recently reported (by groups studying the natural history of hypertension in the medical schools and hospitals associated with Harvard, Columbia, New York University, Minnesota, Michigan and other centers) with follow-up of the same hypertensive groups for periods varying from eight to thirty-four years suggests much lower mortality and morbidity figures for hypertension than current estimates would suggest. Exploitation of the undoubted fact that heart disease is the leading cause of death and disability in the population and that hypertension, arteriosclerosis and rheumatism are regarded as the three major "causes" of heart disease has tended also to magnify the hypertension picture. A certain alteration in the perspective is suggested by the testimony of a student of hypertension, George A. Perera, who observed, 1951, that his group had "never observed an incidence greater than six per cent in any series". This estimate, "so different from previous statistics", was cited by Homer W. Smith as evidence of the need for "larger and more reliable studies".

One of the real problems is to distinguish ill from well hypertensives, an undertaking too complex to be achievable by facile numerical criteria. As upper limits of "normal" blood pressure, above 150/90 mm. Hg in persons over fifty and above 140/90 mm. in persons below forty are rather widely accepted. By other workers, however, the normal range is placed at between 90 and 120 mm. Hg systolic, 60 and 80 mm. diastolic; Heymans, 1950, gave 125 to 130 mm. as an average for the normal range in adult systolic pressure. Hope of learning more about the upper limits of normal blood pressure has stimulated, since 1935, large-scale attempts to correlate changes in blood pressure with other factors: age, sex, race (alone or in combination with geographical environment), genetic and constitutional factors, occupation, economic status, climate, temperature, such physiological variables as posture, exercise, digestion, sleep, weight, such psychic variables as emotion. Although in one such study of more than 11,000 persons Robinson and Brucer concluded (1939) that, except in subjects with evident pathology, the normal levels of blood pressure are established in adolescence and do not rise thereafter, it is maintained by some that average values of both systolic and diastolic pressures do rise with age, especially after sixty-five, although investigators differ as to the age at which the increment begins and its extent. Limited knowledge of normal circulation (Alfred E. Cohn, 1947) justifies only rough correlations between morbid phenomena and pressure levels in some persons; adjustments with age "are far from completely apprehended". Carl J. Wiggers, 1949, defined hypertension as "a state in which arterial pressures exceed normal values, taking into account sex, age, race, activity and temporary psychic states", but "generally, no doubt can exist when pressure relations exceed the values $\frac{150}{100}$ mm. Hg".

Quite as unsatisfactory as attempts to define normal blood pressure are attempts to classify types of hypertension. Hypertension associated with primary renal disease accounts for only from ten to twenty per cent of human hypertension; hypertension without primary renal disease, or essential hypertension, for eighty to ninety per cent. Whether essential hypertension is a disease entity at all, whether it is more than one entity that may arise in more than one way (G. W. Pickering, 1950), whether it is merely one symptom in numerous conditions (William Goldring, 1946) is not yet established. Other questions involve definition of malignant hypertension: whether it is a specific entity (always, or rarely or never) referable to the serious, usually fatal, impairment of renal function; whether it may develop in any type of hypertension provided the level of arterial pressure is sufficiently severe (Pickering, 1952); whether it is simply an accelerated phase of benign essential hypertension; whether it involves some additional factor (F. H. Smirk, 1949). Answers to these questions are the objective of experimental work the direct applicability of which to human disease is still to be confirmed. The trend is to remove from the category of essential hypertension elevated blood pressure recognized as secondary to any nonvascular primary condition or disease; these cases are a comparatively small percentage of the above-mentioned eighty to ninety per cent of cases of essential hypertension. Only increased knowledge of causal factors, Irvine H. Page pointed out, 1951, will change the "current practice of treating hypertension of different causes with the same remedy". Some views envisage hypertension merely as a symptom comparable to fever. The diversity of current remedies for hypertension (sympathectomy, salt restriction, rice diet, psychotherapy, various drugs) and the disparity in their effect (reducing blood pressure in some cases but not in others) seem to indicate (Edgar V. Allen, 1950) that "essential" hypertension is "not one disease but many diseases having in common nothing more than elevation of blood pressure". In human essential hypertension diastolic elevation is generally regarded (Homer Smith, 1951) as the *sine qua non*.

Elevation of either systolic or diastolic pressure or of both may follow disturbance in any one of five circulatory factors involved in regulation of normal blood pressure: cardiac output, circulating blood volume, blood viscosity, elasticity of the large arteries, peripheral resistance. Of these five factors, the values for three, blood volume, blood viscosity, basal cardiac output, are generally held to be within the normal range in human essential hypertension; opinion is divided regarding the state of the large arteries; increase in peripheral resistance is generally held to be the characteristic pathology of hypertension. While noting that "on general grounds and on indirect measurements" the increased peripheral resistance characteristic of hypertension is believed to reside in the small arteries and arterioles, Pickering, 1950, pointed out that too few direct measurements of intravascular pressure have been made at various parts of the total circuit to say with certainty which size of vessel is abnormally narrowed. Wiggers, for instance, expressed the (minority) view that the walls of the larger arteries also participate in the hypertensive process.

Whether the arteriolar constriction has a functional basis (spasm) or an organic basis remains part of a fifty-year controversy as to whether essential hypertension causes or follows arteriosclerosis, or whether the two may develop independently, intensifying each other (Bell, 1951). Goldblatt's view that organic change of renal arterioles (renal arteriolosclerosis) precedes hypertension led him to characterize discovery of the cause of arteriosclerosis as "the number one problem" in solution of hypertension. The relative significance of functional and organic damage remains a therapeutic problem also since if constriction is organic and irreversible, reducing blood pressure by hypotensive drugs may result in insufficient pressure to maintain adequate blood flow to various organs (kidney, brain) to overcome the peripheral vasoconstriction. If, on the other hand, peripheral constriction is functional, then a drop in blood pressure not affecting blood flow will be of benefit in relaxing peripheral constriction. These considerations are pertinent not only in attempts to determine whether peripheral constriction is functional or organic but also in attempts to measure the efficacy of new hypotensive drugs and procedures not merely by their capacity to lower blood pressure but also by their effects (to the degree these are now measurable) on renal, coronary, cerebral blood flow.

Whether the humoral substance sought for more than fifty years as the constricting agent of peripheral arterioles in hypertension is of renal, neural, endocrine origin remains unknown. Belief that the renal pressor system experimentally shown to induce hypertension in animals (1940) might also account for hypertension in man has suffered a decline. It is recognized that disturbed renal, neural, endocrine mechanisms, alone, together, or in alternation, may play a part in maintaining blood pressure within the normal range and in adapting it to most transient emergencies. This view, envisaging hypertension as resulting from exaggerated or protracted activity of the mechanisms that are responsible for vascular homeostasis, is the focus of one line of investigative work. In it, search for a specific pressor substance has been overshadowed by interest in clarifying the mechanisms that regulate normal blood pressure and account for its adaptation to transient rises attributable to physical or emotional stress in normal daily living. Various hypotheses offered between 1947 and 1951 outlining ways in which renal, neural, endocrine, hepatorenal, neuroendocrine mechanisms may work together in initiating or maintaining hypertension include: a "mosaic theory of hypertension" (Page and Corcoran, 1949) explaining how nervous, endocrine, cardiovascular and humoral factors (the last of renal origin) may contribute "in constantly changing interplay to the maintenance of hypertension"; a theory (Raab and associates, 1952) envisaging a balance between adrenocortical and sympathoadrenal neurohormones mediated by the sodium ion; a view that experimental hypertension produced by a renal mechanism is maintained in later chronic stages by a neurogenic mechanism, advanced by Ogden, 1944, and supported (but on different grounds) by Pickering; a "new synthesis" found timely by Eduardo Braun-Menéndez, 1951, viewing hypertension, "even experimental hypertension", as "a metabolic disturbance initiated by different primary causes". He found "untenable" current views that hypertension is exclusively due to secretion of a pressor substance, to exaggerated activity of the nervous system, or to increased or decreased secretion of some hormone. "Whatever the initial or predominant cause of hypertension, a metabolic change occurs which participates in the pathogenesis of hypertension or may even take over the baton and become the conductor of the phenomenological orchestra." Nor do the above exhaust the theories as to primary causes and, especially, as to their many possible interrelations.

## CLINICAL HYPOTENSION AS AN APPROACH TO STUDY OF FACTORS REGULATING BLOOD PRESSURE

Chronic or acute hypotension illustrates as aptly as does hypertension disturbance of the mechanisms that govern blood pressure homeostasis. The shock associated with acute hypotension is, whether in peace or in war, an outstanding medical and surgical problem (which atomic conflict would intensify). Understanding of the shock syndrome "must be firmly based upon a clear and complete concept of the physiological mechanisms which normally maintain and regulate arterial pressure" (Heymans, 1950). These fundamental mechanisms have not as yet been clarified by modern therapies, however effective; for while transfused blood and blood substitutes can reverse early stages of the shock syndrome, they do not serve in so-called irreversible shock. A clear picture of the shock syndrome has not resulted from any of the concepts that, over the years, have served as approaches to investigations on more fundamental levels of circulatory collapse whether envisaged as due to blood loss through hemorrhage or capillary leakage, to derangement of vasopressor mechanisms, to coronary or myocardial failure, to cellular disorganization resulting from anoxia, to toxic factors liberated from injured tissues or cells (revived interest in the toxic hypothesis is illustrated by respectful references to it, 1952, by John Scudder and also by Jacob Fine and associates in the surgery department of Harvard).

Some of the studies over more than fifteen years of Corneille Heymans and associates (University of Ghent) primarily concerned with normal control mechanisms of arterial pressure take into account a possible relation between essentially neural mechanisms that have been demonstrated and chemical factors now dominant in investigative work on both hypertension and acute hypotension or shock. The Belgian group has concentrated especially upon certain vascular areas, the cardioaortic and carotid sinus bodies, the nerve endings in which are both "pressoreceptive" (responding to differences of blood pressure and acting reflexly upon certain nervous system areas, central and sympathetic) and "chemoreceptive" (responding to substances within the circulating blood). Many metabolic substances and drugs, known to change blood pressure and heart rate, have been shown by the Heymans group and others to produce their effects through action of the circulating blood upon the aortic or carotid bodies.

Research programs on shock during the second world war and later at Columbia, New York University, Cornell, Duke, Harvard, Toronto, Vanderbilt, Wisconsin, Yale have led to wide acceptance of two concepts: that the most important alteration in traumatic (as in hemorrhagic) shock is decreased blood volume due largely or entirely to fluid loss at the site of injury; that vasoconstriction in certain sites (the extremities, the kidneys) spares blood for more vital regions. These concepts were confirmed for experimental shock by studies between 1943 and 1945, among others isotope studies by Fine and his group (Beth Israel Hospital, Boston) and studies of J. L. Nickerson (Columbia). Confirmation for human shock was considered to be furnished by clinical measurements, by cardiac catheterization and other techniques, 1943 and later, by Columbia workers in Bellevue (A. F. Cournand, M. I. Gregersen, D. W. Richards, Jr., and associates). These and other studies (during the early war years) seemed at first to explain progressive tissue anoxia in terms of circulatory deficiency, but later it became evident that in addition to disturbed general blood flow there were serious defects in tissue capillary function.

The concept of specific defects in the peripheral vascular system as an essential part of the shock syndrome has been examined in detail over ten years, first at New York University (Robert Chambers, B. W. Zweifach and others), more recently at Cornell (a group, including Zweifach, directed by Ephraim Shorr). Briefly, the experimental studies of these workers center around the view that tissue homeostasis, the primary function of the circulation, depends upon the integrity of the terminal vascular bed to which the heart and large vessels pump the blood. Control of the larger vessels, according to this concept, resides chiefly in the sympathetic nervous system, and, in early shock, adaptive reflexes operate to offset sharp reduction in cardiac output. "These adjustments of the larger vessels" (Zweifach, 1952) "bear no direct relationship to the resultant changes in the peripheral circulation." The terminal vascular bed, to which older concepts assign a secondary role, is regulated by humoral factors (from the adrenals, kidneys, liver): during the initial compensatory stage of shock, a vasoexcitor material, VEM, arising in the kidney which is anoxic because of reduced blood flow, causes heightened vasoactivity and vasomotion; during the second stage of circulatory depression, a vasodepressor principle, VDM (which has been identified as ferritin, an iron-bearing protein arising in the liver), inactivates the pressor principle. It was suggested that these two humoral principles, VEM and VDM, were components of a normally occurring homeostatic mechanism regulating peripheral blood flow under certain circumstances, and in shock acting at maximum capacity. It is recognized that the multiple factors involved in blood pressure readjustments, e.g., the sympathetic nervous system, adrenal secretions, renal and liver mechanisms and others, vary widely under different conditions. What the role of the hepatorenal factors may be in maintaining blood pressure homeostasis under normal circumstances has not yet been projected. The present concept appears to be that ferritin is a physiological principle normally present in the liver and normally converted from the active sulfhydryl form to the inactive disulfide form; in late shock and perhaps in chronic hypertension, the inactivating mechanisms within the liver may possibly be deranged with consequent loss of blood pressure homeostasis.

## RENAL MECHANISMS IN HYPERTENSION

Answers to the questions whether involvement of the kidneys in hypertension is part of generalized vascular disease and whether renal vascular disease plays a part in the origin of hypertension are, as previously indicated, still inconclusive. Even the relation of true sclerosis of the renal arterioles, often associated with essential hypertension, is still debated, although inflammation of the kidneys from any of several causes, interference with their normal blood supply or obstruction of urinary outflow are generally believed to cause hypertension. On the focal question whether renal arteriosclerosis precedes the hypertension or *vice versa*, mention has been made of the view of Harry Goldblatt (who has continued his twenty years' work at Western Reserve at the Cedars of Lebanon Hospital and the University of Southern California), based on evidence from his experimental work and from a few recent studies in other laboratories, that arteriolar sclerosis of the benign phase of hypertension probably precedes elevated blood pressure, and that renal arteriolar necrosis of the malignant phase is terminal. Also mentioned was Bell's conclusion (restated 1951), based on pathological studies and clinical observations on over a thousand cases at the University of Minnesota, that primary hypertension and renal arteriosclerosis arise independently, the hypertension being due to functional (spastic) not structural state of the arterioles. Interpretation of time relationships in arteriosclerotic changes from clinical and autopsy data is admittedly difficult. On the basis of gross inspection of kidneys during life and biopsies from one or both kidneys at operation, R. H. Smithwick and Benjamin Castleman, 1951 (surgery, Boston University; pathology, Massachusetts General), thought that hypertension probably preceded the renal vascular sclerosis noted in fifty-five per cent of their cases of essential and malignant hypertension. Over a decade ago, on the basis of renal blood flow measurements, workers in New York University's hypertension clinic (Goldring, Chasis, Ranges, Smith) characterized the kidney as "the victim, not the culprit" in hypertension, a view reaffirmed on the same grounds by the New York University group, 1951. Reasoning against the concept that hypertensive disease results from "a multitude of microscopic Goldblatt clamps placed upon the renal arterioles", Smith, 1951, conjured a picture of experimental approach to diabetes, before the discovery of the islets of Langerhans, by clamping the pancreatic artery and deducing that pancreatic ischemia was the cause of diabetes. The disagreement has not only had clinical repercussions in prognosis and treatment but has also influenced hypotheses concerning mechanisms by which the kidney produces pressor substances, which react in various ways with other chemical substances, are destroyed by enzymes (sometimes in several alternate ways) in various body tissues, are inactivated by depressor substances, or possibly retained in active state in the body instead of yielding to normal homeostatic controls.

## EXPERIMENTAL RENAL HYPERTENSION

Organic changes reported in the arterioles of the kidney in autopsy material stimulated numerous attempts, beginning 1879, to produce hypertension in animals by damaging the kidney (by X ray, nephrotoxic substances, surgical manipulations) and, after 1918, by occluding partially or completely one or both renal arteries, a procedure resulting in the rapid death of the animals. The first long-sustained experimental hypertension achieved by Goldblatt and his associates in 1932 was induced in dogs, some of which were studied for more than six years. By partially constricting the main arteries of both kidneys with adjustable clamps or constricting one renal artery and removing the other kidney a persistent hypertension was achieved. The benign phase of experimental renal hypertension (studied in dog, rat, rabbit, goat, sheep, monkey) produced by the Goldblatt clamp and allied procedures is conceded to resemble closely the benign phase of human essential hypertension, the dominant functional alteration being a rise in peripheral resistance with no significant disturbance of renal excretory function and little if any gross microscopic change; arteriolar vasoconstriction coincides with increased cardiac effort, and cardiac hypertrophy develops in the left ventricle; cardiac rate and output, blood volume and viscosity, peripheral blood flow, venous pressure remain unaltered. With a greater degree of constriction of both renal arteries followed by impairment of renal excretory function, or with great constriction of one artery and uretral occlusion in the other kidney, pathological changes appear in the small arteries of the kidneys (and other organs) similar to those observed in the malignant phase of essential human hypertension. Although these resemblances have led to many variations in theories of renal origin of human hypertension, Goldblatt's work has served primarily as an approach and a method for studies of the experimental disease during which one (of many) humoral pressor mechanisms dependent upon a substance, renin, secreted by the kidney, was described and elaborated (by Page and associates in 1938, now working at the Cleveland Clinic, and in the same year by Braun-Menéndez and associates at the Institute of Biology and Experimental Medicine, Buenos Aires). Since that time much work has been devoted to analysis of the mechanism by which renin, a substance with properties of a proteolytic enzyme, acts upon a protein, alpha-2-globulin, in the plasma to liberate a third substance, hypertensin (angiotonin), a powerful vasoconstrictor. Studies up to 1951, according to Page, had revealed that hypertensin is a polypeptide, but methods for its quantitative measurement in the blood of hypertensives had not been elaborated. Neither group (Page nor Braun-Menéndez) believes that this pressor mechanism is wholly responsible for any type of human hypertension. Rather, like the Goldblatt clamp, it has provided a tangible mechanism for testing a theory and for measuring in kind and amount factors participating in one of the many influences that raise blood pressure.

## ROLE OF RENAL ISCHEMIA IN PRODUCTION OF EXPERIMENTAL HYPERTENSION

Although production of hypertension by constriction of the renal arteries led to the assumption that ischemia, anoxia or altered hemodynamics within the kidney was a primary factor initiating subsequent mechanisms leading to hypertension, the question whether ischemia is present immediately after clamping of the arteries and therefore involved in starting the vicious cycle was still, 1952, unanswered. The two groups of investigators that developed the hypothesis of the renin-hypertensin pressor system have disagreed. Braun-Menéndez, Leloir and their associates, 1946, regarded ischemia as responsible for the release of renin in experimental renal hypertension in the dog and also as a causal factor in human hypertension. Page and his associates who attributed the release of renin to reduction of pulse pressure considered that if early and extensive renal ischemia is necessary for initiation and maintenance of hypertension then "the experimental method has little in common with human essential hypertension". Many investigators of the experimental disease agree with Goldblatt that there is a transient reduction in renal blood flow immediately after constriction of the main renal artery and also that learning whether the reduction persists will depend on "better and more direct methods than are available at present for frequent determinations of renal blood flow before and after constriction of the renal artery" (Goldblatt, 1948).

While work on the enzymatic activity of normal and ischemic renal tissue had not up to 1951 demonstrated a generally accepted role, primary or intermediary, for ischemia in hypertension, there has been advancing interest (W. Stanley Hartroft, 1952) in the view that constriction of the artery acts "only to alter some essential metabolic function of the kidney which is necessary to keep the level of blood pressure down to normal limits". Homer Smith, while observing, 1951, that ischemia once established does affect pressure, described the mechanism of renal ischemia as still "not clear".

## HUMORAL PRESSOR MECHANISMS OF RENAL ORIGIN

Three of the theories that have oriented investigative work on mechanisms of experimental renal hypertension are outstanding: the first, the theory that the kidney with constricted renal artery is the source of renin which reacts with an alpha-2-globulin in serum to form a vasoconstrictive substance causing increased peripheral resistance; the second, that alteration of intrarenal hemodynamics by constriction of the renal artery results in reducing or destroying the activity of enzymes normally responsible for oxidation of amino acids so that pressor amines that would normally be reduced are not and so accumulate and escape into the blood; the third, that renal injury retains in the body some pressor substance which would otherwise be excreted. The first hypothesis, built around renin, is considered first not so much because renin was historically the first renal vasoconstrictive and pressor substance isolated, and because renin and its reaction product, hypertensin, have been described "as the only agents known which reproduce the circulatory conditions of essential hypertension" (Braun-Menéndez, 1951), but also because most of the problems (site of origin, mechanism of formation and of release) connected with renin apply also to more recently discovered vasoconstrictive and pressor substances isolated from the kidney. Yet emphasis seems to be shifting away from this mechanism as responsible for essential hypertension.

## The renin-hypertensin system

So soon as experimental renal hypertension became available to investigators the question whether renin is the mediating substance became the focus of investigation in a number of laboratories. Two of the major groups (Page, with K. G. Kohlstaedt and O. M. Helmer at the Indianapolis City Hospital; Braun-Menéndez, with Leloir and others in Buenos Aires) reported independently (1939) that renin is not vasoactive in itself but acts like an enzyme on an alpha-2-globulin (hypertensinogen, renin substrate) to liberate the pressor substance hypertensin. All mammalian renin when injected intravenously produces hypertensin with its pressor effect in all animals except in man; only primate renin produces this effect in man, but primate renin can act on hypertensinogen from any animal including man.

Failure (due to lack of a precise and adequate method for chemical assay of renin) to find renin in chronic hypertension, although it has been identified in initial and acute stages of experimental and in a few cases of acute human hypertension, has been subjected to various interpretations: that the methods employed may not be sufficiently sensitive to detect minute amounts of renin in the blood in chronic stages; that renin may initiate renal hypertension but that some other mechanisms may be responsible for maintaining it. Theories concerning cellular changes in the kidneys of hypertensive animals and man that might be evidence of increased formation and release of a pressor substance, presumed to be renin, have been examined chiefly by cytological studies of the juxtaglomerular apparatus of the kidney (N. Goormaghtigh, 1925–1953) and by anatomical and histological studies of the nephron and renal tubules by other workers. Renin determination is under study by immunological methods, the most accurate and sensitive means of detecting small amounts of protein in biological fluids (the Goldblatt and the Wakerlin groups). Page and Corcoran observed, 1952, "the recent almost complete purification of renin points to the probability of a resolution" of the question as to the degree to which the renal pressor system participates in experimental hypertension. Supporters of the view that renin has nothing to do with development and maintenance of experimental renal hypertension include Arthur Grollman and associates (Southwestern Medical College), who, 1951, reported maintenance (up to seventy days) of hypertension in nephrectomized dogs in complete absence of renal tissue.

Limitations in methods used in determinations and assays of other components of the renin-hypertensin system in experimental renal hypertension suggest the need of revising earlier results (Page, 1951). The substrate (hypertensinogen) had not been prepared in pure form, 1951, although it had been identified with the alpha-2-globulin of serum; there was some evidence that the blood level of the substance rises after nephrectomy, that renin injections reduce it. Hypertensin, the reaction product, when infused into animals or men produces a hypertension "differing only in details" from the hemodynamic characteristics of experimental and essential hypertension. Lack of adequate techniques has prevented demonstration of hypertensin in the blood of hypertensive animals (Dexter, 1947; Page, 1951) and elucidation of its chemical and physical nature; results of studies of its destruction by what appears to be a group of enzymes (hypertensinase) carried out by the South Americans and by several groups in this country have not been conclusive. Page, 1951, considered that hypertensin has not been shown to be "the mediator of either renal hypertension in animals or essential hypertension in man . . . nor has it been shown that it is not". Braun-Menéndez also, 1951, stressed the need of suspending judgment as to its role. In the view of Forman and associates, 1953, the fact that pulmonary artery pressures are normal in essential hypertension, but raised by hypertensin in both normotensive and hypertensive subjects, constitutes a strong argument against such a substance in a causative role.

## METABOLIC CHANGES RELATED TO VASOACTIVE SUBSTANCES IN HYPERTENSIVE BLOOD

Altered titers of VEM and VDM in the blood stream (vasoexcitor material produced in the kidney and vasodepressor material produced in the liver) in experimental renal hypertension were attributed by Zweifach and Shorr, 1948, to a shift in kidney and liver metabolism. VEM, being produced normally in the anaerobic kidney, appears in the hypertensive dog and rat under aerobic conditions as well; VDM, later identified as ferritin, and also normally produced in the liver under anaerobic conditions, is, in the hypertensive liver, produced (by a shifted metabolism) under both anaerobic and aerobic conditions. The shift in liver VDM metabolism was attributed to abnormal concentration of VEM liberated into the blood by the hypertensive kidney. The initial renal hypoxia occurring after artery restriction can account for the shift in VEM metabolism but the continuous and unrestrained production of the vasoexcitor material once the renal blood flow is restored with development of hypertension was unexplained, 1951. Shorr, 1951, reported experiments suggesting that the seat of the metabolic disturbance (loss of normal renal capacity to restrict renal formation of VEM to anaerobiosis) appeared to be a "cellular and enzymic lesion in a specific segment of the kidney tubules" (the proximal segment believed by many to be the site of renin release).

That intrarenal amino acids can be converted to pressor amines following interference with the circulation of the kidney *in vivo* and *in vitro* was demonstrated by Richard J. Bing (on the basis of work begun at Columbia, 1941, continued at Johns Hopkins, 1946); but that such conversion is a cause of experimental renal hypertension or human hypertension Bing did not assume or claim. An unknown protein-like principle in blood, probably derived from the kidney and capable of producing a sustained pressor response in nephrectomized cats and dogs, was reported by R. E. Shipley and O. M. Helmer at the Indianapolis City Hospital, 1947. Page, who participated in earlier studies of the sustained pressor principle, considered it possible, 1949, that hypertensin in the body is combined with a protein and occurs as the polypeptide isolated from the hypertensive body only after being split from the protein by extraction procedures. An enzymic mechanism has been proposed for the unexplained pressure-reducing effects of kidney extracts prepared and studied by Grollman in experimental and in some cases of human malignant hypertension; Corcoran, 1948, proposed that the extracts may increase the plasma polypeptidases (enzymes that break down polypeptides, to which class of substances hypertensin is believed to belong) which would increase inactivation of the pressor substance. Enzymic destruction of the pressor polypeptide is regulated by other tissues as well, enzymes that do this (as hypertensinase) having been reported in intestines, blood plasma and other tissues. Eduardo Cruz Coke (physiological and pathological chemistry, University of Chile) maintained, 1946, that normal enzymic destruction of the pressor agent depends upon maintenance of normal respiratory function of the tissues: if conditions (in the kidney or in other organs and tissues) causing renal anoxemia exist "it is most likely that the hypertensin produced will not be destroyed rapidly enough". Henry A. Schroeder (internal medicine, Washington University) and associates, who searched from 1940 to 1950 for pressor substances in human blood, found in the majority of hypertensive bloods a pressor agent that was inactivated by enzymes reacting with amines. By 1950 the pressor material named pherentasin had been purified and reported to contain an amino group essential to activity and also an active carbonyl group. In 175 samples of human blood, presence of the vasoactive material was correlated with cases "having a nephrogenic component". Schroeder's 1952 report noting higher concentrations in renal types of hypertension described pherentasin "as the only pressor substance found in blood of hypertensive patients which is not found in normal blood".

## PERTINENCE OF WORK ON EXPERIMENTAL RENAL HYPERTENSION TO HUMAN HYPERTENSIVE DISEASE

Work on experimental renal hypertension must still be regarded as confusing since, as many investigators have stressed, clinical counterparts of experimental renal hypertension are rare. The danger of oversimplifying complex physiological and chemical mechanisms has led outstanding workers to stress the need of criteria and techniques for examining the relation of different hypertensive syndromes in man to experimental renal hypertension.

As in all biochemical studies involving enzymic mechanisms, methods for study of the renin-hypertensin system are more or less indirect: the renin content of plasma, for example, is measured by rate of formation of hypertensin after addition of excess substrate (alpha-2-globulin); hypertensin is assayed by indirect biological responses. Assays of renin in the blood of hypertensive patients (Braun-Menéndez and associates, 1946) have shown, even in the few positive tests, amounts too small to produce even a minimal pressor effect on intravenous injection. Increased amounts of renin have been reported (Haynes and Dexter, 1944) in the renal venous blood of a small series of patients during acute stages (when pressure was rising) of eclampsia, acute glomerulonephritis, and also in circulatory failure. Pickering regarded the finding of increased amounts of renin in the renal blood in congestive heart failure without hypertension as challenging but not demolishing the renal theory of essential hypertension. Hypertensin injected intravenously in man causes cardiovascular effects similar to those observed in essential hypertension: increase of systolic and diastolic pressures; arteriolar constriction; reduction of cardiac output and increase of venous pressure. There are no subjective effects after moderate pressor doses, as there are no subjective symptoms in early hypertension (Corcoran, 1948). Page, however, considered, 1951, that this testimony needed the support of direct quantitative comparisons from chemical studies.

Under therapeutic motivation, attempts have been made to inactivate hypertensin by an enzyme or group of enzymes called hypertensinase; or by unknown substances contained in kidney extracts. One such renal extract found effective (1940) in reducing pressure in hypertensive rats and in a few cases of human hypertension by Arthur Grollman was related, 1946, to his hypothesis that hypertension is not caused by a renal pressor substance but rather by the absence of "a humoral agent essential for the well-being of the organism, in the absence of which, in the diseased kidney, hypertension results". Results of tests of various kidney extracts in human hypertension include the 1944 finding of Goldring and Chasis that they had no effect on blood pressure and the 1942 conclusion of

Shales, Stead and Warren that the effects were nonspecific. Grollman reported, 1945, striking reductions of blood pressure in a single case of human chronic hypertension following oral administration of oxidized marine oils, the active principle of which he considered resembles his kidney extracts in their chemical and hypotensive effects. Use of quinones (the rationale of which derives from Bing's experiments on production of pressor amines in the anoxic kidney) has been tried clinically with inconclusive results, that is, reduction of pressure in half of those treated (Rosenthal and Shapiro, 1945). Clinical trial of all of these substances (renal extracts, quinones, enzymes, cytochromes, marine oils) was disposed of by Schroeder, 1947, as "only beating around the periphery and not attacking the hub of the problem", exact identification of pressor mechanisms. The following changes in hepatorenal humoral mechanisms, essentially the same as those found in the hypertensive dog and rat, were found (Shorr, 1951) also in human hypertensives: metabolic derangements of renal VEM and hepatic VDM mechanisms; appearance of the two principles in the blood; alterations in reactivity and structure of the capillary bed; lesion of enzymic character in the proximal convoluted tubules. Shorr made it clear that this broad program on circulatory dynamics in relation to human hypertension aimed at testing the validity of an objective experimental approach to further detailed analysis. Immunological methods aimed at producing antirenin in man by injections of animal or human renin, and using immune sera produced in animals to induce passive immunity to renin in man have been explored by Wakerlin's group at the University of Illinois. Wakerlin's 1951 experiments showed high correlation between serum antirenin levels and protection against hypertension in dogs given crude and semipurified renin before simultaneous bilateral renal artery constriction. He considered his most significant experimental results to be reduction to normal levels of blood pressure in a dog having spontaneous (essential?) hypertension after a serum antirenin level of 120 units per cc. was reached. Goldblatt's experimental tests indicated, 1951, production of antirenin to hog renin in human hypertension, but with no lowering of blood pressure. Wakerlin commented that demonstrations of a relation of essential hypertension to renin in a significant number of patients would justify a hope that passive immunization would at least serve to tide over a patient in an acute malignant episode.

Since the halcyon days (Page) when the renal humoral mechanism and experimental renal hypertension were accepted by a majority of the (few) investigators in the field as explaining human hypertension, successive studies of other factors and systems that influence renal mechanisms in the experimental animal have lessened the status of the renal theory and highlighted a "mosaic hypothesis" of hypertension which admits other factors, some of which, however, are envisaged as possibly mediated by renal changes. Influence of the adrenal cortex on blood pressure has been evident from the beginning of systematic study of adrenal cortical insufficiency in patients with Addison's disease and reversal of circulatory shock by administration of desoxycorticosterone acetate (Robert Loeb and associates, 1939). Association of the effects of DCA with renal mechanisms was suggested by the obvious association of both the kidney and DCA with sodium metabolism. Experiments with adrenalectomized animals (in which the effects of DCA and sodium chloride were the same as those in Addisonian patients) and experiments with animals having renal hypertension strengthened the presumption of interrelation between the adrenal cortex and the kidneys; experimental renal hypertension could not be induced or maintained in absence of the adrenal cortex (Goldblatt, 1937; Houssay and Dexter, 1942). Work on so-called (Selye, 1942) hormonal hypertension in a number of laboratories has shown that hypertension produced in the rat by DCA and salt is often accompanied by renal lesions, accounting for description of it (Braun-Menéndez, 1951) as hormonally induced renal hypertension. The adrenal cortex has been implicated in the hepatorenal vasoactive mechanisms described by Shorr and Zweifach. Studies of experimental renal hypertension have from the beginning been concerned with discovering how the nervous system participates. Up to 1951 there had been repeated confirmation of two negative findings: first, that the experimental condition cannot be prevented or abolished by renal denervation, and, secondly, that neural mechanisms regulating blood pressure are not abolished but are active in experimental renal hypertension, as they are also in human essential hypertension. In studies from the other direction, temporary blood pressure rises produced by emotional stress have been correlated in some cases with decreased renal blood flow. Although many have suggested that failure to demonstrate the presence of renin after chronic experimental hypertension becomes established may be due to maintenance of elevated pressures by neural mechanisms, Nickerson, 1951, suggested the reverse, that emotionally initiated sympathoadrenal mechanisms may cause repeated episodes of renal vasoconstriction with consequent permanent changes in renal metabolism. Whatever the role of the kidney in experimental and in human hypertension may prove to be, students of clinical and experimental hypertension, alike, must (Braun-Menéndez) "reckon with this organ as a very important factor in the chain of events". Whether or not the kidney elaborates and liberates vasoconstrictor substances, it is "at the crux of a very complex set of mechanisms concerned with the regulation of body fluids and electrolyte interchanges".

## NEURAL MECHANISMS IN HYPERTENSION

Support for the hypothesis that the vasoconstriction to which essential hypertension is attributed is of nervous origin has been largely due (Pickering, 1950) to the fact that the known role of vasomotor nerves appeals to the student of this disease as one of the "few tangible facts in the circuitous behavior of the circulation". Investigation of blood pressure homeostasis has been concerned with two fundamental neural mechanisms, the activities of afferent nerves that carry impulses to the vasomotor center in the brain; the activities of efferent nerves of the sympathetic nervous system that carry vasoconstrictor and vasodilator impulses to the peripheral arterioles in all areas of the body. Heymans's research dating from the present back to 1929 has been concerned with reflex control of blood pressure (depending upon cardiac output and peripheral resistance) by "intermediation of a pressoceptive innervation of different arterial and venous vascular areas". His work has contributed to knowledge of the cardioaortic area, especially the aortic arch, containing nerve endings sensitive to pressure of the blood coming from the heart and to chemicals carried by the blood through these areas. Since these sensory nerve endings are both pressosensitive and chemosensitive, changes in either the pressure or the chemistry of the perfusing blood influence the impulses carried from them, reflexly regulating arterial blood pressure: when arterial pressure within the carotid sinus falls, vasomotor activity is stimulated; when it rises, the vasomotor center is depressed. The normal function of the moderator or depressor nerves in regulation of blood pressure is to depress the continuous activity of the vasomotor center. The pertinence to hypertension of the normal hemodynamic regulation exerted by the sympathetic nervous system has been increasingly related to findings on the adrenal medulla from converging lines of basic research over the last thirty years: work on mechanisms at the sympathetic nerve endings by which they exert their vasoconstrictor and dilator effects at the neuromuscular junction (in the muscular wall of arterioles); work in the twenties, especially in Cannon's laboratory, on the role of the sympathetic nervous system in adaptation of the organism to stress from within and without, identifying the substance released by adrenergic nerve endings with vasoactive amines also released, in response to stress, into the blood stream by the adrenal medulla and called adrenergic substances. The postganglionic fibers of the sympathetic nervous system are referred to as adrenergic and act, as does epinephrine (adrenaline), on the arterioles (except those of the coronary tree) to increase their tone and narrow their diameter; (all other sympathetic fibers are referred to as cholinergic, acting, as does acetylcholine, as dilators).

An experimental form of neurogenic hypertension became available when Koch and Mies demonstrated in the rabbit, 1929, and Heymans and Bouckaert in the dog, 1931, that sustained elevation of blood pressure could be produced by severing the right and left aortic and carotid sinus nerves (which together constitute the moderator group), releasing the vasomotor center from their inhibitory influence. The operation interferes with one of the chief pathways of afferent depressor impulses to the vasomotor center from which vasoconstrictor impulses are distributed to different segments of the spinal cord, thence over the sympathetic nerves to the peripheral blood vessels. Section of the depressor nerves results in a hypertension "maintained at a high level for months and even years" (Heymans, 1950). Hemodynamic changes regarded as characteristic of this type of hypertension (Braun-Menéndez, 1951; Nickerson, 1951) include increase in heart rate (tachycardia) and increase in cardiac output which Heymans attributed to the associated release from inhibition of centers that bring about simultaneous activation of nerves secreting adrenaline along with release of the constrictor and cardio-accelerator centers. Because the increase in cardiac output was considered to outweigh the slighter increase in peripheral resistance (for which reason this type of hypertension was sometimes described as "cardiovascular"), neurogenic hypertension produced by section of depressor nerves has long been considered irrelevant to human essential hypertension in which cardiac output remains within normal range and peripheral resistance is greatly increased. Heymans, however, suggested that demonstration in dogs of prevention or reversal of this type of experimental chronic hypertension by total excision of the sympathetic paravertebral ganglia may "have some bearing on the pathogenesis of clinical essential hypertension"; a functional deficiency in regulation of the activity of the vasoconstrictor center might be either central or peripheral. Schroeder and Goldman, in a series of experiments aimed at determining, among other things, whether this type of hypertension is "a true chronic diastolic hypertension" or hypertension secondary to increased cardiac output or merely a transitory nervous vasoconstriction, reported, 1952, after a four-year study of twenty dogs made hypertensive by this method, that in three severe hypertension had been sustained for four years and that in these and in nine others "vasoconstriction was demonstrated in local vascular beds". These and a few other reports of the real increase in peripheral resistance in this type of experimental hypertension have revived interest in it (Nickerson, Page, other workers) "as a basis for the intelligent recognition or exclusion of neurogenic factors in human hypertension".

Encouraging to the view that hypertension results from a vasomotor disturbance of morphologically normal arterioles throughout a considerable part of the body was the demonstration (cited by Landis, 1944) of steep rise in blood pressure following stimulation of those sympathetic nerves which terminate in arterioles of the abdominal viscera (splanchnic area) constituting the greater portion of the peripheral resistance in circulation. The more marked response of the splanchnic area, Pickering pointed out, 1950, had led to exaggeration of the importance of sympathetic nerves in control of vascular tone in other areas in which response to stimulation varies quantitatively and qualitatively. He found it "extremely difficult to believe that in essential hypertension the fault lies in the action of the vasomotor nerves. Vasoconstriction of nervous origin there is, but there is no unequivocal evidence that this is abnormal in degree."

Cannon's emergency theory of sympathoadrenal function centered around increased secretion of adrenaline in response to stress left open the nature of the adrenergic hormone which causes both excitatory and inhibitory effects. Cannon separated two factors, the excitatory sympathin E, liberated in structures excited by sympathetic impulses, the inhibitory sympathin I, liberated in structures inhibited by sympathetic impulses. He suggested that epinephrine combined with a hypothetical cellular substance to bring about the transmission of sympathetic nerve impulses. Z. M. Bacq (University of Ghent) when he was working with Cannon in the early thirties advanced the view that sympathin is a mixture of substances liberated by adrenergic nerve action and is itself the transmitter; by 1949, he expressed a conclusion (citing Blaschko's work, 1942) that sympathin E and norepinephrine (a recently identified isomer of epinephrine, occurring in the adrenal medulla and secreted by sympathetic nerve fibers) are probably identical. Goldenberg and associates (Columbia) suggested, 1948, that hypertension may be due to disturbed equilibrium between the two sympathicomimetic substances, epinephrine and nor-epinephrine. Since "the only structural differences between the two substances is a methyl group", according to Braun-Menéndez, 1951, "essential hypertension could possibly be regarded as due to a metabolic disturbance consisting of deficient transmethylation". Goldenberg and Rapport could not, 1951, confirm Holtz's claim that an excessive excretion of nor-epinephrine consistently occurs in essential hypertension. That epinephrine and nor-epinephrine might be involved in hypertension through some mechanism other than constrictive action on peripheral smooth muscle (arteriolar constriction), for instance decrease of resistance to stretch of the arterial wall, was suggested, 1951, by Heymans and van den Heuvel-Heymans. The assumed relation of nor-epinephrine and of other pressor amines to hypertension is another meeting point for work on renal, neural, endocrine factors.

While both sympathectomy and drugs have contributed to what has been called "a vague directional trend" (Page, 1949) toward reopening questions of neurovascular control they have not as yet contributed significantly to elucidation of neural mechanisms in hypertension. Analysis of the result of using these therapies on thousands of patients since 1938 has not, for many investigators, resolved doubts due to: lack of fundamental knowledge of the relation of the sympathoadrenal system to the disease (Nickerson, 1951); lack of real distinction between either sympathectomy or drug therapy and various other nonspecific therapies (Allen, 1950); impossibility of selecting patients for treatment by any reliably objective method (Page, 1951). Even if vasoconstrictor responses to the sympathoadrenal system are blockaded, undefined factors may still maintain normal or elevated levels. Heymans's dogs, deprived by total sympathectomy of reflex regulation of peripheral resistance and blood pressure, recovered, after a time, nearly normal pressures and vascular tone, possibly originating in disconnected sympathetic ganglia, intraneural vascular innervation, or development of primitive autonomic vascular mechanisms. Recovery of high pressure levels and failure of reduction have been noted clinically after sympathectomy.

Sympathectomy procedures in widest use, 1953, included: a one-stage operation removing thoracic ganglia and sectioning splanchnics above the diaphragm, developed by Max M. Peet at the University of Michigan; complete bilateral thoracic-lumbar sympathectomy (regarded as experimental by Page, 1951) developed at Chicago and later at Duke by K. S. Grimson; less extensive lumbodorsal sympathectomy (denervating kidneys, adrenals, splanchnic bed) developed by R. H. Smithwick at Harvard and later at Boston University. From the earliest studies in the thirties these surgeons and others (Adson and Craig at the Mayo Clinic; Crile at the Cleveland Clinic; Page at Indianapolis; Davis and Barker at Northwestern; Heuer at Cornell) have stressed denervation of the splanchnic bed, of the kidneys and of the adrenals. Smithwick, 1953, covering a follow-up ranging from five to fourteen years, compared the results of splanchnicectomy in 1,266 cases of unusually severe essential hypertension with the results of only medical treatment in 467 patients with hypertension of comparable severity. In his view the comparison sug-

gested that "the outlook for hypertensive patients can be improved
by splanchnicectomy even if the basal blood pressure levels are not
significantly lowered postoperatively".    Drugs under study for capacity to block sympathetic pathways have included the ergot alkaloids (dihydroergocornine), beta-haloalkylamines (dibenamine and
its relatives), tetraethylammonium and hexamethonium compounds
and other agents that lower blood pressure and pulse rate through
vagal action without adrenergic blockade (typified by veratrum alkaloids).    Admitting the undoubted capacity of some of the newer
hypotensive drugs to lower blood pressure, an editor of the *Annals
of Internal Medicine* added, 1953, that their ultimate therapeutic value
would depend upon demonstration of their efficacy "in maintaining
a lowered blood pressure in doses which are not disabling and upon
proof that such reduction is advantageous to the patient for a long
time".    Such an evaluation is "not yet available at this early stage
in the use of these drugs".

More attention has been given thus far to study of peripheral postganglionic mechanisms in hypertension than to cerebral centers as a
source of vasomotor impulses.    Functioning of efferent pathways has
been described (Page and Corcoran) as "not sufficiently explored".
Just as definition of the medullary areas from which vasomotor control
emanates gave impetus to investigation of vasomotor mechanisms in
blood pressure (the work of Heymans and of Ranson), so recent work
suggesting mechanisms involving the thalamus and cortex at least
points to the possibility of further knowledge of participation of
cerebral centers in hypertension.

Clinical clues to central nervous mechanisms have come from observations that hypertension is associated with traumatic or neoplastic
damage to the brain affecting either the better defined vasomotor
centers of the medulla in the fourth ventricle or the less well defined
groups of cells in higher areas.    Evidence of pressor activity of central
origin has included (besides Cushing's observations so long ago as
1901, Penfield's 1929 and Page's 1935 reference to diencephalic hypertension) Grimson's 1949 description of hypertension associated with
tumors of the fourth ventricle, description of paroxysmal hypertension
associated with tabes dorsalis by Bennett and Heyman, 1948.    In
animals, hypertension of central origin has been produced by intra-

cranial pressure (intracisternal injection of kaolin and other inert substances, Dixon and Heller, 1932) and by cerebral ischemia following ligation of the carotid, vertebral and spinal arteries (Nowak and Walker, 1939; Fishback and others, 1943).

The assumed relation of intracranial pressure and cerebral ischemia to hypertension has been shown to be more complex than was once believed.  While acute anoxia, cerebral anemia and increased intracranial pressure stimulate the vasomotor center directly and raise blood pressure (Heymans, 1950), "after an initial period of excitation, acute anemia or anoxia provokes inhibition and even paralysis of the vasomotor center with a fall of arterial pressure".  However, even after prolonged and complete interruption of the blood supply, the paralyzed vasomotor center is still able to recover its activity when the circulation is restored even when total anemia has lasted so long as thirty minutes.  Newer methods of measuring cerebral blood flow, developed by Seymour S. Kety and associates at the University of Pennsylvania, 1945, are contributing to clarification of some aspects of cerebral circulation in hypertension (Kety, 1952); studies first reported, 1948 (by Kety with J. H. Hafkenschiel, W. A. Jeffers and others), revealed that cerebral blood flow remained "exactly normal" in the face of nearly double normal values in arterial pressure.  Kety interpreted this as evidence that "the cerebral blood vessels in essential hypertension are markedly constricted", participating in the "generalized increase in vascular tone throughout the body" reported for other vascular areas by other workers.  He considered the cerebral vasoconstriction "at least to a great extent functional" but not of sympathetic origin; this was in agreement with a prevailing view (among physiologists) that cerebral vasculature has no sympathetic innervation (or, if it has, that the vasomotor impulses are too feeble to count in regulation of cerebral circulation).

Establishment of the nature and origin of the constriction of cerebral arteries and arterioles in hypertension is basic to the clinical controversy regarding the relative importance of functional and organic factors in "cerebral accidents".  Pickering, on the basis of clinical and experimental studies over more than a decade, challenged the majority view attributing transient paralysis to functional spasm (in which perhaps local metabolites of a vasodilator nature act in response to transient ischemia) and permanent paralysis to organic obstruction of cerebral arteries (by thromboses). He referred both mechanisms to organic arterial obstruction, the transience or permanence of which depends on the artery obstructed, the site and duration of the ischemia, the efficacy of the collateral circulation in restoring blood flow.

The possibility that some of the increasingly numerous pressor substances reported since the beginning of the century from various organs and tissues arise or act centrally has not been overlooked: Wilhelm Raab reported, 1948, a sympathetic substance in the brain (and in adrenergic nerve endings) which he called "encephalin", the chemical nature of which has not been established. Page, Corcoran and Taylor, 1951, reported liberation into the blood of a vasopressor substance on centripetal vagus stimulation which they thought might be identical with a substance, serotonin, isolated, 1948, by Rapport, Green and Page. Identification of serotonin in various tissues of a number of species and recent successful synthesis of it have stimulated investigation of its possible biological role as a pressor substance without as yet indicating any more specific role for it linking the central nervous system to hypertension than for other pressor substances.

Undocumented debate on the degree to which psychic and emotional factors are a cause or an effect of hypertension is giving way to more precise investigation. Change in diastolic blood pressure in response to nervous and emotional stimulation or to an external stimulus (cold) has been studied by Mayo Clinic workers (Edgar A. Hines, Jr.). Interest in the possible influence of heredity in essential hypertension, manifested in studies of family histories of groups of patients, suggested thirty years ago (1923, Weitz) an hypothesis that essential hypertension is a Mendelian dominant with incomplete (over ninety per cent) expression. Robert Platt (Manchester University) thought it uncertain whether the inherited factor is specific for hypertension or "merely a tendency to arterial or arteriolar change". He favored the view that the majority of cases of hypertension not conforming to the theory of dominance are not essential hypertension but are hypertension secondary to renal or other causes. A 1952 analysis by Caroline B. Thomas (who for many years with Bing and associates at Johns Hopkins has studied experimental neurogenic hypertension) of the family histories of a group of medical students indicated that incidence of hypertension among their parents was twenty-five per cent.  Tests of students by some half-dozen methods for vascular lability, frequently regarded as a precursor of hypertension, showed it to be twice as frequent in the offspring of hypertensive parents as in those whose parents gave no history of hypertension: 39.3 per cent of those with positive parental history of hypertension showed evidence of circulatory lability compared with fifteen per cent of the control group.  Thomas referred to genetic studies as suggesting that hypertension behaves as a single recessive gene.  The tests of vascular lability she employed included the above-mentioned cold pressor test developed at the Mayo Clinic: on the basis of changes in diastolic blood pressure in this test, subjects were classified as hyporeactors, normoreactors, or hyperreactors.  Among hypertensives it was reported that if one parent was hypertensive, forty-three per cent of offspring were hyperreactors; if both parents were hypertensive, ninety-five per cent.  Hines considered, 1951, that combined data from follow-up of the various groups over twenty years "indicate that the majority of patients with essential hypertension are vascular hyperreactors", the vascular reactivity being "largely controlled by neurogenic mechanisms".  He favored the view that neurogenic factors may initiate the rise in systolic pressure which is then sustained by other factors, perhaps humoral.  This view reverses the theory that initial rapid rise in blood pressure is brought about by primary renal metabolic changes and then maintained (after renin can no longer be detected) by neural factors.  Hines found no test as yet which measures vascular reactivity "accurately enough or consistently enough" to make it possible to forecast whether or not a given individual is likely to become hypertensive.  Search for such a test has motivated a few long-term studies in several centers (Columbia, Michigan, Johns Hopkins).

Developing at Cornell over a number of years his theory that blood pressure may respond (as do respiratory, gastrointestinal and other systems) to stress, and that this response may be related to essential hypertension, Harold G. Wolff with Stewart Wolf and others has studied for over five years a group of hypertensives and normotensives. Wolff expressed, 1951, hope that their suggestive findings may stimulate others to seek further evidence of "the effect of man upon man" in the stress of modern life with relation to development of hypertension. After studying over a number of years the detailed life history of twenty-four hypertensives, A. E. Cohn and associates at the Rockefeller Institute Hospital, in cooperation with Carl A. L. Binger and N. W. Ackerman at Cornell, expressed a view, 1945, that, while psychological disorders (prolonged unresolved struggle between dependent strivings and compensatory aggressive drives, with eventual acceptance of defeat of the latter) should not be regarded as causing hypertension, they might be related to it. Some workers repudiate entirely the idea of a personality pattern in hypertension: Weiss, for example, expressed a conviction that there is no pattern but that there is a somewhat higher incidence of various neurotic tendencies in a hypertensive population. Binger, while warning, 1951, against the inference that emotional states can precipitate chronic vasomotor constriction, nevertheless thought that the best hope for some patients with essential hypertension lay in psychotherapy. Various reports of prolonged psychotherapy, however, indicate no cures of hypertension. The patient may be better adjusted, blood pressures may be a little lower, but "the disease is still there" (Perera, 1953).

## ENDOCRINE INFLUENCES IN HYPERTENSION

While influence of thyroid, of estrogens, of pressor and antidiuretic principles of the posterior pituitary in experimental hypertension has been reported only occasionally, adrenal activity in maintaining the functional integrity of the circulatory system has been recognized for nearly fifty years. Early studies suggested that in animals the effect of adrenalectomy on blood volume was associated with altered kidney function. A relation of the adrenal cortex to hypertension was suggested by the finding that in Addisonian crisis adrenal cortical extracts and desoxycorticosterone acetate (DCA) raised blood pressure (Robert F. Loeb, 1939). This demonstration led to experimental production of hypertension in a variety of animals injected with DCA, and to subsequent studies of relations between this type of hypertension and sodium chloride regulation by the adrenal cortex and the kidney. The above-mentioned interest in stress as a factor in hypertension also connotes the adrenal cortex, with which, in the minds of some, stress has unfortunately come to be regarded as synonymous (Perera, 1952). Stress is indirectly implicated also in work on the relation of the sympathoadrenal system to hypertension, in which there is renewed interest in the adrenal medulla.

## THE ADRENAL MEDULLA

A curable and relatively rare type of hypertension caused by single or multiple tumors, pheochromocytoma, of the chromaffin tissue of the adrenal medulla (or the thoracic and abdominal paraganglia) is the only type known to be caused by the medullary hormones, epinephrine and/or nor-epinephrine. Previously noted reports have indicated that the characteristic hemodynamic effects of epinephrine are different from those of human essential hypertension, while the effects of nor-epinephrine, which may be one or the only secretion of these tumors, resemble the changes in hypertension with one exception — increased pulmonary resistance; others have found "no significant difference" in hemodynamic effects of the two compounds (K. G. Wakim and H. E. Essex, Mayo Clinic and Foundation, 1952). The possible relation of disturbance in metabolism of epinephrine and norepinephrine to essential hypertension was suggested by Goldenberg, 1948. While referring to evidence against direct participation of the adrenal medulla in essential hypertension, Perera observed, 1952, "we are not entitled as yet to eliminate the adrenal medulla from further consideration" or to disregard the possibility "that sensitization of blood vessels to normal amounts of nor-epinephrine could account for hypertension". Corcoran and Page pointed to possible interaction (with regard to hypertension) between medulla and cortex, observing, 1948, that while the two glands are very different and "almost accidentally associated in the same capsule", it cannot be said "that the one has no influence on the other". That epinephrine "is capable of exciting the adrenal cortex is now generally accepted" (Long and associates, 1950). Although the mechanism by which this excitation is brought about has been debated (Marthe Vogt, 1944; Sayers and Sayers, 1948), the Yale investigators considered their data to show "without exception" that epinephrine acts directly upon the anterior pituitary to stimulate secretion of ACTH which is the intermediary of epinephrine action on the adrenal cortex.

## THE ADRENAL CORTEX

While the view that the adrenal cortex causes hypertension could not, in Perera's judgment, 1951, be supported, he thought it could be said that "both sodium and the adrenal cortex are related very definitely to the regulation of the blood pressure". Observations on the influence of the adrenal cortex have been made in reports on almost every aspect of experimental renal hypertension: Goldblatt's 1937 report that experimental renal hypertension could be neither induced nor maintained (in the dog and other species) when the adrenal cortex is removed; the 1942 report of Houssay and Dexter that for eliciting hypertensive response in the dog the renin system required the adrenal cortex; Shorr's 1948 report that adrenalectomy abolishes VEM formation in the anaerobic kidney, while DCA restores it. Interpretation of these observations was made difficult (Pickering, 1950) by the well-known fact that adrenalectomy reduces the arterial pressure of normal animals to the point of circulatory failure. The question is whether adrenalectomy in hypertensive animals signifies more than removal of the normal influence of the gland. Contrary to the usual experience, Turner and Grollman, on the basis of studies of the bilaterally nephrectomized and adrenalectomized dog with hypertension, reported, 1951, that hypertension and pathologic tissue changes characteristic of it can develop in the absence of adrenal function. Perera mentioned, 1950, development of abnormal levels of blood pressure in Addisonian patients following renal damage by disease; Abbie I. Knowlton and her group (Columbia departments of medicine and bacteriology) reported, 1947, production of hypertension in adrenalectomized rats.

## RENAL-ADRENAL REGULATION OF SODIUM CHLORIDE METABOLISM

Especially provocative to students of hypertension has been work over fifteen years past on the role of the adrenal cortex in electrolyte balance, notably adrenal-renal relations in sodium retention. Application of fundamental work in endocrinology to an ill-defined clinical condition offers obvious difficulties but also suggestive leads. Robert Gaunt, J. H. Birnie and W. J. Eversole pointed out, 1949, that sodium retention results from most adrenal steroids, of which desoxycorticosterone acetate (DCA) is most active. This synthetic steroid, used as substitution therapy in Addison's disease, has been isolated from adrenal tissue only once, in minute amounts by Reichstein (1938), who synthesized it. Dwight J. Ingle's experiments, discussed in 1950, indicated that other steroids mimic the effect of the salt-regulating steroid, and that under one experimental condition or another the desoxy-steroid can cause either retention or excretion of sodium. In fact, the adrenal cortex is not known "to represent the sole regulatory mechanism for any metabolic process" although it is essential for maintaining normal regulatory and adaptive mechanisms. Understanding of one of these mechanisms (Kendall, 1948), "illustrated in the work of the kidney which depends in a peculiar way upon sodium chloride", and in other physiological functions, requires investigation of the mechanisms by which electrolytes pass through cellular structures. These processes involve all phases of intermediary metabolism.

Study of effects of DCA on blood pressure are concerned, obviously, with certain end results of reactions not yet analyzed in biochemical and cellular detail. An "hormonally induced renal hypertension" reported in rats by Hans Selye and associates, 1943, for example, showed after long-continued overdosage with DCA malignant nephrosclerosis with rapidly progressing hypertension but no conclusion was reached, 1951, regarding the relation between the kidney and the activity of the salt-retaining steroid. Braun-Menéndez, 1950, considered sodium a "sine qua non for the production of renal lesions". However, Friedman and Friedman had, 1948, after producing hypertension and altered renal function in rats by subcutaneous implantation of DCA pellets without sodium, concluded that neither sodium nor renal mechanism was involved. Perera was convinced, 1950, that hypertensive vascular disease is associated with disturbance of salt and water metabolism.

Early in the present century, the assumed role of salt in hypertension stimulated trials of salt-free diets. Grollman and Harrison, 1943, found that drastic sodium restriction without other treatment reduced the blood pressure and prolonged the life of hypertensive rats; in Grollman's view, however, 1951, abnormalities of salt and water metabolism, including change in tissue content, had not been proved to be "the basic dysfunction . . ." Study of tissue electrolytes and water in the renal artery walls of human hypertensives by Louis Tobian and J. T. Binion, University of Texas, 1952, indicated an increase of both, sufficient to cause swelling and narrowing of the lumen of the vessels. They proposed studies to determine whether low sodium diets would lower the sodium and water content of artery walls. Clinical trials of salt-free diet, abandoned earlier, were renewed in 1944 by Walter Kempner (Duke) whose favorable results with the rice diet have been confirmed by some, challenged by others. Clinical trials in a number of centers in which only a few patients have been hospitalized for periods long enough to permit controlled observations (on renal hemodynamics, electrolyte excretion, etc.) have resulted in reports of lowered blood pressure in some patients but understandable disagreement on the question whether salt deprivation is a primary factor in essential hypertension. The 1951 observation of C. B. Chapman, University of Minnesota, on the rice diet probably represents a more or less general view: "To the clinician it provides a temporary means of relieving symptoms attributable to hypertension, but it is a measure that is dangerous in some patients and is curative in none."

The importance of sodium metabolism and the associated water balance in the changes culminating in essential hypertension has been recognized increasingly in what Page referred to as "unifying concepts to provide a more orderly pattern for future experimental work". That the responsiveness of the cardiovascular tissues to humoral pressor agents may determine the degree of hypertension has been pointed out in numerous connections, and among factors influencing this responsiveness sodium is beginning to receive attention. It is well known that administration of desoxycorticosterone acetate is followed by retention of sodium; Braun-Menéndez and Prado reported, 1950, that administration of desoxycorticosterone acetate caused renal lesions, renal hypertrophy and hypertension (in rats) only when sodium chloride was given in the diet or drinking fluid. Explanation of this effect of sodium is still hypothetical. Braun-Menéndez favored the hypothesis that the hormone sensitizes the organism to the action of sodium (rather than the reverse) for which he cited a degree of experimental evidence; he found that all the known factors that favor retention of sodium, whether due to increased ingestion or to decreased excretion, tend to induce hypertension. An hypothesis that sodium is the sensitizer of the arterial musculature to the vasoconstrictive action of the sympathoadrenal hormones (epinephrine and nor-epinephrine), and that desoxycorticosterone acetate enters the picture as the regulator of sodium retention, was proposed by Raab and his associates (University of Vermont), 1952. Page, 1951, discussed a concept, formulated with Masson and Corcoran, relating changes in sodium metabolism to a direct renal-adrenal interaction which becomes a part of the vicious cycle of essential hypertension. A balance between sodium loss and sodium retention was proposed: sodium loss in response to renin and hypertensin, as demonstrated, at least in the rabbit, by Pickering's group, 1949; sodium retention in response to increased secretion of desoxycorticosterone acetate, suggested by observations of hypertrophy of the zona glomerulosa of the adrenal cortex in response to renin (or to the presence of experimental renal hypertension). Since desoxycorticosterone acetate, significant in problems of hypertension and of sodium balance, has been found only once in adrenal tissue, the need for evidence that it is produced and secreted by the gland is a consideration in the studies of the cytology and cytochemistry of the adrenal cortex by Roy O. Greep and Helen W. Deane at Harvard since 1943. Data reported, 1949, were considered to support the view that the zona glomerulosa, a region of the outer layer of the adrenal cortex, secretes desoxycorticosteroids. Hypertrophy of this zone of the adrenal was observed in rats with lowered sodium to potassium ratios in body fluids by Laramore and Grollman, 1950. Page proposed that hypertrophy of the zona glomerulosa in experimental hypertension might be a response to sodium loss; but hypersecretion (of DCA) by the zona glomerulosa would then favor sodium retention and hypertension. The hypothetical vicious cycle would, at the points noted, depend in various ways upon sodium balance. Some of the questions raised by these proposals concerning the interrelated influences of the kidney and the adrenal on sodium balance, and the influence of sodium balance on secretory activities of the kidney and adrenal underlie several current concepts.

## THE PITUITARY-ADRENAL SYSTEM IN RELATION TO VASCULAR HOMEOSTASIS

Theories postulating pituitary-adrenal influences on blood pressure are rarely discussed apart from renal and neural mechanisms. Hypertension, in Peter Heinbecker's hypothesis regarded as a compensatory mechanism designed to increase renal blood flow wherever renal tubular function is reduced or threatened, involves functional influences from the frontal lobes of the cerebral cortex, operating through the hypothalamic nuclei upon the pituitary and eventually upon the adrenal cortex and the renal pressor mechanisms. D. M. Green (University of Southern California School of Medicine), reviewing recent advances in experimental hypertension, considered, 1953, that "experimental evidence points to the hypophysis and hypothalamus as perhaps the most promising areas for future investigation of essential hypertension". That the pituitary-adrenal system may be a pathway through which the sympathetic nervous system operates was set forth by Long and associates, 1947, 1950. How this well-established neural pathway initiated by activation of the sympathetic nervous system and release of epinephrine stimulates, finally, secretory activity of the adrenal cortex which has no nerve supply of its own has been studied by a number of workers (Marthe Vogt, 1944; Long and Fry, 1945; Sayers and Sayers, 1948; McDermott, Fry, Brobeck and Long, 1950). Long raised the question whether epinephrine secretion is a form of stress or the common mechanism by which all forms of stress are carried to the pituitary gland. Selye, 1950, explaining his hypothesis of development of hypertension as a result of increased "defensive" production of adrenal steroids in response to nonspecific stress, thought it improbable that, without associated changes in sodium and protein metabolism and pre-existing renal damage, "hypercorticoidism in itself is responsible for any common type of clinical hypertension".

Clinical studies led Perera, 1952, to leave open the question of adrenal cortical participation in hypertension until chemical methods become available for determination of desoxycorticosterone-like compounds in the adrenal and circulation.  He accorded to the pituitary-adrenal system the role of an important adjunct in the response of the tissues to stress, but to excess adrenal cortical materials no essential part; rather, he suggested an approach through study of the role of the hormones in regulation of normal blood pressure.  That "certain fundamentally important aspects of vascular behavior are appreciated by contemporary science either dimly or not at all" seemed to Pickering, 1950, to account for the *"impasse"* in investigation of hypertension.  Nevertheless, conferences, symposia, critical reviews increasingly reveal a determination to test rigorously each claim and conclusion with the objective of definitively accepting or rejecting it as a sound foundation stone for the ultimate structure.  "Our facts must be correct", wrote Selye, 1950, "our theories need not be if they help us to discover important new facts."

CHAPTER 6

# The Rheumatic Syndromes

*Reflecting connective tissue alterations*

# THE CONCEPT OF CONNECTIVE TISSUE
# DISEASES

The numerous systemic disorders included in the rather miscellaneous group known as the rheumatic syndromes have, in spite of widely differing clinical manifestations, a common denominator: all of them (and various other conditions outside the rheumatic group) involve connective tissue, derived from the embryonic mesenchyme. Many tissues and organs develop from differentiation of the mesenchyme (skeletal and smooth muscle, bone, blood vessels, lymphatic tissue and all the bloodforming organs); in addition there are loose connective tissue elements which form an "edifice" of intercellular substances (fibrillar, elastic, gel-like) supporting the cells of all tissues and organs.  Alterations in this loose connective tissue are considered especially to characterize the rheumatic syndromes.  This orienting concept, developed over twenty years, chiefly by pathologists, was by 1953 widely accepted as reasonably explaining the protean tissue involvement in rheumatic conditions.  Some workers incline to describing the rheumatic syndromes as "collagen" diseases, thus implicating only one of the fibrous proteins of connective tissue, cartilage and bone.  Many workers (as Bauer and Clark, 1953) prefer the more inclusive term, connective tissue diseases, connoting alterations not merely in the collagen fibers but rather in the entire connective tissue complex. Whatever the terminology, it is now clear that the concept of alterations of the connective tissue, varied manifestations of which may possibly be due to individual host and tissue susceptibility, may provide a unifying influence in research on rheumatic conditions (rheumatic fever, rheumatoid arthritis, the arthritis of gout, lupus erythematosus, periarteritis nodosa, scleroderma, dermatomyositis and less clearly defined disorders as bursitis, neuritis, neuralgia) comparable to the unifying influence in cancer research provided by the concept that malignancy is a common potentiality of cells, elicited by unknown metabolic alterations produced by a wide variety of stimuli.

Research on the rheumatic syndromes has suffered from the fact that since no one of them occurs naturally in mammals other than man there is consequent uncertainty as to whether experimental production is possible. There have been experimental approximations: as in reports (Murphy, 1952) of production in rabbits, after multiple focal cutaneous infections with hemolytic streptococci, of valvular, endocardial, myocardial and blood vessel lesions "closely resembling those of rheumatic fever"; as in experimental production in rats (Kerr and Cavelti, 1947), by injections of tissue extracts mixed with killed streptococci, of experimental lesions reported to resemble those of glomerulonephritis and rheumatic fever. Experimental lesions of the periarteritis nodosa type produced in rabbits by serum sickness (Rich and Gregory, 1943) led to active investigation of anaphylactic hypersensitivity as a mechanism underlying periarteritis nodosa and other connective tissue diseases — rheumatic fever, lupus erythematosus, rheumatoid arthritis (Rich, 1947). Similarity between widespread inflammatory connective tissue lesions in rats subjected to a variety of stressful experimental procedures and lesions of the rheumatic and other human diseases (Selye, 1950) led to the hypothesis that permanent disruption of the adaptation mechanism of the pituitary-adrenal system may be a root cause of various human conditions, including the connective tissue diseases. In arthritis (similar to osteoarthritis) produced in adrenalectomized and ovariectomized rats by injection of purified growth hormone of the anterior pituitary, Reinhardt and Li, 1953, noted transient joint swellings which were reduced by cortisone. They pointed out that this inflammatory reaction might be a manifestation of hypersensitivity to an unknown factor, the growth hormone itself being nonantigenic (Li and associates, 1950).

The connective tissue concept has been supported also by clinical observations pointing to apparently common manifestations (not many of which have been proved in humans) in differing syndromes. In separate conditions also have been observed lesions — in addition to those peculiar to the given condition — closely resembling those of other members of the group (Murphy, 1952). These resemblances have suggested that two or more of these conditions may sometimes occur simultaneously or may supersede one another in the same patient (Bauer and associates, 1952). Similarity in sites of tissue damage in the differing syndromes has further suggested a certain association. The tissues involved in rheumatic fever, for instance, and in rheumatoid arthritis are the same: blood vessels, heart, pericardium, skeletal muscles, skin, nerve trunks, adipose tissue, bone, liver, spleen, lymph nodes, eye, the synovia and capsules of joints. Certainly, location of lesions does not appear to be a reliable principle of classification for the rheumatic syndromes. In several conditions, apparent limitation of lesions to certain sites or predilection for single sites remains an unsolved problem. The degenerative joint disease, osteoarthritis, which is somehow associated with the aging process and local stress, is probably a quite different disease from those previously mentioned. Ankylosing spondylitis, marked by peculiar and particularized joint changes, by demineralization of the vertebral bodies and calcification of the lateral spinal ligaments, is sometimes regarded as an especial form of rheumatoid arthritis, sometimes as an independent entity. The more frequent reference to rheumatic fever and rheumatoid arthritis in the present discussion is governed by the more extensive research on rheumatic fever and rheumatoid arthritis and the light this research sheds on the concept of connective tissue diseases generally.

## EXTENT OF THE "RHEUMATISM" PROBLEM
## AND CURRENT STATUS OF CERTAIN
## THERAPEUTIC EXPEDIENTS

Statistical evidence of incidence of the rheumatic syndromes must be speculative because of the lack of fundamental knowledge of etiology, because many of the entities grouped under the rheumatic syndromes are ill-defined, are not reportable, and because there are (notably in childhood rheumatic fever) many cases not recognized at the time and not always recognized later. Partial surveys of a given syndrome (especially rheumatic fever, rheumatic heart disease and rheumatoid arthritis) in a given group or in a particular locality have been, however, suggestive. On the basis of such population samples, a 1952 Public Health Service estimate placed the number of "rheumatism" cases (apparently all forms) in the United States at approximately nine million. In any hundred rheumatism patients seeking medical care it has been estimated (Primer on the Rheumatic Diseases, 1953) that thirty to forty have rheumatoid arthritis. The observed association of antecedent streptococcic infection with many cases of rheumatic fever has suggested an indirect and proportional indication of incidence of rheumatic fever. From three to four per cent of cases of streptococcal infection, according to epidemiological studies of rheumatic fever in the United States armed services (Rammelkamp and associates, 1952) and in various age groups (Rantz and associates, 1952), were followed by rheumatic fever and from twenty to seventy-five per cent of cases of streptococcal infection in rheumatic subjects were followed by recurrence of rheumatic fever. Selective service records showed that half the cases of heart disease for which men were rejected were rheumatic (committee on cardiovascular disease, National Research Council, 1943). Various surveys (1953 Primer) of school children have revealed a one to four per cent incidence of rheumatic heart disease, and autopsy studies have indicated a general incidence of seven per cent. While the death rate from rheumatic heart disease in the vulnerable ages below forty-five has steadily declined, it is estimated that the hearts of fifty per cent of those that have had one or more attacks of rheumatic fever in childhood (Wilson and associates, 1948) are damaged to a degree that constitutes disability. Figures indicating incidence of ankylosing spondylitis (assuming its rheumatoid nature) are not conclusive; in an Army rheumatism center during the last war half the cases diagnosed as rheumatoid arthritis were spondylitis, illustrating predilection of the disease for vigorous and physically active young men.

One index of the unsolved status of the rheumatism problem is the fact that the therapies available for various syndromes remain for the most part empiric. Perhaps an exception — as to clarity of rationale — is prophylactic use of the sulfonamides and penicillin to control the group A hemolytic streptococcic infections generally accepted as predisposing to rheumatic fever. Antibiotics have dramatically changed the outlook in one of the complications of rheumatic heart disease, subacute bacterial endocarditis, which is now considered curable in sixty to seventy per cent of cases, although the damage to heart valves remains (Herrell and Heilman, 1952). For the acute phase of rheumatic fever the use of the salicylates is traditional but the mechanism of their action not well understood. Operation for mitral stenosis for which claims have been made (Varco and Baronofsky, Minnesota, 1952, and earlier workers) in rheumatic heart disease is still to be evaluated. In rheumatoid arthritis, subject to unpredictable remissions and relapses "regardless of therapy", rest, nutrition, analgesics, physical and psychic therapy "seldom do harm", but whether they are effective "is another question" (Ragan, 1951). Evaluation of gold salts, long credited with influencing favorably the course of the disease if used early enough, remained indeterminate after the authors of the Tenth Rheumatism Review, 1953, reviewed American and British literature reporting 7,000 treated cases. It is generally agreed that the toxicity is high (Kling and coworkers, 1952). In spondylitis in which gold is of no value (1953 Primer) roentgen radiation of the spine has been variously reported to produce objective improvement in about half the patients treated (Query, 1949), subjective improvement in sixty per cent and cure in none (Graham, Fletcher and Graham, 1952). The most recent therapeutic agents, adrenal cortical hormones and the adrenocorticotrophic hormone, ACTH, it is generally agreed (as discussed later), temporarily suppress the inflammatory process of connective tissue diseases; but stress has been laid upon the danger of hyperadrenalism, of relapse when the drugs are withdrawn, of flare-up of quiescent infections provoked by the hormones and of the masking of acute infections.

## DIRECTIONS AND SOURCES OF RESEARCH PERTINENT TO CONNECTIVE TISSUE DISEASES

Research on the connective tissue in health and its alterations in disease is gradually converging, however unevenly, from widely separate directions upon those morphological alterations that characterize the rheumatic syndromes. Knowledge of connective tissue formation, its differentiation, its physical and chemical properties, its metabolism is meager (Ragan, 1952). Characterization of its component parts, the ground substance (gel-like, acting as a medium of transport for metabolites and as a shock absorber) and fibrous proteins (elastin, collagen, etc., acting as a means of support for cells and tissues and providing strength, cohesiveness, movement, rebound) is under way, but, as a whole, connective tissue is still "a system whose function we do not know" (Meyer, 1951). Until we do — and new knowledge may be imminent — it is obvious that the rheumatic syndromes cannot be fundamentally understood. Meanwhile connective tissue reactions are a major focus of investigation pertinent to working hypotheses of rheumatic processes: rheumatic fever and rheumatic heart disease as related by unknown mechanisms to antecedent infection of susceptible individuals with group A beta hemolytic streptococci; hypersensitivity, involving antigen-antibody reactions, as a mechanism underlying some or all of the connective tissue diseases; hormone factors including dysfunction of the pituitary-adrenal system leading to abnormal reactions of tissues under stress as a possible mechanism of some of the rheumatic syndromes.

While the above lines of work do not comprehend all active investigative work on the rheumatic diseases, they have given impetus to clinical and also to fundamental investigation in this field. There is a reciprocal influence between the two: for example, the demonstration of powerful effects of cortisone on symptoms of rheumatoid arthritis by the Mayo Clinic workers (Hench, Kendall and associates, 1949) initiated the most active period in the study of adrenal cortical physiology. Conversely, the new developments in endocrine research, drawing together lines of fundamental work in physics and chemistry, in cellular biology and biochemistry, in bacteriology and immunology, have deepened pathological and clinical studies in formerly isolated areas.

### PROGRESS TOWARD ORGANIZATION OF RESEARCH ON THE RHEUMATIC SYNDROMES

Organization of the attack on the rheumatic diseases in the United States, in the sense of stimulating interest in a neglected field, raising and allocating funds for research and for training investigators, planning research through scientific advisory committees, got off to a late start (after interruption by the first world war) with creation in 1930 of the American Rheumatism Association. It has collaborated in eight international congresses on rheumatic diseases organized by the older *Ligue Internationale contre le Rhumatisme*. It set up, 1948, the Arthritis and Rheumatism Foundation which requested the National Research Council to survey work then in progress as a basis for planning and supporting future research. The survey committee (seventeen members representing anatomy, pathology, physiology, physiological chemistry, biology, microbiology and the clinical fields of medicine, orthopedic surgery, psychiatry, physical medicine, public health), reviewing, 1948, work in this field in sixty-six medical schools and teaching hospitals, reported 198 research projects under way in forty-eight schools and an estimated annual expenditure of $950,000. Of this amount, two thirds was designed for research on rheumatic fever, about one third for research on arthritis, $135,500 for fundamental research. Most of the money reported was concentrated in six medical schools. Outside grants (supporting about half the research then in progress) came chiefly from foundations: from the Commonwealth Fund over $800,000 between 1929 and 1949 to three investigators for research on rheumatic fever and arthritis; from the Rackham Fund, 1940, one million for endowment of an arthritis research unit at the University of Michigan; from the Helen Hay Whitney Foundation over $400,000, 1947 through 1949, for rheumatic fever studies in ten medical schools and hospitals. In each of the years between 1945 and 1948, the life insurance industry through its medical research fund contributed about $93,000 for studies of rheumatic fever (of its total appropriation of $1,896,275 in that period for cardiovascular research). Between 1951 and 1953, the Arthritis and Rheumatism Foundation had awarded from public campaign funds $1,133,616 for 150 research projects related to arthritis.

Research on epidemiological aspects of rheumatic fever had by that time been organized by the Armed Forces Epidemiological Board, the American Heart Association, the Children's Bureau of the Federal Security Agency. The national advisory council of the National Heart Institute and other national institutes recommended between 1949 and 1950 grants totaling $350,000 for research on the rheumatic diseases (compared with $80,758 allocated by the Public Health Service in 1948). The National Institute of Arthritis and Metabolic Diseases, created by Congress, 1951, provided a means for planning and organizing research on the rheumatic syndromes and metabolic diseases. For the year 1951, federal agencies, chiefly the Institute of Arthritis and Metabolic Diseases and the National Heart Institute, contributed $993,462 for research in this field, approximately two thirds of which was in grants to university and hospital laboratories outside government.

Groups in medical schools, hospitals and research institutes whose combined clinical and experimental work on rheumatic fever and rheumatoid arthritis over periods of from ten to thirty years has provided leadership in the work of the American Rheumatism Association include: a group under Walter Bauer working in the Harvard medical department at the Massachusetts General Hospital on an arthritis research program set up in 1929; a group working since 1928 in the Faulkner Arthritis Clinic at the Columbia-Presbyterian Medical Center; a group working since 1940 at the Rackham Arthritis Clinic at the University of Michigan; groups of investigators in the departments of pediatrics and medicine at Cornell; a Rockefeller Institute group directed by Homer F. Swift from about 1920 until his death; a group in the medical division, Mayo Clinic, under Philip S. Hench whose interest in rheumatism goes back more than thirty years; more recently a study group on rheumatic diseases organized in 1948 in New York University with representatives from eight departments, and units set up at Northwestern (Alvin F. Coburn), 1947, and at California (Peter H. Forsham), 1952.

Progressive exchange of new knowledge oriented by unifying concepts touched upon above is beginning to integrate clinical research and certain fundamental work in experimental biology and biochemistry (histochemistry, organic, protein, enzyme, physical chemistry, employing electron microscopy, isotopes and other techniques). By new methods of study applied at the base line of connective tissue reactions, investigators are hoping to bring knowledge gradually within the perspective of clinical problems. Papers at a 1951 symposium on rheumatic fever at the University of Minnesota were divided equally between clinical studies and experimental work in cellular physiology, bacteriology, immunology, biochemistry including hormones. A 1953 conference, admitting that therapeutic effects of the adrenal hormones were not yet explicable in terms of the general metabolic effects of the hormones (Pincus and Hechter, 1953), aimed by diverse approaches through discussions of circulatory factors, cellular and acellular tissue changes, inflammation, immunologic and specific infectious processes to shed light on the mechanism of action of adrenal hormones on connective and other tissues.

At the third Macy Foundation conference on connective tissue, 1952, opinion was divided on the questions whether physical or chemical methods of study are more rewarding, whether normal or pathological material is preferable. Electron microscopic studies of collagen have been reported from the National Institute of Arthritis and Metabolic Diseases, Rockefeller Institute, Massachusetts Institute of Technology (biology), Massachusetts General Hospital (medical department), University of Illinois (physiology). Cellular studies (biological, histochemical, including use of enzymes and isotope-labeled compounds) directly or indirectly bearing on connective tissue reactions, include those in pathology departments at Johns Hopkins, Pennsylvania, Yale, Temple, Illinois, Tennessee, Washington University in St. Louis; in anatomy departments in the universities of Michigan, Chicago, Wayne, Washington (St. Louis), Toronto and at Mount Sinai Hospital, New York; in departments of histology, cytology, bacteriology at Yale, Pennsylvania, New York universities, the Rockefeller Institute; in departments of medicine at Harvard, Minnesota, Cornell, Henry Ford Hospital, Mayo Clinic and Foundation. Studies of chemical constitution and metabolism of connective tissue are in progress in departments of physiology, physiological chemistry, biochemistry and medicine at Columbia, Harvard, New York University, Tufts, Minnesota, Wisconsin, Ohio State, Cincinnati, the Rockefeller Institute, the Worcester Foundation for Experimental Biology; in the pediatrics department, Chicago; in bacteriology and immunology departments in the University of Texas, New York University; in pathology departments at Tennessee, Ohio, Wisconsin, Chicago, Wayne; at the National Heart Institute.

The generally accepted significance of antecedent streptococcic infection in many cases of rheumatic fever has focused attention on basic study of the streptococcus. However, only ten per cent of the seventy-odd investigators that reported studies on rheumatic fever to the National Research Council's survey committee, 1949, were engaged "in what might be fairly called fundamental" work on the biology of the streptococcus. Detailed study of the disease-producing streptococci was begun in 1919 at the Rockefeller Institute where successive workers studied the nutrition, cellular composition, extracellular products of the organism together with immune responses to more than fifteen cellular substances to define their antigenic properties; on these and other studies the currently used classification of streptococci (Rebecca C. Lancefield) is based. At New York University, in departments of medicine and microbiology, fundamental chemical and biological studies of the organism were begun more recently. Other work at Northwestern, Stanford, Cornell, Minnesota, Harvard, Yale, Pennsylvania, Ohio State universities, Mayo Clinic and Foundation is concerned with biological and chemical as well as clinical, pathological, immunological aspects of streptococcic infection in relation to rheumatic fever.

Streptococcal antigens are among those used in immunological and immunochemical investigation of hypersensitive reactions, related to at least some of the connective tissue diseases, and, according to some workers, hypothetically to all. Investigators exploring relationships of the immediate and the delayed types of hypersensitive response to the rheumatic syndromes or connective tissue diseases include many workers in departments of cell physiology, microbiology, biochemistry, immunology.  Especially to be noted is work of long standing that has been related by theory or by experimental evidence to problems of the rheumatic diseases: at the Rockefeller Institute, Minnesota (pathology, medicine, pediatrics), New York University (microbiology, medicine, pediatrics), Mount Sinai Hospital, Johns Hopkins (pathology, medicine), Columbia (biochemistry, bacteriology, immunology, medicine), Cornell (medicine), Mayo Foundation (bacteriology, medicine), Stanford (medicine, pediatrics), Yale (anatomy, physiological chemistry), Tulane (pediatrics, medicine). More recent investigations have been reported from Utah (anatomy, bacteriology), Emory, other university centers, Michael Reese Hospital, the National Institutes of Health, the Merck and the Wyeth research institutes.

Reactions in hypersensitive states were among the first shown to change radically in response to cortisone first used in rheumatoid arthritis, and later, with hydrocortisone and ACTH, given in inflammatory conditions of connective tissue.  Experimental studies of mechanisms of the effects of these hormones on normal and pathological tissues have naturally been few; investigators engaged for decades on chemical and physiological studies of the pituitary and the adrenal cortex and their interrelations have probably all contributed to the sharpening picture of the phenomena resulting from action of these hormones on connective tissue.  Pertinent also in studies of connective tissue reactivity has been accumulating evidence of apparently direct effects on joint cartilage of the pituitary without adrenal intervention. Before the concept of connective tissue diseases had been widely considered, endocrine effects on connective tissue had been explored in various laboratories: Institute of Experimental Medicine and Surgery, Montreal; Yale (physiological chemistry, anatomy); Utah (anatomy); California (biochemistry, anatomy); Washington University (pathology); Columbia (medicine); Harvard and later Temple (pathology). Especially to be mentioned in connection with study of effects on pathological connective tissue reactions are the Mayo Clinic and Foundation; the various hospital medical services of Harvard; the Mount Sinai, Henry Ford and Michael Reese hospitals; the Worcester Foundation for Experimental Biology; pathology departments at

Chicago, Minnesota, Johns Hopkins; medical departments of Columbia, Cornell, Southern California, Chicago.

# FUNDAMENTAL WORK ON THE CONNECTIVE TISSUE IN SUGGESTIVE RELATION TO THE RHEUMATIC SYNDROMES

## THE NATURE OF CONNECTIVE TISSUE

The so-called loose connective tissue distributed throughout the body has been morphologically described (Sylvia H. Bensley and A. W. Ham, anatomy, Toronto, 1952) as intercellular fibrous and amorphous substances; or as including a third less well-defined element, the mesenchymal cells which make and secrete at least some of the connective tissue substances (Charles Ragan, medicine, Columbia, 1952). The body might, in the view of Ham and Bensley, be described as an edifice of intercellular substance in which the (gel-like) cells "live as residents" and produce the building materials for the supporting structures. Three kinds of fibrillar connective tissue are distinguished: elastic (yellow) fibers; collagen (white) fibers which form gelatin on boiling and have great tensile strength; the reticulum (believed by many to differ from collagen only in size and not in chemical composition), providing a meshwork for support of the cells. Study by X-ray diffraction and electron microscopy of the fine molecular structure of the kinds of connective tissue elements and the relation between them has as yet resulted in few conclusions (R. W. G. Wyckoff, National Institute of Arthritis and Metabolic Diseases, 1952). The electron microscope has, however, revealed a definitive "fingerprint" for normal collagen in the characteristic periodic crossbanding of the fibril (F. O. Schmitt and associates, biology, Massachusetts Institute of Technology, 1942). The same periodicity was observed by the same method in "almost pure" reticulin, suggesting a functional and morphological continuity between collagen and reticulin which, however, were described by A. H. T. Robb-Smith (pathology, Radcliff Infirmary, Oxford, 1952) as "different". Definitive characterization of collagen was left open at the 1953 Macy conference: "we can agree on our ignorance" (Fremont-Smith).

Studies of normal collagen as a baseline for study of alterations in disease are, in one instance, an outgrowth of fundamental work on fibrous proteins. The twenty years' study by physical techniques of the chain molecules of wool, hair, muscle, epidermis, bacterial flagella, blood fibrin (described, 1950, as nature's own textile business) by W. T. Astbury and his associates in the textile physics laboratory, Leeds University, was extended several years ago to pathological fibrous proteins. With medical collaborators, X-ray and electron microscopic data on fibrous proteins were being used to trace alterations in pathological collagenous tissues, especially from rheumatoid cases.

Formation of fibrillar connective tissue and its regeneration after injury had been debated for almost a century since German pathologists (Virchow, Kölliker) proposed that since these substances do not occur in blood they are formed under direct influence of cells, possibly within the cells (fibroblasts), from which they escape and subsequently consolidate. Tissue culture methods in recent years have resulted in formation of collagen with the characteristic periodic crossbanding and reprecipitated acid-dissolved collagen has shown it in at least some instances (K. R. Porter, Rockefeller Institute, 1951; Wyckoff, 1952). Paul Klemperer (pathology, Mount Sinai Hospital, New York) considered, 1950, that *in vitro* and *in vivo* experiments to date indicate that "not only normal fibroblasts but also a homogeneous ground-substance, adequate in amount and in chemical or physicochemical constitution, is of paramount importance for the formation of collagenous fibers".

Millions of connective tissue fibrils surround the smallest blood vessels, lymphatic channels and other formed structures. The tissue fluid (thirty per cent of the body fluid) is "captivated" on the enormous surface area of the connective tissue fibrils like a film caught between two plates of glass, remaining, however, a liquid capable of transporting ions and diffusing into cells. Between the fibrils is the amorphous gelatinous ground substance (P. D. McMaster and R. J. Parsons, Rockefeller Institute, 1950).

The origin of the ground substance, its metabolic turnover and its function were still, 1952, matters of conjecture (Ragan). From histological and chemical study, some workers have inferred that the fibroblasts developing from embryonic mesenchymal cells deposit the ground substance, then spin off reticulin which is oriented and cemented laterally into collagen from which the white and yellow fibers of connective tissue are built. In most loose connective tissue the ground substance is gel-like; as synovial fluid it is liquid. Walter Bauer and Marian W. Ropes (medicine, Harvard; Massachusetts General Hospital) concluded, 1940 and 1953, that synovial fluid is a protein-containing dialysate of blood plasma (tissue fluid) in which mucin (secreted by the cells of the slightly modified connective tissue surrounding the joint) is responsible for normal viscosity, which is reduced in rheumatoid arthritis because of enzymic destruction of mucin (not demonstrated) or possible hormonal influences on mucin metabolism. Newer knowledge of the ground substance indicates wide variation in its content from tissue to tissue and in relative amounts of its peculiar constituents, acid mucopolysaccharides, soluble collagen, probably other proteins. Its transient constituents derived from the blood and the cells it supports may pass through rapidly or be trapped and stored. Since most tissue cells are not in direct contact with capillaries, their nutrition depends upon passage of substances through the ground substance. Functions of the ground substance, in addition to this nutritive role, include support, repair, protection (trapping of bacteria and other particulate matter, antibody formation) and probably (through its binding power) regulation of the salt and water balance of the body.

While the ground substance cannot be seen under the light microscope (R. D. Lillie, pathology, National Institute of Arthritis and Metabolic Diseases, 1952), some information concerning its physical nature has been obtained by means of the electron microscope (Gross and Schmitt, 1948). Reasons for the retarding of chemical and physical studies include the "extremely small" amount of the amorphous material, consequent difficulty in detecting its reactions and transformations, and the inadequacy of chemical and histochemical methods now available (Karl Meyer, medicine, Columbia, 1952, 1953). Study of the chemistry of the ground substance was initiated by the discovery of "spreading factors" twenty-five years ago by F. Duran-Reynals, followed considerably later by isolation of hyaluronic acid from bovine vitreous humor (Meyer and Palmer, 1934), and more recently from groups A and C hemolytic streptococci, Wharton's jelly of the umbilical cord, synovial fluid, skin and some mesenchymal tumors (Meyer, 1950). The other known mucopolysaccharide in ground substance, chondroitin sulfuric acid, isolated from cartilage over seventy years ago, occurs in loose connective tissue in association with hyaluronic acid, but alone in cartilage. In cartilage and other connective tissue, the presence of the mucopolysaccharides is inferred from histochemical techniques, notably dye reactions and the use of the enzyme hyaluronidase now generally identified with spreading factors.

The frequent association of antecedent hemolytic streptococcic infection with rheumatic fever makes highly pertinent studies of hyaluronic acid and of the hyaluronidases (produced by streptococci among other bacteria) that liquefy it (F. Duran-Reynals, bacteriology and immunology, Yale, 1942; Oscar Hechter, Worcester Foundation for Experimental Biology, 1950; David Glick, physiological chemistry, Minnesota, 1948; D. H. Sprunt, pathology and bacteriology, Tennessee, 1950; Bennett Sallman and J. M. Birkeland, bacteriology, Ohio State, 1950). The mechanisms of synthesis and breakdown of hyaluronic acid in the body are not known. It has been suggested (Ernest Gardner, anatomy, Wayne University, 1950) that the cells of the synovial membrane (and therefore all connective tissue cells) are specifically concerned in hyaluronic acid metabolism. The mechanism of action of the hyaluronic acid-hyaluronidase system in such diseased states as the rheumatic syndromes is the subject of numerous speculations. Meyer, 1947, tentatively outlined the formation of the ground substance beginning with hyaluronic acid, a collagen precursor, and chondroitin sulfate, secreted by young fibroblasts, then precipitated by local acidification into fibers with polysaccharides in a layer on the surface; and hyaluronate progressively replaced, with aging, by chondroitin sulfate. In study of direct effects of the hyaluronidases on connective tissue, Bensley found, 1950, increased permeability of cellular membranes and fraying of collagen fibers in fibrous connective tissue. The hyaluronidases appeared to accelerate a shift from amorphous to fibrillar elements of the connective tissue, a shift occurring in development, aging, repair, suggesting a role in pathological processes. Chemically, the action of the hyaluronidases on hyaluronic acid has been described (Meyer, 1950) as opening of glucosidic linkages in the long-chain molecule of the mucopolysaccharide.

That the primary lesions or changes in the rheumatic syndromes are chemical derangements of the ground substance of the mesenchyme (Klemperer, 1948; C. H. Altshuler and D. M. Angevine, pathology, Wisconsin, 1949; Meyer, 1952; Ragan, 1952) is not as yet demonstrable (Albert Dorfman, pediatrics, Western Reserve, 1952). The concept has, however, oriented investigation of the rheumatic syndromes as systemic in nature (Bauer and associates, 1952) and as related by common connective tissue alterations. Studies of these alterations (which may be degenerative, proliferative, inflammatory, with frequent overlapping of these processes, according to Bauer and Clark, 1953) must be accompanied by studies of normal connective tissue (Angevine, 1951).

## CONNECTIVE TISSUE MANIFESTATIONS OF RHEUMATIC SYNDROMES
### CARDIOVASCULAR, JOINT, NEURAL, NEUROMUSCULAR LESIONS

While in rheumatic fever practically any connective tissue in the body may be involved (Ragan, 1952), lesions of heart and blood vessels are regarded as most serious, and the typical Aschoff body or node, described in 1904, is generally considered to have diagnostic significance. The cellular origins of the Aschoff node have been debated for fifty years. At a 1951 symposium the view that its original cells are microscopic muscle fibers derived from the myocardium was supported by George E. Murphy (Rockefeller Institute) who left open the possibility that damage to the muscle cells might result from a primary chemical disturbance within the ground substance surrounding the muscle and collagen fibers, as suggested by many, including Dorfman, 1952. This latter or "classical" view describes this peculiar lesion as occurring in the interstices between the bundles of myofibers, and near arteries and veins. Other heart lesions in rheumatic carditis have been described as containing a central core of swollen collagen. In any case, the myocardium is eventually involved (Murphy). Of clinical significance in connection with rheumatic fever is the fact that myocardial cells, in common with cells of the nervous system and the glomeruli of the kidney, do not regenerate; "once destroyed they are not replaced" (A. E. Cohn, Rockefeller Institute, 1949).

Production of Aschoff bodies as essential in the rheumatic fever picture has been a natural aim in the long effort to achieve an experimental model. Lesions resembling those of rheumatic carditis were among those described in animals subjected to serum sickness (Arnold R. Rich, pathology, Johns Hopkins University, 1946; H. C. Hopps and R. W. Wissler, pathology, Chicago, 1946). Murphy, however, reviewing reports of experimental work, 1952, thought that "the tissue hallmarks of rheumatic heart disease have not been produced in animals by foreign serum or its fractions". Renewed attempts by the Rockefeller Institute workers to produce typical lesions of rheumatic fever in animals subjected to repeated infections with hemolytic streptococci resulted (in a few animals) in myocardial lesions "closely resembling human Aschoff bodies" of the type described as developing from injured myofibers (G. E. Murphy and Homer F. Swift, 1950; Murphy, 1952).

The Aschoff body and rheumatic subcutaneous nodules are believed by many workers to be histopathologically identical with rheumatic nodules throughout the body. Cells contained in inflammatory foci in the heart (in loose connective tissue adjacent to blood vessels and under the endocardium) were considered by Bauer and Clark, 1953, to be similar to the cells of the Aschoff nodule, if not identical with them. These foci and the subcutaneous nodule were all described as consisting of swollen, fragmented collagen fibers (fibrinoid degeneration) interspersed with characteristic cells (having granular cytoplasm and conspicuous nuclei). The rheumatoid subcutaneous nodule shows necrosis of connective tissue, usually absent in the nodule of rheumatic fever. Artificial induction of subcutaneous nodules in rheumatic fever patients by subcutaneous injection of the patient's own blood as a means of studying the mechanisms, carried on since 1935 at the House of the Good Samaritan, Boston, at first suggested that "an unidentified nodule-stimulating substance" may be present in the blood of active rheumatic fever patients but not of recovered or normal individuals. Continuing studies were considered, 1952, to lend less support to the former theory than to a theory (based on use of a traumatizing technique for injections) that nodule formation is an expression of generalized susceptibility of connective tissue to trauma (B. F. Massell, W. B. Coen, T. D. Jones, 1952). The nodules in rheumatoid arthritis, while clinically similar, show histological differences that may be diagnostic (Bauer and associates, 1952). Reports of rheumatic fever-like lesions in hearts of rheumatoid arthritis patients are conflicting. According to Bauer, 1954, a certain percentage of patients with rheumatoid arthritis have rheumatic heart disease.

Fibrinoid, a component of rheumatoid nodules, has not been shown to be collagenous in origin (Bauer, 1951). Absence in fibrinoid of the characteristic amino acid of collagen, hydroxyproline, suggested that the two are unrelated (J. H. Kellgren, Manchester, 1952). Lesions of blood vessels in rheumatic fever involving connective tissue include hyperplasia of the elastica of the vessels. Lesions in the small blood vessels "nearly always in the proximity of circulating arterial blood" have been described as reversible but not evanescent (Alvin F. Coburn, rheumatic fever unit, Northwestern, 1950) and as heightening need for further knowledge of the chemistry of arterial tissue. In rheumatic pneumonitis, the primary injury was described as focal damage to the alveolar capillaries (Rich and Gregory, 1943). Hemorrhagic manifestations are common to all connective tissue diseases (Bauer and Clark, 1953). The theory that hemorrhagic phenomena involving permeability or rupture of capillary walls are referable to changes in capillaries themselves was not supported by B. W. Zweifach and Robert Chambers (medicine, Cornell, and biology, New York University, 1950). They considered that capillary hemorrhage produced by hyaluronidase results from effects on intercellular cement rather than on the endothelial cell itself and that the mechanism acting primarily on the structures surrounding and supporting the capillary wall, finally resulting in increased outward filtration, does not operate under physiologic conditions but may develop in certain pathological states. Attributing to vitamin C deficiency a role in the hemorrhagic tendency in rheumatic fever, William J. Kerr (medicine, California, 1948) thought that supplemental intake of the vitamin might control the hemorrhagic manifestation. Over the years questions have been raised as to whether the hemorrhagic effects in rheumatic fever might result from the traditional salicylate therapy (Karl Paul Link, biochemistry, Wisconsin, 1945; Armand J. Quick, pharmacology, Marquette, 1944). Evidence not favoring this theory includes a 1945 controlled study of prothrombin levels in large numbers of young adults in the rheumatic fever unit of the Corona naval hospital, showing no hemorrhagic manifestations following salicylate therapy. In pathological studies of rheumatoid arthritis, proliferation and degeneration have been described in all coats of the smaller blood vessels (G. D. Kersley and H. J. Gibson, Royal National Hospital for Rheumatic Diseases, Bath, 1952).

Involvement of the joints in the rheumatic processes naturally follows the fact that "the highly vascular synovial tissue lining the capsule is slightly modified connective tissue" (Ropes and Bauer, 1953). Bauer's group considered that changes in the synovial fluid in disease reflect "alterations in the synovial tissues and intra-articular metabolism". The arthritis of rheumatic fever (usually described as inflammatory and involving swelling and edema of connective tissue fibers, laying down of fibrin) generally subsides rapidly and completely, rarely if ever evolving into rheumatoid arthritis (Bauer, 1954). The earliest changes in the synovial tissues in rheumatoid arthritis have been described as "indistinguishable from other joint inflammations and, with other changes, involving the interfibrillar elements" (Ragan, 1952).

Histological studies in a few laboratories in this country and England most frequently refer neural lesions, including degenerative processes in the brain in rheumatic fever, to associated blood vessel damage. Some of these studies are oriented toward problems arising from Sydenham's chorea as a manifestation of rheumatic fever, and, in some views, "presumptive" of it, although it has been observed also in patients with lupus erythematosus (Bauer and Clark, 1953). Murphy's 1952 observations included, in a case of severe chorea with rheumatic carditis, occlusion by platelet masses of small arteries and arterioles of the brain, myocardium and other tissues. Obliterating arteritis in the brain was described by Walter L. Bruetsch (psychiatry and neurology, Indiana, 1947) as a not infrequent "late cerebral sequel" in rheumatic cardiac patients. Severe mental changes (without the motor phenomena of chorea) associated in some cases with focal brain lesions were described as "rheumatic encephalitis" by H. A. Warren and John Chornyak, Veterans Administration, Chicago, 1947.

Feeling that pathology of the joints, the heart and the subcutaneous nodule does not represent the pathology of a systemic disease, and that muscular changes may be accounted for by neural lesions, Hugo A. Freund and associates (medicine, Wayne University) began, 1938, a study of the entire nervous system in rheumatoid arthritis. Discrete nodules in the epineurium and perineurium of peripheral nerves, not connected with involved joints, were described, 1942 and 1945. It was not possible to say whether the nodules found in muscles in almost all cases studied preceded the joint involvement or were primarily connected with blood vessel or with neural lesions. Occurrence of these lesions has been confirmed by others (Joseph J. Bunim, Currier McEwen and others, in the study group of rheumatic diseases, New York University, 1948; Kersley and associates in England, 1948). To determine the specificity and the diagnostic value of the cellular nodules in muscle and any associated biochemical changes in the muscle, the New York University group studied biopsy specimens from normal controls and from several hundred patients with rheumatoid arthritis, numerous nonrheumatic diseases. Their findings, 1952, were positive in percentages of fifty-six in rheumatoid arthritis, forty in spondylitis, twenty-five in other diseases. Freund, discussing these findings, 1952, thought that lesions in normal persons might indicate latent disease. Findings in essential agreement with those of the New York University group were reported, 1952, by Bauer and associates, on the basis of biopsy and autopsy specimens of muscle, peripheral nerves, the sympathetic chain, the spinal cord from cases of rheumatoid arthritis, lupus erythematosus, dermatomyositis, periarteritis nodosa, scleroderma, rheumatic fever. In rheumatoid arthritis these lesions were found both in muscles and in nerves. The muscle lesions were always found in the interstitial connective tissue, usually in relation to a blood vessel and not always in relation to joints. The nodules in nerve sheaths were described as similar to those in muscle; accumulations of cells occurred in the meninges of the central nervous sytem; the scattered alterations, sometimes severe, found in the nervous tissue of the cord were obviously related to the focal inflammatory connective tissue lesions; foci of lymphocytes, plasma cells and other cellular reactions were found in the sympathetic nerves. Focal collections of cells were found in muscle and nerve sheaths of the other connective tissue diseases studied.

## METABOLIC CHANGES IN CONNECTIVE TISSUE AND BODY FLUIDS IN THE RHEUMATIC SYNDROMES

Intensive study of the cellular, biochemical, or metabolic alterations in the connective tissue that precede demonstrable pathology in the rheumatic syndromes is only beginning. While chemical constituents of the connective tissue itself do not appear to participate in marked degree in the breakdown and synthesis of the general metabolic continuum, a dynamic equilibrium nevertheless exists between the interstitial fluid, the fibers, the ground substance and products of the cells and substances transported by the blood (Edward W. Dempsey, anatomy, Washington University, formerly Harvard, 1952).

### METABOLISM OF CARBOHYDRATES, CHIEFLY THE POLYSACCHARIDES OF THE GROUND SUBSTANCE

"Reduced tolerance for carbohydrate" was noted by the Research Council's survey committee among physiological alterations characteristic of rheumatoid arthritis. Of fundamental work illuminating the intermediary metabolism of carbohydrates in the rheumatic syndromes, notably of the polysaccharides of the mesenchyme, there is as yet little. While chemical structure of the most widely studied of these polysaccharides, hyaluronic acid, was recognized, 1953, as still unknown, its basic unit was known to be "a disaccharide composed of acetylglucosamine and glucuronic acid", and chondroitin sulfate was also known to contain glucuronic acid (Meyer, 1950). Liver glycogen is considered a source for synthesis of glucuronic acid (believed to be involved in metabolism of steroid hormones), maintained at constant levels in the blood by an unknown homeostatic mechanism which is apparently disturbed in rheumatoid arthritis. W. H. Fishman and associates (cancer research unit, departments of surgery, medicine, biochemistry, Tufts, 1951) raised the question whether the lability of blood glucuronic acid concentration in rheumatoid arthritis could be related to its presence in hyaluronic acid and chondroitin sulfate in cartilage and joints, and whether disordered glucuronic acid metabolism may characterize this condition. Ragan and Meyer, 1950, noted the suggestive finding that excretion of glucuronic acid was strongly influenced by salicylates.

### WATER AND ELECTROLYTE METABOLISM IN RHEUMATIC PROCESSES

Water and electrolyte balance is obviously involved in inflammatory processes. Most body cells, as previously noted, depend for their nutrition upon connective tissue surrounding the capillaries and receiving nutritive substances through their semipermeable membrane. The tissue fluids escaping from the capillaries return to the blood stream by way of the venous ends of the capillaries or by way of the lymphatics. Alteration of any one factor in this process results in excess tissue fluid (Bensley and Ham, 1952). One factor, studied by C. I. Reed and associates (physiology, Illinois, 1947, 1949), was autonomic control of normal fluid and electrolyte balance in the joint cavity and possible relation of this factor to pathological changes in the joints preliminary to arthritis. Study in England (James Reid, 1951) of correlated clinical and biochemical changes occurring in acute rheumatic fever treated with salicylates indicated removal of excess water from the body by diuresis, increased excretion of sodium and chloride, decreased excretion of nitrogen and potassium, effects identical with those following cortisone and ACTH therapy. Reid suggested that acute rheumatic manifestations might be expressions of an abnormal fluid shift resulting from disorders of electrolyte and protein metabolism.

### PROTEIN METABOLISM IN CONNECTIVE TISSUE IN RELATION
### TO RHEUMATIC PROCESSES

The undifferentiated cells of mesenchyme are associated with intercellular substance containing scattered proteins, the differentiated fibroblasts with fibrous proteins oriented into fibrils and fibers.

An hypothesis that the syndrome of rheumatic fever results from uninhibited proteinase activity on mesenchymal tissue, developed by I. A. Mirsky (when in Cincinnati) and tested experimentally, proposed, 1945, "that these proteolytic enzymes are either activated *in vivo* by streptococcal fibrinolysins or result from the release of intracellular proteinases consequent to the cellular damage produced by infection, trauma, or 'anaphylactoid' reactions. Further, it was assumed that the individual who is susceptible to the development or recurrence of rheumatic fever is one who cannot inhibit adequately the proteinases thus activated."

Most studies of protein metabolism in the rheumatic states have been carried out in terms of spinal fluid and blood proteins. Ludwig, Short and Bauer, 1943, found increased concentrations of protein in the spinal fluid four times as often in patients with "rheumatoid spondylitis" as in patients with the peripheral form of rheumatoid arthritis. Since the ventricular fluid is normal as regards protein content, the protein "leak" from the blood plasma to the spinal fluid must be lower down. It would follow that the source of the increased protein in spondylitis does not necessarily need to be the inflamed spinal meningeal tissues. Available evidence favors this view.

Protein metabolism is a fundamental aspect of every approach to the rheumatic syndromes. The National Research Council's survey committee stressed the need to study the proteins of ground substance of loose connective tissue, and "the more highly organized mesenchymal tissues", cartilage, bone, blood vessels. Mentioned illustratively was a study at the DuPont Institute in Delaware of the protein content of bone, in its relation to arthritis. Especially needed is exact knowledge of changes in serum proteins in rheumatic diseases and of changes in protein utilization and turnover; contributions toward such knowledge include studies of urinary excretion of specific amino acids in rheumatoid arthritis (W. Paul Holbrook, Southwestern Clinic and Research Institute and A. R. Kemmerer, nutrition, University of Arizona, and coworkers, 1952).

# ROLE OF INFECTION IN THE RHEUMATIC SYNDROMES

## SEARCH FOR MICROORGANISMS PRESUMED TO BE DIRECTLY INVOLVED

Search for a microorganism *directly* involved in rheumatic processes (more than a hundred have been suspected at one time or another) has been renewed by work on the still unclassified group of pleuropneumonia-like organisms (filtrable, species specific, occurring naturally in man), one of which was reported to produce in mice lesions resembling those of both rheumatic fever and rheumatoid arthritis (A. B. Sabin, Children's Hospital Research Foundation, Cincinnati, 1941). Since this demonstration these organisms have been under continuous study at Harvard by Louis Dienes (bacteriology) and by Bauer in the arthritis clinic at Massachusetts General. Organisms of this group differ from the viruses and rickettsiae in growing in cell-free media, some even in protein-free media (Sabin, 1952). A certain significance has been attached to the *in vitro* susceptibility of strains of these organisms to gold salts, one of the therapeutic expedients in rheumatoid arthritis. By similar reasoning, Thomas M. Brown (medicine, Johns Hopkins), 1952, thought that prolonged clinical trial of aureomycin might clarify the possibility of a relation between pleuropneumonia-like organisms and human rheumatic disease.

Various pyogenic cocci (gonococcus, meningococcus, pneumococcus, staphylococcus, streptococcus) and various bacilli (tubercle, brucella, etc.) and other organisms appear to be responsible, by direct infection of synovial tissues, for the so-called acute infectious arthritides. While grouping these with the rheumatic syndromes has a certain justification because of their common connective tissue involvement, the pathology, in the acute stage, of the joints infected with these organisms appears to be quite different from that of rheumatoid arthritis.

The hypothesis, previously supported actively in England, that a virus is the etiologic agent of rheumatic fever rests chiefly upon agglutination by rheumatic fever sera of minute particles obtained by ultracentrifugation of rheumatic pericardial and pleural fluids (Schlesinger, Signy and Aimes, 1935). The particles were described as morphologically similar to elementary bodies of vaccinia, varicella, psittacosis viruses. Repetition of these experiments in patients with rheumatoid arthritis and chorea by a group at the Lister Institute (Eagles, Evans, Fisher and Keith, 1937) seemed to confirm the agglutination phenomenon in about half of a large number of rheumatic sera. No correlation could be detected between positive agglutination and clinical phase of any of the diseases. The agglutination phenomenon was described by Swift, 1936, as not necessarily either specific or of etiological significance.

Attempts to produce lesions and symptoms of rheumatic diseases by injection of ultrafiltrates from fluids and tissues of rheumatic fever patients or injection of viruses have all failed, although myocarditis and valvular lesions had been reported in rabbits inoculated with virus III, vaccinia, fibroma, myxoma, pseudorabies viruses (John M. Pearce, pathology, Long Island College of Medicine, 1939, later Cornell). Protection tests with rheumatic fever convalescent sera have been negative (Joseph E. Smadel, Army Medical School, 1947). Mervyn Gordon (St. Bartholomew's Hospital, London), who, since 1939, has attempted experimental production of rheumatic fever with viruses combined with streptococci or other agents, regarded, 1948, myocarditis induced in rabbits by psittacosis virus as supporting his belief that the "rheumatic granuloma of Aschoff is almost certainly a virus". One explanation offered for failure of human materials to induce rheumatic lesions in animals is the well-known species specificity of viruses. One of the major arguments against the virus hypothesis is that whereas viruses are *intra*cellular parasites, it is the *inter*cellular ground substance that is the site of rheumatic fever lesions; whether these lesions are primary or secondary is, however, an unanswered question. Since Schlesinger's early work, numerous workers have suggested that the hypothetical virus is able to gain ground only in host tissue that has been rendered susceptible by streptococcal infection.

## The Streptococcus, in Indirect Relation to Rheumatic Fever

### The heightened reactivity hypothesis

Relation between upper respiratory tract infections with group A hemolytic streptococci and rheumatic fever was described, 1948, by the National Research Council's survey committee as "well-grounded", although mechanisms of the relationship are still (1954) unknown. The 1953 Primer on rheumatic conditions described rheumatic fever as "an acute or chronic inflammatory process initiated by a preceding group A hemolytic streptococcic infection". Most investigators, however, now agree that environmental and host factors have a determining part in this "initiation". Current work on the relation of antecedent streptococcic infection to rheumatic fever reflects newer concepts of infection in terms of interrelated metabolism of invading microorganisms and of host cells, and in terms of biochemical studies of group A hemolytic streptococci and the effects of the many soluble products of these organisms on tissues remote from those directly infected. Approaches to the problem of the rheumatic syndromes and the role of the streptococcus through the above routes were described by the survey committee as "more inviting" than the traditional bacteriologic approaches. They appear also to be more rewarding.

The host factor in rheumatic fever was envisaged by Coburn, 1950, as combining a genetic "metabolic defect and a sensitization to group A streptococcus". The idea of hypersensitivity to an infectious agent goes back at least so far as Koch's (1891) discovery of hypersensitivity to the tubercle bacillus. The apparently hypersensitive manifestations of tuberculosis and syphilis were compared by Swift in 1925 to those of rheumatic fever. He expressed, 1952, the view that successive antecedent group A streptococcal infections lead in some persons to "heightened irritability of their tissues to subsequent infections with group A streptococci heterologous in type to those with which they had previously been infected; and that when this heightened reactivity reaches a certain degree it may manifest itself as rheumatic fever". This hyperreactivity hypothesis has greatly broadened the investigative field, introducing many variables and requiring study of different types, degrees and sites of tissue damage.  The few available studies in terms of cellular alterations and the more numerous studies of streptococcal antigens by chemical methods have not altered the truth of the statement that, as yet, no one component or metabolic product of any strain of hemolytic streptococcus (Maclyn McCarty, Rockefeller Institute, 1952, listed seventeen) has been identified as the cause of rheumatic fever and rheumatic heart disease, acute nephritis, erythema nodosum, all of which are recognized sequelae of group A streptococcal infection of the upper respiratory tract (Swift, 1952).  The conservatism of Swift's statement is in itself an index of the present state of ignorance.  Concrete studies from year to year add substance to this or that hypothesis.  For instance, Swift's reference to a "possibly inherited" tendency in the tissues of certain persons to overreact to streptococcal infections was considered to be supported by a genetic study of rheumatic families, using statistical methods of analysis, carried out between 1940 and 1946 at the New York Hospital (May G. Wilson, pediatrics, Cornell, 1947).

In whatever way infection may operate in the rheumatic syndromes — as a trigger mechanism, as a hypersensitive reaction, as the result of a derailed defense mechanism — investigative work is now at least oriented by the concept that susceptibility and resistance to infection are largely matters of bacterial and host metabolism.  Susceptibility may be determined by modification of the host's response to the organism by gene-controlled metabolic defects, which may be influenced by nutrition, by endocrine states, by chemicals, by psychic trauma.

## THE BIOLOGY OF THE STREPTOCOCCUS

Great importance attaches to work on the biology of the streptococcus.  The Lancefield (Rockefeller Institute, 1940) serological classification of streptococci, based primarily upon elaboration by hemolytic streptococci of carbohydrate substances known as C, subdivided the hemolytic organisms into twelve groups each having a group-specific C substance.  Among group A hemolytic streptococci, responsible for ninety-five per cent of streptococcal disease in man (Swift, 1952), at least forty serological types have been differentiated.  The nonhemolytic or viridans streptococci (for some years discussed in relation to rheumatic fever on the basis of their isolation from rheumatic fever hearts showing bacterial endocarditis attributed to the nonhemolytic streptococcus) cannot be serologically grouped because no demonstrable C substance occurs in these organisms. Classification of strains in a genus of bacteria, essential for determining their natural habitat, their disease-inducing propensities, depends in large part on study of the cellular and extracellular substances, especially the enzymes and antigens. The enzymes, in breaking down more complex molecules (of the media in which they grow, which may be tissues of the host) into simpler ones, probably make nutriment available to the bacteria. Knowledge of the antigenic substances of streptococci has been used in support of the theory that these organisms play an important role in etiology of rheumatic fever. Among other group A streptococcal substances, either contained in the cells or produced during their *in vitro* growth, that act as antigens and stimulate formation of antibodies are enzymes (streptokinase, streptodornase, hyaluronidase), hemolysins (streptolysin O and S which disrupt red blood cells and release hemoglobin) and toxins (erythrogenic toxin produced by many strains and responsible for the rash of scarlet fever). Hyaluronic acid, usually classed as an extracellular substance produced by certain strains (under certain cultural conditions it surrounds the cell as a capsule, responsible for the mucoid character of these strains), has not been shown to provoke antibody formation. With these and other developments, techniques for study of group A streptococcal infections of man have yielded considerable information, which still, however, falls far short of elucidating the biology of the streptococcus; only beginnings have been made in study of the role of that organism in the pathogenesis of disease (McCarty, 1952). Because hyaluronic acid is an important component of the ground substance of the connective tissue assumed to undergo chemical alteration during streptococcic infection, its presence in streptococcal capsules has suggested the possibility that it is related to pathogenesis of rheumatic fever, but the relationship has not been proved. Also unproved is a role for the hyaluronidase enzymes produced by these organisms in initiating damage of the ground substance (spreading effect).

## EPIDEMIOLOGICAL AND CLINICAL DATA BEARING ON THE
## ROLE OF THE STREPTOCOCCUS

During the last war, epidemiological studies of rheumatic fever conducted under the auspices of the Armed Forces Epidemiological Board included a three-year study at the Warren Air Force Base, Wyoming (with the cooperation of the staff of the streptococcal disease laboratory at the Public Health Service communicable disease center and the Army Medical School), under the direction of Charles H. Rammelkamp (medicine, Western Reserve) and with other medical school investigators (Colin M. MacLeod, bacteriology, New York University; John H. Dingle, preventive medicine, Western Reserve; Floyd W. Denny, pediatrics, Minnesota). This group considered, 1952, outstanding epidemiological factors revealed by their rheumatic fever study (latitude, altitude, crowding, dampness, etc.) "important only because they are related to the preceding streptococcal infection which initiates the attack of rheumatic fever". Lowell A. Rantz and associates (medicine and pediatrics, Stanford), continuing their wartime investigations in a three-year study of streptococcal infections in children, reported, 1952, further evidence that repeated infections with hemolytic streptococcus, possibly with different types within group A, affect susceptibility to rheumatic fever. Summing up, 1952, other epidemiological evidence, Swift considered it well demonstrated that streptococcic and "no other infections, either respiratory or nonrespiratory, acted as forerunners of rheumatic fever". Decreased incidence of rheumatic fever in Baltimore and other cities since the war, although unexplained, paralleled decreased incidence of streptococcal infections resulting from antimicrobial therapy (Francis F. Schwentker, pediatrics, Johns Hopkins, 1952).

Especial interest has been focused on the so-called latent phase, a period between active infection and appearance of rheumatic symptoms, varying from more than two weeks up to six weeks (Swift), or, in some cases, from forty-eight hours to under a week (Rantz). Rantz found in his young adult subjects not actual latency but "active development of a process which apparently begins as soon as the streptococcal infection has taken place". The length of the "latent" period has become important in antibiotic therapy in streptococcic infections as prophylaxis against rheumatic fever. Early and vigorous treatment (penicillin, aureomycin) of upper respiratory tract infections for prevention of first attacks and of recurrences of rheumatic fever is supported by clinical evidence.

## SEARCH FOR A SPECIFIC STREPTOCOCCIC COMPONENT

Extensive work on the known intracellular and extracellular components and products of the streptococcus has provided no evidence that any one of them is a specific rheumatogenic substance. Identified *in vivo* activities of these substances were limited, 1952, to the well-known production of skin rash in scarlet fever by the erythrogenic toxin, and to inhibition of phagocytosis by capsular hyaluronic acid and the M protein, demonstrated by Sidney Rothbard, Hospital of the Rockefeller Institute, 1948. Chemical and biological analyses carried out on soluble and insoluble products of viable organisms obtained from lesions and on extracts of infected tissues (Dennis W. Watson and William J. Cromartie, bacteriology, immunology, medicine, Minnesota) have indicated, 1952, that group A organisms produce more hyaluronidase during active infection in the host than *in vitro*, a finding that may account for demonstration of antibodies against the enzyme in almost all sera in the normal population, attributed to exposure to hemolytic streptococcic infection. Other unknown enzymes and antigens produced *in vivo* may play an essential part in pathogenicity, or responsibility may lie with antigenic materials remaining at certain sites in the heart after the organisms have disappeared, or with a combination of such substances with material derived from the host. An approach to the question of distribution of antigens in tissues by exposing sections of tissue from mice injected intravenously with the antigens to antibody labeled with fluorescein suggested that (at least in the mouse) two types of polysaccharide antigen and three types of protein antigen can escape from the blood stream and invade the connective tissue, especially that supporting the blood vessels (A. H. Coons, bacteriology and immunology, Harvard, 1952). Such an approach might be extended, it was suggested, to search for a possible rheumatic fever streptococcal component in inflammatory areas, although the presence of such a hypothetical substance, and of antibody against it, would not of itself establish the etiology of the disease. The possibilities of this approach emphasize the need for regular production of the syndrome in animals.

## Serological Studies of Reactivity to Streptococcic Infection

In about one third of rheumatic fever patients, hemolytic streptococci have disappeared by the time the rheumatic symptoms appear (Swift, 1952) and even when they are found their classification requires serological techniques. Laboratory studies of the theoretical relationship have, therefore, been confined chiefly to immunological evidence of antecedent infection, sometimes detectable only by careful serological studies. Detailed studies (Stanford, the Rockefeller Institute, Naval research units, Yale, Pennsylvania) have "thoroughly established the exaggerated antibody response to streptococcal infection in those developing rheumatic fever compared with patients suffering uncomplicated infections" (McCarty, 1952). One suggested explanation of this difference is that the rheumatic subject may be "an immunologically queer fellow" who makes "more antibodies than many other people" (Rantz, 1952). Studies of several antibodies are required since one or more of four antibodies show rises in practically all rheumatic fever patients. Further application of physical and chemical techniques to immunology will, it is hoped, lead eventually to precise description of the role of surface antigens in microbial virulence, of hyaluronic acid in tissue immunity, of phagocytes in cellular immunity in terms of enzymic or other chemical reactions (Henry P. Treffers, immunochemistry, Yale, 1952).

## Immunological Reactions in Terms of Metabolism of Bacteria and of Host

While immunology has for years been dominantly associated with practical aims in medical and veterinary science, advancing chemical concepts (the work of Arrhenius and his Danish pupils, of Svedberg and associates in Sweden, of Michael Heidelberger at Columbia, of Oswald T. Avery and Karl Landsteiner at the Rockefeller Institute) have now established the discipline of immunochemistry. Chemical concepts were extended to the nature of antigens and antibodies long before the advances in protein chemistry and in enzyme chemistry were made available in the immunological field. The protein nature of antibodies was established and it was shown that antibody synthesis and destruction took place at the same speed as that of other serum proteins. Dubos's observation that bacteria utilize the multiple and complex biocatalysts that govern and integrate the metabolism of all living cells touched on the essential fact that all reactions concerned in infection and resistance, the host-parasite relationship, are metabolic. "Inhibition of growth, enzymic decomposition, agglutination, lysis, etc. are only the secondary manifestations of primary reactions which depend upon the union between the cellular receptors, on the one hand, and the biological reagents, be they antiseptics, antibodies, enzymes, bacteriophages, on the other."

Immunological reactions against hyaluronidase, demonstrable in rheumatic fever patients, have been interpreted by some as evidence of a role for this enzyme, produced by some group A streptococci. It was described, 1950 (Bennett Sallman and Jorgen M. Birkeland, bacteriology, Ohio State), as an "important factor", in hemolytic streptococcic infection, at least in the chick embryo, and hyaluronidase production was assumed to be related to the virulence of certain strains for man. Higher titers of specific inhibitor of streptococcal hyaluronidase in sera of rheumatic fever and scarlet fever patients than in sera of patients with uncomplicated streptococcic infections were reported by George J. Friou, 1948–1950 (studies at the Georgia naval medical research unit and later at Yale), T. N. Harris, Children's Hospital, Philadelphia, 1950. Challenging the hypothesis that rheumatic fever is a manifestation of enzymic action of streptococcal hyaluronidase on the hyaluronic acid of connective tissue, some workers have pointed out that the streptococcal types at present known to produce largest amounts of hyaluronidase (group A types 4 and 22) either have not been identified in association with rheumatic fever or have caused epidemics without recurrences in rheumatic patients; other potent producers of hyaluronidase, such as pneumococci and clostridia, have never been associated with infections antecedent to rheumatic fever (Swift, 1952).

## The Streptococcus in Relation to Rheumatoid Arthritis

Association of the streptococcus with rheumatoid arthritis has been suggested from time to time largely on the basis of a high titer of agglutinins against living beta hemolytic streptococci in sera of rheumatoid arthritis patients. The survey committee, 1948, considered that, although the reaction appeared to be nonspecific, it deserved further study. A nonspecific agglutination test (agglutination of sheep red cells pretreated with antisheep cell serum) developed in the Columbia laboratories was considered a useful aid in differentiating rheumatic fever, rheumatoid arthritis and degenerative joint disease (R. H. Boots, M. O. Lipman, J. A. Coss, with Ragan, 1952). Unfortunately, the test is rarely positive in patients that have had rheumatoid arthritis for less than a year (Bauer, 1948). Coburn, 1945, referred to immunologists for solution the question whether this agglutinin may be not a primary process but rather part of a secondary mechanism following tissue damage. The conclusion that in rheumatoid arthritis neither antecedent infection nor abnormal immunity mechanism is etiologically significant was expressed, 1952, by L. S. P. Davidson (medicine, University of Edinburgh) following the finding (from a controlled investigation of etiological factors, sponsored by the Empire Rheumatism Council) that more than eighty per cent of over four hundred rheumatoid arthritis patients had not suffered from any infection within three months of onset. A thirteen years' study of streptococcal antibody titers in the sera of patients with early and late rheumatoid arthritis in the medical department, Columbia, led, 1952, to the conclusion that the hemolytic streptococcus is not an etiologic factor in rheumatoid arthritis; many of the early cases suggesting rheumatoid arthritis have been diagnosed later as adult rheumatic fever.

# HYPERSENSITIVITY MECHANISMS IN CONNECTIVE TISSUE DISEASES

Most known disease-producing agents are to a greater or lesser extent "conditionally acting pathogens", according to Hans Selye,

1952 (experimental medicine and surgery, Montreal), the condition being "special circumstances of sensitization" in the host. The hypersensitive reaction describes host reaction to antigens that provoke antibody formation, with cellular and tissue changes including inflammation. The fact that inflammation involves the connective tissue furnishes one basis for the suggestion made decades ago that rheumatic fever and certain other rheumatic syndromes are hypersensitive reactions. These reactions, important in developing concepts of tuberculosis as well as of the rheumatic syndromes, are indeed being increasingly considered in most pathological states. The specific altered capacity to react implied in hypersensitivity ("allergy" in more popular usage) usually reflects "prior contact (although not always evident) with the same material or one closely related to it chemically" (as phrased by Merrill W. Chase, Rockefeller Institute, 1952). Aside from formation of antibodies in response to (or in recognition of) substances previously encountered, there may be other basic mechanisms as yet unknown.

The hypersensitive reaction is of two major types, immediate and delayed. The reactions of the immediate type (asthma, hay fever, "hives", gastrointestinal disturbances) develop soon after contact or absorption of the specific "allergen", and circulating antibodies are demonstrable. The reactions of the delayed type (poison ivy, most drug sensitivities, reactions from certain products of microorganisms as tuberculin) begin several hours after introduction of the "allergen", show progressive changes over several days or longer, and antibodies are rarely found. Rich, 1951, deploring current confusion in terminology (and consequently in thought), advocated dropping the term allergy. It had been, in his view, "debauched" by being used indiscriminately to describe all types of hypersensitivity to all types of antigens and all types and degrees of antibody response. Rich favored classification of hypersensitivity in two types: the anaphylactic or immediate reaction which includes several variants; the tuberculin or delayed reaction usually considered to be typical of bacterial hypersensitivity. Distinction between these two types has proved a logical preliminary to investigation of them by immunological methods. The delayed type of hypersensitivity has been studied extensively since Koch described the tuberculin phenomenon in 1891 because it is responsible for the skin reaction used as a diagnostic test for tuberculosis, and because hypersensitivity in tuberculosis is believed by many to be responsible for the protean tissue destruction in the disease. Although newer techniques such as cellular transfer, microdissection, use of labeled antibodies and other methods of cytochemistry have renewed hope of understanding bacterial hypersensitivity, controversy persists regarding its significance in pathogenesis of tuberculosis (and, by analogy, other diseases) and in resistance. As a reasonable explanation of bacterial allergy generally, Chase proposed, 1952, "that the invading microorganism carries its antigens into a locus which becomes a special environment as host cells mobilize, and that the character of these cells and the manner in which they deal with the slowly liberated protein antigens, being in some way different from the usual mechanism that leads to antibody production, determines the predominating, delayed type of sensitivity". Recent recognition of basic relationships between certain immediate reactions and the tuberculin type of hypersensitivity has suggested that both may share in a common cellular mechanism. This might explain why connective tissue reactions in man that are lessened by cortisone and ACTH appear to have features of the delayed type of reaction (Stoerk, 1953) and also of the immediate or anaphylactic type. Investigators working with a chronic type of anaphylaxis in animals for more than twenty years have been animated by hope of illumining mechanisms of certain diseases of man, especially the joint involvement in rheumatic fever.

## RELATION OF ANAPHYLACTIC HYPERSENSITIVITY TO CONNECTIVE TISSUE DISEASES

The vascular and other connective tissue lesions described in animal anaphylaxis are, as noted above, suggestive of the pathology of certain human diseases. Study of possible relation of chronic anaphylactic type of hypersensitivity to human disease was intensified after Klinge's (1933) production of inflammation and degeneration of soft tissue, especially collagen, and of similar alterations in the heart muscle and valves, blood vessels, muscle, tendons by serum-induced anaphylactic hypersensitivity in rabbits. Repeated injection

of the antigen (horse serum) into the same joint resulted in a destructive and deforming arthritis. These experiments, focusing attention
upon changes in intercellular components of the connective tissue,
especially the ground substance, were the basis of the conclusion
that rheumatic fever and rheumatoid arthritis are systemic diseases
affecting the connective tissue, and that the changes represent
hypersensitive reactions (Klemperer, 1950).

   While Klemperer and his colleagues were expounding (1942) their
concept of "diffuse collagen disease", Rich and his associates published experimental and clinical findings on which they based the
conclusion that periarteritis nodosa is a syndrome of hypersensitivity of
the "serum sickness" type. In the tissues of seven patients who had
died after showing anaphylactic reactions following serum and
sulfonamide therapy, Rich, 1942, reported vascular lesions — necrosis, fibrinoid alteration, hyalinization of the arterial media and
perivascular infiltration with mononuclear and polymorphonuclear
leukocytes — similar to those of periarteritis nodosa. Experimental
confirmation followed, 1943: ". . . periarteritis nodosa has been reproduced in all of its essential details in the experimental animal by
creating conditions similar to those obtaining in serum sickness in
the human being". During the next two years, Rich and Gregory
reported finding unexpectedly in some of these animals cardiac
lesions "basically similar to those of human rheumatic carditis". In
his 1947 Harvey lecture, Rich noted as characteristics of both rheumatic fever and anaphylactic reactions: focal injury to the connective tissue; carditis in some individuals, periarteritis in others;
skin lesions, purpura, tissue eosinophilia; focal lesions, of which the
Aschoff body and periarteritis nodosa are both examples; finally,
capacity (first reported by Swift, 1928) of salicylic acid to relieve the
arthritic symptoms of both serum sickness and rheumatic fever.
Rich also noted that the anaphylactic pulmonary lesions produced in
experimental animals by serum sickness "are of the same basic type
as those seen in rheumatic pneumonitis", sometimes an accompani-
ment of rheumatic fever. He considered that rheumatoid arthritis,
rheumatic fever, periarteritis nodosa and disseminated lupus erythematosus exhibit, in addition to collagen and vascular damage,
many clinical and pathological features in common with the pro-

tracted type of anaphylactic reaction represented by serum sickness and drug hypersensitivity. William E. Ehrich, Joseph Seifter and C. Forman (Graduate School of Medicine, Pennsylvania, and Wyeth Institute, Philadelphia), 1949, thought the constellation of lesions produced in rabbits by large injections of horse serum resembled those of human rheumatoid arthritis rather than of rheumatic fever.

## ROLE OF THE STREPTOCOCCUS IN THIS CONCEPT

If hypersensitivity is the actual pathogenic mechanism of rheumatic fever and also of other syndromes not shown to be associated with antecedent streptococcic infection, what role in this concept is to be assigned to the streptococcus? Rich, 1947, thought that certain streptococci (as hemolytic) might simply "contain a substance that is particularly active in producing hypersensitive reactions of this type" in the same way that egg white, strawberries and shell fish are more active than certain other foodstuffs in causing urticarial anaphylactic lesions.

To explore the role of hemolytic streptococcic infection in producing anaphylactic hypersensitivity and also to develop a closer approximation to rheumatic fever in animals, some investigators have turned from soluble antigens to whole streptococci used as antigens in study of specialized types of hypersensitivity (Arthus and Shwartzman reactions) resembling anaphylaxis and reported to occur in man. In a possibly useful experimental model of rheumatic fever, Lewis Thomas (pediatrics and medicine, Minnesota), 1952, produced a generalized reaction in rabbits by repeated intradermal injections or single intravenous injections of live streptococci (as the preparing procedure) followed by the (provoking) intravenous injection of small amounts of gram-negative bacterial toxin. Profound alteration in susceptibility of the heart, kidney and other tissues to damage by bacterial toxins which would cause no damage in normal animals free of infection could not be compared to rheumatic fever in man without imagining an event equivalent to intravenous injection of large amounts of bacterial toxin. However, Thomas pointed out that, in man, prolonged or repeated streptococcic infections may heighten susceptibility to small amounts of other bacterial toxins which could account for tissue damage in human disease. The tissue damage produced in rabbits by similar use of bacteria and bacterial products included (Chandler A. Stetson, streptococcal disease laboratory, Warren Air Force Base, Wyoming, 1952) vascular lesions similar to those found in the hearts of patients with early active rheumatic fever (occlusion of capillaries and small veins by masses of leukocytes and platelets, followed by necrosis and hemorrhage).

### Hypersensitivity to tissue antigens

Coburn, 1950, posed a question raised repeatedly by various workers, as to whether early and late rheumatic manifestations are due to a common mechanism "or whether the damage to the tissue incurred in primary lesions gives rise to a secondary mechanism, such as an auto-antigen-antibody reaction". So-called autoantibodies (to the host's own tissues presumably altered by disease) were interpreted by Chase, 1952, as examples of "cross-reacting" antibodies. Other studies (Kerr and Cavelti, 1947) have been carried out to test the theory that human rheumatic lesions may be caused by antibodies produced by the body against "certain tissues, such as perhaps heart or connective tissue", which had been activated or rendered antigenic by the streptococcus. Immunization of animals with homologous connective tissue and killed streptococci was reported to produce widespread lesions of the perivascular connective tissue (Cavelti, 1952).

### Unsolved problems of the anaphylactic hypersensitivity mechanism

Investigators who consider that the hypothesis of anaphylactic hypersensitivity best explains rheumatic disease have nevertheless asked whether this explanation would be much more than the substitution of one riddle for another. "Why is it that one individual becomes immunized under the antigenic impact of a foreign substance, while another is sensitized, the antibodies being exclusively or predominantly located in the cells? Only a convincing answer to this question would offer a real solution of the etiological problem of rheumatism" (Leventhal, 1943). Relation between the immunity-producing antibody (the so-called blocking antibody) and the sensitizing antibody in connection with hypersensitivity was explored (Jacques J. Bronfenbrenner, bacteriology and immunology, Washington University, 1948) in terms of the possibility that there are two kinds of antibodies (heightened resistance; heightened susceptibility) but he found no evidence to support this hypothesis. To him the available evidence, in terms of enzyme reactions and reaction rates, led to the conclusion that while, in response to any one antigen, there is produced only one antibody, the antibodies may vary in individual molecules, some being imperfect in combining power, some in specificity. According to his reasoning, heightened resistance records the consequences of the union of antigen with antibody as they affect the antigen, and heightened sensitivity records the consequences of the union as they affect the host. The dominance of one set of consequences depends upon secondary factors.

From various experimental approaches to the anaphylactic type of sensitivity emerges the concept that the essential element is damage to tissues, especially the vascular endothelium, either by antigen-antibody interaction or nonspecific toxic materials. Especial importance attaches, therefore, to work on sites of antibody formation (Elvin A. Kabat, bacteriology, Columbia, 1947; T. F. Dougherty, anatomy, Utah, 1953) and to work on sites of antigen-antibody reaction and of possible selective accumulation of antigens in certain tissues, studied by tracer methods (A. H. Coons, bacteriology and immunology, Harvard, 1952; Samuel C. Bukantz and coworkers, medicine and pathology, Washington University, 1951; Felix Haurowitz and C. F. Crampton, biochemistry, Indiana, 1952). Coons pointed out, however, that presence of antigens and probably also of antibodies in connective tissue is not proof that rheumatic fever results from antigen-antibody reactions at that site, for any substances present in the blood would be found in an area of inflammation.

Simultaneous or associated occurrence of anaphylactic and tuberculin types of hypersensitivity has long been known in bacterial infections, including streptococcic and tuberculous. Relation between different types of hypersensitivity might (Chase, 1952) be referable to a common cellular mechanism.  Such a mechanism is at least suggested by the close resemblances (after the marked differences of the first three days) found by P. G. H. Gell, 1953, in histological studies of skin lesions produced by the anaphylactic reaction and by tuberculin in sensitized animals.  He inclined to the view that both types of immune reaction-pattern may be involved, "the explosive anaphylactic reaction masking the more persistent manifestations of tuberculin-type allergy".  Relation of types of hypersensitivity to manifestations of the connective tissue diseases is under study by use of the pituitary and adrenal cortical hormones on experimental hypersensitive states and reactions, stimulated in part by transient suppression by these hormones of analogous symptoms in humans.

## HORMONE INFLUENCES IN CONNECTIVE TISSUE DISEASES

The importance of the new approach furnished by the adrenal hormones — cortisone (E), hydrocortisone (F), the hypothetical salt-regulating hormone (DCA), the pituitary adrenotrophic hormone (ACTH) and the growth hormone — in investigation of connective tissue diseases is indicated by the extent of current studies on the effects of these hormones on antibody production, on inflammatory response to traumatic, bacterial, chemical and hypersensitive stimuli.  The weight of opinion appears to favor the view that the effects of the hormones on connective tissue are nonspecific.  Essential to these hormone studies, phenomenally extended in the six years since the first clinical trial of cortisone in rheumatoid arthritis (1948) and subsequent rapid purification and production of the adrenal and pituitary substances, is the concept of the axial principle governing the anterior pituitary and its target endocrine glands (thyroid, gonads, adrenal cortex).  This concept envisages a two-way pathway: the pituitary sends out its stimulating trophic hormones, and each target gland, by producing increased amounts of its hormone, raises the blood level of that particular hormone; on the return journey, the increased supply of each hormone inhibits or lessens secretion by the anterior pituitary of the respective trophic hormone.  In addition to this well-established axial principle, there is increasing evidence of antagonism, probably operating at the peripheral tissue level, between ACTH or the cortical steroids under its control and the growth hormone of the anterior pituitary (Selye, 1950; William O. Reinhardt and Choh Hao Li, 1953; others). The ascendency of the anterior pituitary over the endocrine system has been likened (James H. Means, internal medicine, Harvard, 1951) to that of the cerebral cortex over the nervous system; the pituitary, by means of direct action of its hormones on organs and tissue or indirect action through other endocrines (gonads, thyroid, adrenal cortex), plays a dominant role in the adjustment of the organism which is health and, it follows, in the maladjustment which is disease. Studies over the years of the influence of the hormones, generally, on rheumatic processes indicate that sooner or later the pituitary-adrenal system comes dominantly into the picture. Sex hormone influence, for instance, once considered to account for differing sex susceptibility to gout was shown by later work to be mediated by the adrenal (W. D. Robinson, Jerome W. Conn and associates, medicine, Michigan, 1949, 1952; Peter H. Forsham, George W. Thorn, F. T. G. Prunty and A. G. Hills, medicine, Peter Bent Brigham Hospital, 1948).

## Mechanisms of Pituitary-Adrenal Action on Connective Tissue and Connective Tissue Diseases

Clinical use of cortisone and ACTH in rheumatoid arthritis and other conditions affecting the connective tissue was based upon conclusions and conjectures arrived at between 1929 and 1940 partly as the result of "various clinical observations and partly as the result of numerous experimental failures" (Philip S. Hench, medicine, Mayo Clinic, 1952). The idea of potential reversibility of rheumatoid arthritis was based upon relief of symptoms observed during jaundice and pregnancy and attributed to "substance X", possibly a bisexual, possibly an adrenal hormone. Events following the 1948 trial in the first rheumatoid arthritis patient of compound E at that time prepared in minute amounts by partial synthesis in the Merck laboratories collaborating with Edward C. Kendall (biochemistry, Mayo Foundation, later at the Forrestal Research Institute, Princeton) are well known. Early clinical observations confirmed the "group-specific" rather than disease-specific nature of the ameliorating effects of the adrenal hormone, the effects being upon the same types of tissue (muscular, fibrous, collagenous). Clinical use of the hormones by the Mayo workers and then by others was extended early to disseminated lupus erythematosus and acute rheumatic fever. It was found also that the hormones were effective in various other conditions, notably those showing chemical and other types of nonspecific inflammation.

Among obstacles (pointed out by Hench) to study of the mechanisms of hormone action on connective tissue have been: lack of knowledge as to how much cortisone (or hydrocortisone, compound F) or ACTH is produced daily by the normal body and as to whether or not this production is altered during the diseases in which the effects have been studied; uncertainty as to how much cortisone is produced by the adrenals in response to administered ACTH, as to what is the suppressive effect on the pituitary when excess cortisone is given, as to how many hormones are actually secreted by the adrenal cortex.

## THEORY OF RELATIVE RATHER THAN ABSOLUTE HORMONE DEFICIENCY IN CONNECTIVE TISSUE DISEASES

Opinion is divided on the first two of the above-mentioned questions. Means put strongly, 1951, his warning that administration of excess amounts of a hormone in diseases not "simply due to deficiency of these hormones" must be looked upon, aside from immediate asymptomatic benefit, as "disintegrating". The suppressive effect of the hormones, in bringing about in connective tissue diseases temporary symptomatic benefit not specific to any tissue, has been interpreted by many investigators as a conditioned deficiency. In this interpretation, Selye, 1953, questioned whether in spite of apparently "normal" production or excretion of corticoids, rheumatic patients might be producing "an insufficient amount of corticoids for the condition of disease in which they are. If I may use an analogy: a man running fast will unfailingly develop circulatory disturbances if his heartbeat continues to remain perfectly 'normal' during strenuous exercise." According to Hench, 1952: "The administration of cortisone may correct a relative, not an absolute deficiency, and satisfy an increased tissue requirement for the hormone. Thus current opinion is that the hormones act at the tissue, or cell, level. But this tentative conclusion must be the subject of much further study."

## EMPIRICAL STUDY OF EFFECTS OF PITUITARY-ADRENAL HORMONES IN CONNECTIVE TISSUE DISEASES

Early clinical trials of cortisone and ACTH, later hydrocortisone, showing the temporary nature of the often dramatic beneficent effects and reversion of them when hormone administration was stopped, left no doubt that the disease processes themselves were not changed and provided no clues to what initiates these processes. The hormones, in Hench's phrasing, 1952, dampened rather than extinguished the fire, providing "as it were, an asbestos suit behind which the patient, like some Biblical Shadrach, Meshach or Abednego, protects his tissues from the fire. If this protection is removed prematurely, before the fire has spent itself, the patient and his tissues will react again to the burning. But if the protection is not discarded until the natural duration of the fire is over, the patient remains largely free of symptoms and apparently 'well'." This, however, is a rare outcome (Bauer, 1954). That use of these substances is still empirical was emphasized by Angevine at a 1951 conference on connective tissues: "We are putting coins in the music boxes and out comes the music, but we have no idea of what we are doing. The reason is that we are in the wrong dimension. We missed the most important one which connects anatomy and chemistry."

## MORE FUNDAMENTAL STUDY OF MECHANISMS

Investigation of mechanisms of action and interaction of these hormones, about which little more was known in 1953 than in 1948 (Kendall), has included attempts to describe the phenomena most intimately allied with adrenocortical action. The first metabolic studies (protein, electrolyte, diabetogenic effects, white blood cell and lymphocyte destruction) attempting to correlate biological activities with therapeutic effects seemed to refer the therapeutic effects not to these phenomena but rather to more "specific", "direct" action, chiefly upon connective tissue (Randall G. Sprague and M. H. Power, medicine, Mayo Clinic, 1951). Effects of the pituitary-adrenal axis or system on tissues have been studied in relation to many concepts including those discussed in foregoing sections: the nature of connective tissue and alterations of it in disease; immune reactions and the poststreptococcal state; hypersensitivity.

Explanation of the connective tissue diseases as examples of maladaptation to prolonged stress (Selye) was described as worthy of consideration by Bauer and Clark, 1953. Whether or not the theory that derangement of the adrenocortical adaptive mechanisms may produce such diseases as arthritis, periarteritis, carditis of the rheumatic type, among others, is proved to be correct, it has "awakened or revived the interest of many in the dynamics of illness and its many component parts, disease susceptibility, the polymorphic nature of disease, the possibility that seemingly heterogeneous disease states may represent common pathogenic situations, and other facets of illness. The concept, if correct, would not be without its preventive and therapeutic implications" (Bauer and Clark, 1953). While considering it impossible to conclude that a pituitary-adrenal anomaly plays a basic etiologic role in rheumatoid arthritis, Bauer expressed "no doubt that stimulation of the anterior pituitary and the adrenal cortex can influence the disease favorably". The adrenal cortex, as pointed out, 1951, by George A. Perera (medicine, Columbia), may "teach us many hidden metabolic secrets through its ability to exaggerate normal regulatory activities in health, in stress and during disease". Adaptations of tissues, metabolic rates, etc. may require increased amounts of adrenal cortical hormones, which (D. J. Ingle, 1953) may *permit* rather than *cause* the alterations following prolonged stress. "The hormones of the adrenal cortex are essential for the development of certain disease processes just as they are essential for processes of normality." Increased hormone secretion in stress "may represent a normal homeostatic response and not derailment of function" (Ingle and Baker, 1953).

Work on the hormones, recently extended, seems to justify hope that it may prove definitive as an approach to study of the nature and reactivities of connective tissue. By 1953 there was no doubt of the powerful effects of the pituitary and adrenal hormones on all tissues of mesenchymal origin. Approaches to study of these effects on connective tissue deal with the ground substance, with cells and tissues. Direct effects *in vivo* of ACTH and cortisone on permeability of the ground substance, involving the mucopolysaccharides but not the hyaluronidase enzymes, were interpreted by Seifter, W. Ehrich and coworkers (Wyeth Institute, University of Pennsylvania, Massachusetts Institute of Technology), 1953, as "probably an alteration of the mucopolysaccharides" toward resistance of attack by the enzymes. That permeability of the ground substance is related to the concentration and molecular state of the mucopolysaccharides was considered a reasonable assumption (Dorfman, 1953) but this permeability may also be related to the physicochemical state of tissues generally, as influenced by rates of salt and water metabolism. In inflammation, for example, the sequence of events and of hormonal effects is gradually being outlined, but changes in the circulatory system and its tissues are certainly also involved. Effects of the hormones on vascular aspects of inflammation (William R. Barclay and Robert H. Ebert, Chicago, 1953), of hypersensitivity (Rich and associates, 1950) illustrate use of the hormones for study of mechanisms.

Although mechanisms of formation and laying down of acellular connective tissue elements are unknown, Dorfman considered effects of the cortical hormones on cells of the fibrous elements to be indirect evidence of participation of these fibroblasts in production of the ground substance, known to be affected by the hormones. Inhibition of growth and differentiation of fibroblasts by ACTH and cortisone was demonstrated by Ragan and associates, 1949. In the view of various workers, effects of the hormones on single cells may eventually shed light not only on fibroblasts but also on many aspects of normal connective tissue, on inflammation and other disease processes, on mechanisms of therapeutic response (Ragan and associates, 1949), on cellular division and other activities as phagocytosis (L. M. Leonard and D. D. Rutstein, Harvard, 1953; J. W. Rebuck and R. C. Mellinger, Henry Ford Hospital, 1953; Valy Menkin, Temple, 1953; Matthew Taubenhaus, Michael Reese Hospital, 1950; A. S. Gordon and G. F. Katsh, New York University, 1949).

As for hormonal effects on lymphocytes and on tissues in which these cells are formed, extensive studies have indicated an intimate relationship with inflammation, immunity, hypersensitivity (Dougherty, 1952, 1953; Stoerk, Merck Institute, 1953). The reticuloendothelial cells have long been implicated in antibody formation, and their differentiated offspring, the lymphocytes and plasma cells, which are at least one site of antibody formation, are markedly affected by adrenocortical hormones (Dougherty, 1953). As to the influence of the hormones on the two types of hypersensitivity reactions, there are different findings, as suppression in guinea pigs of the delayed or tuberculin type but not of the immediate or anaphylactic type (Edward E. Fischel and associates, medicine, Columbia, 1951; Stoerk, 1953); and as inhibition of tissue damage in anaphylactic hypersensitivity without removing the state of sensitization (Dougherty, 1952; Rich and associates, 1950; Gregory Shwartzman and S. S. Schneierson, microbiology, Mount Sinai Hospital, 1953).

## POSSIBLE IMPLICATION OF ADRENOCORTICAL INFLUENCE IN SALICYLATE THERAPY

Similarity between effects of salicylates and of adrenocortical hormones on manifestations of rheumatic fever, inflammation and hypersensitivity has suggested that their mechanisms are also similar, or at least similarly nonspecific. That the effect of sodium salicylate may be dependent upon its intermediary action on the adrenal cortex was suggested by Forman, Seifter and Ehrich, 1949, by W. Smith and J. H. Humphrey in England in the same year, and later explored further by this group and others (Shwartzman and associates; Stanley Marcus and D. M. Donaldson, bacteriology, Utah, 1952). The Pennsylvania workers concluded, 1953: that massive salicylate therapy had little effect on rheumatic fever after antibodies have been formed; that its effectiveness early in the disease was due to suppression of antibody formation by a stressor action of its own; that colchicine was a more potent stressor and was effective by the same mechanism in experimental serum disease; that the mechanism in both cases was toxic stimulation of the adrenal cortex. Shwartzman and Schneierson reported, 1953, that of a long list of substances tested for power to inhibit or modify the hypersensitive reaction by their effect on blood coagulation, release of histamine, on central and peripheral nervous systems, only a combination of sodium salicylate and calcium pantothenate (considered to enhance the effect of salicylate) inhibited the reaction in all animals tested.

## CURRENT RESEARCH VISTAS — IN ELUCIDATION OF CONNECTIVE TISSUE REACTIONS

The unsolved problems of connective tissue reactions in the rheumatic syndromes meet, as do all the unsolved problems of medicine, in the area of intermediary metabolism where the fine chemical details of disturbed mechanisms must eventually be identified. And in fundamental metabolic work on the rheumatic syndromes, as on any other condition, major investigative emphasis may shift from time to time from one technique to another, from one process to another, from one substance to another, featuring polysaccharides, lipids, proteins, as any one of these, by the fortunes of discovery, happens to reach the front of the investigative stage, catching the limelight from converging rays of developing work. At present the unsolved problems of connective tissue reactions seem especially to reflect the unsolved problems of protein metabolism. One of the mucopolysaccharides of the ground substance is firmly bound to protein to form a true mucoid and the hyaluronidases (and all enzymes) are proteins. Problems of formation, growth and reactivity of fibrous connective tissue are "in all biological fairness" (Astbury) attracting attention of chemists long interested in problems of structure and synthesis of fibrous protein molecules. All investigations of infection, immunity, hypersensitivity on fundamental levels increasingly draw upon and contribute to the pool of knowledge of protein chemistry in studies of cellular growth, mutation, antigenic activity of specific proteins, antibody formation involving cellular metabolism and serum globulins, antigen-antibody interaction and its effects on the cells of the host. Further, one day, as C. N. H. Long put it, 1951, investigators will have to resolve the questions of factors that regulate release of the anterior pituitary hormones and, eventually, those that regulate formation of these powerful protein entities.

# CHAPTER 7

# Tuberculosis

*Illustrating metabolic mechanisms of*
*infection and resistance*

## INTRODUCTORY

Hans Zinsser once observed that man is very susceptible to tuberculous infection but capable of becoming remarkably resistant to it. Even in parts of the world showing the lowest mortality rates, R. J. Dubos said, 1949, man lives, in relation to tuberculous infection, in a

309

state of unsteady equilibrium which can be "readily disturbed in favor of the disease". The ability of the tubercle bacillus to live as a parasite for long periods without causing disease in the infected host has been interpreted by one school of thought to mean that a "biological equilibrium", reached where populations have attained a level of "civilization" affording favorable hygienic conditions, will, in time, be sufficient to eliminate the disease. Esmond R. Long, reviewing, 1940, the natural history of tuberculosis, described in all communities subjected to infection a progressive trend from acute generalized tuberculosis to chronic generalized tuberculosis, to chronic pulmonary tuberculosis. No way has been worked out, however, for defining or stabilizing favorable environmental factors capable of influencing the equilibrium between man and the tubercle bacillus. Notable advances in control have not meant "conquest" of tuberculosis. Koch's discovery of the tubercle bacillus in 1882, far from expediting the answer to the major question, what enables tubercles to grow, may even have put the clock back. The organism, Dubos wrote, 1949, is still in our midst, "as ubiquitous and as virulent as ever". After more than fifty years' study, we are ignorant of "the means used by the bacillus to behave as a parasite" and also of "the nature of the components and products of the bacilli which may elicit protective mechanisms". We are equally ignorant of the "mechanisms by which the host attempts to protect itself against invasion or injury". With these central metabolic problems still unsolved, there is little cause for complacency about progress in control of a disease which is attended by economic and social loss and suffering probably equaled only in mental illness.

## EXTENT OF THE TUBERCULOSIS PROBLEM

James B. Amberson, 1950, referred to an estimated five million deaths each year among fifty million tuberculous people in the world. The United Nations International Children's Emergency Fund, 1949, described tuberculosis as the chief cause of death among children throughout the world. Esmond Long, 1948, cited figures showing that the rise in death rates was greatest in the countries most ravaged by the war. Studies by the World Health Organization based on seventeen per cent of the world population showed, however, in 1953, a fifty per cent drop in tuberculosis death rates since 1945, Sweden showing a sixty-eight per cent and the United States a forty-seven per cent decline. Reduction in extrapulmonary forms of tuberculosis in this country has been influenced by almost complete elimination of infected dairy cattle and by pasteurization of milk, leaving chronic pulmonary tuberculosis as the central problem in the United States. The National Office of Vital Statistics noted tuberculosis as the seventh ranking cause of death in the United States in 1951, as it had been also from 1946 to 1948.

### Research Associated with Control Programs

The expert committee on tuberculosis of the World Health Organization had recommended, by 1948, integration of international and national control programs, fellowships for training physicians, surveys for case finding, evaluation of BCG vaccination. These recommendations reflect the usual initial emphasis on preventive measures antedating support of scientific investigation of fundamental problems. The National Tuberculosis Association of this country did not set up its research committee until 1921 although it had assumed leadership in tuberculosis control since the date of its founding, 1904. Early research projects led to a cooperative study of the chemistry of the tubercle bacillus, development, production, standardization and clinical testing of purified protein derivative of tuberculin. In this program the Public Health Service, the Henry Phipps Institute, University of Pennsylvania, and thirty-four other research centers collaborated. The American Trudeau Society, the medical section of the national association, founded in 1905, instituted in 1946 a coordinated program primarily to explore integration of streptomycin with other therapeutic procedures in pulmonary tuberculosis. The national association appropriated approximately $100,000 for studies of streptomycin therapy and other research projects, 1947–1948, and in 1951 supported thirty-five projects and eighteen fellowships.

Recognizing that tuberculosis is a major health problem during and after war, the association had in 1919 advocated activity in control and research by the federal government, but action was delayed until the United States entered the second world war when the Public Health Service established a tuberculosis control section, expanded,

1947, to the division of tuberculosis. By 1950, the division had developed a program of assistance to state and voluntary agencies in casefinding (the Public Health Service reported, 1950, approximately fourteen million chest X rays in 1949), treatment, rehabilitation and a coordinated study of chemotherapy. In 1951, the division of tuberculosis became part of the division of chronic diseases in the Bureau of State Services, and by 1953 federal appropriations for tuberculosis amounted to $8,414,280 ($5,307,800 in grants-in-aid to the states for control programs, and $1,314,000 for research). For fundamental research on the tubercle bacillus and host reactions, on chemotherapy, the National Microbiological Institute, in 1953, made grants of over $260,000. The cooperative pattern has been evident in integration of the Trudeau Society's streptomycin program with a similar study initiated in 1946 by the Veterans Administration with the Army and Navy. Cooperation of the National Research Council and of the Council on Pharmacy and Chemistry of the American Medical Association has been directed toward defining problems, organizing investigative procedure, assuming responsibility for exchange of ideas and results, publicizing of data and evaluation of therapeutic procedures. Centers in universities, research institutes and hospitals that have carried on experimental and related clinical investigation of tuberculosis for a number of years have included: the Henry Phipps Institute of the University of Pennsylvania; the department of pathology, Johns Hopkins; the departments of pathology, medicine, public health and preventive medicine, Cornell; the pathology and chemistry departments of Yale; the bacteriology department, Northwestern; the department of medicine, the division of clinical pathology, Mayo Clinic, and the division of experimental medicine, Mayo Foundation; the Rockefeller Institute for Medical Research; the Saranac Laboratory, Trudeau Foundation; and the research laboratories of the Massachusetts General Hospital, the National Jewish Hospital at Denver, the Maybury Sanatorium, Michigan, the Olive View Sanatorium, California, the Montefiore Hospital, New York.

Illustrating the substantive interest in a few of the *university* centers: investigators at the Phipps Institute began their long series of studies on the chemistry of the tubercle bacillus, of tuberculin and of the nature of the skin reaction to it in 1932 when Esmond R. Long became director. In development of the purified protein derivative of tuberculin, Florence B. Seibert's studies (begun in 1924 at Chicago) of the components of the tubercle bacillus were still under way, 1950, with studies of the nature of allergic and immune reactions. Long's work has been concerned with epidemiological and pathological studies with PPD, the life history of the tubercle bacillus, chemotherapy. E. L. Opie (who later returned to the Rockefeller Institute) carried on from 1931 his studies of the mechanisms of infection and immunity in tuberculosis in the Cornell pathology department other members of which, cooperating with the streptomycin project of the American Trudeau Society, have reported upon modifications of tuberculous lesions, cellular pathology in the nervous system and changes in the tubercle bacillus following streptomycin administration. Clinical studies, oriented especially toward the phenomenon of streptomycin resistance and toward toxic effects, have been carried on under the direction of Walsh McDermott of the department of medicine. Interest in experimental tuberculosis as part of broad investigative concern with immunology and bacteriology has been illustrated by the work of A. R. Rich in the pathology department, Johns Hopkins, of G. P. Youmans in the bacteriology department, Northwestern and of Sidney Raffel in the bacteriology department, Stanford. Rich has continued since 1921 studies of the mechanisms of hypersensitivity and immunity, concentrating during part of this period on distinction between the tuberculin type and the anaphylactic type of hypersensitivity. Since 1935 studies of Youmans have been concerned with the life cycle of the tubercle bacillus, and, since 1945, with experimental chemotherapy. For more than ten years, Raffel's work has been concerned chiefly with the relation between immunity and hypersensitivity in tuberculosis and, recently, relations between the metabolic requirements of the bacillus and its virulence. Studies begun, 1927, by R. J. Anderson in Yale's chemistry department, on the lipids of the mycobacteria were being continued, 1951, with cultures grown in isotopically marked medium in a cooperative project with the Phipps Institute, the Columbia medical school, the Office of Naval Research. Fluctuations in the chemical composition, especially mucoproteins, of the blood of patients with tuberculosis were being studied, 1951, by R. J. Winzler of the biochemistry department,

University of Southern California, as an extension of his investigations in the field of enzyme chemistry, intermediary metabolism, blood proteins.

Tuberculosis research in certain endowed *research institutes* and *hospitals* not directly associated with medical schools has included work at the Mayo Foundation by W. H. Feldman, whose interest in veterinary pathology has led to study of the relations between bovine, avian and human tuberculosis, and of chemotherapy in tuberculosis, the latter including collaboration with H. C. Hinshaw of the Mayo Clinic (later of Stanford) in the streptomycin research project of the American Trudeau Society. Experimental tuberculosis (tissue reactions to various fractions of the bacillus and cellular reactions in defense) was a leading interest from 1925 of Florence R. Sabin and of investigators trained in her laboratory at the Rockefeller Institute. Dubos, whose twenty years' work on the bacterial cell is well known in relation to early development of antibiotics from bacteria, began, several years ago, with his associates at the institute, re-examination of methods of study of experimental tuberculosis with particular attention to factors affecting the growth of the bacillus *in vitro* and *in vivo* and influencing virulence. The Saranac Laboratory of the Trudeau Foundation was for many years a center of research on silicosis and other industrial diseases in relation to tuberculosis, under the direction of the late L. U. Gardner; in recent years, William Steenken, Jr., and F. H. Heise have concentrated upon various aspects of experimental chemotherapy. The many other specialized hospitals and sanatoria that have made investigative contribution include the National Jewish Hospital, Denver, where H. J. Corper carried on for more than twenty years studies on diagnosis, pathology and therapy of tuberculosis; tax-supported centers include the Chicago Municipal Tuberculosis Sanatorium now cooperating with the University of Illinois to supply BCG vaccine for long-range clinical studies directed by the Public Health Service; the division of applied immunology, Public Health Research Institute, New York City (Jules Freund, Hubert Bloch and others), engaged in experimental studies of virulence, chemotherapy and a cooperative study with the Public Health Service and the World Health Organization on immunization.

Among *scientific societies*, the National Tuberculosis Association, with its numerous state and local affiliated associations, has, as previously mentioned, assumed leadership in control and later in cooperative research. Its medical section, the American Trudeau Society, has followed the pattern of cooperation in its streptomycin research project, and in surveys of the status of various surgical therapies. In the streptomycin programs, other scientific societies through committees of the National Research Council and of the American Medical Association have contributed their experience, techniques and counsel. The New York Academy of Sciences aided the streptomycin tuberculosis research program by organizing the 1949 conference on chemotherapy of tuberculosis with the aid of grants from twelve manufacturers of streptomycin. The national association publishes *The American Review of Tuberculosis* with summaries in Spanish and French, the chief journal in this field in America, and has financed a culture bank at the Trudeau laboratory from which standard strains of the tubercle bacillus are supplied to investigators in all parts of the world. Contributions from *industry* traditionally aid the development of new chemotherapeutic agents; the thirty-six participants in the 1949 conference on chemotherapy included eighteen investigators from six industrial laboratories. Six pharmaceutical firms contributed to the streptomycin program of the American Trudeau Society drugs worth over a million, and, with six others, reported to the society a total of $1,208,900 spent during 1947–1948 for research on chemotherapeutic agents, almost $700,000 for other types of tuberculosis research including a few fellowships. Twelve manufacturers of X-ray equipment reported spending during the same period $276,250 for tuberculosis research. Of $3,636,250 spent for tuberculosis research, 1947–1948, by the *federal government* (Public Health Service, Departments of Agriculture, Interior, Army, Navy, the Veterans Administration), more than three millions supported chemotherapeutic studies.

An outstanding contribution to the cooperative attack from a *state government* was the appropriation in 1947 of $361,250 by Illinois for the construction and maintenance of an institute at the University of Illinois College of Medicine, to be a center for production and study of BCG vaccine.

## METABOLIC PHENOMENA IN BACILLUS AND HOST

Two general concepts derived from many approaches to bacterial metabolism are now influencing research on the infectious diseases: the concept of bacterial metabolism as essentially similar to the metabolism of the cells of the host; the concept of parasitism as a metabolic process possibly expressed in terms of enzyme adaptation made necessary because the bacteria having lost some of their powers of synthesizing substances essential to their growth have become dependent upon the substrates provided by the host. The concept of the versatility of microorganisms in fulfilling their energy requirements has been extended by innumerable findings showing bacteria, once regarded as the simplest forms of living matter, to be one with all living cells in their metabolic complexities. "The mechanisms of energy transfer and of intermediary metabolism," according to Dubos, 1948, "are essentially as complex in the least exacting bacteria as they are in the most fastidious organism." Many parasitic bacteria appear to require as nutrients essential amino acids, vitamins used for synthesis of many enzymes and other compounds needed as nutrients by host cells (Dubos, Monod and Pappenheimer, 1952). The metabolism of bacteria and of the host cells are both involved in the capacity of microorganisms to cause disease. Whereas bacterial metabolism was first thought of as a problem of cultivation of these organisms *in vitro* (and in this respect paralleled the early nutritional orientation of the study of animal metabolism), this metabolism is being grasped in terms of Lipmann's "reversible reaction continuum". The function of any compound, or of any radical even, in metabolism is seen to be not merely that of an ingredient in a biological recipe but rather that of an element taking part in some essential reaction. Knight said, 1945, "It is the metabolic process which is the essential thing and the compounds used in carrying it out are essential metabolites, *i.e.*, the substrates used for the process, or the substances which form parts (prosthetic groups, etc.) of the enzyme systems which carry out these essential reactions." With this concept kept to the fore, reaction processes are studied with an objective important to the understanding of the infectious process, *i.e.*, the discovery whether or not the substances necessary to essential processes can be synthesized rapidly enough by the organisms to eliminate the necessity of acquiring them from the environment. This "complementary interrelation between nutritional requirements and the organism's own synthetic abilities" is the basis of the use proposed by Fildes, by Knight and others of the term "essential metabolite". It is in terms of essential metabolites or of identified cellular components that investigators are looking for differences between strains of organisms, differences in virulence and biological characteristics, differences in reactions with cells of the host, with immune bodies and other reagents produced in the host's body, and finally with antibacterial substances introduced into the host's body. Dubos, 1950, emphasized that analysis of the nature of the factors that determine virulence lies at the center of the study of the pathogenesis of tuberculosis. A recent trend is the study of components of the tubercle bacillus directly in terms of structure by means of ultraviolet and electron microscopy and indirectly in terms of chemical morphology. This architecture is being analyzed in terms of proteins, lipids, polysaccharides and related substances, in terms of enzymes and enzyme activity, and finally in terms of essential metabolites which are necessary for enzymic reactions.

The chief lines of research have been conducted on the so-called H 37 strain which was isolated at the Saranac Laboratory in 1906 and has maintained its virulence, according to Steenken and Gardner, 1946, through continuous transplantation on suitable media up to the present. This organism is naturally pathogenic for man, apes, monkeys, slightly for dogs and parrots, but not for other birds or cattle. The bovine strain, pathogenic for both man and cattle, has not been studied to a comparable degree. The recent interest in BCG vaccination, by which living bacilli of an attenuated bovine strain are injected on the assumption that a nonprogressing primary infection with tubercle bacilli induces immunity which protects against subsequent infection with a virulent strain, is stimulating fundamental work on the chemistry and metabolism of the Pasteur Institute bacillus of Calmette and Guerin, as at the Microbiological Institute of the National Institutes of Health. The human and bovine strains have similar acid-fast staining qualities, protein constituents, biological effects when inoculated into susceptible animals, and sensitivity to physical agents. As the work on the chemistry and metabolism of the human bacillus matures, its significance for bacteriology and for biology in general becomes clearer, particularly in relation to virulence and its significance in the epidemiology of infection. Virulence as applied to the tubercle bacillus is acquiring meaning in terms of specific morphological and metabolic characteristics possessed by some organisms but not by others. This approach has been made possible by the development of new cultural methods, and by the exploration of the capacities of the laboratory mouse and other small animals as hosts for experimental tuberculosis.

By the addition to a simple synthetic medium of two classes of wetting agents, Dubos and his associates reported, 1947, that the hydrophobic character of the surface of tubercle bacilli could be overcome, this characteristic being responsible for the typical slow growth, in the usual liquid media, in clumps and heavy pellicles. Studies of these cultures have revealed effects of various types of lipids and other nutrients on the rate and abundance of growth of the bacilli, leading to the hope that the peculiar affinities of the bacilli for various types of lipids, demonstrated in these studies, may point to the significance of lipids in the pathogenesis of tuberculosis. To accumulation of lipid material around virulent bacilli growing in the newer media has been attributed the peculiar microscopic "serpentine cord" formation of these (bovine and human) strains observed by Middlebrook, Dubos and Pierce, 1947. The cord formation appears to be associated with the spreading method of growth on the surface of media, and may also "play a significant part in the pathogenesis of tuberculosis" (Middlebrook and Freund, 1952).

Rich's 1951 statement, which he considered to be supported by extensive studies over a period of fifty years, that the action of the tubercle bacillus in the animal body is not to be attributed to either an endotoxin or an exotoxin is apparently in agreement with the prevailing view. He referred to studies by many investigators which have failed to show that the proteins, lipids and carbohydrates present (as complex substances and in complex combinations) in the tubercle bacillus exert an appreciable toxic effect on the normal body. In addition, the tubercle bacillus itself when injected into normal animals or into tissue cultures is phagocytized by macrophages, but has been shown to live in symbiosis with these cells and in cultures with other virulent bacteria. In other words, Rich maintained, no substance is liberated by the bacillus growing *in vitro* or *in vivo* that is capable of explaining the destruction of tissue that occurs in the tuberculous body. His contention is that substances derived from the bacillus and capable of inducing the state of hypersensitivity account for the highly toxic systemic effects of the tubercle bacillus and its components in the tuberculous hypersensitive body. In work on the chemical constituents and metabolic products of the bacillus (Seibert, 1941), the proteins produced during *in vitro* growth or released from dead bacilli into the surrounding medium have claimed the larger share of investigative interest. It is these compounds, known collectively as tuberculin, that are believed by many, with exceptions to be noted, to be responsible for the hypersensitive state. The more extensive studies have dealt with a search for the active principle of tuberculin.

Because the tuberculous host develops an altered tissue reactivity (hypersensitivity) to the several different *protein* fractions of tuberculin, the tuberculin skin test has been used since 1907 (von Pirquet) in diagnosis. Early work on the tuberculin proteins, aimed at production of a stable, highly potent, standardized tuberculin devoid of impurities for use in diagnosis, resulted in Purified Protein Derivative of tuberculin (Seibert, 1941). Since PPD is separated by ultrafiltration and pressure dialysis from liquid nonprotein medium (Long) on which tubercle bacilli have been grown for ten weeks, it was concluded that the proteins in the filtrate are products of the organism's metabolism. Another view, that the active principle is a bacterial protein liberated upon the death and autolysis of the organism, has been supported by other workers. Rich stressed, 1951, that this purified protein is innocuous for normal animals and for cells from normal animals growing in tissue cultures; a tuberculous guinea pig is killed by one mgm. whereas 100 to 150 mgm. are required to kill a normal guinea pig.

It should be emphasized that bacterial components that give rise to hypersensitivity in the animal body are not identical with components that act as antigens to stimulate the formation of protective antibodies. "Of the multiple antibodies which result from the injection of a suspension of bacteria, or of extracts of them", Dubos said, 1945, "only one or a very few afford protection against infection while all cause different types and degrees of hypersensitiveness." Heidelberger and Menzel showed that two separate and distinct antigens exist in the proteins of the tubercle bacillus, but the significance in clinical tuberculosis of the antibodies produced in response to the antigens of the bacillus is still undetermined. Zinsser said that the possession by a protein of antigenic function giving rise to hypersensitivity is correlated with the body's inability to eliminate the protein promptly by ordinary mechanisms of excretion. It is supposed that such proteins remain in the circulation and form a slow union with the body cells. It is also assumed that immunological specificity is a function of chemical structure but, although there is considerable evidence of correlation, immunological techniques have so far proved to be more sensitive indicators of differences than have chemical techniques. The active Purified Protein Derivative of tuberculin exhaustively studied in the Phipps laboratory (and in Svedberg's laboratory in Sweden) was found by recently developed physicochemical techniques to be a relatively small molecule in comparison with certain active substances prepared from unheated tuberculin. A difference in biological activities also exists between the two, the larger molecule being antigenic and the smaller molecule being practically nonantigenic. It was thought that any correlation found between the molecular size and the biological activity of the active fraction would be significant for immunology and for protein chemistry in general, especially since the fraction, which maintains its potency unchanged for years, appears to be a remarkably stable protein among those having biological activity. Data on molecular size so far obtained by Seibert leave open the possibility that potency and antigenicity may be inherent in different parts of the same protein molecule.

The hypersensitivity resulting from infection of animals with tubercle bacilli or injection with killed organisms or their extracts is of such degree that subsequent injection of small amounts of extracts or of tuberculin is followed by violent reactions, often by death. A prevalent view is that the symptoms of general toxicity are largely a result of acquired hypersensitivity to "metabolic products of the parasite" (Middlebrook and Freund, 1952). Knowledge of the identity of the components or metabolic products of the tubercle bacillus having direct or indirect toxic effects in the body, of the mechanisms of these reactions in terms of the cellular structures or the metabolic processes destroyed or inhibited, of factors controlling the production and activity of these substances is still to be established. These unknown mechanisms are regarded as basic to understanding the nature of tuberculous infection and the host's reactions to it.

The view that the protein stimulating the hypersensitive reaction is a normal component of the bacillus which is liberated by autolysis was put forward by Raffel and by Corper, 1946. Lurie's observation, 1949, that with moderate numbers of inhaled bacilli resistant rabbits develop tuberculin sensitivity more rapidly than susceptible rabbits led him to conclude that only bacilli that have been destroyed can liberate sensitizing antigens. Raffel and Forney, 1948, reported that a protein fraction mixed with a "purified wax" fraction induced sensitization to "old tuberculin" but that neither fraction alone had that effect. If further study should prove such a component to be the antigen responsible for producing the hypersensitive state, which so far has resulted only from the presence in the body of tuberculous infection or the injection of the whole killed bacilli or their unfractionated extracts, the way would be open for study in fine chemical detail of the complex reactions of this hypersensitivity which can now be studied only in the biological terms of skin sensitization exhibited in response to the purified protein derived from tuberculin.

Quantitative determinations of the amino acid composition of proteins have been made by chromatographic methods by Stein and Moore of the Rockefeller Institute, who used tubercle bacilli to explore the possibilities of this method for determining the composition of proteins in fractionated biological materials. Hydrolysates of virulent and avirulent tubercle bacilli were reported, 1950, to show no differences in amounts of sixteen amino acids and of ammonia. In the tubercle bacillus, as in other microorganisms that have been studied by cytochemical techniques, the proteins are intimately associated with nucleoproteins and polysaccharides. The nucleoproteins of various species of acid-fast bacilli have been examined by chemical, physicochemical and serological techniques in a long series of studies by Heidelberger and Menzel who reported only slight immunological differences between the human and bovine nucleoproteins.

Avery and Heidelberger and associates (1931–1934) found *carbo-*

*hydrates* extracted from the human type of tubercle bacillus to be integral parts of lipid and protein molecules. Sabin and co-workers, who studied the cellular reactions in animals to these fractions, found no evidence of toxicity for the normal body, no power to evoke hypersensitivity or to elicit local reactions in the tuberculin-hypersensitive body. Experiments reported, 1944, by Kropp and Foley were thought to demonstrate that a pure polysaccharide extracted from virulent bacilli and lethal for tuberculous but not for nontuberculous guinea pigs had significance in the metabolic alterations in the disease. Localized skin reactions in human subjects were correlated with the presence of active or arrested infection, and the serum of tuberculous patients contained antibodies against the polysaccharide. Choucroun reported, 1949, a precipitin test for carbohydrate antibodies in human tuberculosis and concluded that the carbohydrate as well as lipocarbohydrate fractions play an active part in resistance. Rich suggested, 1951, that the high degree of *in vitro* reactivity exhibited by certain tuberculocarbohydrates demonstrates that these components "are highly active in the process of antibody-stimulation during the development of acquired resistance to the tubercle bacillus".

The *lipids* of the acid-fast bacteria have been regarded as being somehow responsible for the peculiar staining qualities and the peculiar resistance of these bacteria to penetration by antiseptics and other cell poisons, from the time of the earliest chemical investigations of the tubercle bacillus. These lipids studied for nearly twenty-five years by Anderson were described in his 1940 Harvey lecture as composing from twenty-five to forty per cent of the dry weight of the cell and containing a series of new fatty acids, including the extensively studied tuberculostearic and phthioic acids. The long-held view that the bacillus is surrounded by a waxy capsule was challenged by Dubos, 1947, who suggested that the surface of the bacillus "possesses an exposed protein component". With Middlebrook and Pierce he investigated the "hydrophobic substance" of the cell as an approach to the old problem of virulence, a problem that has occupied many investigators since 1920 when Calmette secured an avirulent variant of the bovine strain now used in BCG vaccination. The Rockefeller Institute workers have shown that acid-fastness varies from a high degree in virulent to a low degree in avirulent cultures. The hydrophobic substance or substances retard or inhibit contact with anti-bacterial substances (p-aminosalicylic acid, streptomycin), and the hydrophobic quality is modified by various lipids and lipid derivatives. The authors suggested, therefore, that the marked affinity of these bacilli for various types of lipids may be of significance in the pathogenesis of the disease and in its chemotherapeutic treatment.

The isolation by Choucroun, 1943, of a substance contained in paraffin oil extracts of dead tubercle bacilli which, in minute amounts, produced in normal guinea pigs a fatal reaction involving extensive lung involvement led her to question whether this substance is an important antigen of the bacillus, or a peculiar component of the bacillus responsible for at least a part of the pathological manifestations of the infectious process. Choucroun thought the paraffin oil-soluble complex may be the antigen capable of stimulating resistance so far observed only in animals injected with living bacilli. It is consonant with what is known of infection and resistance that a single bacterial substance may be the most powerful toxin responsible for protean manifestations of infection, and at the same time may be the antigenic substance capable, under favorable circumstances, of stimulating acquired immunity. The previously mentioned cord formation of virulent tubercle bacilli growing *in vitro* was thought by Middlebrook, 1950, to be caused by lipid material which holds the bacilli together and also contains "virulence factors". Virulent but not avirulent bacilli were shown by the same workers to inhibit the migration of leukocytes of normal, susceptible hosts *in vitro* and *in vivo*. Extraction of young virulent bacilli with paraffin oil or a lighter hydrocarbon by Bloch at the Public Health Research Institute, New York, 1950, left viable organisms having reduced virulence for experimental animals and lacking the power to inhibit the migration of leukocytes *in vitro*. The lipid material extracted, however, exerted an inhibitory effect on leukocyte migration and a toxic effect for mice upon repeated small injection. After a period in which sensitization occurred, the lipid material produced extensive hemorrhagic lesions. Virulence and the consequent chain of events called infection are interrelated metabolic activities of the invading organism and of the host cells which can hardly be considered separately.

# SUSCEPTIBILITY AND RESISTANCE IN TUBERCULOSIS

A dominant view in the 1950 discussions of the British Tuberculosis Association was that infection, though important, is "not the major factor in the prevalence of tuberculosis"; the individual's reaction to infection is determined by hereditary factors, age of infection, non-specific resistance influenced by nutrition and other environmental factors, and specific resistance or immunity. The characteristics of tuberculous infection are dependent upon the cellular response of the host which changes during the progress of infection and provides modified conditions for the multiplication and dissemination of the organisms. The host reaction is regarded as a dominant factor in determining the outcome of the first infection type of tuberculosis, which may be either a rapidly progressing fatal disease or a benign lesion that heals by resolution or undergoes caseation and calcification.

It has long been known that tuberculous infection is not confined to those having symptoms. Present estimates are somewhat lower than those current at the beginning of this century when the findings offered by a number of pathologists from unselected autopsy material were accepted as proof that over ninety per cent of all adults had either healed, inactive or active tuberculous lesions in the lungs. The idea that universal primary infections act as a natural control measure has been challenged by certain epidemiological studies. Whether the "reinfection" or adult type of infection is an exacerbation of the benign primary infection, the quiescent first lesion, or is newly acquired, its characteristics, according to Freund and Middlebrook, 1948, depend upon "preceding immunological status, *i.e.*, the existence of a prior tuberculous infection". The unanswered questions are: "Do the tubercle bacilli in the healed lesion survive and thus maintain the immunological status of the host? Are they dead but not destroyed and eliminated?" Studies by numerous investigators have shown no viable bacilli in many of these healed lesions, and first infection type of disease has been acquired by persons whose lungs contain a healed primary lesion. Freund and Middlebrook suggested that tuberculin sensitivity may be maintained by "casual contacts" with tubercle bacilli that cause no demonstrable lesions in persons recovered from a benign infection. Whether the infection is of the primary or reinfection type, the bacillus initiates a struggle in which, according to Dubos, if the natural resistance of the host is overcome, the acquired resistance is unlikely to gain a decisive victory. In this struggle, as Rich has pointed out, the main recourse of the host is his natural resistance for, aside from the possible but highly uncertain effects of BCG vaccination, none of the methods for producing active or passive immunity has been found applicable to immunization against tuberculous infection. Dubos concluded, 1949, that the views attributing the decline of epidemic tuberculosis during the last century to an increase in inherited resistance by a process of natural selection, to a process of immunization resulting from subclinical infections in the more resistant population and to improvements in living standards accompanying the growth of industrialization are plausible but are based on assumptions for which objective evidence has not been found. While the decline has been attributed in part (Long) to removal from the population of numerous sources of infection, almost 180,000 of the 500,000 cases in the United States were classed (Birkhaug, 1948) as infectious and not hospitalized.

## Factors in Natural Susceptibility and Resistance

Little closely focused experimental work has been done on the host factors of race, age, sex, although beginnings have been made through the use of the mouse and rabbit. There is obvious difficulty in separating *race* factors from social and economic factors associated with standards of living and hygienic levels. Parran attributed the fact that mortality among the Negroes in the United States stood at a higher rate in 1944 than the rate among the whites in 1919 chiefly to the influence of poverty and ignorance. The idea prevails that races or population groups gradually acquire a degree of resistance after exposure to infection for many generations. Great potential importance in certain unexplained aspects of *age* incidence in tuberculosis has been realized by both fundamental investigators and clinicians. The high resistance and low death rate in the age group from five to fifteen (evident in 1900 when infection was almost universal) must be (Dubos, 1951) "the expression of some general biological law". Whether a direct, metabolic influence of *sex* can account for National Office of Vital Statistics figures showing that the higher death rate for white males over white females was increased twenty per cent in 1910 and ninety per cent in 1948 is not known.

The interconnection of age, sex and endocrine factors in susceptibility to tuberculosis is recognized if not understood. The question whether the sex *hormones* might be a factor in susceptibility and resistance was raised by Lurie in the course of his studies of constitutional factors. Rabbit experiments reported by him and his collaborators, 1949, showed that estrogen retards "progress of tuberculosis at the portal of entry in the skin and diminishes its dissemination to the internal organs in highly inbred animals, chiefly by reducing permeability of the connective tissue". The hormones appeared to have no effect on multiplication or destruction of tubercle bacilli in the tissues, on antibody formation, or on development of hypersensitivity. While no clear evidence was obtained that the sex hormones used affect the progress of tuberculosis in rabbits *via* the adrenals, tuberculosis, as such, caused marked hypertrophy of these glands. These findings, and the evidence that has been accumulating of a role of the adrenal cortex in phagocytosis (Gordon and Katsh, 1949) and in hypersensitivity and antibody production through its influence on the lymphocytes (Dougherty, 1948) have led to investigations in Lurie's laboratory, 1950, of the role of the adrenals in constitutional resistance.

Rabbit experiments reported, 1951, were interpreted as evidence that cortisone "markedly and fundamentally affected the essential mechanism of the pathogenesis of tuberculosis". Similar observations on clinical pulmonary tuberculosis reported (Le Maistre, Tompsett, Muschenheim, Moore, McDermott) at the 1951 clinical ACTH conference were interpreted as "an example of modification of the host-parasite relationship mediated entirely through an action on the host". The modification ceased abruptly when hormone administration was stopped. Although loss of cutaneous hypersensitivity occurred in about half the patients with slow return at the end of treatments, no evidence of alteration in the tubercle bacillus by the treatment was obtained.

Lurie, discussing, 1941, the experimental approach to *genetic factors*, referred to clinical studies by Diehl and Verschuer comparing the behavior toward tuberculosis of thirty-seven identical twins and sixty-nine fraternal twins. Tuberculous infection in twenty-six, or seventy per cent, of the identical twins pursued a similar course; in the fraternal, *i.e.*, genetically different twins, tuberculous infection of the same nature was found in seventeen, or only twenty-five per cent. Heredity was considered the deciding factor in resistance. In continuation of earlier studies at the Henry Phipps Institute by Lewis and his associates, who used inbred families of guinea pigs, Lurie's six families of inbred rabbits, in their response to natural respiratory infection, which is believed to parallel the conditions of human exposure, fell into three groups, and the pulmonary tuberculosis acquired, generation after generation, differed among the groups in features similar to those observed in different racial groups in man. The response of rabbits to immunization varied according to the genetic constitutions, no immunity developing in highly susceptible strains, and high immunity developing even after vaccination with killed bacilli in resistant strains. The rabbits of some families were intermediate in their behavior and it was suggested that the mixed type of tuberculosis which occurs in the American Negro is a human counterpart of the varying susceptibility to tuberculosis in these rabbit families having varying genetic characters, rather than varying environmental determinants. Long, 1941, reviewing the evidence for hereditary determination of susceptibility in the Negro, suggested that, in a group having mixed hereditary factors for resistance, the influence of natural selection toward elimination of the more highly susceptible requires either a long time or an intense epidemic within a homogeneous population.

While genetic factors cannot be ignored ("we must not forget the guinea pig, the elephant, the Negro and the twin"), Day pointed out, 1951, that psychological ("psychosomatic") factors, not susceptible to scientific analysis, appear to operate also in the onset of tuberculosis, and in recovery (often, "it is the patients who heal each other").

## FACTORS IN ACQUIRED SUSCEPTIBILITY AND RESISTANCE

Although *nutrition* is a major principle in the nonspecific treatment of tuberculosis, Dubos, 1948, considered that the possible influence of nutrition has not been effectively separated from the influence of other nonspecific factors.  He and his colleagues studied the influence of Schneider's diets on susceptibility of three strains of mice to infection with known amounts of virulent human tubercle bacilli and suggested that absence of an unknown factor in wheat germ, found by Schneider, 1946, to increase resistance and survival in infected mice, causes a "nonspecific physiologic disturbance" influencing susceptibility. Hart and Rees, 1950, citing studies to test the effects on experimental tuberculosis of diets deficient in protein and vitamins, high in egg yolk or various lipids, concluded: "No nutrient or class of nutrients, or even a general reduction in caloric intake, has been incriminated."

There is a growing body of knowledge (not specific to tuberculosis) of the effects of protein depletion on production of antibodies which, however, have not been proved to be the crucial mechanisms of resistance.  According to Cannon, 1948, protracted depletion of protein reserves in animals leads to atrophy of tissues of the reticulo-endothelial system, generally regarded as essential to the building up of reserve leukocytes.  Coordinated investigations measuring protein requirements for restoration of tissue synthesis in protein-depleted animals seem to indicate that in mammals dietary lack of any one of nine indispensable amino acids (arginine being the exception) can be corrected only by specific replacement therapy.  In the absence of a single essential amino acid in the diet, tissue synthesis comes to a standstill, all other amino acids becoming useless for tissue synthesis and evidently being converted into glucose, or deaminated and excreted. If this concept that the synthesizing mechanisms "operate on a 'perfectionistic' or 'all or none' principle to the extent that if they cannot build a *complete* protein when it is required they will build none at all" holds for man, its significance in treatment of tuberculosis is obvious, since the dietary aspects of therapy in tuberculosis are based upon the objective of fortification of natural resistance and tissue repair.

The susceptibility of the tubercle bacillus to any one or any group of *chemotherapeutic agents* has been related to various factors as the nature and property of its membrane — its permeability, its acid-fastness, its hydrophobic character.  The inevitable emergence of the cell surface as an area of especial significance in the tubercle bacillus recalls a general observation of Dubos, 1945, that phospholipids, several types of which are capable of protecting living cells against many toxic agents, are commonly present in biological materials, and the possibility that these substances may become adsorbed at the cell surface of the tubercle bacillus may be worth investigation. In the recent studies at the Rockefeller Institute of factors determining virulence of tubercle bacilli, referred to previously, it has been shown, according to Middlebrook, 1950, that the chemical structure of the surface of all virulent strains of mammalian tubercle bacilli differs "in a special way" from that of the avirulent strains. Bloch's finding, in virulent strains, of lipid material which alters the permeability of the cellular surface is an example of knowledge that may eventually guide the search for bacteriostatic agents active against the tubercle bacillus. Water solubility or high polar molecular structure associated with water solubility rather than fat solubility characterizes, however, all the effective chemotherapeutic agents capable of inhibiting growth of the tubercle bacillus (Fox, 1952). In chemotherapy of tuberculosis, studied intermittently for a century, "certain specific questions still unanswered today were being asked at least sixty years ago" (Donovick, Rake and Titus, 1950), as why many types of compounds active against the bacillus *in vitro* fail to affect the disease *in vivo*. The problem appears to be not only penetration of the bacterial cell but also penetration by drugs of tissues altered by hypersensitivity with its concomitant inflammation, and by caseation, penetration of the drug into phagocytic cells before and after they acquire a population of tubercle bacilli (Florey, 1952).

Of the tuberculostatic drugs, the most thoroughly studied have been streptomycin and its derivative, dihydrostreptomycin. The general conclusion resulting from treatment of approximately 7,000 patients (all types of tuberculosis) under different streptomycin regimens, reported, 1950, by the streptomycin committee of the Veterans Administration to the Council on Pharmacy and Chemistry, was that, in itself, "streptomycin can never (or hardly ever) be counted on to cure tuberculosis". Relapse rates within twelve months in tuberculosis of the alimentary tract and of draining cutaneous sinuses, in which the drug has been particularly successful, were about five and ten per cent, in pulmonary tuberculosis thirty-five per cent. Reports of identical effects, by both laboratory tests and clinical trials, of streptomycin and dihydrostreptomycin in a series of studies organized by the American

Trudeau Society were thought by Hinshaw, 1953, to raise confidence in the methods used for solution of problems arising from clinical use of streptomycin — an endeavor, in his view, not matched in medical history.

Problems raised by administration of drugs in relatively high dosage over long periods include that of acquired resistance of the tubercle bacillus and that of toxic effects in the host. These problems were serious obstacles to use of streptomycin (which on prolonged administration damages the vestibular branch of the eighth cranial nerve) and of dihydrostreptomycin, regarded as less toxic, to both of which the bacillus becomes resistant. Para-aminosalicylic acid (PAS) had by 1950 (Hinshaw) become widely accepted as an auxiliary drug to replace streptomycin when resistance has been established, or as an alternate in prevention of streptomycin-resistance and toxic effects of the drug. A new category of synthetic antituberculosis drugs, pyridine and pyrazine carboxylic acid derivatives closely related to nicotinamide (which was found to have tuberculostatic activity), includes the isonicotinyl hydrazines (isoniazid) and pyrazinamide. The vitamin activity of the nicotinamide is not related (Fox, 1952) to its tuberculostatic activity and the pyridine structure of these compounds is, at least theoretically, responsible for the chemotherapeutic effect. The committee on therapy of the American Trudeau Society concluded, 1953, that, although the toxicity of isoniazid as compared with that of streptomycin and dihydrostreptomycin is relatively minor, the rapid appearance of resistance to isoniazid made it a less valuable chemotherapeutic measure than combined streptomycin and PAS. Early reports indicated that, although the antituberculous action of pyrazinamide-isoniazid was "superior and qualitatively different from that of current antituberculous drugs used either singly or together", their use, in the dosage required, resulted in high incidence of hepatitis in man (McDermott and associates, 1954). Nevertheless, sustained reversal of infectiousness (in ninety per cent over six months) was regarded (Campagna, Calix and Hauser, 1954) as justifying use of pyrazinamide-isoniazid as a public health measure in far-advanced ambulatory cases. A 1954 progress report on a Public Health Service cooperative study with twenty-two state and private sanatoria described isoniazid and PAS as quite as effective as isoniazid and streptomycin. Hinshaw and many others have pointed out that one of the greatest benefits of chemotherapy in tuberculosis is in preparation of patients for thoracic surgery, in preventing postoperative infections and reactivation of quiescent lesions.

Thoracic surgery substitutes local tissue rest for the generalized rest of older therapies. During recent years it has, especially in its most recent developments, dramatically changed the picture of tuberculosis; in some of its uses it has, for many patients, reduced the traditional ten or twelve years of bed rest to one or two years. It has become, for suitable cases, routine in many hospitals and sanatoria. Collapse therapy, the rationale of which lies in aiding healing and preventing spread of infection by relieving tension upon cavities and scar tissue in the lungs by reduction of motion and pull, has been achieved chiefly through thoracoplasty. New bone formation within the periosteum of the removed ribs maintains permanent collapse of the affected lung tissue. Tissue rest without thoracic surgery (regarded as too dangerous in some cases of bilateral or widespread involvement) has been attempted by various expedients: by pneumothorax (injection of air into the thoracic cavity); more rarely by pneumoperitoneum (injection of air into the peritoneal cavity); by diaphragmatic paralysis resulting from crushing of phrenic nerve (waning in popularity). The more radical pneumonectomy (removal of an entire lung) and lobectomy (removal of individual lobes), first tried for tuberculosis in 1937, have become much more general with modern developments in anesthesia and antibiotics. Wedge resection of individual lesions or processes from infected lungs, in 1950 reported from a few centers in small series of cases, had, by 1952, become the practice in more than half the number of resections reported. During 1952 sixty-three lesions were resected (wedge) from twenty patients at the Trudeau Foundation. Reports by 1953 indicated for resection (except pneumonectomy) such low mortality that problems in need of research are no longer confined to survival and control of disease but extend to urgent problems of the patients' postoperative cardiovascular and respiratory physiology (Woodruff and associates). Follow-up studies, after resection (1.6 per cent positive for tubercle bacillus after eight months, Steenken, Trudeau Laboratory, 1953; seven per cent reactivation of infection after an average of twenty-seven months, D. O. Shields and associates, Veterans Administration, 1952), showed no major surgical complications, no operative mortality. Postoperative administration of antituberculosis drugs appeared to be general practice, with some patients discharged from hospital three months after surgery; the minimum period for preoperative drug therapy was four months. At a 1951 conference, fourteen cases of thoracoplasty were reported; there was no defense of pneumothorax or of diaphragmatic paralysis through phrenic nerve crushing. As to resection of residual lesions after chemotherapy, the committee on therapy of the American Trudeau Society, 1954, thought that no decision could be made until more is known of the bacteriology of these necrotic lesions. The committee re-emphasized "the valuable role of surgical collapse in the treatment of pulmonary tuberculosis". Current evaluations of thoracic surgery point to a justifiable hope that with progressive improvements in anesthesia, further development of antibiotics and of chemotherapeutic possibilities, the changes wrought in the tuberculosis picture may be permanent.

Although *specific acquired immunity* against tuberculous infection can be demonstrated, according to Freund and Middlebrook, the role of humoral antibodies has not been revealed. Dubos's 1949 statement noted previously is unqualified: "Nothing is known of the immune mechanisms by which the host attempts to protect itself against invasion or injury by the bacillus." The nature of hypersensitivity induced by the living or killed bacillus, the relation of hypersensitivity to immunity or to mechanisms of specific resistance, the relation between avirulent and virulent organisms as antigens and the application of certain facts and assumptions to prophylactic immunization are the chief problems under investigation. In addition, there is renewed interest in the nature of the cellular reactions of the host in resistance.

Although immune responses in animals were demonstrated by Koch, it was much later that Römer elaborated the theory that specific immunity and hypersensitivity in tuberculosis are essentially a unified phenomenon. The view that *hypersensitivity* is associated with resistance, although not necessarily with immune antibodies, was re-examined, 1942, by Woodruff and Kelly, whose experiments (guinea pigs) led them to conclude that there is a quantitative relationship between allergy and pulmonary resistance. Among those that abandoned the view that acquired resistance is dependent upon hypersensitivity are Opie (1932) and Calmette (1933). Rich, on the basis of his experiments and observations and those of others, has continuously supported the view (as stated by him in 1951) that "hypersensitive inflammation has never been satisfactorily shown to be necessary for the successful operation of acquired immunity at any stage of any infection under any condition". Avoiding the extremes of the two opposed views, he proposed that hypersensitivity may be regarded "as a condition which, under some conditions, is decidedly deleterious and, under some conditions, exists without any appreciable deleterious or beneficial effect". The protein nature of the active principle of tuberculin which evokes the hypersensitive skin reaction has been established, as noted previously, although sensitization to tuberculin has been produced only by active infection or by introduction parenterally of living or dead bacilli. Rich held the view that bacterial hypersensitivity typified by the reactions of the body to tuberculin (used to mean any preparation containing protein components or products of the tubercle bacillus) is distinctly different from anaphylactic hypersensitivity, produced by any foreign protein introduced into the tissues. The differences include: a delayed local and systemic reaction compared with the prompt and acute reactions in anaphylactic hypersensitivity; a "focal reaction" at sites of infection; failure of passive transfer of hypersensitivity by injection of serum from a hypersensitive to a normal animal; a lethal effect of the specific bacterial protein on cells from the hypersensitive body *in vitro;* the necessity for introduction parenterally of living or dead bacteria or filtrable viruses to establish bacterial hypersensitivity as contrasted with the establishment of anaphylactic hypersensitivity by the proteins alone; frequent absence of anaphylactic hypersensitivity in a body with a high degree of bacterial hypersensitivity. Hypersensitivity is so uniformly present in the tuberculous body and is so widespread among body cells, even in tissue culture and in wandering individual cells (Heilman, Feldman and Mann, 1944), that positive skin reaction to the tuberculin test is interpreted as an index not only of hypersensitivity but also of infection (Rich, 1951). While a positive tuberculin skin test indicates that the reactor is infected, it does not (since it may occur in the absence of lesions recognizable by X ray) necessarily mean tuberculous disease.

The diagnostic significance of serological tests measuring specific resistance in terms of *humoral antibodies* was investigated by Middlebrook and Dubos, 1948, who described an agglutination test carried out with a water-soluble component of tubercle bacilli and of old tuberculin adsorbed on sheep red cells, which were agglutinated by sera from immunized rabbits and from patients with active tuberculosis. An apparently specific precipitin test for antibodies elicited by a carbohydrate component of the tubercle bacillus was reported by Choucroun, 1949. The antigen used in this test is a pure water-soluble carbohydrate split by hydrolysis from the antigenic lipo-carbohydrate fraction of the bacillus which, according to Choucroun, plays a part in active resistance.

Specific resistance in terms of *cellular reactions* including the role of body cells in determining the fate of tubercle bacilli in the body and the role of body cells as sites of antibody production is under investigation by Hubert Bloch, who pointed out, 1948, that since the tubercle can be produced by the injection of dead bacilli, of fractions of bacilli, and of some synthetic fatty acids, its formation cannot depend upon the action of living, virulent bacilli. Living, virulent bacilli are, however, essential to the production of progressive tuberculosis. Experiments reported led to the suggestion that virulent bacilli (but not the avirulent variants) can exert on the leukocytes that have phagocytized them a "lytic effect which results in the release of the bacilli into the extracellular fluid". The initial reaction of the leukocytes to both virulent and avirulent bacilli occurred at the same rate, and it was concluded that the problem returns to the property of virulence of the bacillus. Lurie reported to the fourth international congress for microbiology, 1947, experiments using subcutaneous injection of virulent tubercle bacilli suspended in melted agar. Body fluids readily penetrated the solidifying agar islands but the cells invaded them slowly so that the action of cells and of body fluids could be observed separately *in vivo*. It was found that, in the normal animal, bacilli in acellular agar islands and also bacilli in colloidin-coated silk bags containing agar multiplied rapidly. In the immune animal multiplication of bacilli was markedly inhibited in both preparations into which the body fluids could enter, and the bacilli were agglutinated rather than dispersed. The extracellular factors, however, were regarded as secondary to the phagocytic activity of the mononuclear cells of the immune animals which increased in response to nonspecific particles and tubercle bacilli. Active tuberculosis, also, conferred on the mononuclear phagocytes themselves bacteriostatic properties for tubercle bacilli which were independent of humoral immunity.

That certain body cells can be tuberculin-"sensitized" and can carry hypersensitivity from a sensitized to a new host was indicated by injection of living, undamaged (mononuclear) white cells from peritoneal exudates, spleen, lymph nodes or blood from hypersensitive animals into new animals which became sensitized for a limited time (Chase, 1945; Cummings and associates, 1947; others). The transfer of tuberculin sensitivity in man by injection of leukocytes from venous blood of tuberculin-positive patients into tuberculin-negative persons was reported by H. S. Lawrence (Bellevue), 1949. The problem of antibodies involved in tuberculin sensitivity (an antibody of an especial sort may be concerned, Chase, 1952) was approached by studies of lymphocytes, based upon the role claimed for these cells in antibody production, by Favour who with Miller, 1951, reported dissolution of lymphocytes in the blood of tuberculous animals and man *in vitro* following addition of tuberculin and complement. Further, a "factor" released from tuberculin-sensitive lymphocytes apparently confers on normal plasma, in the presence of tuberculin and complement, ability to cause dissolution of normal lymphocytes. Favour speculated that loss of hypersensitivity in tuberculosis could be explained by loss of effective lymphocytes from the blood stream; the effect of cortisone and ACTH, known to cause lysis of lymphocytes, might also be explained by this phenomenon. These studies are among many indications that the controversy concerning the relation between allergy and immunity in tuberculosis is leading to investigation of fundamental mechanisms.

These mechanisms and their interrelations are important in view of the world-wide programs of *BCG vaccination* now under way. By May, 1951, over thirty-seven million persons had been tuberculin-tested and over sixteen million vaccinated with BCG under the auspices of the World Health Organization. Anderson and Palmer of the

Public Health Service stated the view, 1950, that the adoption of BCG programs in countries unable to employ the usual control measures, while understandable, is not based upon "any recent demonstration of the vaccine's value in the prevention of tuberculosis". Neither research nor clinical experience has resolved the controversy. The unsolved problems include: the actual character of the vaccine including the number of viable organisms in it and their survival rate; standards for selection of persons eligible for vaccination which depend, by present methods, upon arbitrary criteria of tuberculin reactivity; standards of successful vaccination which rest upon the unknown relationship between allergy and immunity in tuberculosis; the duration of tuberculin sensitivity produced by vaccination and its significance; clinical effectiveness of vaccination as judged by statistics of incidence and mortality. In many parts of the world, effectiveness of vaccination is judged by the duration of hypersensitivity as measured by the tuberculin test, but Rich pointed out, 1951, that whereas hypersensitivity and acquired resistance ordinarily develop together, the two states are not necessarily parallel in duration and degree. The division of tuberculosis, recognizing the need "to prove, before it is too late", just what BCG vaccine could do in the population, organized three large evaluation programs and stressed the need of further fundamental research. Dubos and his associates, 1950, who discussed the application of their experimental analysis of virulence of tubercle bacilli to problems of BCG immunization, pointed out that the immunizing effect of BCG vaccination depends upon a certain degree of multiplication of the attenuated bacilli in the vaccinated host. This *in vivo* multiplication has been found by them to be conditioned by a number of independent factors, including: the receptivity of the host, which may be influenced by malnutrition or toxic factors; the number of living bacilli injected; the intrinsic virulence of the BCG culture. Standardization of BCG vaccination was concluded to require control of the "enormous differences" found in various vaccines in the content of living cells and in the biological characteristics of those isolated. At a 1948 seminar on BCG, Sweany of the Chicago Municipal Tuberculosis Sanitarium mentioned as shortcomings of vaccination with living cultures: "the dangers of contamination or mixing cultures with virulent strains, the difficulty of applying it to great masses of people, the false security that may be engendered by its use", and its failure to afford the complete protection that smallpox vaccination insures. Attempts to develop an immunizing vaccine prepared with killed bacilli were reported, 1947, by workers at the National Institutes of Health who used a newly-developed apparatus for the ultraviolet irradiation of bacteria in masses. Birkhaug, now working at the laboratories of the New York state health department, reported, 1951, that one-year-old vaccines, either dry glucose BCG or frozen glucose BCG, were as good antigenically, i.e., produced as many positive tuberculin tests, as fresh living vaccine which maintains its antigenic activity unchanged for only ten days.

The value of BCG as a research tool for study of factors influencing susceptibility and resistance is beginning to emerge in planned studies of familial variations in acquired hypersensitivity (C. E. Palmer and S. N. Meyer, Public Health Service, 1951), of possible effects of climate, sunlight on persistence of hypersensitivity (J. D. Aronson, University of Pennsylvania and Office of Indian Affairs, 1951).

The present picture of the tuberculosis problem registers confusion as well as progress. Mass X-ray surveys organized with the desirable aim of discovering every early case continually raise new problems concerning care and treatment of the discovered cases. Traditional therapies are increasingly subjected to sterner challenge; the sanatorium, for instance, has been described by some students of the problem as already outmoded in that new therapies require the equipment and services of the large general hospital. Dubos suggested, 1951, that we are probably "reaching the point of diminishing return in what can be expected from application of knowledge". This makes more than ever urgent the pursuit of fundamental knowledge of tuberculosis and its epidemiology, guided constantly by new concepts and new points of view, including bold recognition of the value of unorthodox approaches.

CHAPTER 8

# The Nature of Viruses
# and of Virus Diseases

*Illustrating metabolic interaction of*
*invading agent and invaded host*

# INTRODUCTORY

The observations that follow, ranging far over the virus field, have only one, and a limited, purpose — to throw light on the nature of viruses generally by collating concrete findings in investigative work on individual viruses for whatever generalized value these may suggest. It is likely to be a long time before simple generalizations on viruses as a whole can be justified. The virus field is unevenly developed; there are still viruses or suspected viruses about which practically nothing is known, and there is doubt of the adequacy of presently available principles of virus classification. As competent studies of individual viruses and virus infections increase in number and in depth, they will become the constituents of that generalized and ordered knowledge of viruses that will some day be arrived at. This was the animating principle on which the 1950 international congress of microbiology appointed five expert study teams, each to study a different group of viruses in an attempt to discover or uncover general principles that might justify classification in the near future of at least the better known viruses. Meanwhile, at the risk of seeming to group entities not in all ways coordinate, of comparing things only distantly comparable, the present discussion has brought together findings, observations, even speculations, stimulated by fundamental work on individual viruses when they seem to furnish leads toward that basic knowledge which may some day provide the biological key to viruses of plants, animals, man, regarded not merely as pathogenic organisms responsible for some of the most troublesome human diseases but also as strategic structures in the biological hierarchy.

## Multiple Disciplines Involved in Virus Research

In outstanding centers of virus research throughout the world — the Rockefeller Institute for Medical Research, the International Health Division of the Rockefeller Foundation, various divisions of the United States Public Health Service, the National Institute for Medical Research in England, the Pasteur Institute in Paris, the Walter and Eliza Hall Institute for Medical Research in Australia, university centers in many countries — virus workers include zoologists, botanists concerned with problems of the cell and genetics, plant and animal physiologists and pathologists, chemists, physicists and physical chemists working in biology and medicine; among medical men, specialists in internal medicine, pediatrics, bacteriology, pathology, public health. Some years ago, W. M. Stanley, in a Harvey lecture, suggested that the chemical concept of a virus as a nucleoprotein molecule interests pathologists as a cause of disease; bacteriologists because viruses possess properties that have long been regarded as characterizing living organisms; chemists because viruses have properties that have not hitherto been ascribed to molecules; physicists because of the properties of viruses as macromolecules and because some virus nucleoproteins show the layering phenomenon that has been called a new property of matter; biologists because viruses seem to have properties characteristic of both living and nonliving things; geneticists because viruses in some respects appear to parallel genes; philosophers because viruses, in their postulated borderland relation to the living and the nonliving, involve the perennial question, "What is life?"

The complex and individual nature of viruses has been stressed by the fact that the brilliant results obtained in therapy of certain bacterial and protozoan diseases by chemical agents and antibiotics has not been paralleled in treatment of viral diseases. The difference in response may be attributable (Thomas M. Rivers, 1952) to fundamental differences in the nature and metabolic activities of the two groups. In contrast to bacteria which are in most instances killed by adequate concentrations of therapeutic substances, viruses are themselves not inactivated or injured, as shown in work on the chemotherapy of experimental viral diseases, by such substances: all that happens is that further multiplication ceases. Death of bacteria is attributed to interference with certain of their enzyme systems or metabolic processes; as intracellular parasites, viruses are believed not to possess complete enzyme systems essential for multiplication. "If this is true, then such systems are supplied wholly or in part by their host cells and therapeutic agents can have no direct, deleterious effect on them through disruption of such systems. Nevertheless, their activities can be interfered with and their multiplication inhibited indirectly through the action of therapeutic agents which disturb enzyme systems and metabolic processes of their host cells." Hope of combating virus diseases continues to lie less in the direction of chemotherapy than of vaccination.

FACTORS THAT INHIBIT AND FACTORS THAT ADVANCE VIRUS RESEARCH

The always difficult question as to how far experimental results are applicable to human disease has outstanding current pertinence in virus investigation. Stanley, 1941, expressed the view that there is no fundamental difference in virus properties and that the chemical properties of plant viruses are, therefore, pertinent in the study of animal viruses. In the other direction, Thomas Francis, Jr., while conceding, 1947, that virus diseases of plants present "many interesting aspects", felt that the reported absence of antibodies, the limited conditions under which infection can be instituted and other features of plant virus diseases, far from being helpful, might even be confusing factors in interpreting human virus disease. Frank L. Horsfall, Jr., of the Rockefeller Institute, observed, 1952, that, in spite of the absence of antibodies in plants, the mechanisms of infection and of recovery from viruses in plants and in animals (but not in bacteria) appear to be so similar that in all probability "the underlying mechanisms may not be dissimilar". C. H. Andrewes of the National Institute for Medical Research described similarities between the animal, plant and bacterial viruses as "so striking that I cannot but believe that they are creatures of the same nature". N. W. Pirie observed, 1946, that before significance is attached to differences between plant and animal viruses it should be borne in mind that a properly representative sampling of either group has not yet been studied: selection of plant viruses for study has been governed by economic considerations, selection of animal viruses largely by pathological considerations, in particular hope of developing prophylactic vaccines. In applying to man the results of experimental work with animals, there is obvious need to bear in mind possible qualifying factors, for instance, how different portals and routes may vary susceptibility in certain species and how much error might result from concluding that, because a monkey from India had been shown to contract poliomyelitis after the virus was sprayed into its nose, the "human animal" develops the disease by passage of the virus through the nose and by that method alone. On the other hand it remains true that ability to reproduce in primates most of the aspects of human poliomyelitis with a high degree of fidelity (Bodian, 1952) made possible much of present knowledge of the pathogenic mechanisms of poliomyelitis and current tests of poliomyelitis vaccines in man.

For some viruses there is still no satisfactory experimental animal. Efforts to find it for given viruses have resulted in many failures and also in progressive successes. A decade ago workers realized the unsatisfactoriness for influenza study of the hamster and the ferret (expensive, difficult to handle, highly susceptible to infection with distemper virus) and the advantage of mice and chick embryo. Experimental study of poliomyelitis virus was advanced by Charles Armstrong's success (Public Health Service, 1939) in adapting the Lansing strain of human poliomyelitis virus, pathogenic for monkeys, to cotton rats and mice, making it possible for a number of laboratories without funds or facilities for maintaining monkeys to engage in studies of rodent-adapted poliomyelitis virus. Use of the fertile hen's egg and various tissues of the chick embryo for isolation and cultivation of an increasing number of viruses steadily expands virus research and reduces its cost by lessening the need for animal colonies. This "experimental animal" has proved a source of materials for large scale production of vaccines (for seventeen virus infections by 1952), has facilitated diagnosis of several virus infections (influenza, mumps) by making possible direct inoculation with infectious material, has served for testing the efficacy of chemotherapeutic agents.

Impetus was given to research in laboratory, clinic and field on certain poliomyelitis problems, notably the problem of producing sufficiently large amounts of the virus for vaccines, by propagation in test tubes of the three known serological types of poliomyelitis by tissue culture methods, 1949, by John F. Enders, Thomas H. Weller, Frederick Robbins, of Harvard. A killed virus vaccine, development of which (by Jonas E. Salk and associates, University of Pittsburgh) was made possible by this propagation had, by the summer of 1954, been tested for protective power in almost a half million children. Tests in animals and human volunteers of nonvirulent variants of existing viruses, developed in the hope of achieving a living virus vaccine for oral administration, were, 1954, reported by several laboratories. As a result of replacement of animals by tissue culture cells, the kidney tissues of a single monkey (costing $35, in 1954) formerly required to demonstrate, by inoculation of the animal, existence of the disease in one case, provided, 1954, tissue culture cells sufficient for 3,000 diagnostic tests or for three injections of vaccine for a thousand persons. Perhaps the most important result of the success of tissue culture propagation of large amounts of the virus has been the impetus to research in unexplored areas with application of newer techniques to study of other animal and human viruses. Study of the behavior of poliomyelitis viruses in tissue culture had led by 1953 to possibilities of critical investigations of the host-virus system comparable to those carried on with bacterial viruses. Maintenance of single virus particles and their progeny led to hope of further genetic studies with animal viruses, of study of biosynthesis of animal viruses and the metabolism of virus infected cells, of variations in behavior of different strains of the same virus.

Cultivation of a virus, however, represents only one stage in making the virus available to investigators. Methods have still to be developed for separating it from tissues and fluids without loss of virus activity, without admitting contaminants and, if the objective is a virus for use in vaccine, without loss of antigenicity. So long as few viruses are available in comparatively pure form, as now, the nature of a virus must be studied largely through study of its effects. This limitation conditions the tempo of advances. Isolation by Stanley of a chemical fraction from plants with tobacco mosaic disease, its purification and characterization, the demonstration that virus infectivity is associated with the nucleoprotein particle have proved a great stimulus to chemical work on the nature of viruses, leading to the first attempt to classify plant viruses on a systematic basis related to their chemical and serological properties. Nevertheless only twenty of the approximately 200 known plant viruses had, according to Pirie, been so studied up to 1946.

Efforts to facilitate study of virus properties have led to progressive improvement, since 1930, of serological methods for identification of viruses and to application to viruses of chemical and physical techniques for determination of purity of proteins, as chromatography, counter-current distribution, diffusion, sedimentation, electrophoresis, ultrafiltration, high speed centrifugation. Within the past ten years the electron microscope (which can project sharp images of objects so small as one ten-millionth of an inch) has made it possible to recognize certain characteristic molecular changes in cells attacked by viruses. Although biochemical reactions cannot be observed (since the necessary high vacuum in the electron microscope makes it impossible as yet to use living cells), R. W. G. Wyckoff considered that it would some day be "entirely feasible" to observe these reactions. Important advances in the electron microscopy of viruses (Backus and Williams, 1949; Porter and associates, 1947 and 1948) were cited, 1952, by Stanley and Lauffer as reasons why not only the larger but also many other viruses not yet examined by means of the electron microscope should now be studied in both purified and unpurified form. Light on the basic problem of virus multiplication within the host cell is expected from use of stable and radioactive markers in virus research, to determine whether tagged substances in injected viruses appear in newly formed virus (C. A. Knight at the Rockefeller Institute, 1948; Kozloff, Putnam and associates, 1950 and 1951, in work with bacteriophage).

## SCOPE OF THE VIRUS PROBLEM IN BIOLOGY AND MEDICINE

The difficulties of conveying the scope of the swiftly moving virus problem are obvious: only sixty years ago viruses were unknown; by 1950, five of the seventeen leading communicable diseases reported weekly by the National Office of Vital Statistics were known to be virus diseases. New viruses are still, as Peyton Rous once put it,

to be found for the looking. "It is no exaggeration," according to
the president of the Rockefeller Foundation, 1949 (in referring to
eighteen "new" tropical viruses discovered accidentally in the course
of tests for yellow fever), "to say that virology stands today about
where bacteriology stood in the early 1900's". Rivers's comparison,
a decade ago, of the realm of viruses and virus diseases with a boom
town is still pertinent. Not only is the number of viruses multiplying
with boom town rapidity but also, just as construction in such a town
is on various levels, so degrees of knowledge of the various viruses are
still notably uneven. The unevenness bears little relation to whether
the given virus is old or new or to the volume or the intensity of the
investigative work upon it. The history of poliomyelitis research over
a half century aptly illustrates the fact that every progressive achievement further complicates the problem. The profound changes in
conception that have followed successive gains in knowledge of poliomyelitis were set forth by Paul, 1952: "A disease, originally regarded
as limited to infants, is no longer confined to infancy; a disease originally considered mildly contagious is now regarded as almost as
contagious as measles; a disease in which the clinical picture was originally thought to be limited to acute paralysis is now regarded as a
disease in which only one in a hundred or more of those infected
become paralyzed and, when the Lansing strain is involved, perhaps
one in a thousand; from an endemic disease it has tended to become
epidemic; from a curiosity it has become a common and periodic
scourge." In spite of many advances since Rous, a decade ago,
closed the Messenger lectures at Cornell "on a note of uncertainty",
the state of scientific thought concerning the viruses in general still
largely reflects the "uncertainties" he reviewed: "The natural scope of
these agents has still to be mapped, though it is realized that they
may exist wherever life does and that they do strange things to this
life, which in turn can influence them, altering their capability. No-
body can yet say whether they constitute a biological group or merely
have in common a few physical attributes, small size in special. Their
primary source is not known nor the character of most of them. It
seems likely that some of them exist habitually in a harmless association with cells; perhaps some even aid in the functional activities of
living things."

While measurement of the scope of the problem in terms of numbers of viruses has admittedly only temporary validity, the figures are suggestive: of plant viruses there were (Holmes, 1948) 139 recognized types with hundreds of strains of some of these, as approximately 400 for tobacco mosaic (Kunkel, 1947); twenty-eight bacterial viruses have been recognized, with many strains; approximately a hundred virus diseases of insects (Steinhaus, 1953); several hundred animal viruses. As to the number that attack man, Horsfall, 1949, mentioned "at least forty"; Henry Pinkerton, 1952, raised to "about sixty" human diseases "of proved or strongly suspected viral etiology". A virus investigator once referred to the tendency, throughout the years, to toss into the "virus wastebasket" conditions of uncertain etiology, to be sorted out or retained with advancing knowledge. Illustrative of conditions removed in comparatively recent years from the "wastebasket" are whooping cough, and diseases due to pleuro-pneumonia-like organisms. In some quarters the view is entertained that the psittacosis-granuloma group should also be removed and considered intermediate between rickettsia and virus, or even in some views (Rake, 1953) as belonging with rickettsia. Pretibial or Fort Bragg fever, tossed into the wastebasket during the war, was removed by 1952 on identification of the leptospiral organism. In the rapidly changing virus world, the above totals have little significance; the cumulative picture of the scope of the virus problem derives rather from the emerging truths and/or hypotheses toward which investigative work on single viruses points at this time.

## RANGE OF THE ENCEPHALITIDES

The list of viruses roughly grouped together because they cause encephalitis in man and animals has grown steadily since 1930. Among the newcomers is "Murray Valley encephalitis" recovered by F. M. Burnet from a 1951 outbreak (thirty-nine cases, ten deaths) in Australia and thought to have an animal reservoir since horses and dogs were found naturally infected. Among the encephalitides three broad groups have been loosely distinguished by various workers: primary encephalitides, those having primary affinity for the central nervous system, especially those assuming epidemic proportions; secondary encephalitides, considered to include those caused by or associated with viruses not ordinarily considered encephalitogenic but in which a virus may be recovered; postvaccinal or postinfection encephalitides (following infection by viruses not ordinarily encephalitogenic), from which the primary virus is not ordinarily recoverable (for which reason viral etiology remains in doubt).

The agents of the primary encephalitides, commonly grouped in this country as epidemic, acute infectious, arthropod-borne, include viruses isolated during epidemics of St. Louis encephalitis (1933), Japanese B encephalitis (1936), Russian Far Eastern (1937), equine encephalomyelitis in eastern United States (1933 from horses, 1938 from man), in western United States (1931 from horses, 1938 from man) and Venezuelan equine encephalitis (1938 from animals, 1943 from man); viruses primarily encephalitogenic but not epidemic, as lymphocytic choriomeningitis, endemic in lower animals, especially mice, louping ill, a natural disease of sheep, capable of causing a mild nonfatal encephalitis in man. In this list perhaps belongs B virus of which there are only four known cases, all fatal, since Sabin and Wright first isolated the virus, 1934, from a fatal infection following a monkey's bite. Estimations of the incidence of the various encephalitides, except in widespread epidemics in which a coherent clinical picture or isolation of the virus provides a basis of conclusions, are difficult because smaller outbreaks or scattered individual cases are frequently associated with a number of viruses having interrelations not yet clarified. The clinical resemblance among the encephalitides is great, and pathological and epidemiological similarities are sometimes sufficiently marked (as between St. Louis encephalitis and western equine encephalomyelitis) to cast doubt on figures primarily dependent on the clinical signs. In any case, the geographic distribution of the various epidemic encephalitides is now known to go beyond the boundaries of the areas that originally furnished their names, eastern, western, St. Louis, Japanese, Russian, Venezuelan, West Nile. A 1951 release from the National Office of Vital Statistics, in noting an increase in encephalitis cases from 575 in 1948 to 1,651 in 1950, implied that the figures might be too low in any case since "many thousands are believed to have gone unrecognized or to have been erroneously diagnosed as poliomyelitis". Incidence in epidemic years has been higher. In the first serious St. Louis epidemic, 1933, 1,130 cases were reported in all ages with highest incidence in those over forty-five; the case fatality was reported by W. McD. Hammon, 1945, to range from five to thirty per cent. In the thirty-eight human cases in the 1938 epidemic of eastern equine encephalomyelitis in Massachusetts (in which 200 horses died), twenty-five deaths occurred, chiefly in children ten years old and younger. In an explosive 1947 epidemic in Louisiana ninety per cent of the 14,000 horses afflicted died; of fifteen persons that contracted the disease, nine died. Experience has indicated, according to K. F. Meyer and B. Eddie, 1947, that morbidity due to both the eastern and western equine viruses is highest in children under five years in whom the permanent effects (spastic paralysis, deformities, idiocy) were described by Hammon and Gordon Meiklejohn, 1942, as "fearful". High incidence of western equine encephalomyelitis in epidemics in Manitoba (1941) and in the San Joaquin Valley, California, was observed in infants although P. K. Olitsky and J. Casals, 1952, described this virus as attacking chiefly adult males that work out of doors. Mortality rates for western are similar to those for eastern equine encephalomyelitis, from seven to twenty per cent. Olitsky and Casals described Russian Far East encephalitis as appearing most frequently in May and June among forest workers in lumber camps and villages, rarely in children under five. Japanese B encephalitis (July, August) caused thirteen epidemics in Japan between 1871 and 1929, the most serious in 1924 with 6,000 cases and sixty per cent mortality. A research project on this virus has been conducted in Japan under the United States Army. Hullinghorst, Burns, Whatley (United States Army) and Young Tai Choi (chief, Bureau of Preventive Medicine, Seoul, Korea) reported, 1951, an epidemic of Japanese B encephalitis during the summer of 1949 in Korea.

Encephalitis lethargica (von Economo's disease, sleeping sickness, type A encephalitis), regarded as a primary encephalitis, appeared in epidemic form throughout the world between 1915 and 1925 (and, according to Josephine Neal, 1942, in this country in New York City, Iowa, and West Virginia, in 1918); epidemic outbreaks have, for some unknown reason, ceased since 1926, and only occasional single cases are now reported. Since a causative agent has never been isolated, opinion differs as to whether this encephalitis is to be attributed to a virus at all and whether, if it is, the virus is specific to this condition.

Of potential significance for human encephalitis because they have been demonstrated to be neurotropic in laboratory animals, because antibodies against some of them have been found in man and because at least two of these viruses, West Nile and Bwamba fever viruses, have been recovered from the blood of man, are six of the previously mentioned eighteen tropical viruses collected from East African and South American yellow fever laboratories between 1937 and 1949. One virus (Mengo) has been recovered from mosquitoes, from one monkey, one human; three (Semliki Forest virus, 1944; Bunyamwera virus, 1946; and Ilhéus virus, 1944) had been recovered up to 1949 only from mosquitoes, as have also four others isolated, 1944, from mosquitoes in South America and shown to be encephalitogenic in experimental animals, and the California (Hammon-Reeves) virus (found, however, only three times in two species of mosquitoes).

Secondary encephalitis has been reported following or in association with such ordinarily nonencephalitogenic viruses as herpes simplex, lymphogranuloma venereum, mumps, measles. Casals and Olitsky, 1952, distinguished this group from postinfection (and postvaccinal) encephalitis not only because the virus is ordinarily not recoverable from the latter group but also because of the difference in basic pathology, that of the first group being primarily that of the virus implicated; the dominant pathology of postinfection encephalitis (which may appear during convalescence from nonviral infections also but which has been more frequently reported after such viral infections as measles, influenza, vaccinia, mumps, varicella, variola, infectious hepatitis, dengue, yellow fever) is perivascular demyelination. In reviewing five of the theories that have been advanced to explain postinfection encephalitis, these authors, 1952, after noting that this encephalitis has not been transmitted to experimental animals, considered it "safe to say that no one has definitely shown the direct action of a virus to be the cause of postinfection encephalitis". Dependable incidence figures are not available for postinfection or postvaccinal encephalitis.

Because of their encephalitic manifestations and pathology, rabies and poliomyelitis are sometimes included by those attempting a comprehensive picture of viruses that produce encephalitic symptoms. Among recently recognized encephalitogenic viruses is encephalomyocarditis. In the lengthening list of infections with encephalitic manifestations in which virus etiology is suspected is infectious polyneuritis.

## SIGNIFICANCE OF POLIOMYELITIS IN THE VIRUS FIELD

Poliomyelitis and measles were the only two communicable diseases to reach epidemic proportions throughout the nation between January 1948 and July 1949. Whether increase in poliomyelitis cases in recent years is an actual increase or rather the result of better reporting, or of including other viruses simulating poliomyelitis, is not conclusively known. Prevailing opinion supports the view that the rise is real.

After sixty years of experiment and discussion, we still do not know (National Foundation for Infantile Paralysis, 1947) "where the virus causing it comes from, how it enters the human body, what is its course once inside an individual, how it grows and affects nervous tissue". Conclusive answers to these questions were still not available in 1954. Over the years various attempts at informal classification of the poliomyelitis viruses have raised many questions, as, recently, whether with the group of viruses causing human poliomyelitis should be included certain viruses that produce some poliomyelitis-like effects (as Theiler's encephalomyelitis of mice, the recently discovered Teschen virus of swine still imperfectly known), rodent strains, as the Columbia-SK and M viruses of C. W. Jungeblut, and other neurotropic viruses. The National Foundation for Infantile Paralysis, through its 1951 committee on typing, decided that on the basis of definitions set forth by the foundation's 1948 committee on nomenclature there are three immunologically distinct types of poliomyelitis virus, Brunhilde, Lansing, Leon, presumably "world-wide in distribution" (H. A. Howe, 1952).

## MEASLES — THE COMMONEST OF EPIDEMIC VIRUSES

The other major threat among epidemic virus diseases especially affecting children, measles, was described by Rake, 1952, as endemic in all large communities, major epidemics appearing at about three-year intervals. For one week in 1951 the National Office of Vital Statistics cited 23,253 cases of measles reported in the United States as against seventy-one cases of poliomyelitis, 2,140 cases of scarlet fever, 1,454 cases of whooping cough. According to Rake, by the age of twenty approximately eighty-five per cent of persons in civilized countries have had the disease. Mortality differs greatly as between ordinary and epidemic years; the number of deaths (472) reported in an epidemic year, 1948, in the United States was almost double the number in 1947.

## Smallpox Exemplifying a Measurably Controlled Virus

It has been a truism in virus comment that the discovery of Jennerian vaccination in expediting control stymied research on the variola virus. Metropolitan Life Insurance Company statistics, 1948, described smallpox as rapidly approaching extinction in the United States, the number of cases dropping from 110,000 in 1921 to 378 in 1944, to thirteen in 1951. There have been, however, reminders sufficiently recent that actual conquest on a world-wide basis has not been consummated: reporters to the *Lancet*, 1951, including a member of the department of infectious diseases, University of Glasgow, described an outbreak of smallpox in Glasgow in March, 1950; A. W. Downie (University of Liverpool), 1951, described a recent outbreak of smallpox in the Brighton area (132 cases, no reported deaths, between December, 1951 and April, 1952) as "another reminder of the continuing hazard of the introduction of virulent smallpox into this country from parts of the world where it is endemic". An inland outbreak in England of alastrim (described as a mild but highly infectious disease, sometimes indistinguishable from mild or modified smallpox) was reported, 1952, to be apparently traceable to raw materials from parts of the world where alastrim smoulders persistently. Smallpox is a continuing Middle East problem and a release from our National Office of Vital Statistics, March, 1951, noted it as "presently occurring in epidemic form in Burma and India". The high mortality rate justifies fear of even small outbreaks.

## The Influenza Viruses

Horsfall once observed that the name influenza, suggesting the influence of the stars, would better be retained until we know more about the virus that is responsible for human influenza. There have now been many advances, some of them at least pointing to the possibility of ultimate control. Influenza occurs in three manifestations, endemic, epidemic, pandemic. Of influenza pandemics, the worst was that of 1918 in which it has been estimated that twenty millions died, 400,000 in the United States. Most of the investigative work on influenza has been done on epidemic influenza (chiefly on influenza A, isolated by Smith, Andrewes and Laidlaw in England in 1933 following the first isolation of an influenza virus of swine by R. E. Shope in 1931; influenza B, isolated in this country by Francis and by T. P. Magill, 1940). A third serologic type, influenza C, was isolated by R. M. Taylor, 1947, by Francis and his associates, 1950. The apparition of antigenically different strains has been a confusing factor in attempts to develop effective prophylactic vaccination, although a vaccine containing three strains of two types (A and B) now has widespread use in the United States.

Observations of various workers over the last two decades indicate cyclical recurrence of influenza A every two or three years, of influenza B every four or five years. Epidemics of influenza (in general of mild character) were practically world-wide in 1950–51. While epidemic influenza is not comparable to pandemic in gravity or in mortality, it is responsible for a great deal of temporary incapacity in the whole population and tremendous absenteeism in industry. Mortality in epidemic influenza is rather generally referred to fellow-traveling pneumococci, streptococci, staphylococci.

Certain of the theories advanced to explain the pandemic of 1918 pose interesting questions concerning the true relation of endemic, epidemic and pandemic manifestations, and other fundamental unsolved aspects of influenza viruses, including the relation between human and animal strains. The appearance of the new epizootic disease of swine in October, 1918, and the similarity between its pathological manifestations and those of the human influenza epidemic just getting under way led Shope (1936) to views shared by many veterinarians and farmers that swine might have been infected, in the first instance, from man, although no virus from either disease had been identified at that time. The beginning, 1933, of studies of a virus-like agent isolated from human influenza cases led to Laidlaw's 1935 suggestion, which Shope thought reasonable, "that swine influenza virus represents a surviving form of that pandemic in man in 1918"; that is, the same virus may be a surviving form of an extinct or temporarily quiescent human influenza virus.  Both may be diseases of complex etiology involving both virus and some indispensable bacterial agent. The reverse possibility — that human infections have arisen from a swine host — was left open by Francis, Quilligan and Minuse, 1949, who discovered antigenic resemblances between a swine strain isolated in Korea and human strains such as the A-prime group first encountered in human disease in 1947.  Various workers since 1936 have mentioned the possibility that antibodies to swine virus in human sera might be explained on the basis of the common antigen demonstrated for human and swine influenza strains.  The relation of strain variation to the severity of epidemic influenza has become a focus of international study.  Accumulated studies since 1935 (under the Army's Commission on Influenza, the work of which is now integrated in an international program under the World Health Organization) of national and international centers that are collecting and comparing strains may enable investigators to put together knowledge concerning the appearance of certain strains, at different times and different places throughout the world, in small but periodic epidemics of varying virulence, and to arrive at an explanation of pandemics as a mounting wave of these epidemics.  Somewhat challenging a tendency to consider sporadic, endemic, epidemic and pandemic influenza "as different diseases presenting somewhat similar clinical syndromes", Francis, 1950, observed that possibly "the same influenza virus may be encountered in any of these stages of distribution".  As supporting evidence he mentioned the sharply different manifestations of influenza A at various times: its world-wide distribution in 1936–37 in sharp and characteristic waves; its appearance only in isolated and limited minor flurries (sometimes in subclinical form) in the spring of 1943; its appearance in the autumn of that year as a widespread and abrupt epidemic.  Accumulated knowledge of small epidemics in various parts of the country has somewhat strengthened the concept of influenza as an endemic disease with epidemic peaks depending, in the view of Francis, 1950, less on the appearance of antigenically different strains than on variation of biological characteristics accounting for an agent's pathogenicity and virulence, which may or may not be associated with antigenic variation. Francis, Salk and Brace commented, 1946, on evidence tending to support "the concept of influenza B as a disease with widely varied epidemiologic appearances but one which behaves commonly as an endemic disease with epidemic peaks at intervals of four to five years". The Andrewes hypothesis of gradation of virulence of influenza virus from a basic virus adapted "to perpetuating itself as a latent infection" through seven mutant stages to virulent pandemic virus of the A type would, if proved, explain many difficulties: failure to find a virus between epidemics; occurrence in outbreaks of mixtures A, B and other viruses; variations in biologic properties of viruses isolated at different times; anomalies in the relation between antibody titer and active immunity.

## RELATION OF THE COMMON COLD TO THE TOTAL VIRUS PICTURE

Although up to 1953 a virus had not been isolated, chiefly because no susceptible animal had been found, the concept that the inciting agent of the common cold is a virus has had, according to Horsfall, "strong support" (Dochez, Kneeland and Mills, 1930–36; Andrewes and his associates of the Common Cold Research Unit, British Medical Research Council, 1946–53). Horsfall, 1952, estimated the incidence of the common cold, a condition of "reasonably well defined features", in the United States as approximately two to four attacks per person annually. Since these colds average about five days each, the American people suffer one and a half billion days of discomfort and reduced efficiency, if not of actual disability (1947 bulletin of the Metropolitan Life Insurance Company). Various studies suggest that from forty to fifty per cent of all days lost from work are attributable to colds; the announcement a few years ago of a drive sponsored by the American College of Chest Physicians and the American Association of Industrial Physicians and Surgeons for funds for research on the common cold indicated that it costs American industry "an estimated billion dollars annually".

## PRIMARY ATYPICAL PNEUMONIA

The chairman of the commission on acute respiratory diseases of the Army's Epidemiological Board, John H. Dingle, remarked,

1948, that primary atypical pneumonia has within the past ten years become the commonest form of pneumonia. Primary atypical pneumonia was described by Army sources, 1944, as one of the most important causes of man days lost from military duty. Hobart A. Reimann, 1950, referred to a once prevalent idea that increase in "virus pneumonia" of late years was due to decline of the bacterial pneumonias (a decline attributable largely to the sulfa drugs), unmasking the virus pneumonias by removing the bacterial superinfection. He did not, however, regard this as the true explanation of the increase in virus pneumonia, considering the increase to be real. "The epidemics of mild disease of the respiratory tract, of which virus pneumonias represented the severest forms as reported in 1938 and 1939, were forerunners of the pandemic of 1941–43. Pneumonia was present in ten per cent of such cases and outnumbered pneumococcic pneumonias in the proportion of four to one. Similar outbreaks have not occurred since then . . ." In addition to the epidemic forms, there occur "severe, sporadic, nonseasonal virus pneumonias. Whether the epidemic forms and the sporadic forms are etiologically the same still cannot be said since the cause of neither is known. Clinically they are identical." Frequently the extent of pulmonary involvement is revealed only by roentgenographic examination; because of this, earlier studies had related the disease largely to nose, pharynx and larynx, extending only occasionally to trachea, bronchi and, even more rarely, to bronchioles and lungs. Dingle, 1948, on the basis of experiments with human volunteers (Army commission on acute respiratory diseases) concluded that the disease is at least initiated by a filter-passing agent, presumably a virus. M. D. Eaton and his associates, then at the virus and rickettsial laboratory of the California health department, pointed out, 1944, that during the preceding five years primary atypical pneumonia had been ascribed to "at least eight separate and distinct infectious agents", including psittacosis (ornithosis), the rickettsia of Q fever, the virus of lymphocytic choriomeningitis, in all of which occur certain forms of pneumonia. Whether the infection is merely a syndrome definable in terms of clinical features or a specific disease entity attributable to one or more infectious agents remains to be established (Horsfall, 1952) since there is not as yet agreement among investigators as to the nature and

# 358     UNSOLVED CLINICAL PROBLEMS

identity of the causal agent. The mechanism of one of the diagnostic expedients (aside from X ray) in this condition, cold hemagglutinins, has been described as unknown (Peterson, Ham and Finland of Harvard, 1943); they and others have suggested that cold agglutination has occasionally been demonstrated in conditions unrelated to primary atypical pneumonia and may be "no more than a laboratory curiosity". Dingle, 1948, described diagnosis of primary atypical pneumonia as "still one of exclusion", adding that two laboratory tests that may be of "some help" are the cold hemagglutination test and the agglutination of streptococcus MG. If both of these tests are positive, there is a high probability that the diagnosis is correct but if both are negative "it may be very difficult to establish a diagnosis" (Horsfall, 1952).

## Mumps Virus — Still a Problem as to Tissue Specificity

Until recent years progress in the study of mumps was delayed by inability to cultivate the agent. Gordon of Harvard set forth, 1940, alternate conceptions prevailing at that time: mumps as (1) a primary local disease of the parotid gland; (2) a rather generalized systemic infection, the virus penetrating the blood stream and localizing in various glandular structures, especially the parotid; (3) a primary disease of the central nervous system, followed by secondary localization in salivary glands, pancreas and gonads. On no one of these concepts has general agreement yet been reached, in spite of considerable progress during the last few years in experimental work on cultivation of mumps, and in experimental trial of prophylactic vaccine. Enlargement of the parotid gland was described by Enders, 1952, as the most constant feature but "involvement of other organs is not uncommon". Increasing attention has been given in recent studies to the degree to which mumps virus attacks the central nervous system, even if it is, according to a 1946 Army group, "basically a systemic disease which has a special predilection for the salivary glands, mature gonads, pancreas and breasts".

## Herpes Simplex and Herpes Zoster

Herpes simplex virus, one of the commonest infectious agents of man, causes clinical conditions variously classified as diseases of skin, mucous membrane, eye, central nervous system. Characteristics of the virus include preference for tissues of the embryonic ectodermal layer, vesicle formation in the epithelial lesions from which intranuclear inclusion bodies have been isolated (Scott, 1952). The protean manifestations of herpes simplex infection range from the ordinary fever blister to acute inflammation of brain and meninges. Present concepts distinguish, without reference to site of infection, between primary herpetic infection (occurring in persons without neutralizing antibody), more common in the young than the old, usually associated with a systemic illness, often severe and sometimes fatal, and recurrent attacks (in persons who possess neutralizing antibody) without systemic symptoms however severe the lesions. The behavior of the virus somewhat accounts for Doerr's description fifteen years ago of herpes simplex as not an infection at all in the ordinary sense but rather "a queer physiological response of the cells concerned to the stimulus of fever and certain types of external irritation", and as rather a product of human cells than a descendant of pre-existing virus. Burnet found this view out of key with the Pasteurian doctrine, that all pathogenic microorganisms are descendants of similar organisms, but suggested that it might account for the way in which herpetic lesions appear, without infection from the environment; he advanced an hypothesis postulating infection in infancy, life-long carrying of herpes simplex, manifestations of which are evoked only by trigger mechanisms.

Herpes zoster ranges (*Lancet*, 1950) from a banal painless rash "calling for no treatment other than a shake lotion" to a gangrenous secondarily infected eruption with severe and persistent pain. Craver and Haagensen pointed out, nearly twenty years ago, that secondary or symptomatic herpes zoster has been caused by a variety of processes, may appear in the course of such common infectious diseases as varicella, pneumonia, influenza, diphtheria, meningitis and pulmonary tuberculosis, is not uncommon in the generalized stage of cancer and may accompany lymphosarcoma, Hodgkin's disease and the leukemias. In some such cases, clinical data suggested that herpes zoster might be due to involvement of nervous structures by tumor processes. Joseph Stokes, Jr., observed, 1952, that herpes zoster may be secondary to an insult to a susceptible dorsal nerve root and may accompany any one of numerous conditions.

## TRACHOMA AND INCLUSION CONJUNCTIVITIS

Trachoma is a problem of notably lesser proportions in this country than in the Near East, Africa and southern Europe. Phillips Thygeson pointed out, 1952, that while ninety per cent of the Egyptian population is affected, incidence in the American regions in which trachoma has been best known is decreasing rapidly. The "peculiar belt of incidence" in the United States, according to Julianelle's 1938 volume, runs through West Virginia, Kentucky, Tennessee, southern Illinois, Arkansas and Missouri, in which state Julianelle studied it intensively for a decade, and in which the Missouri Trachoma Hospital was still, 1952, assessing the relative therapeutic value of sulfonamides and antibiotics. The federal government has long supported investigative work on trachoma because of its incidence among Indians. Disposing of various theories that trachoma might be due to protozoon, fungus, bacterium, or to an agent intermediate between rickettsia and virus, Thygeson, 1952, while noting that the agent filters with difficulty, because of its large size, described it as a virus. He considered inclusion conjunctivitis and trachoma distinguishable by involvement, in trachoma, of the cornea in which it inevitably produces cicatrization, while inclusion conjunctivitis (a benign form of conjunctivitis in the newborn) never affects the cornea significantly and heals without scarring. Earlier work had pointed to a maternal genitourinary factor in the ocular inclusion blennorrhea of newborn infants. Such genitourinary aspects led Thygeson, in his earlier studies of it, to characterize as an "occupational disease" ocular infections in obstetricians and gynecologists. On the basis of size, susceptibility to chemotherapy, staining and morphologic characteristics, Thygeson, 1952, included trachoma and inclusion blennorrhea viruses with the "transitional group, midway between the typical large viruses and the rickettsia" (the lymphogranuloma-psittacosis group).

## "OLDER" VIRUSES NOT EXHAUSTIVELY INVESTIGATED

Among viruses on which, until recently, comparatively little work has been done in the United States is lymphogranuloma venereum or inguinale, described as a specific venereal disease affecting chiefly the lymphatic tissues of the iliac and inguinal regions and attributed to a virus. Investigative attempts in recent years, particularly in American laboratories, have been concerned with systemic effects, possibly hereditary aspects, improvement of diagnosis by complement-fixation, therapy with the sulfa drugs and with antibiotics, notably aureomycin and terramycin. The susceptibility of this virus to chemotherapy, its broad antigenic relations to the agents causing psittacosis and certain pneumonitis infections in animals have led to the suggestion (previously mentioned) to remove it with other large viruses from the virus wastebasket and place it, until more exact classification becomes possible, in a group intermediate between rickettsia and virus, or frankly with rickettsia (Rake, 1953).

Rubella or German measles is another virus on which, until recently, little work was done (partly because the disorder attributed to it had not been considered serious). Rake, 1952, observed, "apart from filterability, pointing to a virus, little is known about the causative agent". The report of the Massachusetts state health department covering the years from 1942 to 1949 observed: "This disease which tends to be quiescent for long periods of time reached epidemic proportions in 1943 for the first time since 1935. Two minor waves were observed in 1946 and 1949." Gregg's extensive studies in Australia, 1941, substantiated by Swan and his associates, 1943, and more recently by American workers, have centered interest on the part played by rubella in production of congenital malformations in children born of mothers that have had rubella in the early months of pregnancy. The congenital anomalies most frequently reported have been heart disease, cataracts, deafness and, more recently, malformed teeth, mental retardation, underdevelopment. According to Rake, 1952, the Australian surveys (1944, 1946, 1949) indicate that the percentage of serious defects ranges from eighty-three per cent following rubella in the first month of pregnancy to sixty-one per cent in the fourth month. American statistics suggest a defect rate of about fifty per cent following rubella in the first three months. Investigating the possibility of defects associated with other virus diseases during pregnancy, Michael Reese Hospital workers, 1953, found in 154 cases of virus diseases other than rubella during early pregnancy twenty-one per cent of anomalies not, however, following the rubella pattern. Twenty-six cases of congenital defects collected, 1943, by the American Academy of Pediatrics, summarized by M. H. Bass, 1952, included thirteen attributed to maternal infection with measles, mumps, chickenpox, infectious mononucleosis, poliomyelitis. Maternal rubella accounted for only seventeen among 1,366 cases of congenital heart disease studied by Stanley Gibson, 1953.

Among other viruses which are not new but on which little work has been done is molluscum contagiosum, the elementary bodies of which, however, have within recent years been studied in the electron microscope (by Yale workers, Melnick, Strauss and associates, 1949–51; by Rake and Blank, 1950).

## Viruses Restudied under War Stress — Sandfly Fever, Dengue, Hepatitis

Among viruses owing to war renascence of interest is the virus causing sandfly or pappataci fever, also known as phlebotomus. In early 1943, a commission was sent to North Africa to investigate this condition known (through transmission to human volunteers by Shortt, Poole, and Stephens, in India, 1934) to be caused by the bites of infected sandflies. According to Sabin, Philip and Paul, 1944, adult native populations in endemic zones are in general immune, but new populations, as troops moving in, are susceptible.

According to Sabin, 1952, some of the largest epidemics of dengue, a mosquito-transmitted virus, have occurred in the United States, Australia, Greece and Japan since 1920. He cited Chandler and Rice as estimating that between 500,000 and 600,000 cases occurred in Texas during the 1922 epidemic. In Sabin's view, the total number of cases in the Army during the last war was much larger than the 84,090 reported. Investigations thus stimulated by wartime hazards led to cultivation, purification, characterization of the agent and development of a dengue vaccine which Sabin and Schlesinger, 1945, found safe in tests with human volunteers but which they regarded, 1952, as still to be tested in epidemics.

Infectious hepatitis has had a long association with military history, "contagious jaundice" having been recorded as a scourge of Napoleon's armies, of the Union forces in the Civil War, and as a "regular camp follower" of the Allied armies in the Mediterranean campaigns of the last war.  W. Paul Havens, Jr., and John R. Paul, 1948, observed that in the absence of specific diagnostic tests its exact distribution and prevalence remain poorly defined.  Within recent years outbreaks have been reported in widely separated parts of the world.  The same workers, 1952, in noting that there are probably several forms of viral infections of the liver which are variants of one general group, named as the two major members of the group infectious hepatitis and serum hepatitis.  In 1945 the filterability of the agent causing infectious hepatitis was established, together with some of the characteristics of the agent, its transmissibility in a series to man. Continuing this work, Henle, Stokes and their associates, in Pennsylvania's pediatrics department, reported, 1950, cultivation of the agent in tissue culture and in the embryonated hen's egg, and production of the disease in human volunteers with the propagated agent. Havens and Paul, 1952, noted that of the numerous attempts since 1942 to induce the disease in various laboratory animals, some had failed, others had not been confirmed.  Serum hepatitis, they thought, could be described "arbitrarily" as a disease ordinarily produced by parenteral inoculation of human blood or its products obtained from persons carrying the causative filterable agent although not apparently ill.  They referred to "many thousands" of cases resulting from injections of human convalescent serum, vaccines containing human serum, plasma and, rarely, whole blood, containing the agent. While methods have been devised which "appear to be effective" for certain individual fractions (especially gamma globulin), "there is no practicable way to treat all products of human blood to render them safe".  Although clinically and pathologically the two kinds of hepatitis "are almost indistinguishable", certain differences (in incubation period, in experimental infection by the oral route, in duration of the blood-borne phase) have been observed, notably that the two viruses are immunologically distinct.

## AMONG THE NEWER VIRUSES

The lengthening list of newer viruses includes the eighteen tropical viruses isolated in the Rockefeller Foundation's South American and African laboratories in the course of routine tests of human serum, mosquitoes, monkeys, for detection of yellow fever virus. Another addition within the last decade is the agent of Colorado tick fever, at first regarded as rickettsial, later described as a tick-borne virus after the 1944 demonstration (by Florio and his associates) that filtered infectious substances could be serially transmitted in man and animals. Hilary Koprowski and Herald R. Cox (1946–47) adapted the virus to the mouse and chick embryo and have prepared an experimental vaccine which, in 1952, had been tested in twenty-four volunteers. One of the causative agents of epidemic viral gastroenteritis, a disease or, according to Joel Warren, 1952, a family of diseases of man, has been shown to be a virus (Irving Gordon and associates, 1949). Whether this infection is related to the more severe epidemic diarrhea of the newborn (from which two "presumably virus" agents have been isolated) had not been established, 1952.

New, at least to continental United States, is the agent causing epidemic keratoconjunctivitis, described as acute and highly contagious. A 1951 bulletin of the National Office of Vital Statistics estimated the total number of cases for all the Hawaiian Islands at from 5,000 to 6,000. Ten years earlier there had been various reports of epidemic outbreaks during the summer, first in Oahu, Hawaii, San Francisco, where chiefly shipyard workers were involved, later in Schenectady, Hartford, New York City.

The encephalomyocarditis virus is one of a group of four viruses isolated from the chimpanzee or monkey (encephalomyocarditis, Columbia–SK, Columbia–MM, Mengo encephalomyelitis) designated (by Warren, Smadel, Russ, 1949, in the Army graduate school's virus laboratory) as the encephalomyocarditis family because, according to the findings of the several laboratories concerned, they are immunologically indistinguishable. These workers regarded the four as probably different strains of a single virus with no relation to the Lansing, Yale-Sk and Brunhilde strains of poliomyelitis, or to strains of mouse encephalomyelitis virus. The 1949 report of the International Health Division stated as a prevailing opinion that this group "rarely infects man". The reported human infections (encephalomyocarditis and Mengo strains) have, according to Warren, 1952, in all instances occurred in close proximity to rodents which "probably serve as reservoirs" for all four viruses.

Also among new additions is the Coxsackie or C group of viruses, the first of which was isolated by G. Dalldorf and G. M. Sickles (division of laboratories, New York State health department) from the feces of two children with paralysis in the course of investigating 1948 poliomyelitis outbreaks in Coxsackie, New York. A similar but not identical strain (isolated, 1948, reported 1949) by Curnen, Shaw and Melnick (Yale medical school) was recovered from one boy with pleurodynia and from five patients with pleocytosis of the cerebrospinal fluid (but without paralysis) during the summer of 1948 when aseptic meningitis was prevalent in Connecticut and Rhode Island. Other strains were isolated later in other parts of the United States, and associated with three clinical entities: pleurodynia (or Bornholm disease), herpangina, aseptic meningitis. The Connecticut-5 type of C virus was identified as the cause of a Massachusetts outbreak of pleurodynia by Enders, Weller and their associates at Harvard, 1950. By 1952 the virus had been identified in Europe, Asia, Africa, Australia. J. L. Melnick, who, with his associates, classified over 160 strains into fifteen different immunologic types, considered, 1953, the virus global in distribution. He and E. C. Curnen, 1952, tentatively characterized the C viruses as a loosely assembled group causing "a variety of acute, self-limited diseases", and having in common certain biologic and physical properties but distinct antigenic differences and unusual pathogenicity for infant mice and hamsters. On the relation of the Coxsackie group to poliomyelitis virus with which the C group had at first been confused, Curnen and Melnick pointed out, 1952, lack of evidence "that poliomyelitis viruses are related to C viruses even when both are recovered from the same source".

## HYPOTHETICAL VIRUSES

It must be said at the outset that in connection with any condition of unknown etiology, virus origin may be, and usually has been, suggested, not merely as a guess but as an hypothesis explored by scientific techniques, as in the case of schizophrenia. The following illustrations represent only a few of the conditions as to which virus origin has been more tenaciously held or made the subject of more persistent work. The virus hypothesis in the etiology of rheumatic fever received no support in the "regularly reproducible" myocarditis that can be induced in mice by all four viruses of the EMC group (Columbia-SK, MM, Mengo encephalomyelitis, encephalomyocarditis). Smadel expressed the explicit view that the myocardial lesions produced in mice by the encephalomyocarditis virus were definitely "not the lesions of rheumatic fever". Based on experimental cardiac lesions produced by viruses, a virus theory of rheumatic heart disease is, however, still entertained by some workers. "In spite of evidence to the contrary", J. M. Pearce observed, 1950, "during the past several years it has been possible to show that a filtrable virus when introduced into the animal body by a peripheral route can specifically infect the heart and there produce anatomical lesions and functional derangement, that this ability is not the property of a single virus but is common to several, and finally that an important factor in inducing the cardiac localization of virus is decrease in the amount of oxygen supplied to the heart." He added that the similarity in morphology of the "pancarditis" that can be produced by experimental viral infection to human rheumatic heart disease and to other inflammations of unknown etiology "suggests again . . . that these lesions too may be of viral origin". In his view, failure of repeated attempts to recover a virus by means of animal inoculation from the tissues and fluids of individuals suffering from rheumatic fever "does not preclude the possibility of viral etiology".

Infectious polyneuritis could, in some views, be grouped with the encephalitides. It occurs after bacterial infections, after infections of unknown etiology involving the respiratory or intestinal tracts, and, according to Olitsky and Casals, 1952, occasionally without recognizable antecedent infection. Mortality rate is about twenty per cent and fatal cases in children have been wrongly diagnosed as poliomyelitis. Olitsky and Casals, 1952, described the agent as unknown, "perhaps a virus".

The same workers described infectious mononucleosis as "probably" caused by a virus; Rivers, 1952, characterized its etiology as "not definitely known, although a virus is suspected".

One phase of the ancient controversy as to whether Hodgkin's disease is neoplastic or infectious (before there was any general promotion of the idea that perhaps there is no fundamental antithesis in the two concepts) included the suggestion that Hodgkin's disease may be caused by a virus. Preliminary work on an active, ultra-filterable agent extracted from chest-fluid and lymphoid tissue of patients having Hodgkin's disease was reported to the Fourth International Cancer Research Congress, 1947, by C. G. Grand of the biology research laboratory at New York University. The University of California pathologist, Warren L. Bostick, enumerated, 1952, characteristics of Hodgkin's disease suggestive of virus infection, or at least consistent with it: "the state of relative anergy; the granulomatous type cellular reaction; the occurrence of morphologically acceptable inclusion bodies in the Reed-Sternberg cells; the high fever and cyclic behavior of the disease; and the tendency to attack relatively younger adults." He cited the failure of many efforts, his own with Hanna, 1951, and those of others, using a large variety of animals and "every conceivable route of administration", to produce Hodgkin's disease experimentally. Three groups of workers have however reported changes in cells growing in tissue culture upon exposure to cell-free and apparently bacteria-free fluids from Hodgkin's disease tissues. Reports that Hodgkin's disease material can interfere with growth of influenza virus and that hepatitis virus influences favorably the progress of the disease, suggesting virus factors, have not been confirmed. "What research for a virus in Hodgkin's disease has not yet done is to conclusively demonstrate that these agents are present only in Hodgkin's disease tissues, that they are demonstrable in every case of Hodgkin's disease, and that they are capable of producing the disease." That proof awaits production of the condition in an experimental animal.

Attitudes toward the moot question whether viruses may be a cause of human cancer or a factor contributing to it have changed radically since Peyton Rous's 1911 description of transmission of a chicken sarcoma by injection of cell-free filtrates of the tumor. Skepticism has been measurably replaced by what has been called a perfectly respectable speculation that "cancer may be caused by self-duplicating virus-like agents" (Henry Pinkerton, 1952). The list of bird and animal tumors from which transmissible agents with virus characteristics have been obtained includes: the chicken sarcoma of Rous; at least one type of fowl lymphomatosis (B. R. Burmester and others); the rabbit papilloma of Shope from which carcinomas develop under certain circumstances; mouse mammary carcinoma shown by J. J. Bittner to be transmitted by the milk agent, later isolated as a virus; kidney carcinoma in the leopard frog (Balduin Lucké); wound-tumor disease of plants (L. M. Black); various tumors of fish in which evidence is only circumstantial (R. F. Nigrelli); mouse leukemia (Ludwik Gross); a transmissible venereal tumor in dogs (A. G. Karlson and F. C. Mann); molluscum contagiosum and warts of human skin (Harvey Blank). In view of the gaps in knowledge of the action of viruses in tumor formation, Rous, a decade ago, discouraged extending the concept of virus causation to cancer generally. F. Duran-Reynals described, 1950, the virus theory of cancer as "intellectually satisfying" because properties of the filterable virus meet requirements of a cancer cause, i.e., cells are indispensable to viruses; cell growth may be stimulated along with virus infection; virus action is conditioned by the most varied stimuli and strict genetic background; viruses are highly tissue-specific and tumor-type-specific yet may induce lesions in other tissues; virus infections acquired at an early age may remain latent, becoming active in an adult or old host; and viruses may exist frankly or be masked, undetectable by ordinary means. Latency, variation and masking are among the attributes of known viruses that have been studied in relation to tumor agents. A phase of latency has been described in Rous sarcoma and mouse mammary cancer. Variation has been induced in the Rous chicken tumor virus by passage through other bird species. Masking has been studied intensively to explain the behavior of the Shope papilloma virus, which is recovered from papillomas in the natural host, the wild cottontail rabbit, but which apparently disappears and cannot be recovered from experimentally produced papillomas of domestic rabbits and in resulting cancers of domestic rabbits and wild hares. Presence of the virus has been inferred since Shope in 1933 showed that domestic rabbits bearing virus-induced papillomas from which the virus could not be recovered still developed neutralizing and complement-fixing antibodies against the virus, and were relatively resistant to reinfection. Many have pointed out, as Shope, 1950, that if the papilloma virus were unknown the etiology of these tumors, in which the virus is demonstrated by immunological means, would remain unknown; apparent absence of virus from the generality of cancers could, therefore, be explained by lack of an antigen for testing. Induction of neoplasms by injection (or, in the case of mouse mammary cancer, by nursing) of cell-free filtrates of tumors does not (C. P. Rhoads, 1952) prove viral origin. It does, however, establish the importance of "cellular components of less than cellular size". The concept of "the spectrum from plastid to plasmagene to virus" would explain much otherwise incomprehensible in cancer research; Pinkerton thought well-established the assumption that malignant cells "contain abnormal self-duplicating constituents of some type which are responsible for their continuous aggressive behavior". Some British workers agree with Gye's view, 1945, that autonomous growth is the central problem in neoplastic growth, and that, so far, only one agent, intrinsic and intracellular, capable of stimulating uncontrolled growth has been found, the cancer viruses.

## Viruses Studied Rather as Research Tools than as Agents of Disease — Vaccinia, Bacteriophage

While most of the information obtained from detailed study of vaccinia during the thirties (Craigie at the Connaught laboratories; Rivers, Hoagland and Smadel at the Rockefeller Institute) has been, as Burnet observed, 1945, "at the present time curiously irrelevant to human problems or to any understanding of the biological relationship of vaccinia to the natural pox diseases", the vaccinia work has nevertheless had distinct potential and actual bearing on the study of the nature of viruses generally. The physical and chemical characteristics of vaccinia are known with a fair degree of accuracy, and analyses have been made of its immunological behavior in experimental animals. (Since 1945, Downie's studies in England of the naturally-occurring cowpox has thrown new light on this virus.)

Work on bacterial viruses, bacteriophages, first described by Twort, 1915, d'Herelle, 1917, has been one avenue through which virus investigation has been carried to fundamental biological areas remote from the clinical field but involving mechanisms essential to understanding clinical virus disease. Intensive bacteriophage studies are being conducted in this country (M. Delbrück and R. Dulbecco at California Institute of Technology; E. A. Evans, Jr., L. M. Kozloff, F. W. Putnam, University of Chicago; S. E. Luria, University of Illinois; A. H. Doermann and A. D. Hershey, Carnegie Institution, Cold Spring Harbor; Philip B. Cowles, Yale; Seymour S. Cohen, University of Pennsylvania; Gunther Stent and Dean Fraser, University of California virus laboratory) and abroad (in France by André Lwoff, Pasteur Institute; and in England, Denmark, Sweden). Increasing work with bacteriophages is now less concerned with the hope of utilizing them therapeutically for destruction of certain bacteria than with discovering a model for virus-host relations. Delbrück, 1946, and others have described bacteriophages as experimentally the most accessible group for studying not only the relationship of virus with the cell host and virus reproduction but also the chemical composition of viruses, the phenomenon of virus interference, virus mutation and other fundamental virus problems. "In this perspective bacterial viruses may well come to occupy a key position in biology."

## SCOPE OF THE VIRUS PROBLEM CONVEYABLE ONLY IN FUNDAMENTAL BIOLOGICAL VALUES

From the foregoing review emerges the superficiality of any attempt to convey the scope of the virus problem in terms of increasing numbers of viruses or extent and epidemiology of virus diseases (even if the data on incidence and the reporting mechanisms were dependable). Theobald Smith's concept of infectious disease as a manifestation of parasitism has been described as broadening the explanation of infectious disease in man from a medical to a biological base. In Smith's concept, parasitism is a biological phenomenon, normal rather than pathological, a "compromise or truce between two living things accompanied by predatory processes whenever opportunity is offered one or the other party". The efficient parasite, Francis commented, 1952, is one that does not kill its source of maintenance or deplete it. The stepwise "work" of the efficient parasite involves gaining entrance to the host, reaching tissues in which it can establish a "suitable residence" in which to develop its capacity to infect, multiply, meet the defensive reactions marshalled by its host, find, in the event of the death of the host, a satisfactory portal of exit (as in respiratory or fecal excretion) since the materials and agencies involved in this escape represent the virus's resources for transmission to a new host, a critical step in the biological progression. In this progression the determining factor, the degree of adaptation between virus and host, involves many uncertainties: the virus may fail to adapt to the host at all; it may be modified by the host; it may settle down perhaps to living amicably with the host; or there may be a fight to the death. Smith pointed out that the degree of equilibrium accounts for the difference between endemic and epidemic disease, and that epidemics must be studied in terms of "host-parasite relationships and the environmental factors which modify them". Knowledge of these relationships and evaluation of these factors require background knowledge of plant and animal viruses, of reservoirs, intermediate hosts, the biological cycles that link virus diseases in animals to infection in man. Man may be the obligate host for a virus which depends on human cells for its propagation; he may be a principal host; or he may be only an occasional host, "an accidental interloper, as in rabies". For a rational explanation of the behavior of an infectious disease in human populations, it becomes requisite to understand the extent to which man is involved in the continuous propagation of the causative microparasite or shares this biological role with other species — animal, bird, or insect.

## ILLUSTRATIONS OF ANIMAL VIRUSES SIGNIFICANT IN HUMAN DISEASE

The social and economic cost to man of virus disease in animals and plants would justify a treatise on its own account. There is little need to demonstrate the economic loss caused by plant viruses that attack potatoes, beets, tomatoes, peas, peppers, spinach, wheat, clover, sugar cane, peaches, tobacco, cucumbers, etc.; or by animal viruses, causing loss of horses by equine encephalomyelitis, of fowl by Newcastle disease, of livestock by foot-and-mouth disease. Between 1946 and 1952, the United States spent approximately $123,000,000 for slaughter of infected animals in Mexico to prevent the spread of foot-and-mouth disease to the huge livestock population of the United States. In 1952 northern United States was threatened by epidemics in Canadian herds. Numerous outbreaks, 1951 and 1952, in England, Holland, France, Belgium, western Germany led to research in government laboratories in all these countries. Development of this theme, however, goes beyond the boundaries of this discussion. Concern here is with possibilities that animal viruses may be transmissible to man; and that animal viruses may adopt man as a permanent host. Up to the present not many animal viruses have been conclusively shown to be transmissible to man on a large scale. Included in the list of virus infections of animals to which man is susceptible, besides rabies, equine encephalomyelitis, foot-and-mouth disease (rarely transmitted to man), Newcastle disease of fowl, psittacosis are: lymphocytic choriomeningitis, louping ill, Rift Valley fever (reported in man only from Africa) cowpox, vesicular stomatitis of horses, ovine pustular dermatitis of sheep (three cases reported in 1946), infectious anemia of horses (rare in man). Mentioned also as known or suspected to be transmissible to man (naturally or experimentally) have been canine and ferret distemper, acute feline infectious agranulocytosis, mouse and fox encephalitis, swinepox, fowl leukosis, fowl laryngotracheitis, fowl coryza. As to many of these viruses, little is known, even of their extent among animals. It is known, however, that certain animal viruses that produce only subclinical infection in the original host are capable of setting up severe infections in man. The biological cycle is not necessarily from animal to man but may on rare occasions (W. A. Hagan, Cornell veterinary college, 1947) be from man to animals. "Recently vaccinated persons have been known to cause outbreaks of vaccinia in cattle."

There were fewer than fifty human cases of rabies in the United States in each of the years from 1938 to 1945 inclusive, according to H. W. Schoening (Bureau of Animal Industry, Department of Agriculture), although the number of cases (chiefly in dogs but also in other animals, domestic and wild), ranged between 7,000 and 10,000 annually. Only thirteen of the approximately 8,000 cases of rabies reported for the country in 1948 occurred in man. Foxes, skunks, coyotes, bobcats, among which epizootics of rabies have been known to occur, have all been known to give the virus to man. Harald N. Johnson, 1948, described fox rabies as so widely distributed as to preclude any immediate prospect of eradicating the disease from this vector. Demonstration (1950, 1951) that the vampire bat transmitted rabies that proved fatal in a number of human cases in Trinidad and Mexico and in large herds of cattle led Joseph Bernstein in *Natural*

*History* magazine, 1952, to describe rabies of humans and livestock as "a major public health and economic problem of the American tropics". The Florida board of health reported, 1953, rabies infection in six (two Seminole, four yellow) of ninety bats shot.

The suggestion that "serological surveys in the field would probably bring to light cases which have hitherto escaped detection, thus providing a truer picture of the incidence of louping ill in man", was made by British workers, 1949. The virus which causes meningoencephalitis (and cerebellar ataxia) in sheep has been known (rarely) to induce in a few laboratory workers a mild nonfatal type of encephalitis.

Transmission of psittacosis to man has been traced (Meyer, 1952) to parakeets, to turkeys. According to Meyer, close to fifty species belonging to five large orders in the class *Aves* may spontaneously be infected with the psittacosis virus, which may be, for taxidermists and meat packers, a not inconsiderable occupational hazard. Data on the spread of this virus among humans, without the avian intermediary, include at least twenty-three instances, in which contact with sick birds was excluded: a 1945 epidemic in Buenos Aires with thirteen deaths in twenty-six cases; a 1941 report of the transmission of psittacosis virus by one man to three nurses; a 1943 epidemic of severe pneumonitis in the bayou region of Louisiana in which eight deaths occurred in nineteen recognized infections among nursing attendants. These and other recent observations favor the hypothesis that nonavian, and possibly human strains, play a part in the spread of psittacosis. Burnet suggested that we are at present "probably witnessing the adoption by psittacosis virus of man as a permanent host".

There is suggestive interest in Armstrong's report, 1941, that eleven per cent of 2,000 sera collected at random from persons who offered no history of an attack of lymphocytic choriomeningitis showed neutralizing antibody to this virus. This endemic virus infection of lower animals, especially mice, was accidentally discovered (1934) by Armstrong and Lillie in a monkey used in study of the virus of St. Louis encephalitis; Traub (1935) established the mouse as the natural host. After Rivers and Scott (1935) recovered the virus from the cerebrospinal fluid of human beings ill with acute aseptic meningitis, Lépine and his associates (1937) demonstrated transmission to man by experiments with human volunteers. Since then the disease has been recognized in man, in a mild phase as grippe, in severe phases occasionally fatal, as meningitis. Olitsky and Casals, 1952, described the important public health aspect of a virus "present in certain lower animals commensal with man, such as the gray or house mouse".

The expressed intention of the International Health Division to conduct an international survey of the incidence of the previously mentioned eighteen neurotropic viruses isolated from animals and mosquitoes in the tropics in the last decade, to discover the extent to which they may constitute a hazard to man, represents one of several indications of a tendency to explore more closely the relation of animal viruses to human infection. Illustrative of possibly numerous, as yet unclarified, connections between agents of similar animal and human diseases is an apparently human form of jagziekte or driving disease of sheep. First recognized in South Africa, the sheep disease is now prevalent in many parts of the world, is epidemic in Iceland where loss of sheep is "enormous", and was lately recognized in western United States. Evarts A. Graham described it as a primary carcinoma of the lung attributed by pathologists that have studied it to an unknown virus. Graham described, 1951, three human cases of pulmonary carcinoma which appeared to be morphologically and clinically identical with the sheep disease. The role of man and, indeed, the role of sheep in the whole biological cycle is, as suggested earlier, by no means defined by the mere finding of human cases (assuming that in this instance the animal and human disease are the same). Establishing which is the obligate, which the accidental host, which other animals, birds, or insects may function in the cycle, identifying the reservoir of the virus is a quest of great complexity. Slowly theories and speculations achieve a degree of support in cumulative observations. The concept that yellow fever is primarily a virus infection of animals, and man only an accidental host, is suspected of applying also to dengue; and increasingly (on the basis of serological surveys of wild and domestic birds, fowl, in various parts of the western United States) to equine encephalomyelitis, which some believe to be a primary infection of birds and only accidentally of horses and of man. The suspicion that poliomyelitis may be, if not rodent-born, perhaps in some indirect way related to several rodent neurotropic viruses has been repeatedly urged as a reason for further work in this direction. The increase in virus pneumonias in man throughout the last decade has called attention to respiratory viruses in animals, resulting in the identification throughout the last decade of pneumonitis virus of mice (PVM), pneumonitis in cats, calves, ferrets, hamsters.

It is clear that fundamental understanding of the viruses that cause human disease involves understanding of animal and plant viruses, which indeed, as Burnet pointed out, 1950, may prove the better experimental material for work on the fundamental biological questions. "One must take knowledge where one finds it." Separation of viruses into plant, bacterial, animal, human may after all, it has been pointed out, be an artefact, resulting from methods of study. It may be a necessary condition of stepwise investigative work but the fixations that go with it may constitute a threat to the unity of the biological picture.

*The following section dealing with virus workers and centers of virus work (page 375 through page 393) is not a necessary preliminary to the discussion of the nature of viruses which is resumed on page 393. Identification of virus workers may, however, be helpful in orienting readers of the sections that follow.*

# VIRUS WORKERS AND CENTERS OF VIRUS WORK

## INTRODUCTORY

Fewer than a half-dozen of the research laboratories maintained by various governments, by endowed research institutes, by universities and medical schools in the United States, in the British Empire, in France, in the Soviet Union, Japan, Sweden, Switzerland, in several South American countries have attempted, in their virus investigations, to include representatives of the full range of viruses that attack plants, insects, bacteria, animals, including man. One obvious explanation is that the significant dates in virus knowledge are comparatively recent: 1892, recognition of the first virus disease in plants, tobacco mosaic; 1896, recognition of the first virus disease of animals, foot-and-mouth disease; 1901, demonstration of the first virus disease of man, yellow fever. The amount of attention given particular viruses has often depended upon the stage of development of necessary tools and techniques. Research in poliomyelitis began to expand so soon as Karl Landsteiner and E. Popper demonstrated, 1908, that the monkey is susceptible to human virus infection. But since monkeys are expensive, certain poliomyelitis research was limited to the few laboratories that could afford to buy them until Charles Armstrong (Public Health Service) succeeded, 1939, after systematic testing of many animals, in adapting a strain from a fatal case in Lansing (since known as the Lansing strain) to cotton rats and mice. Virus research expanded more rapidly after development, by E. W. Goodpasture in America (1931) and F. M. Burnet (1933) in Australia, of the chick embryo technique, eliminating animals and animal quarters entirely for some kinds of virus research. Provision of adequate supplies of virus (following cultivation of viruses in chick embryo and in tissue culture and improved techniques of purification) for quantitatively significant studies was a large factor in advancing knowledge (of yellow fever, influenza) and in progressing toward control by vaccines. Isolation of a chemical fraction from tobacco mosaic, its purification and crystallization in 1935 by W. M. Stanley at the Princeton Laboratories of the Rockefeller Institute, and demonstration that virus infectivity is associated with that particle not only stimulated chemical work on the nature of plant viruses (leading to the first attempt to classify them systematically on the basis of chemical and serological properties) but also intensified efforts to purify and characterize the particles of many other plant and several animal, human and bacterial viruses.

The degree to which progress depends on availability of a susceptible experimental animal and of adequate quantities of the purified virus is excellently illustrated by the recently expanded research in influenza and the nation-wide trials of new influenza vaccines. It took the British workers several years of systematic testing of a variety of animals to discover, 1933, the susceptibility of the ferret to human influenza infection. Not until 1933 did Wilson Smith, C. H. Andrewes and P. P. Laidlaw, in the British laboratories, isolate influenza A virus and not until 1940 was influenza B virus isolated in this country by Thomas Francis, Jr. and by Thomas P. Magill. The ferret, however, was not found to be a perfect animal: its response was not uniform; ten to fourteen days were required for the development of antibodies, the index of infection. Chick embryo techniques first applied by Burnet at the Hall Institute in Australia, 1940, to cultivation of influenza virus became the method not only for primary isolation of virus from human cases, but also for adequate production of virus for vaccine and for research. Discovery (by G. K. Hirst, then in the International Health Division's laboratories, and, independently, by Ronald Hare and Laurella McClelland in the Connaught Medical Research Laboratories, University of Toronto, 1941) that influenza virus possesses the power of agglutinating red blood cells of domestic fowl and that after adsorption of the virus on the red cells it can subsequently be eluted into saline made it possible to harvest ten times the quantity of virus produced by earlier methods; availability of greater quantities of virus made practicable large-scale production of vaccine; subsequent discovery that immune serum inhibits the hemagglutination reaction proved useful not only as a swift *in vitro* method for measuring antibody levels against influenza in diagnosis and in immunological studies but also as a research tool in identifying strains and in studying virus-host cell relations. Before 1940, the few major centers of influenza research included: the National Institute for Medical Research, England (Andrewes), the Rockefeller Institute for Medical Research (Francis, Horsfall, Rickard, in the New York laboratories; until 1948, Shope, Stanley, Knight in the Princeton laboratories); the Rockefeller Foundation's New York laboratories (Lennette, Hirst and others); in France, the Pasteur Institute (many workers since 1900, including Levaditi, Lépine, Lwoff); the Connaught laboratories, University of Toronto (Craigie, Hare, McClelland); the Walter and Eliza Hall Institute for Medical Research, Melbourne, Australia (Burnet, Lush, others). Government-supported influenza research has notably expanded. In the United States the Army's wartime Influenza Commission (using chiefly civilian workers under Francis) has continued studies supplemented in its own virus research laboratories under Joseph E. Smadel; the Navy has supported influenza research in Research Unit No. 1 at the University of California; the Public Health Service has supplemented research in its Microbiological Institute and in the nation-wide coordinated program for collection and identification of influenza strains under Magill by grants to investigators in universities and medical schools. In the latter, departments of biology, biochemistry, bacteriology, medicine, pediatrics, public health, physics, chemistry have contributed steadily to influenza research, notably in the universities of Michigan, California, Pennsylvania, Pittsburgh, Illinois, Utah, Harvard, the California Institute of Technology.

## MONEY SPENT FOR VIRUS RESEARCH

It is not always possible to separate amounts designed for research from amounts designed for control or after care. This applies to the $8,428,119 spent by the International Health Division of the Rockefeller Foundation in the twenty-four years between 1913 and 1936 for research in the field and home laboratories on yellow fever (chiefly), influenza, rabies, and for related large-scale control experiments. Even less readily identified as virus research expenditures are funds for investigating fundamental cellular mechanisms which may ultimately reveal how the virus multiplies. Grants for this purpose (to laboratories of biology, physics, chemistry) often contain no reference to virus; for instance, the $126,434 given by the Committee on Growth of the National Research Council in 1951–1952 to seven universities, four other laboratories for virus studies (nine for studies of animal tumor viruses, two for plant tumor virus studies, one for studies bearing on virus infection as a cause of cancer, two for bacteriophage, four for study of virus-cell relationships) does not take into account funds (more than $300,000) from the same source for fundamental cytochemical and metabolic studies. These funds distributed by the Committee on Growth are collected by the American Cancer Society in annual nation-wide campaigns. From the public also (the March of Dimes) come the funds of the National Foundation for Infantile Paralysis which, between 1938 when it was established and 1953, had distributed 696 research grants (totaling approximately eighteen millions) to 111 institutions. While the federal government has spent considerable sums to keep foot-and-mouth disease from crossing the Mexican border, it has spent little for investigation of this disease since the discovery that slaughter of infected animals and quarantine could control it. Congress, 1950, refused a Department of Agriculture request for funds to construct a foot-and-mouth disease research laboratory, instructing the Department to look further into use of foreign laboratories. In 1952, however, after an outbreak in Canada, Congress appropriated ten millions for a laboratory, the first in this country. While total figures for the federal government's expenditures for virus investigation are not available, rapid increase in these is evident in the Navy's medical research grants for virus work; in the Army's support of research conducted by members of the Influenza Commission working in various universities or in field units; in Public Health Service grants for studies of influenza, the common cold, measles, mumps, encephalitis viruses; for research on genetic, cellular and metabolic aspects of virus. These federal grants are in addition to the steadily expanding intramural work in government laboratories. The state of California, with an estimated annual loss of $100,000,000 from virus diseases of plants and animals, appropriated approximately $2,000,000 in 1948 to construct the biochemistry and virus research laboratory now directed by Stanley on the Berkeley campus of the state university.

### VIRUS RESEARCH CENTERS ABROAD

International cooperation among agencies of virus research, a part of the upswing of international scientific activity since the close of the war, is represented by world-wide distribution of the influenza typing laboratories organized by the World Health Organization, by the proposal of its committee of poliomyelitis experts, 1954, that a similar network be established for identification of poliomyelitis viruses, and by the second international poliomyelitis conference (the first having been sponsored by the National Foundation for Infantile Paralysis, 1948), held, 1951, in Copenhagen. Approximately a thousand persons, including about six hundred physicians, attended from thirty-seven countries.

Virus work under way for many years in the Pasteur Institute in *France* (now concentrated in the virus research division directed by Lépine) has included since 1910 work on poliomyelitis, rabies, vaccinia, variola, mumps, yellow fever, psittacosis, influenza, lymphogranuloma venereum, herpes zoster, the encephalitides, the Coxsackie viruses, infectious tumors in fowl, work on the role of viruses in cancer, lymphocytic choriomeningitis, a number of virus diseases of animals and also continuous fundamental investigations of the nature of viruses, of mechanisms of host-virus relations (Lwoff's bacteriophage studies). In 1948, Levaditi and Lépine published, with twenty-six collaborators, a second edition of their 1938 volume on human virus infections.

In *Great Britain*, the Rothamsted Experimental Station has, under the leadership of a plant pathologist interested in genetics, F. C. Bawden, and a chemist, N. W. Pirie, become, since 1936, one of the major centers for research on the biophysical and biochemical properties of purified preparations of plant viruses. At the Animal Virus Diseases Research Institute, Pirbright (forty miles from London), problems under study have included the relation of strain differences to virulence, epidemiology, immunity, control of animal virus diseases; the director, Ian A. Galloway, and associates were intensifying, 1952, their study of strain differences of foot-and-mouth disease virus (conducted since 1941) in response to hundreds of outbreaks of this infection in 1951–52 in England and throughout Europe. British virus research has been largely centered since 1920 in the laboratories of the National Institute for Medical Research (C. H. Andrewes and associates), supported by government funds through the British Medical Research Council. Besides conducting its own research, the National Institute makes grants for integrated virus research in universities, medical schools and their associated hospitals, agricultural stations, outside the institute, and now maintains a world influenza center at Hampstead, to which, in 1949, strains of influenza virus were being sent from recent epidemics in western Europe and other parts of the world for typing and for W. J. Elford's structural studies with the electron microscope. Viruses studied in the laboratories of the National Institute throughout the last twenty years include: bacterial and plant viruses (through cooperative research); among viruses that attack animals, foot-and-mouth disease, distemper, rabies, psittacosis; among viruses pathogenic to man, herpes, vaccinia, influenza, the common cold, lymphogranuloma inguinale. Other English centers of virus research include the Lister Institute, University of London (basic work on vaccinia by the former director, J. C. G. Ledingham), the Wellcome Laboratories of Tropical Medicine (basic work on mechanism of virus multiplication by D. J. Bauer, 1952), the Agricultural Research Council's plant virus research unit at the Molteno Institute, Cambridge (Roy Markham), the London School of Hygiene and Tropical Medicine (F. K. Sanders), the Virus Reference Library, London (F. O. McCallum).

In *Canada* earlier work of the Connaught Medical Research Laboratories, University of Toronto, was concerned with vaccinia (James Craigie), with influenza (Hare and McClelland, 1941), more recent work with the Coxsackie viruses and (A. J. Rhodes) with poliomyelitis, including development of methods for mass production of some of the virus used in the United States in the 1954 vaccine trials.

In *Australia*, mention has been made of the work of Burnet, director since 1944 of the Walter and Eliza Hall Institute of Medical Research in the Royal Melbourne Hospital, and his associates, including the veterinarian, W. I. B. Beveridge, in developing the chick embryo technique. The nature of virus, the nature of immunity in various virus diseases, the mechanisms involved in host-virus reactions, have, in these laboratories, provided a connecting thread for research on many viruses: fowl pox, vesicular stomatitis, psittacosis, herpes, rabies, pseudorabies, vaccinia, infectious ectromelia, Newcastle disease of fowl, poliomyelitis, mumps, influenza and bacteriophages.

Ten governments in *Latin America* and two in *Africa*, aided by the International Health Division of the Rockefeller Foundation, have conducted research in field and laboratory, on the epidemiology, pathology, immunology and control of yellow fever.

*Sweden* has been for nearly a half century a major source of epidemiological studies of poliomyelitis, including Sven Gard's studies for the League of Nations' health organization. As director of the department of virus research in the Karolinska Institutet, Gard, in 1952, was continuing work looking toward effective vaccination against poliomyelitis. In *Japan*, research on Japanese B encephalitis, now conducted by American investigators borrowed by the Army's Epidemiological Board, originated more than ten years ago in the Government Institute for Infectious Diseases in the Tokyo Imperial University. Before the war virus work in these laboratories included studies of rabies, lymphogranuloma inguinale, vaccinia. Early work on plant viruses in *Russia* antedated the government-supported centers of virus research which include, in Moscow, the Institute of Microbiology of the Soviet Academy of Sciences where V. L. Ryzhkov has studied plant viruses, especially tobacco mosaic, since 1927; the filterable virus department of the All-Union Institute of Experimental Medicine, in which A. A. Smorodintseff has conducted experimental studies of influenza in animals and human volunteers since 1934; and in Leningrad, the Pasteur Institute.

## Virus Research Centers in the United States

In the United States, research institutes, foundations, universities, medical schools, industrial laboratories, government laboratories have contributed to virus research for varying periods throughout the last half century. Only illustrative mention of institutions and workers is possible here; there are many omissions, notably of the growing number of virus workers in veterinary and plant centers.

In the Rockefeller Institute for Medical Research, the department of the laboratories (which now includes the former department of animal and plant pathology situated at Princeton for thirty years) and the department of the hospital have conducted virus research; Simon Flexner's poliomyelitis research was begun when the institute opened its first laboratories (bacteriology and pathology) in 1902. The institute's virus research represents one of the few programs that include a fair sampling of viruses that attack man, plants, animals, insects, bacteria. Viruses studied in one or the other of the institute's laboratories since 1902 have included: poliomyelitis, the pox viruses (variola, vaccinia, swine pox, fowl pox), influenza (of man and of swine), the encephalitides (eastern and western equine, Japanese B, St. Louis, Russian Far East, Venezuelan equine, West Nile, Sabin's B), other neurotropic viruses (rabies), fowl tumor and rabbit papilloma viruses (both discovered by Rockefeller Institute workers), vesicular stomatitis, dengue, lymphocytic choriomeningitis, herpes, mumps, infectious hepatitis, foot-and-mouth disease, psittacosis, Newcastle disease, Coxsackie viruses, viruses associated with pneumonia of mice, cats, calves, the virus of primary atypical pneumonia of man. Pseudorabies, louping ill of sheep, rinderpest, swine influenza, hog cholera, various animal poxes have been studied in the laboratories of animal pathology, along with the generally neglected insect viruses (as the virus of silkworm jaundice). Plant viruses studied in the plant pathology laboratories have included mosaic viruses of tobacco, alfalfa, cucumber, white clover, also potato yellow-dwarf virus, aster yellows, tomato bushy stunt. Recent workers on the neurotropic viruses have included Isabel M. Morgan, R. W. Schlesinger, P. K. Olitsky, J. Casals, the late L. T. Webster (rabies). The relation of viruses to tumors in birds and animals has been a major investigative interest in several of the institute's laboratories since Peyton Rous demonstrated, 1911, that sarcomatous growth in fowl could be caused and transmitted by a cell-free filtrate of a naturally occurring fowl sarcoma. The institute's virus research has included biological studies of virus-induced chicken tumors, with the late J. B. Murphy and others, chemical and cytochemical studies of chicken tumor viruses, with Albert Claude (later continuing cytochemical studies in Belgium) and with a succession of workers, including F. Duran-Reynals (later continuing studies of virus tumors at Yale). At the Princeton laboratories in 1933 Shope obtained from papillomas occurring in the skin of wild cottontail rabbits a virus capable of inducing in other rabbits papillomatous growths which frequently progress to malignant carcinomas. Chemical and biological studies of this virus have been conducted by a succession of workers in the New York laboratories, including J. G. Kidd (later at Cornell) and are a part of present studies by Rous seeking light on mechanisms of malignant change "through intensive scrutiny of the cellular changes set in train by the virus". J. H. Northrop's studies in the general physiology laboratory (at Princeton, later at the University of California) have been concerned with the relation between the chemical structure and the physiological activity of certain proteins (enzymes, antibodies, viruses). Mechanisms of the formation of these active substances from precursors led to investigating the formation of bacterial viruses and the relation between growth of the host cell and synthesis of bacteriophage. Virus studies in the hospital bear in large degree upon diseases being investigated there, the common cold, influenza, primary atypical pneumonia, infectious mononucleosis. The vaccinia work of Rivers, the hospital's director, (including development of a smallpox vaccine employing not the traditional calf lymph but suspensions of chick embryo cells) deriving from research at the institute on vaccinia initiated by Hideyo Noguchi so long ago as 1915 has, with similar studies it has stimulated elsewhere, been significant in illuminating the nature of viruses generally.

In the laboratories of plant pathology, L. O. Kunkel's work has been animated by concern with host-parasite relationships in plants in inheritance of susceptibility and resistance to disease. The attempt to translate these genetic concepts into chemical terms that will explain the mechanism of mutation is reflected in the amino acid analyses by Stanley and Knight of strains of tobacco mosaic virus, 1940. Stanley's isolation, 1935, of a characteristic particle shown to possess virus infectivity, and to be a nucleoprotein, has had wide repercussions in biology among those concerned with the role of proteins in the synthetic mechanisms responsible for self-duplication of the cell. During the war years, 1942 to 1945, Stanley and his associates suspended work on plant viruses to undertake, under government contracts, development of methods for concentrating, purifying and inactivating influenza virus leading to production of a centrifuge-type vaccine now in use in the United States and other countries. Studies of Japanese B encephalitis and also of dengue viruses and vaccines were conducted (in collaboration with Sabin) in response to war needs.

Investigators that have carried virus research programs from the Rockefeller Institute to other centers include: G. P. Berry, who, until 1949, directed the bacteriology department at the University of Rochester; J. G. Kidd, later in Cornell's pathology department; F. Duran-Reynals, later in Yale's microbiology department; J. W. Jobling, in Columbia's pathology department; M. A. Lauffer, Jr., and W. C. Price, at the University of Pittsburgh; H. S. Loring, in Stanford's biochemistry department; Joseph E. Smadel, scientific director, department of virus and rickettsial diseases, Army graduate school; J. W. Beard, at Duke; Isabel M. Morgan, at the Johns Hopkins Poliomyelitis Research Center; A. B. Sabin, at the University of Cincinnati; Stanley, since 1948 directing a virus laboratory at the University of California; J. T. Syverton, in the bacteriology department at the University of Minnesota; T. P. Magill, director of the bacteriology department at the Long Island College of Medicine; T. F. MacNair Scott, in the pediatrics department of Pennsylvania; W. F. Friedewald, at Emory; Thomas Francis, Jr., director of the virus laboratory at Michigan; G. K. Hirst, director of research on infectious diseases at the Public Health Research Institute, New York; several institute workers, later directors of virus research in large pharmaceutical houses (H. R. Cox, at Lederle Laboratories; Geoffrey W. Rake, in the Squibb Institute).

The Rockefeller Foundation's International Health Division's studies in its New York laboratories have supplemented far-flung epidemiological studies on a few viruses: yellow fever (reaching to three continents over thirty-five years); influenza and a group of pneumonitis viruses found in animals and in man; recently on the previously mentioned group of insect-borne viruses (neurotropic for mice) isolated by workers in the tropics between 1937 and 1948. The division's workers were responsible for isolating the yellow fever virus in 1927, for discovery and development of a modified strain, for employing it in a campaign of vaccination (in Uganda in East Africa, in Nigeria in West Africa, in Brazil, Colombia, Panama, British Guiana, Peru, Bolivia, Ecuador, in South and Central America) in the course of which many millions were vaccinated in cooperation with governmental agencies which are now continuing this work independently. The systematic campaign on two continents identifying the principal insect vectors and vertebrate hosts led to new concepts of the biological cycle of yellow fever infection. On a considerably smaller scale than the yellow fever program has been work conducted in the home laboratories or supported in others (at Columbia, Michigan, Pennsylvania, Ohio State universities, and in the California state health department) on virus infections of the respiratory tract, influenza, the common cold, the pneumonitis viruses. In recognition of increasing contributions to this field from other agencies, the division has withdrawn support of research on the respiratory viruses, but has continued the influenza work in the home laboratories. The division has conducted, independently, and in cooperation with the Army's influenza commission during the war, widespread tests of progressively improved vaccines. Past or present contributors to progress in influenza research — Francis, Magill, Rickard, Horsfall, Hirst — have since 1935 participated in the influenza work of the division's laboratories on both the practical prophylactic level (nation-wide tests of vaccines) and the fundamental level (work on mechanisms of virus multiplication, and of host cell-virus relations generally). Expanding concern with mechanisms involved in the growth of viruses within the cell has brought into the virus field biologists concerned not primarily with infectious aspects of viruses but rather with genetic and nuclear mechanisms involved in virus reproduction (A. H. Doermann and A. D. Hershey, working on intracellular growth of bacteriophages, genetics department, Carnegie Institution of Washington).

It is in the universities and medical schools that the most significant changes in volume and continuity of virus research have occurred. In 1950, the virus research proceeding on a more or less continuous basis in fifty-five departments of thirty-four universities (in thirty-one of which the work was centered in the medical school; in three in university biology and physics departments) was not altogether concerned either with the nature of virus or with virus diseases. At least seven of the medical school programs have been dominantly concerned with ways and means of dealing with after effects (nerve and muscle damage) of poliomyelitis. In only twenty of these programs does the research go back more than a decade; in eight it was initiated after 1940. Of the twenty programs representing continuous work on one or more viruses for from ten to twenty years, fourteen were in bacteriology and pathology departments (traditionally concerned with infection), six in pediatrics departments (traditionally concerned with communicable diseases of children). The work in bacteriology departments included: at Ohio State (N. Paul Hudson) since 1935, work on methods of cultivating viruses, on poliomyelitis, vaccinia, herpes simplex, more recently influenza; at the University of Rochester (G. P. Berry from 1932 to 1949, from 1949 Howard B. Slavin), work on virus tumors, psittacosis, western equine encephalomyelitis, more recently work on lymphocytic choriomeningitis and herpes and on immunological relationships of viruses; at the University of Southern California (John F. Kessel and associates, since 1934), exploration of the infectivity, virulence, pathology and antigenic relationships of different strains of poliomyelitis virus isolated in southern California epidemics. Recent virus programs under federal grants include study of physiological effects of influenza by J. E. Kempf, since 1946 in the bacteriology department of the University of Illinois; immunological and epidemiological studies of mumps and influenza by G. R. Leymaster, since 1948 in Utah's department of preventive medicine; research on psittacosis-lymphogranuloma viruses by M. F. Shaffer, since 1947 in Tulane's bacteriology department. Research on influenza in Cornell's bacteriology department by John Y. Sugg continued work on this virus begun in 1938 with Magill, who later went to Long Island's bacteriology department, and who has directed the national influenza strain study center. Aided by a five-year grant of $18,370 from the National Foundation for Infantile Paralysis, Charles A. Evans, director of the bacteriology department in the University of Washington's new medical school, continued earlier virus work (on fox encephalitis, canine distemper, herpes, poliomyelitis) in studies directed toward increasing the yield of virus by cultivation in non-nervous tissue. Under Colin M. MacLeod, head of New York University's bacteriology department, a five-year grant from the National Foundation was being used, 1950, for investigation of the relation of metabolic changes in nerve tissue to resistance to viruses and to multiplication and spread of virus in the destruction of nerve cells.

Systematic attempts by John F. Enders and associates in Harvard's bacteriology department to improve tissue culture methods of propagating viruses (since 1940, vaccinia, mumps, herpes, poliomyelitis) originated in work begun more than twenty years ago. Propagation of one type of poliomyelitis virus in tissue cultures, announced by Enders, Weller and Robbins, 1949, was followed in 1950 by announcement that the two other known immunogenic types had also been cultivated and the changes seen during propagation of one type suggested that an attenuated strain useful for a vaccine might be developed. By 1953 Enders and his associates were applying tissue culture methods to other viruses that have long proved resistant to cultivation with the ultimate aim, in the case of measles, of producing a vaccine if propagation should prove successful.

The list of viruses studied in Columbia's bacteriology department has grown steadily since its former director, Frederick P. Gay, began studies of herpes simplex ending with his death in 1940. Poliomyelitis studies begun in 1930 by Claus W. Jungeblut included, 1948, work on mechanism of infection of rodent-adapted poliomyelitis in relation to age and portal of entry. Other contributions from this department have included: work on methods of cultivating viruses (Murray Sanders); studies of the common cold (A. R. Dochez with Yale Kneeland, Jr., and K. C. Mills, of the department of internal medicine), aided by the International Health Division since 1921, by federal grants from 1946 to 1949; studies of pneumonitis in mice, of atypical pneumonia and influenza in man. Attempts to isolate and purify the infective agent of Rous sarcoma were pursued for more than fifteen years in the pathology department by a group working with James W. Jobling; the viral nature of the "milk factor" as a cause of mammary cancer in mice has been the subject of a long-term collaborative study by Cushman D. Haagensen and associates in the surgery department with Samuel Graff of the biochemistry department.

Fundamental concern with tissue and cell specificity of certain viruses, with host-virus relations, with mechanisms of immunity underlies histopathologic studies on a lengthening list of viruses — herpes simplex, smallpox, fowl pox, vaccinia, rabies, mumps, canine distemper, poliomyelitis, stomatitis — conducted in Vanderbilt's pathology department since 1925 by Goodpasture, G. J. Buddingh (who after 1948 continued his work on dermatotropic viruses at Louisiana State University School of Medicine) and others. Goodpasture's early experiments with O. Teague on the neural transmission of herpes simplex from the periphery to the central nervous system provided the working hypothesis that axones are the transport media for neurotropic viruses, notably for rabies and poliomyelitis. Goodpasture's series of studies on fowl pox which led to use of the chick embryo in cultivation of viruses influenced, as previously indicated, the whole picture of virus research thereafter.

In connection with more than two decades' work on the virus of rabbit papilloma, the late R. G. Green, in Minnesota's bacteriology department, outlined some of the major concepts regarding the nature and origin of virus. Other studies dealt with fox encephalitis (control of epizootics), a virus disease of owls, canine distemper, herpes simplex. Green collaborated with J. J. Bittner, director of the division of cancer biology, in studies of the virus nature of the milk influence in mammary cancer of mice.

Research on St. Louis encephalitis has been conducted, since the 1933 epidemic, in Washington University's departments of medicine, pathology, bacteriology and pediatrics. In the bacteriology department, bacteriophage has been a continuing interest since 1928, first of the department's former director, J. J. Bronfenbrenner, more recently of A. D. Hershey, later in the genetics laboratory of the Carnegie Institution.

In a number of pediatrics departments virus research has owed its origin to concern with control of children's infections. A. B. Sabin's poliomyelitis research (chemical and biochemical factors influencing susceptibility, 1952) as professor of pediatric research at the University of Cincinnati and fellow of the Children's Hospital Research Foundation followed wartime investigations of dengue, sandfly fever, Japanese B encephalitis. At Yale for many years, beginning 1932, field and laboratory research on epidemiology, immunology and strains of poliomyelitis were a joint project under James D. Trask in the pediatrics department and John R. Paul in the department of medicine, later director of its section on preventive medicine. Continuing these studies in the poliomyelitis study unit established 1945 (and since then supported by two five-year grants from the National Foundation for Infantile Paralysis), Paul has also conducted research on infectious hepatitis (with W. P. Havens, Jr., later at Jefferson). Other contributors to experimental work on poliomyelitis have included Dorothy M. Horstmann, Edward C. Curnen, Joseph L. Melnick, the two latter having since 1948 made intensive study of the Coxsackie viruses. Other virus programs at Yale include previously mentioned studies of Duran-Reynals on virus tumors in the microbiology department in which Philip B. Cowles has investigated bacteriophages since 1930; in the department of medicine, R. H. Green's studies of respiratory viruses, supported by federal grants between 1946 and 1950. Since 1935, Joseph Stokes, Jr., head of Pennsylvania's pediatrics department, and associates have been continuously engaged in research leading to development and testing of vaccines for influenza, measles, mumps, and to studies of the virus of infectious hepatitis. From the associated Children's Hospital, contributions have included fundamental studies of the nature of the influenza viruses with relevance to mechanisms of infection (at the cellular level) and control (Werner Henle, bacteriologist), of herpes simplex (T. F. MacNair Scott), studies of the role of metabolic mechanisms of host cells in virus synthesis (Seymour S. Cohen, physiological chemist), of the role in multiplication of viruses of nucleoprotein particles of bacteriophage (Thomas F. Anderson). Virus tumors have been studied in the pathology department by Balduin Lucké since his description, 1932, of the transmission, by a cell-free extract, of renal tumors occurring in the leopard frog, and by D. R. Coman.

Four divisions of the University of California are contributing to virus research. The work of W. N. Takahashi, plant pathologist, on the ability of certain substances to inhibit multiplication of plant viruses is considered to bear on mechanisms of chemotherapy in virus infections. Research conducted since 1924 on psittacosis and ornithosis, by Karl F. Meyer and his associates in the Hooper Foundation for Medical Research, has, during the last decade, been supplemented by laboratory and field studies of the encephalitides, including epidemiological studies which, under the direction of W. McD. Hammon (later at the University of Pittsburgh) and W. C. Reeves, have sought, over eleven western states, the insect vectors and animal reservoirs for various viral encephalitides. In the bacteriology department, A. P. Krueger's current research (begun in 1934) on bacteriophage aims to shed light on cell-virus relations. The new virus research laboratory opened in 1952 and directed by Stanley is equipped for research and advanced training in virology, with a center for electron microscopy under Robley C. Williams, with facilities for use of stable and radioactive isotopes, for ultracentrifugation and electrophoretic studies; it is one of few virus centers dealing with all types of viruses, plant, bacterial, animal. Viruses under investigation, 1953, included poliomyelitis, influenza, certain tumor- and cancer-producing viruses, several virus diseases of domestic animals, bacteriophages, several plant viruses. The fundamental concern here is the chemical, physical and biological characterization of the properties of viruses. A report on purified preparations of Type II poliomyelitis, including the first unequivocal isolation of this virus, its characterization (morphology, size) in the electron microscope, was published from this laboratory (Stanley, Bachrach, Schwerdt) in 1953.

Influenza was the first virus selected for research in the University of Michigan School of Public Health when Francis became, 1941, chairman of its department of epidemiology. The experimental program on epidemiology of poliomyelitis, systematically developed in this department during recent years, included a study, begun 1945, on possible reservoirs of poliomyelitis virus in various environments (rural, urban). Grants from the National Foundation for this work have also provided funds to train virus workers. Epidemiological studies of equine encephalomyelitis (Gordon C. Brown) have been included, and work has been done on hepatitis, herpes, atypical pneumonia. Studies (employing poliomyelitis, herpes, influenza viruses) reported from the virus research laboratory since 1950 (W. W. Ackermann, Francis, others) are concerned with the possibility that blocking of cellular metabolites by antimetabolites might inhibit intracellular multiplication of virus.

Research on poliomyelitis going forward, 1948, in several Stanford departments included: in the bacteriology department, Edwin W. Schultz's work (since 1931) seeking approaches to prophylaxis through studies of portal of entry and of immunological aspects of virus; in the pediatrics department, H. K. Faber's work exploring in monkeys and in man, since 1933, the possible paths by which the poliomyelitis virus gains entrance, reaches the nervous system, is excreted; in the pharmacology department, work (aided by Public Health Service grants) testing the efficacy of more than 150 antibiotics, dyes, sulfonamides, biologic and metabolic compounds against various experimental virus infections; in the chemistry department, H. S. Loring's work on the degree and methods of inactivating virus that will produce an effective agent for active immunization.

Poliomyelitis is the major current virus interest at the Johns Hopkins center for research on poliomyelitis and related viruses, established, 1942, under K. F. Maxcy in the school of hygiene and public health, with two five-year grants ($732,500) from the National Foundation. Epidemiological studies have been added to the neurocytological research in this center, in monkeys and in man, conducted since 1943 by H. A. Howe and David Bodian, who before that year conducted these studies, with grants from the Commonwealth Fund, in the medical school's anatomy department. Other Johns Hopkins virus programs included T. B. Turner's studies (aided by federal grants) of influenza and the common cold, in the bacteriology department of the school of hygiene; and Frederik B. Bang's work in the department of medicine, on pathological changes revealed by the electron microscope in cells infected by viruses (between 1946 and 1952, fowl pox, eastern equine encephalomyelitis, herpes simplex, vaccinia, influenza, Newcastle disease).

In Western Reserve's pediatrics department, the late John A. Toomey, for twenty years, in the face of differing general opinion (later reversed), accumulated evidence for the gastrointestinal tract as the portal of entry for poliomyelitis virus. In the department of medicine, vaccinia and other viruses were studied by R. F. Parker who brought these interests, 1936, from the Rockefeller Institute.

The role of protein synthesis in virus reproduction was under investigation (with a five-year grant of $26,000 from the National Foundation) in Chicago's biochemistry department by Frank W. Putnam, Lloyd M. Kozloff and Earl A. Evans, Jr.

At the University of Pittsburgh, 1945, virus research was introduced into departments of biology, chemistry and physics, through workers formerly at the Rockefeller Institute: Max A. Lauffer (physical and chemical studies of influenza A virus particles); W. C. Price (genetic study using bean mosaic virus). In 1951–52, Hammon, in the university's graduate school of public health, organized field tests of the protective value of gamma globulin against poliomyelitis in a half million children, during epidemics in three states. In 1954, nation-wide trials were made of the experimental poliomyelitis vaccine developed in the virus research laboratory of the medical school's bacteriology department by Jonas E. Salk and his associates (and tested for three years in monkeys, in human volunteers and in small groups of children in the Pittsburgh area). Continuing studies were concerned with typing of strains, with simplified tests for diagnostic use and for testing duration of immunity following vaccination with killed virus vaccines (influenza, poliomyelitis) and the ability of adjuvants to increase the efficacy and duration of immunity induced with such vaccines.

In the California Institute of Technology, Max Delbrück has been continuously concerned with theories of virus replication, using bacteriophages because they are assayable with a high degree of accuracy, because they are stable, because their host cells (various types of bacteria) can be simply cultivated under well-defined conditions, and because the bacteriophage in a culture of actively growing cells is accurately reproducible. These theories are a major interest also of R. Dulbecco, who came to the institute in 1950 and who before that worked with S. E. Luria. Luria, formerly in the bacteriology department of Indiana University, later in the same department in Illinois University, has continued his work on the genetics of bacteriophage.

Among other virus programs in medical schools is work conducted since 1937 in Duke's department of experimental surgery to which J. W. Beard brought (from the Rockefeller Institute) his work on virus tumors, since 1949 directed to fowl leukosis virus; this work has gradually expanded to include studies on isolation, purification, chemical and physical characterization of influenza A and B, swine influenza, the equine encephalomyelitis viruses. Collaborators included D. G. Sharp, Dorothy Beard and the department's biochemist and research associate, A. R. Taylor, who in 1947 identified a new antigenic type of influenza, tentatively named C. Other contributions to virus research include: studies of the cytology and cytochemistry of viruses at St. Louis University (Henry Pinkerton, pathology department); studies of influenza and the common cold at Emory University (W. F. Friedewald). Federal grants have assisted studies of dermotropic viruses at Wayne University and of Kansas reservoirs of encephalitis at the University of Kansas; substantial grants from the National Foundation for Infantile Paralysis have aided poliomyelitis research since 1947 in several schools of medicine not previously mentioned in this connection (Bowman Gray, Emory, universities of Colorado, Utah, Oregon, Indiana), in the departments of botany and biochemistry of Washington University, St. Louis.

Federal agencies engaged in virus research include, in addition to the Public Health Service, the Army, the Department of Agriculture, with their more extensive programs, the Department of the Interior (trachoma studies in the Bureau of Indian affairs), the Navy (continuing wartime research on respiratory viruses).

The Army's virus research, under *ad hoc* Army medical research boards, began with the yellow fever commission of 1900–1902. The role of insect vectors, established by that commission for yellow fever, became an orienting interest in later investigations of dengue, equine encephalomyelitis, St. Louis encephalitis, by F. II. K. Reynolds, R. A. Kelser, J. S. Simmons, from 1930 to 1945. Dengue has been the subject of three separate Army programs: in 1907, in Manila; in 1930, by Reynolds and Simmons; in the second World War on the Pacific islands. However, the wartime vaccination experiments were conducted by civilian investigators (Sabin, Schlesinger) on loan to the government "for the duration". Essentially civilian also (although financed by the Army during and since the war) was the work of several commissions (neurotropic virus commission, headed by Paul; commission on measles and mumps, headed by Stokes; commission on influenza, still, 1953, directed by Francis, which conducted the nation-wide trials of influenza vaccines). However the Army also now maintains its own previously mentioned department of virus and rickettsial diseases in the Army medical service graduate school under Smadel. With the aid of the Society of American Bacteriologists and the National Research Council's committee on American type culture collection, the Army has established a viral and rickettsial registry to receive and distribute animal viruses (thirty-four in 1953) commonly used in teaching and research.

For so long as thirty years some of the plant and animal virus diseases and human diseases due to viruses harbored or transmitted by domestic animals have been under investigation in the Department of Agriculture's bureaus of animal and of plant industry, including foot-and-mouth disease. H. W. Schoening, lately retired as director of the Bureau of Animal Industry's pathology department, has, with other investigators since 1930, studied several other animal viruses: rabies, Newcastle disease of fowl, equine encephalomyelitis (for which, in horses, in 1934, L. T. Giltner and M. S. Shahan of the bureau developed a vaccine). New insect and avian vectors of encephalomyelitis have been sought by the bureau with state experiment stations, state and federal health authorities. For many years the department's Bureau of Plant Industry maintained coordinated investigations on plant viruses, including extensive tobacco mosaic studies, begun by H. A. Allard, 1916, continued by H. H. McKinney (whose observation of the association of yellow mosaic with ordinary green tobacco mosaic from a different source led him to suggest, 1926, "virus may become altered locally in the plant, thus producing mutations"). Research on plant and animal viruses has also been conducted in the various federal regional research laboratories, as the Regional Poultry Research Laboratory, Lansing, Michigan (Ben R. Burmester's investigation of fowl leukosis). Virus research programs on plants and animals in state experiment stations and agricultural colleges have dealt with: serology of plant viruses, 1949, Oklahoma Agricultural College; fowl virus infections (an interest of F. R. Beaudette's since 1923), New Jersey Agricultural Experiment Station which also, in S. A. Waksman's program, has been testing antibiotics against viruses; Newcastle disease of fowl, in Illinois, California, Wisconsin and other states. Other virus studies in state colleges and stations have been concerned with: a virus disease of potatoes studied (T. P. Dykstra, 1942) through the coordinated work of a number of experiment stations; a virus disease of red currants (Ohio Experiment Station); stone fruit viruses (George W. Cochran, Utah State Agricultural College); a virus suspected of causing a group of diseases attacking citrus fruit (California Citrus Experiment Station since 1943); a new mosaic disease of beans (reported, 1943, by the Cornell Agricultural Experiment Station).

The virus research of the Public Health Service, although occasional as compared with continuous federal cancer research, although not concentrated in a single virus laboratory and not supported by basic appropriation, has nevertheless expanded steadily to include studies (epidemiological, clinical, experimental, bacteriological, biological, chemical, physical, pathological, immunological) on poliomyelitis, influenza, the common cold, dengue, mumps, rabies, vaccinia, Rous sarcoma virus, pneumonitis, yellow fever, postvaccinal jaundice and infectious hepatitis, the encephalitides (eastern and western equine, choriomeningitis, St. Louis), rabies, the psittacosis-lymphogranuloma and the Coxsackie groups. Most of this work has been centered in the division of infectious diseases, now a unit in the Microbiological Institute. Since 1950, however, it has been supplemented by contributions from regional laboratories established by the service's communicable disease center to increase facilities in many state health departments for diagnosis of virus infections and to serve as "listening posts" for potential epidemics, as through collection of influenza strains in local outbreaks. Significant contributions from Public Health Service officers include: adaptation to rodents of the three known types of poliomyelitis virus (the Lansing type by Armstrong; the Leon virus by Karl Habel and Li, 1951, at the National Institutes of Health; in 1953, transfer to mice of the Brunhilde type by Li and Schaeffer of the communicable disease center's regional virus and rickettsia laboratory in Alabama); discovery, 1933, by Armstrong and R. D. Lillie of the virus of lymphocytic choriomeningitis; cultivation in the chick embryo of mumps virus by Habel and preparation of a killed-virus vaccine tested, 1947, in human epidemics.

In the National Institutes of Health, the National Cancer Institute, since 1938, has included virus studies in connection with various experimental virus cancers, of Rous sarcoma and the mammary tumor agent (particular interests of H. B. Andervont). From the laboratory of physical biology, R. W. G. Wyckoff has reported electron microscopic studies of plant, animal and bacterial viruses. A study section on virus and rickettsial diseases was included in the division of research grants and fellowships, organized 1946; forty projects recommended by this section received sixty-five grants amounting, through August, 1948, to $803,784, a small sum, however, as compared with $29,669,905 given for cancer research and $13,195,225 for heart disease projects, 1946–49. The influenza information center, established 1949 within the National Institutes, continued, 1950, to serve as headquarters for the western hemisphere in the world-wide network of influenza laboratories (fifty-five in forty-four different countries, 1953) initiated by the World Health Organization's influenza study program, 1947. The international program had been preceded in the United States by a national network of influenza laboratories (sixty-two by 1953) sponsored by the armed services commission on influenza. The present sponsorship is now shared by all the armed services and the Public Health Service which, besides its center in the National Institutes of Health, maintains at Long Island University the influenza strain study center for the Americas. To this center, suspected influenza viruses are sent by eight regional laboratories which also supply antigens and antiserums to collaborating laboratories in their respective areas.

Few state, county and city public health laboratories have the funds, trained staff or equipment required for virus research. However virus divisions have been established or extended in a number of state health laboratories. Illustrating the truth that diagnosis of virus infections is often in itself a research procedure, several of the state laboratories that have been made centers for collecting and identifying influenza strains, for recognition of poliomyelitis, identification of Coxsackie viruses, have initiated modest investigative programs. Older research programs include several aided by the International Health Division of the Rockefeller Foundation (in Alabama, Georgia, California), others developed with state funds (Michigan, New York). Virus work (not voluminous) at the local level is illustrated by early epidemiological and pathological studies (of the poliomyelitis epidemics of 1916 and 1931) made by the New York City Board of Health, which, for some years, maintained a poliomyelitis research bureau. A serum center, established later, explored the possibilities of convalescent serum against poliomyelitis and mumps. Experimental work on bacteriophages, on immunological aspects of St. Louis encephalitis, on influenza vaccination, and studies of the nature of antigen-antibody reactions in viruses were also carried on, from 1936, in the bureau of laboratories of the Health Department under Ralph S. Muckenfuss until the bureau's investigative activities were merged with those of the tax-supported Public Health Research Institute established by New York City. At this institute, Hirst since he came, 1946, from the Rockefeller Institute to direct research on infectious diseases, has continued his work on influenza, on mechanism of the hemagglutination reaction; and Schlesinger's studies here have dealt with virus interference, variation, cellular resistance to viruses.

In addition to the continuous fundamental research, mentioned illustratively above, in university, medical school and government laboratories, contributions have been made by national voluntary societies (the National Foundation for Infantile Paralysis, the American Cancer Society); by a few hospitals (Michael Reese Hospital Research Institute); by industrial laboratories (the American Cyanamid Laboratories; the Lederle Laboratories with their section of viral and rickettsial research under Herald R. Cox which, under the direction of Hilary Koprowski and associates, contributed to a collaborative test, 1952–53, of poliomyelitis vaccination in human volunteers; the Squibb Institute's virus laboratory under the direction of Geoffrey Rake; the Merck Institute to which Shope took his virus studies in 1949).

## THE NATURE OF VIRUSES

### ATTEMPTS AT CLASSIFICATION

Definitive groupings of viruses, according to morphology, serological reactions, method of transmission (including type of vector), tissue tropism, whether particular (neurotropic, viscerotropic, dermotropic, pneumotropic) or general (pantropic), have not been possible in the present state of knowledge. Nor has an adequate basis of classification been found in the nature of virus action (degenerative, hyperplastic) on the host cell. Various workers have stressed the point that present knowledge of all viruses is insufficient even for establishing common principles of classification and that fixed groupings and nomenclature may, therefore, be a danger, particularly to research. Others feel (Burnet, 1953) that a "beginning must be made somewhere", that it may be better to make tentative classifications and then revise them as knowledge accumulates. Francis O. Holmes of the Rockefeller Institute (who was responsible for the Bergey classification of 1948) stressed the useful purpose served (in his own field of plant viruses) by classifying certain plant viruses according to known properties with regard to insect vectors, thus making it possible sometimes to predict the expectable type of vector for a given virus. This and other evidence favoring attempts at classification were taken into account at the Fifth International Congress for Microbiology in Rio de Janeiro, 1950, at which a committee of sixteen virus investigators from various countries appointed study sections to consider five of the most extensively studied groups: the psittacosis-lymphogranuloma group (section headed by Rake); the pox group (Buddingh); the influenza group (Burnet); the insect-pathogenic viruses; the arthropod-borne encephalitis viruses (Hammon, Lépine). The criteria adopted as a basis for tests of classification and for discussion at the succeeding international congress (Rome, 1953) included: (1) morphology and method of reproduction; (2) chemical composition and physical properties; (3) serological and immunological properties; (4) susceptibility to physical and chemical agents; (5) natural methods of transmission; (6) host, tissue and cell tropisms; (7) pathology, including inclusion-body formation; (8) symptomatology. Subsequent discussions, notably at the 1952 conference held (under the chairmanship of Burnet) by the biology section of the New York Academy of Sciences, disclosed considerable difference of opinion concerning the weight to be attached to some of the above criteria. Hammon, for instance, found most of the criteria inapplicable (in the present state of knowledge) to the arthropod-borne encephalitis viruses. These, he observed, could be grouped only because they produce one type of disease, encephalitis, because they happen to have an arthropod as one of a series of hosts and possibly also because "man is an occasional victimized host". On the basis of immunological relations, members of the group were, with few exceptions, completely unrelated; of chemical composition of many members of the group "little or nothing is known"; studies of physical properties, aside from morphology, have proved completely inadequate for most of the members of the group "as are studies on susceptibility to physical and chemical agents"; although "encouraging progress is being made" in knowledge of natural methods of transmission, inadequacies exist in the data; although host tropisms have been extensively studied for some members of the group, there are great variations; in tissue tropisms these viruses "vary from pantropism to what appears to be relatively strict neurotropism"; while pathology in the brain of laboratory animals appears strikingly similar, symptomatology varies widely. In sum, Hammon considered classifications "premature". Similarly, Lépine considered that the rapid tempo of virus research would make it necessary to revise a few years hence any framework now adopted: "In the field of virus research, we are still at the stage of explorers entering the virgin forest." A more hopeful view was expressed with regard to the pox, the poliomyelitis, the Coxsackie groups, bacteriophages.

Discussions of classification revealed a cleavage between the school that attaches greater significance to the effects of viruses on the host and the school that regards as more important the intrinsic nature of viruses ("we need a classification of viruses, not of diseases"). Increasingly, virus investigators — biologists, biochemists and chemists, medical men — recognize that the heart of the problem lies in dynamic interaction between host and virus, and in the host-cell mechanisms involved in virus reproduction. In reviewing "important gaps in knowledge" that must be filled before any sound classifications of viruses can be achieved, Burnet, at the end of the 1952 conference referred to above, described as "the most interesting of all problems of classification" the question "whether plant, animal and bacterial viruses have a common evolutionary origin or whether, even within the three great groups of known viruses, there are diverse evolutionary origins". While to this pragmatic session Burnet described this most fundamental of all virus questions as "too remote from present-day knowledge to justify discussion", the nature and origin of viruses is at some point involved in study of every particularized aspect of viruses and of virus diseases.

## Various Concepts of the Nature and Origin of Viruses

Developing knowledge has shown that the earlier oversimplified controversy as to whether viruses are living microorganisms ("modified living parasites"), or "nonliving" chemicals (autocatalytic proteins) may be rather a matter of relative emphasis than of essential antithesis. That a different approach rather than a quite different school of thought is involved in what remains of the cleavage was explained, 1952, by Andrewes (at the second international poliomyelitis conference): those, he said, that have studied viruses from the widest point of view, focusing on their properties, their reactions with the host cell they infect, incline to consider viruses as organisms, while those that look at them "from perhaps a more restricted point of view" (chemists, physicists, geneticists) are more likely to "toy with other hypotheses". Andrewes, inclining to the first group, proceeded to offer "six strong reasons" for considering viruses as organisms: they multiply; they vary, and the variants are heritable; most of them are definitely complex in chemical composition; they are antigenically distinct from constituents of the cell of the host they invade; at least the animal-pathogenic viruses (Andrewes deprecated the extent of his own knowledge of other than animal viruses) apparently form a regular gradient from the smallest (the viruses of foot-and-mouth disease and of poliomyelitis) up to the large (psittacosis); they have host-parasite relationships similar to those of bacteria and other parasites.

Exemplifying the second group, Stanley, at the same conference, repeated his reasons for regarding the tobacco mosaic virus as a molecule: "Organisms are characterized by protoplasm with its attendant water, by metabolic activity, and by size, shape and organizational inhomogeneities. Tobacco mosaic virus, on the other hand, appears to consist of rather rigid nucleoprotein rods, essentially devoid of internal water, exhibiting no metabolic activity and possessing a remarkably uniform size and shape and an internal structure of great regularity . . ." Stanley added — without doubt in some recognition of the comment frequently made by his critics that findings in tobacco mosaic cannot be generalized for all viruses — "no inference is intended that all viruses are molecular in nature; on the contrary the evidence indicates that certain viruses are organismal in nature."

The historical development of relative emphases on organism and molecule, which represent — but only in a way — biological versus chemical slant, has more than academic interest in any approach to the whole virus problem. It was natural that with the first identification of virus with human disease, at the opening of the present century (yellow fever, 1901), the traditional concepts of bacteriology should be transferred to viruses, then regarded as merely submicroscopic microbes. It was also natural that the influence of more recent work in biology and biochemistry directed toward the mechanism of cell duplication should draw the two originally divergent views together toward a concept that abandons the controversy as to whether or not a protein molecule is "lifeless" and focuses rather on virus multiplication as a problem of protein synthesis. The compromise view that perhaps the smaller viruses may be protein molecules with capacity for self-duplication while the larger and more complex viruses may be "the midgets of the microbial world", multiplying as bacteria multiply, does not, on the whole, satisfy biologists. With their instinct for the homogeneous nature of life, however diverse its expressions, they reject the concept of duality, preferring to consider viruses as one, even though the differing degrees of life shown by the wide range from the smallest to the largest viruses are not yet susceptible to precise definition by chemical, physical, genetic studies.

Describing, 1935, viruses as "the smallest units showing the reproductive property considered typical of life", R. G. Green, in Minnesota's bacteriology department, outlined alternate ways in which viruses might evolve from living microbes of the past: they might be surviving parasites that had evolved from free-living ultramicrobes that, although now extinct, had once inhabited the earth; they might be "parasitic forms of life developing by retrograde evolution from visible microbes similar to the visible forms now existent". He rejected the first hypothesis on the ground that there is no way of substantiating it; he accepted the second, or retrograde-evolution, theory as following naturally from "our knowledge of evolution in the visible world". Many workers have stressed the point that capacity to reproduce, as a definition of living, leads logically to the view that viruses have evolved from visible microorganisms.

Whatever the biological views concerning the nature and origin of viruses, however, accumulated studies of purified viruses (plant, bacterial, animal) during the past decade have led to general belief that they may be described by their chemical and physical properties, their biochemical behavior. "No one now doubts that viruses have properties that can be described in biochemical terms" (Pirie, 1946). Biochemical study led Beard, after more than a decade's work on the chemical and physical properties of virus proteins, to abandon his advocacy of the molecular hypothesis; "few", he observed, "have had the temerity to include the large vaccinia virus among the molecules". While admitting, 1948, the possibility that all viruses may not be of the same nature, he regarded the hypothesis that any virus consists of a single compound "made up of the same number of atoms arranged in the same way" as not only not established but also as "incompatible with the known variability and adaptability of viruses with changing conditions". He found, 1951, "no chemical or physical basis in either theory or fact for the supposition that any viruses are too small to support the degree of organization required for living matter".

Of obligate parasitic nature, as the outstanding criterion of virus, its tendency progressively to transfer its work to the host, exponents have included Green in this country, 1938, and, in England, P. P. Laidlaw, who, also in 1938, stressed the view that viruses arise from higher forms of microorganism now extinct by a process of progressive adaptation to a parasitic existence in which the parasite is finally reduced to a bare nucleoprotein molecule capable of self-replication but relying on the host cell entirely for the necessary materials and energy. Parasitism or "laziness" might, in his view, be pushed to such an extreme that eventually the virus would lose all independent metabolic activity and "live a borrowed life, truly the supreme summit of parasitism". The virus would consist merely of specific nucleoprotein possessing the power of reproduction; outside the susceptible cell it would appear to be inanimate. The large viruses would be those that had lost the power to synthesize one or two factors essential to their growth. The small viruses would be those that had lost all auto-synthetic power, possessing only ability to transmit the characters of the species, such as the crystallizable plant viruses and possibly the very small animal viruses. Between these two extremes would be viruses that had achieved specialization in parasitism to varying degrees, progressive loss of enzyme activity being attended with corresponding decrease in size. Burnet, whose views of virus incline to those of Laidlaw and Green, and who stressed the "pragmatic necessity" of regarding viruses as living organisms which have evolved by parasitic degeneration from larger microorganisms, many of them in all probability from bacteria, considered that his 1950 preferred definition of virus (". . . a parasitic microorganism considerably smaller than most bacteria, which is capable of multiplication only within living susceptible host cells") was "elastic enough to allow one to include or exclude the rickettsial and psittacosis-type organisms as circumstances require!" He envisaged viruses as presenting "an unbroken series, proceeding from the smallest and simplest to the largest and most complex, and from them to the rickettsia", with no sign of fundamental difference between the members of this series. The viruses evolve, in his view, from a series of mutations by loss of power of chemical synthesis associated with progressive adaptation to an environment (intracellular) in which such ability is not required for survival. The existent viruses represent various stages on this path. The virus picture must be "fitted into the pattern of evolutionary change that has been worked out for higher organisms . . ." Work still to be done will, he thought, probably show that protein synthesis, a strictly biological activity, will eventually be understood in terms of replica production by subcellular, essentially living entities. "The production of virus protein in the infected cell will then represent only one special example of protein synthesis in general." The material atoms and the energy necessary for replica production are drawn in some way from the metabolic activities of the cell.

The concept that emphasizes the nonliving nature of virus and dependence upon host-cell mechansims for virus multiplication also goes back practically to the time of "discovery" of virus and has been associated chiefly with work on plant, bacterial and a few animal viruses, largely with the chicken tumor virus. There is not a great deal left of the thoroughgoing "lifeless chemical" theory of virus, little tendency to revive what Francis, 1948, called "the battered corpse of spontaneous generation". Woods, 1899, believed virus to be an oxidizing enzyme; Twort, some fifteen years later, suggested among other possibilities that bacteriophage virus might be an enzyme with capacity for propagation; Vinson and other plant virus workers (who from the beginning have emphasized the chemical nature of virus) suggested, 1931, that virus might be a lifeless chemical, an autocatalytic protein of ultimate host-cell origin. Work on the chicken sarcoma virus suggested, as previously indicated, that it might have intrinsic origin in the host cell. During the thirties, several workers (Krueger, Northrop) explored two hypotheses long associated with the work on bacteriophage: first, that virus multiplication results from autocatalytic transformation, by infecting virus, of a precursor (proteinogen) that exists in the host cell prior to infection; and, secondly, a modification of this hypothesis, suggesting that a trace of precursor (proteinogen) in the host cell is synthesized in increasing amounts after infection by progressive conversion of the original supply of proteinogen to virus. Recent work on purified preparations of bacteriophage viruses (chiefly $T_2$ strain), exploring the influence of the entering virus on host-cell mechanisms has tended to change the perspective of the old controversy regarding invading microorganism and host-cell mechanisms of protein synthesis. Most of this work has been focused on desoxyribonucleic acid the presence of which in bacteriophage Hershey characterized, 1952, as reinforcing the notion "that a virus particle possesses the minimum of genetic and reproductive functions".

Using radioactive markers (incorporated in bacteriophage virus, in bacterial host-cell components, in elements of the medium on which the bacterial host cell draws for synthesis of its own substance, especially of protein and nucleic acids) various workers have sought in the virus and in the materials and synthetic mechanisms of the host cell to discover the sources of desoxyribonucleic acid from which "progeny" virus are formed during intracellular multiplication. Cohen observed, 1946, that when bacterial cells were infected with bacteriophage virus they synthesized three times as much of the virus type nucleic acid as of ribonucleic acid which had dominated in the host cell before virus invasion. Since bacteriophage (and other viruses) are not conclusively known to possess enzymes for synthesis of their own materials, these experiments "strongly suggested" to Cohen (1947; 1953) that "a host is prevailed upon to supply the metabolic enzymatic equipment and energy supply for the multiplication of the virus which invades it". Cohen concluded that a generalization emerges from which virus may be defined as "a parasite which organizes a specific enzymatic environment for its own multiplication". Reflecting prevailing theories on the mechanism of duplication of genes, antibodies, adaptive enzymes, viruses, he suggested (1947; 1953) that virus is not a self-duplicating substance but that on entrance into the cell the virus nucleic acid provides a model (template) followed by the host cell which is thus diverted from synthesis of its own type of nucleic acid to synthesis of viral type nucleic acid.

Many parallels have been drawn between virus and gene, emphasizing in varying degrees similarities in size, protein nature, biological capacity for duplication. Geneticists, Francis pointed out, 1948, have been attracted "by the analogies which exist in the problem of the gene and its method of multiplication, reduplication and aberration". It has been suggested that viruses may be particles escaped from the nucleus; more recently (with the developing biological and medical interest in extra-nuclear particles) that they may be aberrant or mutant cytoplasmic particles capable of continuing reproduction independently of the nucleus or dependent only on the cytoplasmic substance for production. Lauffer, Price and Petre, 1949, considered it increasingly clear that viruses are not like genes themselves but may resemble

groups of genes, such as may be found in the fragment of a chromosome. Kunkel pointed out, 1947, that whereas multiplication of genes
ordinarily is not faster than rates of nuclear division, viruses far exceed
those rates; that viruses pass from cell to cell, while genes do not
(except from sperm to ovum during fertilization); dividing (growing)
somatic cells simply begin with a full complement of genes exactly
like those of the parent cell: "viruses are autonomous; genes are part
of the hereditary mechanism. A gene represents a single factor in
reproduction and may be of simple structure. A virus, like that of
tobacco mosaic, which has been shown to carry a series of factors
capable of varying independently in mutations, must possess sufficient
organization to permit such variety. In this respect tobacco mosaic
behaves more like a chromosome than a gene." Beard, 1948, found
"no evidence confirming the belief that viruses may represent or be
similar to genes". J. H. Mueller observed, 1945, that perhaps the
"crucial difference" between the transplanted gene and the smallest
virus may lie in the specificity of the protein which is present in the
virus or to which the transplanted gene probably attaches itself in the
cell. "In the one case the protein heterologous to the cell renders the
particle a completely foreign parasitic molecule which eventually becomes injurious as it accumulates. In the other instance, the cell's
own protein combines with the new nucleic acid, and the resulting
homologous nucleoprotein takes its place in the normal economy of
the cell and confers a new property upon it."

It is in the "cancer viruses" that C. D. Darlington, 1944, found close
comparison with the plasmagene, the ultimate distinction between
them being "the accidental one of transmission by heredity or by
infection", both having a high frequency of mutations. He suggested
that mutations may make plasmagenes pathogenic or that plasmagenes
in the wrong host may be viruses. Alexander Haddow of the Royal
Cancer Hospital in London, 1944, observed that in certain cases
"similarity of behavior becomes identity", and that, for the Rous
agent at least, no real distinction can be drawn between its typical
activity and that of a mutant plastogene. T. M. Sonneborn, 1946, in
Indiana University's zoology department (investigating plasmagene
action in certain strains of paramecia), described as "amazingly like
that of the viruses" the behavior of a cytoplasmic factor or plasmagene

(known as Kappa) inherited cytoplasmically independently of the nuclear constitution of this single cell protozoan.  It resembles the gene in determination of a hereditary unit, in self-duplication, in chemical composition, in mutability.  It differs from the gene, however, in various respects: in its location (cytoplasm); in occurring in large numbers in the cell; in its multiplication and distribution in the cell independently of cell division.  The Kappa factor, capable of killing other strains, was compared to a virus by Rhoads, 1952, who saw encouragement in the demonstration that Kappa can be killed selectively within the cells.  Burnet, 1950, said that the possibility that virus-like agents might arise within cells without previous infection requires "more serious consideration in the light of the plasmagene concept which may find a place in the elucidation of the cancer viruses", a problem of the first importance for the future.

Occurrences of apparently spontaneous origin of animal viruses are almost unheard of in G. M. Findlay's view, expressed, 1946, at a meeting in England of the Society for General Microbiology.  If such spontaneous origin were possible, why, he asked, does it not occur when viruses are eliminated from a population by destruction or quarantine.  He cited the fact that quarantine had been of undeniable efficiency in keeping out such viruses as rabies, foot-and-mouth disease and rinderpest as evidence that these gave no sign of arising *de novo* in fresh hosts.  G. W. Beadle's concept, 1945, arrived at by genetic studies on *Neurospora*, implies a similarity between genes and the enzymes through which their action is mediated; the genes produce replicas of themselves and also "partial replicas" which pass into the cytoplasm and produce the functioning enzymes.  Ludwik Monné's concept of "purposefulness" inherent in the organization of living substance (which, if severely disturbed, is replaced by nonpurposeful and detrimental processes — disease) envisaged, 1948, as the ultimate units of life not the cell, which is "an organized system of several types of self-perpetuating nucleic-acid-containing bodies", but these bodies which include genes, microsomes, viruses.  He regarded the simplest viruses (pure nucleoprotein) as the simplest form of protoplasm, and the more complex viruses (the more highly organized vaccinia, for example) as comparable to cytoplasmic fibrils and chromosomes which are organized units made up of the ultimate units.  These ultimate units contain all the nucleic acid, which is not diffusely distributed and which increases in all kinds of cells during growth. In rapidly growing cells, the synthetic power of the nucleoproteins prevails, and in disintegrating cells the hydrolyzing power of nucleoproteins prevails. In organized protoplasm, according to Monné, nucleic-acid-containing elements, the self-perpetuating granules (viruses, genes, chromidia) are arranged into self-perpetuating fibrils (such as chromosomes) and these are arranged into self-perpetuating cells.

It is clear that the views of most fundamental virus workers, whatever their particular slant, recognize, as one worker put it more than a decade ago, the need of "some broader and more flexible explanation" than either the microorganism or the autocatalytic enzyme theory, and at least envisage the possibility that viruses, in Northrop's words, may "bridge the gap between free-living bacterial cells and the simplest chemical structure carrying the vital impulse to divide. . . ." For the virus, according to Mueller, while deficient in many of the functions essential to growth and reproduction is "living" in the sense that it divides when placed in a suitable environment. In his chemical, medical and philosophical concepts of virus, already frequently mentioned, Stanley invoked Aristotle's suggestion that nature makes so gradual a transition from the nonliving to the living that the boundary line is doubtful, possibly nonexistent. The problem resembles an attempt to determine the exact point at which one color blends into another in a color spectrum; or an attempt to establish just where acid becomes alkaline. One can, of course, set up arbitrary points of division but the difference is still a matter less of fundamental nature than of degree. "I believe that the work on viruses has provided us with new reasons for considering that life as we know it owes its existence to a specific state of matter and that the principle of the vital phenomenon does not come into existence suddenly but is inherent in all matter." William Seifriz of Pennsylvania's botany department, in some of his discussions of protoplasm, pointed out that reactions which we are in the habit of associating with living things are, upon analysis, often found to be characteristic of nonliving systems as well. Charcoal, for instance, "respires", crystals "grow", a kind of "memory" exists in jellies where a previous event determines present action. We can distinguish living matter from nonliving only by selecting a number of properties all of which living matter possesses, but only one or two of which are possessed at a time by any one nonliving system. It is, in Seifriz's view, a question of complexity; and it is in this sense that viruses may constitute "a link between the living and the nonliving".

# CHARACTERISTICS OF VIRUSES AND THEIR BEHAVIOR IN THE CELL

## Progress in Cultivation of Viruses

Since investigative work on the physical qualities, chemical composition and behavior of virus in the cell depends upon the availability of a sufficiently large quantity in relatively pure form, work on cultivation of viruses has been considered a strategic prerequisite to analysis of their intrinsic properties. Cox pointed out that since the chick embryo has not been proved to be a natural carrier of any virus infection and since the embryo cannot produce antibody, the statement of Beveridge and Burnet, 1946, that this method more closely resembles test tube cultivation of bacteria than it does animal inoculation is still valid. By 1952, Cox noted that with a few exceptions practically all of the known viruses affecting animals and man had been propagated in one or another of the tissues of the developing chick embryo, some multiplying in all, others only or better in one. Twelve viruses were described as multiplying readily on the chorio-allantoic membrane and producing easily visible foci, nine as multiplying but producing only weak foci or requiring adaptation to produce them; five viruses, including measles and rabies, were listed as multiplying without causing lesions; eight viruses (including mumps, influenza, Newcastle disease) as multiplying readily in the allantoic sac. Of these, sixteen have been cultivated for production of live or killed vaccines. More recent additions to the list include the viruses of atypical pneumonia (1944), foot-and-mouth disease (1948), mumps (1945), dengue (1950), infectious hepatitis (1950), Lansing type poliomyelitis (1952).

The other method of propagation, tissue culture, originated as did the chick embryo method in embryological work in biology. Marked advances in propagation of viruses in tissue culture date from development by Maitland and Maitland in England (1928) of methods and media leading (with some modification) to cultivation of a number of viruses. The previously mentioned propagation of the three known types of poliomyelitis virus in non-neural tissues of the human embryo by tissue culture methods, stimulated intensive research on tissue culture methods of propagating these viruses in various centers (Harvard, Minnesota, Toronto, Western Reserve, Oregon, Duke, Yale) and on viruses that have thus far resisted cultivation. Impetus was given to research on many especial poliomyelitis problems: development of rapid methods for diagnosis; study of strain differences. Other studies have been directed toward development of a homogeneous host population of animal cells in which relation of virus particle to host cell may be critically analyzed by the quantitative and genetic methods that have stimulated research on these problems with bacteriophage since 1940. Tools for a similar attack on animal viruses have only recently become available through work of investigators long primarily concerned with behavior of cells in tissue culture (among others, G. O. Gey, Johns Hopkins; W. R. Earle, National Cancer Institute). By development of a "pure" line of a single type of mammalian cell (Gey), a host-cell population for study of animal viruses has been provided that compares favorably in homogeneity and "purity" with the bacterial populations advantageously used in bacteriophage work (Younger, 1953). A technique developed (Dulbecco and Marguerite Vogt, 1953) for isolation and maintenance of single virus particles and their progeny opened the way for genetic studies not heretofore possible for animal viruses and for investigations of biological properties of animal viruses which up to 1953 could be studied only indirectly by their effects on animal and human hosts.

Changes that occur in virulence or pathogenicity of viruses for susceptible hosts in the course of serial passage of viruses in tissues of the chick embryo or in tissue cultures have provided the viruses of modified virulence now used in several vaccines. Both methods are being currently employed to explore a fundamental virus problem, interaction of virus and host cell; tissue culture methods are used in study of the basic problem of the cellular site of virus reproduction and in study of metabolites essential for virus synthesis.

Viruses not (as of 1952) cultivated by either method, or cultivated so rarely or with such difficulty that they were not yet available for laboratory procedures, include those of measles, varicella, rubella, primary atypical pneumonia, common cold, infectious hepatitis, phlebotomus fever, herpes zoster. Progress in cultivation of infectious hepatitis viruses (in the chick embryo and in tissue cultures) was reported, 1950, from the University of Pennsylvania, by the Henles, Stokes and their associates. In September, 1953, Andrewes and his associates in the Common Cold Research Unit published a preliminary report citing evidence that "the common cold virus had been propagated" through ten serial cultures of embryonic human lung tissues; and in 1954, Enders and his associates were applying tissue culture methods in attempts to propagate the measles virus.

## PURIFICATION OF VIRUSES

By 1952, the number of viruses that had been sufficiently purified to make possible elementary chemical analyses did not exceed twenty. Rivers, 1952, thought it probable that fifty, possibly up to ninety, per cent of the preparations advanced as purified contain impurities. Bawden, 1952, characterized some of the purified preparations of plant viruses as "demonstrably mixtures of infective and noninfective nucleoproteins". The purest preparations of virus by available physical and chemical tests may, according to Andrewes, "still be far from homogeneous" by the more sensitive biological techniques. Animal viruses are so intimately bound to the cells on which their multiplication depends that separation, especially of the smallest, has been described as a "formidable task". Indeed, the inability of expert investigators to separate influenza virus completely from host protein has given rise to the hypothesis (Wilson Smith, 1952) that the host protein may be built into the virus in the infected cell, serving as a framework that alters both the structure and the virulence of subsequently formed virus following this model. The properties of some of the tissue substances (notably protein components usually, according to Stanley and Lauffer, 1952, carried down in such preparations) so closely resemble viruses as to confuse estimations of virus size and weight; some such estimations have later been shown to be or to include measurements of the tissue contaminant. The approach to purification of animal viruses is in transition, according to Joel Warren and associates, 1949, through broadening methodology, involving the electric drive centrifuge, chromatography, ion exchange resins, radioactive tracers, replicas for electron microscopy, the micro-complement-fixation test, digestion with crystalline enzymes and methods of cytochemistry. Warren, 1950, noted progress (at differing levels of achievement) in purification of thirteen viruses on the basis of the work reported between 1932 and 1949: vaccinia, rabbit papilloma, influenza A, influenza B, swine influenza, eastern equine encephalomyelitis, murine encephalomyelitis, Columbia SK, polio-myelitis (Lansing), Newcastle disease, mumps, Japanese encephalitis, encephalomyocarditis. In addition, certain types of bacteriophage have been described in purified form. In November, 1953, Stanley announced that Lansing type poliomyelitis virus had been purified to the extent that it has up to 20,000 times the infective power of the original infected tissue; the same methods were expected to result in similar purification of the other two poliomyelitis types in Stanley's laboratory.

## Physical and Chemical Properties of Virus

It has been frequently stressed that no one property may yet be taken as a single virus criterion. Establishment of protein structure in virus does not, for instance, as Stanley pointed out, define virus since protein structure is attributable also to hormones, enzymes, toxins, respiratory materials and perhaps genes; since "practically nothing is known about protein structure, the addition of viruses to this diverse group aided but little in the establishment of their true nature". No one of the physical properties — size, shape, density, weight — has been found to constitute a valid criterion of virus character. In size, for instance (and practically every known virus has now been measured by ultrafiltration, ultracentrifugation, the electron microscope), viruses range in a continuous spectrum, from the virus of foot-and-mouth disease with a diameter of ten millimicrons to the virus of psittacosis with a diameter of 450 millimicrons (Stanley, 1952). In shape, viruses show no greater uniformity; they may be spherical, ovoid, cuboid, sperm-shaped, rod-shaped. Beard, 1951, distinguished certain broad groupings, finding that the plant viruses, with one exception, are spheres or long rods, the bacterial viruses are chiefly tadpole-shaped, animal viruses vary from spheres to tadpole shapes, insect viruses (with the exception of one group that is tadpole-shaped) are (Bergold, 1953) chiefly rod-shaped.  Robley C. Williams, of Stanley's laboratory, after using improved methods of microscopy, 1952, considered it "most probable that the intact particle of tobacco mosaic virus is that of an elongated hexagonal prism".  It has been observed that this is the first time an individual virus has been found to have external crystalline shape suggesting that it grows in molecular form and that its structure is not accidental.  Williams, Stanley and Schwerdt, 1953, described purified particles of Lansing type poliomyelitis as spherical in shape with a diameter of approximately one ten-millionth of an inch.  Williams emphasized the significance for theories of virus multiplication of the physical characteristics reported from such studies on the ground that any acceptable hypothesis about modes of reproduction must explain why particles of the tobacco mosaic virus are shaped "like lead pencils with constant diameter and uniform length", while influenza virus is "approximately spherical and non-uniform in diameter".

Relatively few virus preparations have thus far been obtained in sufficiently high purity to permit dependable analysis of their chemical composition.  Results of elementary analyses of different viruses have often been very similar, apparently (Stanley, 1952) because "many viruses are nucleoproteins".  Stanley compared, 1943, the exacting task of analyzing tobacco mosaic nucleoprotein to an attempt to learn "the inner workings and structural details of the Empire State Building by means of casual inspection", the first step being to take apart the structure and learn the number and kind of the various building materials.  Ordinary proteins (none of which so far has yielded to complete analysis or to more than theoretical blueprints of structure) vary in molecular weight from thirty to a few hundred thousand; tobacco mosaic nucleoprotein has a molecular weight of about fifty millions, and is a conjugated protein in which the six per cent nucleic acid is attached as a prosthetic group to the ninety-four per cent protein moiety.  The tobacco mosaic nucleoprotein is, moreover, of relatively simple structure compared with the animal viruses.  How far from adequate as yet are some of the methods for separating virus components is suggested by Stanley's 1952 reference to the degree to which the "rather drastic" methods employed to secure the nucleic acid components of viruses probably alter most of these preparations, nucleic acid of tobacco mosaic virus giving a molecular weight of about 15,000 when obtained by one method, and about 300,000 when obtained by another.

The finding in Stanley's earlier studies that, although all strains of tobacco mosaic studied contained the same amount of nucleic acid, they possessed different chemical properties, led to a search to determine whether the chemical differences between the strains might reside in the protein components.  Studies of amino acid composition of purified preparations of tobacco mosaic protein, begun by Stanley and Ross, 1939, were supplemented by improved methods of analysis applied by Knight, 1942 to 1948.  Analysis of eight strains of tobacco mosaic protein with reference to sixteen amino acids led Stanley to conclude, 1946, "the mutation of a virus can be accompanied by changes in the amount of one or more amino acids, by the introduction of a new amino acid, or by the elimination of an amino acid".  Slight differences in chemical composition affecting structure could be accompanied by marked changes in virulence.  Summarizing amino acid determinations on purified preparations of the PR8 strain of influenza A, and the Lee strain of influenza B, Knight, 1947, reported that while the two strains contained approximately equal amounts of twelve amino acids, significant and characteristic differences occurred in the amounts of five others.  Stanley raised the question, 1948, whether these differences might be partly responsible for lack of immunologic relationship between the strains; for different pH stability ranges shown by Miller, 1944; for difference in red cell agglutinating capacities shown by Knight, 1946; for widely divergent heat stabilities reported by Salk, 1946.  While not overestimating the value of these merely preliminary results on amino acid composition, Stanley observed, 1948, that mutation of a virus to form a new virus strain is "not so mysterious as it was a few years ago".

Other viruses that have been analyzed for these recognizable components include, besides several other plant viruses, rabbit papilloma, equine encephalomyelitis, Newcastle disease, $T_2$ bacteriophage and vaccinia. Observing that the viruses of all types investigated thus far "possess the chemical common denominator of nucleic acid and protein", Knight, 1950, thought the most consistent difference between animal and plant viruses to be absence of lipid from plant viruses, and "invariable association" of lipid with animal viruses; of the animal viruses investigated, "the Shope papilloma virus most closely resembles the plant viruses in composition since it is almost solely nucleoprotein".

That nucleic acids have been found in all viruses thus far examined "cannot be ignored" (Stanley and Lauffer, 1952). Indirect evidence of various kinds of the biological importance of nucleic acids includes indications that they are essential elements in the chemical mechanisms of cell division and growth, of heredity, and in the nature and growth of viruses and in inheritance, at least of bacteriophage. By 1945, according to W. T. Astbury (University of Leeds) study of the nucleic acids had arrived at only "a blurred recognition of their status". Since 1950, progress has been rapid in examination of their external structure, by X ray (Astbury and associates since 1936; M. H. F. Wilkins, R. F. Franklin and associates, King's College, London), by electron microscopy (S. Furberg in Sweden; Robley C. Williams, California); in their chemical analysis (Alexander R. Todd, Cambridge University; Erwin Chargaff, Columbia). Models of the internal structure of nucleic acids, in the sense of spatial arrangements of atoms within the molecule, were proposed, 1953, by Linus Pauling (on the basis of studies of protein structure, since 1936), by J. D. Watson and F. H. C. Crick (Cambridge University), in 1954, by Watson with Alexander Rich (National Institutes of Health).

Study of the physical and chemical properties of viruses is in a manner preliminary, looking toward study of their biological properties, as their capacity to multiply in living cells, their host range, their specificity for certain tissues, certain cells, their capacity to agglutinate erythrocytes, their antigenic constitution, their immunologic properties, their capacity for variation, their virulence. In invasiveness and virulence are involved not only the above-mentioned properties of viruses but also the metabolic peculiarities of host cells, which live by virtue of a "complex symbiotic equilibrium" of their intracellular components, largely nucleoprotein, including genes, mitochrondria, enzymes (Pinkerton, 1952). These cellular properties may be a suitable environment for an invading virus which by its growth may injure the cell and start a process ending in disease, or these same properties may be a defense against some invaders, not others. Degree of infectivity — whether by virus, bacterium, or other infective agent — is determined by balance between "devices of aggression of an agent and mechanism of host defense" (Maxcy, 1952). Investigation of virus infectivity thus rests upon the principles that govern the processes of parasitism, whatever the infecting agent.

## THE NATURE OF VIRULENCE AND THE MECHANISM OF INFECTION

Andrewes, 1947, projected a process by which "in the simplest conception", the "ideal perfectly virulent virus", if unimpeded, reaches a susceptible cell, multiplies in it rapidly, disrupts it and is effectively conveyed to other susceptible cells, the result being maximum damage to the host. He pointed out, as have others, that it is not certain whether mere rapid mass-production of virus particles is enough to make a virus virulent. Direct destruction of the infected cells must be important. Possibly also the presence of dead or less perfectly adapted virus particles may slow down the whole proccss. Lauffer, Price and Petre, 1949, regarded as primary the question whether all the particles of which a virus is made up are active, whether one of them "if active and favorably situated with respect to the host" can induce infection or whether more than one must be present. In their view, only one particle is required. Bryan and Beard thought that the required number of particles is variable, "depending upon the susceptibility of the host". Luria, 1950, thought it safe to assume that the material carrying virus activity is differently organized in its intracellular, replicating dynamic state and in the extracellular, static condition. For this reason he thought it unlikely that even intensive work on properties of extracellular virus particles could "throw much light on the fundamental problem of virology: virus reproduction. The limitation appears to be an operational one — the alteration, upon infection, of the very properties that the physicochemist analyzes."

Some workers (as Wilson Smith, 1951) have felt that "undue preoccupation" with virus particles as the seat of infectivity has, over the years, resulted in neglect of other biological virus properties influencing virulence. Howe, 1952, discussing newer knowledge of poliomyelitis, observed: "It is now apparent that differences in virulence are independent of antigenic type." Andrewes mentioned, among factors that may affect virulence, differences in the lethal dose; affinity for certain tissues or organs (if poliomyelitis attacks the medulla, the disease is more frequently fatal); differences among the neurotropic viruses in ability to reach the central nervous system from the periphery (tissue culture may change the properties of a virus so that it can no longer pass to the central nervous system and kill); aptitude for synergism with secondary bacterial invaders (the influenza pandemic of 1918); changes in antigenic constitution (in the case of a community that has a certain level of resistance to, for instance, influenza virus, a mutation affecting the antigenic structure of the virus may render it capable of attacking people immune to ordinary strains. Smith, on the basis of his own work with 1951 influenza strains, as well as findings by Francis, 1947, of changed biological behavior of certain influenza virus strains when heated, advanced, 1952, the hypothesis that differences in virus architecture may play a dominant part in virulence, and that changes in virulence of strains with supposedly stable antigens may result from a change in growth environment (including either changes of host species or of host tissues) through effects on the surface architecture of virus, the change deriving from the host protein in the course of virus duplication with consequent enhancement of virulence. The mechanisms responsible for modification of virulence that follows passing of certain virulent strains through animals, chick embryo tissues, or tissue culture (a procedure valuable in securing variants for vaccines) have not yet been clarified, although the view that such passage in some way provides an environment that favors propagation of a chance mutant has recently gained ground. While, as Enders observed, 1952, "the production at will of pathogenically modified variants is not yet feasible", the possibility that strain modifications may ultimately be controlled and beneficently directed is a research objective. The finding that virus virulence can remain constant for one plant host but be modified with respect to a different host upon formation of a given chemical derivative of the virus led Stanley, 1946, to express the hope that eventually heritable structural changes in a virus will be achieved by means of known chemical reactions. The undesirability of depending upon chance mutations for modified strains needed for vaccines should, he thought, stimulate work on chemical modification through alterations in structure.

The influence of host "spreading factors" in infection generally, whatever the agent, is pertinent in virus investigation. Spreading factors were indeed discovered, 1928, by Duran-Reynals, in a study of the effects of spreading factors contained in testicular extracts on a typical virus, vaccinia. The spreading factors, acting upon the ground substance or mesenchyme, are considered to determine whether, after an infective agent, virus or other, has passed the portal of entry, the infection remains localized or becomes disseminated. In bacterial infections, according to D. H. Sprunt, 1950, spreading of the infection through the ground substance and thence to organs and the circulation may actually decrease the chance of establishing infection; spreading of viruses, however, according to Duran-Reynals, 1942, always enhances the infection, a view supported by Sprunt, who explained his experiments as indicating that spread of a virus increases the chance of its contact with a susceptible cell, which it enters immediately. The mechanism of the spreading process in infection has been described as action of the enzyme hyaluronidase in liquefying and destroying the function of hyaluronic acid, a mucopolysaccharide of the connective tissues. That function is to bind water in the interstitial spaces, help hold cells together, be permeable to metabolites, and, even more importantly, according to M. Stacey, 1946, to offer "resistance to penetration by foreign matter including agents of infectious disease". The effective agent in destroying these functions, hyaluronidase, has been found in extracts derived from certain bacteria and venoms, but whether viruses produce hyaluronidase, as do, for instance, hemolytic streptococci, has not been established.

## INVESTIGATIVE APPROACHES TO THE HOST CELL-VIRUS RELATION

### NATURE OF THE HOST CELL-VIRUS RELATION

"What we need to understand", Burnet pointed out, 1950, is that "delicate balance within the cell which determines whether or not an entrant virus will flourish." Beard, 1948, compared the considerable progress made in understanding the virus outside the cell with the little known of "the processes within the cell where the relatively inert particle enters the enormously dynamic stage of reproduction and growth". Certainly, there is no easy, constant, simple story of how the virus behaves within the cell, what it does to the metabolic mechanisms of the cell or what such mechanisms do to the virus. Differences already mentioned in the viruses, in the cells and tissues which they parasitize in differing degrees, in the infecting dose (unknown in the natural disease unless it causes death and permits some assumptions from observed tissue damage, varying widely even in experiments with the same virus, the same animals), and many other factors complicate the host cell-virus story. Illustrating the wide variation in known effects produced by viruses in the cells which they select, Francis, 1948, observed: "Yellow fever virus destroys hepatic parenchymal cells, poliomyelitis virus destroys the motor cells of the spinal cord, influenza virus destroys the epithelium of the respiratory tract, encephalitic viruses destroy ganglionic cells of the brain." The viruses causing chicken tumors may act upon cartilage, bone, connective tissue. Illustrations of known variation in effects could be greatly extended.

Almost twenty-five years ago, Rivers had summarized three primary pathologic changes in virus diseases, hyperplasia alone, hyperplasia followed by necrosis, necrosis alone. "The balance between the stimulative and destructive tendencies of a virus determines whether hyperplasia alone or necrosis is the predominant part of the pathologic picture." In 1952 he observed that virus tumors in animals (Shope's papilloma and Rous's sarcoma), in which chiefly proliferation and progressive multiplication of cells occur, are at one end of the spectrum; at the other end are those virus diseases in which the infected cells are incapable of multiplication (nerve cells or neurons), and in which the first evidence of infection is lysis of infected cells (rabies, poliomyelitis, louping ill). In other viral diseases (Rift Valley fever, yellow fever, foot-and-mouth disease) the active agents produce their effects so rapidly that there is insufficient time for hyperplasia to occur, "or, if it does, it plays a minor role in the picture". He referred in 1952 to the still "lengthy discussions" as to whether inflammation is a primary response to the presence of virus or is rather secondary to cellular injury. From direct observations made possible by electron microscopic studies, Frederik Bang, 1952, described three general differences of cellular reactions to specific viruses: "(1) Certain viruses, influenza and Newcastle viruses in particular, may so alter the surface of some cells that a variety of spicules replace and/or dominate the normal microvilli. Virus may be released into the allantoic fluid through this process. (2) Certain other viruses characteristically cause a ballooning of both cytoplasm and mitochondria with subsequent degeneration of the latter. (3) Smaller viruses, such as encephalitis, may destroy cells by a piecemeal effort, with no visible general effect on the cell, and then proceed as if by replacement of the ground substance."

About half of the sixty known or suspected virus diseases of man are associated with development of structures, inclusion bodies, which are hallmarks of the specific agent and some of which, as the Negri bodies of rabies, are diagnostic criteria. Some inclusions appear in the nucleus, some in the cytoplasm, a few in both. Their nature, "not well known" (Rivers, 1952), has been an objective of renewed investigation by modern methods (cytochemistry and electron microscopy) as in the above-mentioned studies of Bang with G. O. Gey, at Johns Hopkins. Use of these methods led Scott and associates, on the basis of studies of the intranuclear inclusion body of herpes simplex, to describe, 1952, the inclusion body as a "dynamic occurrence" rather than a pathological end result of viral activity. Pinkerton, 1952, referred to these bodies as "the most obvious indication of disturbed intracellular metabolism", and thus a logical starting point for study of the complex biochemical lesions caused by viruses. He considered it "not clear" whether the substance of such bodies derives from virus or host cell; he thought it likely that a part might be derived from the metabolic pool on which the cell draws for normal synthetic activities, one of the several hypotheses currently advanced to explain the intracellular mechanisms responsible for virus growth generally.

Referring to only two of the various hypotheses as to what the interaction between cell and virus may be, Francis queried, 1947: "Is it a specific enzymatic reaction of the virus with a cellular substrate ordinarily required for the cell's maintenance, thus diverting to the use of the parasite an essential metabolite of the cell?  Is it a disturbance of one or more of the genes of the cell, even to the extent of promoting a lethal gene?"  To these he might have added, on the basis of recent work with influenza, is the reaction between the virus and the cell surface always a part, the initial step, in invasion?  Or is it a normal metabolic process within the cell diverted from its usual course by multiplying not the normally existing protein within the cell but the protein particle provided by the invading virus?  Other hypotheses offer different combinations of the possibilities — and additions to them.  Host-virus relationships range, various workers have suggested, from a type of parasitism which results in the death of a cell to an equilibrium in which cell and virus survive together for a period.  Biochemical studies of infected host cells and tissues seeking the mechanisms involved in the host cell-virus relation include: those of Ackermann and Francis, 1950, aimed at clarifying "some of the biochemical changes which characterize the host tissue" during herpes infection by measuring "the rate of growth of the tissues, of two of the respiratory enzyme systems, of changes in the nucleic acid composition, and of the protein content"; work on experimental influenza, by Burnet's group, 1951, the result of which seemed to indicate two major steps in initiation of infection by influenza virus, "(1) physical adsorption between two complementary surfaces of colloid dimensions (the virus particle and the cellular 'receptor area') — something like an antigen-antibody combination; (2) ingestion of the adsorbed virus by the cell (viropexis) — something like phagocytosis."  Current research, especially in laboratories employing bacteriophage and influenza as models for study of host-virus relations, is directed to analysis of five steps in the relation of the virus to its host cell: attachment of the virus to the cell, penetration, a latent stage during which the virus cannot be detected and during a part of which it has been demonstrated to be noninfectious (in bacteriophage), growth or multiplication of the virus, emergence of the fresh virus.  Knowledge of these five stages is as uneven as the amount of investigative interest thus far accorded each.  Current interest is marked in the third, or latent, stage, most fully demonstrated for bacteriophage but also reported for influenza (Hoyle, 1948; Henle, 1949), vaccinia and mouse encephalomyelitis viruses (F. K. Sanders, 1952), pneumonia virus of mice and mumps virus (Horsfall, 1950), western equine encephalomyelitis virus (Schlesinger, 1951) and other viruses. Sanders, 1952, raised the question whether loss of infectivity of vaccinia virus during the latent period might be associated with loss of nucleic acid from the entering virus particle, resumption of infectivity appearing only with the addition of nucleic acid when newly formed virus particles are being completed toward the end of the intracellular phase. The experiments with bacteriophage (Hershey; Anderson; Herriott; Stent; others), however, suggested that the addition of infectivity may wait on protein synthesis and that its loss during the latent period of bacteriophage may be explained by the fact that on entry into the host cell, bacteriophage virus leaves its protein "coat" behind. To the protein component of the virus is attributed the first step of virus invasion: attachment of the bacteriophage to the host cell. Dalldorf, 1950, in expressing the view of various leading workers that adsorption of virus — the union of virus with cell — is "quick and final", referred to the 1935 finding of Rous's group that isolated cells mixed with vaccinia and fibroma viruses "combined so quickly it was impossible to mix and separate". In intensive investigation of the mechanism of adsorption of viruses, the hemagglutination phenomenon (the adsorption of virus, especially influenza virus, onto red corpuscles) has proved a powerful tool.

## THE HEMAGGLUTINATING PROPERTY OF VIRUSES IN STUDY OF CELL-VIRUS RELATIONS

More than ten years' study of influenza virus with its capacity to agglutinate red blood cells has revealed that the first step in the process of cellular infection by influenza and related viruses is "the interaction of the virus with certain cell-surface components of mucoprotein or mucopolysaccharide character" (Burnet, 1951). When suspensions of red cells are mixed with virus and allowed to stand, the virus is first adsorbed by the red cells which are then agglutinated in visible red-cell clumps; after several hours the combination undergoes spontaneous separation and the virus is eluted. This virus property — in the form of capacity of influenza viruses to agglutinate red blood cells of chickens — was discovered, 1941, by Hirst in this country, independently by Hare and McClelland in Canada, and subsequently found to apply to the red cells of at least twenty-two animal species. Although each virus has its own "spectrum" of the various species of red cells which it will agglutinate, the hemagglutination reaction is the same for all viruses for which it has been demonstrated. Expanding study of the phenomenon may lead to much wider implications than are at present justified. At present virus hemagglutination has been studied largely *in vitro* as a model of the mechanism of union of virus particles with host cells. An example of possible wider implications was the suggestion of Moolten and Clark, 1952, that the red blood cell may be a vehicle of virus transport from the portal of entry to the tissue of predilection, and (on the basis of isolation of several viruses from patients manifesting autohemagglutination or acquired hemolytic anemia) that serological procedures involving red cell agglutination may be a practical means for rapid detection of viremia (preclinical infections, healthy carriers). At present, however, the major focus of investigative work is the mechanism of the attachment of virus to cell in the hope that it will shed light on the mechanism by which host cells are infected, by clarifying the nature of the hemagglutinin and of the cell substance with which the virus unites. Hirst, 1952, characterized the mechanism as "obscure" and probably different for different groups of viruses. On the basis of present (rapidly changing) knowledge, viruses fall into three tentative groups with reference to hemagglutination: the influenza, mumps, Newcastle group (in which hemagglutination is considered a property of the intact particle of virus); the variola, vaccinia, ectromelia, meningopneumonitis group (in which the hemagglutinin is separable from the intact virus particle); a third group (requiring rather exacting laboratory conditions to demonstrate hemagglutination which apparently occurs with only a few species of cells for each virus) including certain neurotropic viruses (Japanese B, St. Louis, Russian spring-summer encephalitis; the encephalomyocarditis group, mouse encephalomyelitis, West Nile fever), mouse pneumonitis, fowl plague, foot-and-mouth disease.

Studies and theories explaining the mechanism of virus-cell union refer chiefly to the influenza, mumps, Newcastle group. Viruses of this group, eluted from red blood cells, retain their original capacity to agglutinate fresh red blood cells, but the loss of capacity by the agglutinated red cells to adsorb fresh virus of the same strain or type is "presumably due to the loss of virus receptors". According to Hirst, 1952, this occurrence is best explained "on the assumption that the virus possesses an enzyme which is capable of attacking a surface component of the red cell called the receptor group".

Work concerned with identification of the cell receptor substances and of the receptor-destroying substance of the virus in several laboratories (Burnet, Lind, Horsfall and Hardy, Hirst) suggested that receptor substances for influenza are mucopolysaccharides (Burnet; Hirst, 1952) or polysaccharide-protein complexes (Henle, 1950). Receptor substances, in the case of influenza, have been found not only in red cells of chickens but also in cells susceptible to infection by influenza virus, as in J. D. Stone's demonstration, 1948, that intact receptors were necessary for infection of the chorio-allantoic membrane of the living chick embryo and of the excised mouse lung. The latter experiments, Hirst observed, 1952, indicate that intact receptors on host cells "are probably necessary for or, at least, greatly facilitate influenza infection".

The receptor-destroying substance of the virus was described by Burnet, 1953, as an enzyme. In 1951, on the basis of experiments indicating that mucinous bronchial sputum is actively inhibitory against infection by influenza A (PR8) virus, he suggested that the enzymic activity of the virus may be a mechanism for its release from the respiratory mucin trap. To the question "whether the necessity of an initiating enzyme action on a cell surface component is a prerequisite for the infection of appropriate cells by other viruses", he had answered, 1948, "I feel that this may well be the case and the idea may provide a useful working hypothesis for future research." Hirst, 1952, referred to the function of the receptor-destroying substance of influenza as of especial interest "since it is the only complete enzyme known to be closely associated with a virus". Apart from the specific significance of such an enzyme in the infectious cycle of influenza, the concept is relevant to the biological activity of other viruses: Ludwik Monné, 1948, referred lack of catabolic activity in the simplest viruses to the fact that they contain no enzymes while the more complex viruses (among which he cited vaccinia) contain some enzymes and are, therefore, endowed with "a certain catabolism".

The ability to inhibit the hemagglutination reaction by specific antiserum containing antibodies to the particular strain of influenza virus, first thought to represent a specific immune response against the virus, was found later to be a property shared, in low concentrations of the inhibitor substance, by "almost any tissue suspension" (Hirst, 1952) and in high concentrations by various tissues and body fluids (Burnet and Beveridge, 1945), notably normal red blood cells (Hirst, 1948), human urine. Experiments with influenza virus have shown the inhibitors to be nonspecific (Friedewald, Miller and Whatley, 1947) and mucoprotein (Burnet). Tamm and Horsfall, 1952, described inhibitor substance obtained in a highly purified state from normal human urine as a single homogeneous mucoprotein substance. The demonstration that mucinous bronchial sputum is actively inhibitory against hemagglutination by influenza virus led Burnet to suggest, 1951, that the intact film of mucus over the bronchiolar epithelium may represent a first line of defense against influenza infection. Little is known, however, of the function of inhibitor substances (Hirst, 1952). Recent reports that in the course of influenza infection both inhibitor and cell receptor substances are destroyed (Fazekas de St. Groth, 1950; Schlesinger, 1951; Liu and Henle, 1951) led Hirst to observe, 1952, that it is not yet clear whether the ability of a virus to destroy inhibitors is a factor enabling the virus to free itself from firm combination with mucopolysaccharides in body secretions in order to proceed to susceptible cells (as Burnet suggested), or whether the destruction of host-cell receptors is preliminary to penetration of the cell by the virus. Although it is not clear at what point in the infectious cycle receptor destruction may be important, no one, he pointed out, has yet succeeded in inactivating the receptor-destroying property of a virus without destroying its ability to infect. The concept of blockade or destruction of cell receptors by virus, illustrated by the work on the hemagglutinating property of viruses, has also been invoked as one of several explanations of the capacity of one virus to interfere with the simultaneous propagation of a second virus.

### THE INTERFERENCE PHENOMENON AS AN APPROACH TO INTRA-CELLULAR PROCESSES

As a possible means of throwing light on intracellular processes, various virus workers (Burnet; Schlesinger; Henle; Delbrück; Luria,

Horsfall) have studied the so-called interference phenomenon, by which one virus, or virus strain, "interferes" with the growth of a second virus or virus strain within the cell and, in effect, "protects" the cell against infection with the second virus or second strain. Henle, 1950, stressed the difficulty of knowing "whether the various instances of interference described are all based upon related mechanisms, or whether several entirely different reactions are involved in the various observations". Schlesinger noted that interference in animal viruses may be complete or partial and may occur at various stages in the infectious cycle. Referring to well-known examples of "interference" among animal, plant and bacterial viruses, he emphasized the difficulty of drawing a sharp line between "interference" and "dual infection", of which interference is only a specialized aspect.

The interference phenomenon was first observed in plants: more than twenty years ago, McKinney reported that a yellow mosaic virus would not propagate in tobacco plants in which the common light green mosaic was already present, and several plant workers reported that feebly pathogenic viruses protected a plant from more virulent strains, provided the two strains were generically related. In 1935 Hoskins demonstrated that an intramuscular injection of a neurotropic strain of yellow fever virus (which ordinarily produces little or no obvious disease) could protect animals against simultaneous infection with the highly pathogenic viscerotropic strain. In extending these observations, Findlay and MacCallum concluded (1937) that the interference was not caused by production by the first strain of antibody assumed to protect against the second and they demonstrated this by showing interference between two immunologically unrelated viruses, Rift Valley fever and yellow fever viruses, when introduced simultaneously.

Since that time investigators have multiplied illustrations of interference, demonstrating not only exclusion by one strain of an immunologically related strain (with different tissue tropisms, different degrees of virulence, or different degrees of adaptation to the host in which interference is being demonstrated) but also interference between antigenically unrelated active agents (as mumps excluding western equine encephalomyelitis; yellow fever excluding influenza A); and between active and inactivated virus (as exclusion by inactivated influenza A of active influenza A or B, active mumps, western equine encephalomyelitis). Bodian, 1949, reported interference between virulent Lansing type strains of poliomyelitis and strains of other types. Interference of mouse-adapted strains of human poliomyelitis virus with propagation of simian virus in rhesus monkeys was confirmed by Jungeblut, 1948, who concluded that active, unmodified virus is required and that, since inactivated viruses failed to prevent paralysis, it would not be possible to apply the phenomenon to human prophylaxis. Other illustrations of interference have included: the finding of Findlay and MacCallum (1937) that monkeys inoculated subcutaneously or intraperitoneally with a mixture of neurotropic and pantropic strains of yellow fever usually survive, while control monkeys inoculated with either virus alone usually succumb; apparent interference between fixed virus and street virus in rabies; interference in experimental infection (reported by Dalldorf and Douglass, 1938) between poliomyelitis and canine distemper or lymphocytic choriomeningitis viruses; interference (in man and monkeys) between dengue and yellow fever (Sabin and Theiler, 1944); interference between human and swine influenza viruses (Ziegler and Horsfall, 1944); interference in tissue culture between yellow fever and West Nile, influenza A and Venezuelan equine encephalitis viruses (Lennette and Koprowski, 1946). Since 1944 various workers (Horsfall, referring to influenza, 1952; Delbrück, in connection with bacteriophages; Henle, 1950, and Schlesinger, 1952, referring to various forms of interference) have commented on numerous variables (strains, host species, route of inoculation, virus dosage, timing and amount of challenge virus) that may make generalization difficult. "Which member of the virus pair will grow and which will be excluded depends on the nature of the viruses, on chance, and on the interval of time between the adsorption of the first and the second. . . . At present there is no adequate theory of the mechanisms of these viral interactions" (Hershey and Bronfenbrenner, 1952).

Hypothetical mechanisms of interference include several considered by Jungeblut and Sanders: the possibility (1940) that the first virus exhausts host metabolites needed for propagation of the second; the possibility (1942) that antiviral activities of one virus, or of some product resulting from the primary infection, interferes with multiplication of the second; the possibility that the excluded virus is prevented from spreading by the inflammatory tissue response induced by the interfering agent, a theory that would not be applicable if inactivated virus is employed as the interfering agent.

The question whether interference occurs on the surface or within the cell is raised in several of the theories. The so-called penetration hypothesis of Delbrück, 1945, predicated on the mutual exclusion effect when one cell is simultaneously infected with two serologically related bacteriophages, proposed that the second virus is prevented from penetrating the host cell by changes induced on the cell surface by entrance of the first bacteriophage particle; since subsequent demonstration (Hershey, 1946) that dual infection of one cell by closely related strains of bacteriophage can occur, the penetration theory, according to Henle, 1950, has been abandoned. On evidence obtained in bacteriophage experimentation, C. E. van Rooyen and associates proposed, 1951, that the excluded virus is rapidly broken up after being adsorbed at the surface of the infected cell, and probably never gains entrance. The hypothesis of blockade or destruction of receptors on the cell surface, to which either virus has to become attached in order to gain entrance into the host cell, is based on previously described work on the hemagglutinating property of viruses. Schlesinger, 1951, showed that receptor destruction plays no role in interference between active influenza and equine encephalomyelitis viruses.

Increasing interest, support and work are being directed toward the concept that the mechanism of interference involves not surface components of the host cell but its intracellular metabolic machinery. Illustrative is the theory advanced by Delbrück and Luria, 1942, ascribing interference to competition for a key enzyme system or systems necessary for the synthesis of each of the opposing viruses. J. Fong, 1949, inclined to the view that, "since infection leads first to alterations in the metabolism of the host, it seems likely that the interference phenomenon results from changes in host functions". This view, that the intracellular metabolic system of the host, rather than the cell receptors or the metabolic requirements of the viruses (which may be different), is the major factor upon which the phenomenon of interference depends, was expressed, 1949, by Ginsberg and Horsfall.

Dalldorf, 1950, in referring to his own search for evidence indicating that the phenomenon of interference has epidemiologic importance, noted that Findlay and MacCallum, in reporting interference between Rift Valley fever and yellow fever, mentioned the difference in distribution of the two diseases in Africa. Dalldorf also recalled Stephens's description of an epidemic of atypical pneumonia in an area in which infectious hepatitis was endemic; "no new cases of hepatitis were seen during the epidemic, although they recurred once it ceased". He reported, 1951, that, in epidemics studied during 1947–1949, isolation of Coxsackie viruses had been more frequent where paralytic poliomyelitis had been less frequent. Proof in man being difficult or impossible to secure, results of experiments, using immature (*i.e.*, susceptible to Coxsackie) mice and withholding the challenge dose of poliomyelitis virus for some days, were offered as indicating that "combined infection is less lethal than either alone". Rhodes and Melnick, at the second poliomyelitis conference, rejected the concept of interference between Coxsackie and poliomyelitis viruses.

While work on the interference phenomenon has been significant chiefly for the light it throws on host-virus interrelations and virus multiplication, it could ultimately (Henle, 1950) lead to "immensely practical results". Horsfall found (1950, 1951) that, when an infectious virus is used to produce interference, multiplication of a second virus or of the same virus added anew may be prevented so long as multiplication continues. He proposed, 1952: "Both in plants and animals, the enduring immunity which follows numerous viral infections appears to be more readily explained on this basis than by the presence of specific antibodies . . ." He added as a factor improving the prospect of chemotherapy in virus diseases that interruption of viral multiplication (without inactivation of the virus) within the cell by a few substances could be explained in a similar manner; capsular polysaccharide of *K. pneumonia* specifically interrupts intracellular multiplication of two viruses that show interference, and fails to interrupt multiplication of three that show no interference.

## SYNERGISM OF VIRUS AND BACTERIUM

Perhaps related to the interference phenomenon is combined activity of virus and bacterium, resulting sometimes in aggravated disease. Illustrative of instances in which fellow-traveling bacteria have greatly complicated virus infection is smallpox, the secondary toxic stage of which Burnet, 1944, associated with streptococcal infection of the mucosal lesions and to a lesser extent of the skin pustules. Findlay suggested (1936) that the real difference between alastrim, in which the toxic stage is practically absent, and smallpox may consist less in differences between the viruses than in the presence (in smallpox) or absence (in alastrim) of streptococcal infection. Possible relationship of a nonhemolytic streptococcus, designated MG, with a (possible) viral agent of atypical pneumonia was raised, 1943, by the Rockefeller Institute workers. Horsfall and associates, who isolated this organism from the lungs in fatal cases, found, 1945, agglutinins in the sera of approximately fifty per cent and in severe cases seventy-five per cent. The relationship of streptococcus MG may be coincidental, secondary, or etiological in combination with a virus. In clinical medicine, certain therapies (antibiotics) are often hopefully directed rather at the bacterial fellow-travelers than at the virus as in atypical pneumonia, feline enteritis and other virus conditions. Described by Smadel, 1951, as a "preview" of the usefulness of antibiotics in an influenza pandemic was the abrupt ending of fatalities by penicillin (to which certain bacterial fellow-travelers are notably responsive) given to every case in an influenza epidemic in the Canadian Arctic resembling the 1918 pandemic. Viruses isolated were identical with A and A prime strains which had caused mild epidemics at the same time in more populated areas. Experimentally, multiple intramuscular injections of the bacterium, *H. influenzae suis*, into swine harboring latent swine influenza virus will provoke severe, perhaps fatal, attacks of influenza. Shope's interpretation, 1950, of this mechanism was that bacterial infection is one of many stimuli (*e.g.*, cold, wet weather) capable of starting a violent outbreak of influenza (present in masked form) in susceptible swine. Shope's hypothesis of interepidemic survival of the swine influenza virus in nonsusceptible hosts (worms) and of the role of bacterial infection in provoking epidemics in swine has been the basis of theories to account for the high rates of communicability and death in the 1918 pandemic. Fellow-traveling bacterial agents mentioned as responsible include the hemolytic cocci and human strains of *H. influenzae*.

### HYPOTHESES ON THE BASIC PROBLEM — VIRUS REPRODUCTION

Horsfall, 1949, described virus multiplication as "unquestionably ... the most important problem in the virus field". Present evidence, he added, seems to indicate that multiplication of viruses within cells (usually within the cytoplasm, occasionally perhaps within the nucleus) "is mediated by a perversion of the normal metabolic processes of the host cell which become oriented in the direction of fostering viral synthesis". The metabolic processes of the virus-invaded cell have become measurably accessible through new methods: electron-microscopic observation of changes in infected cells suggesting the site of virus multiplication; introduction into the host cell of two genetically different strains of bacteriophage to see what combinations of these are later released by the cell; tagging of substances in the infecting virus and host cell to discover which of these appear again in the "progeny" liberated later; use of antimetabolites of various kinds known to inhibit particular enzyme systems of the normal cell with a view to determining, in tissue cultures, which cellular substances and systems may be critical for virus growth.

Observations, such as Zinsser's (so long ago as 1937) that the rate of virus increase (equine encephalomyelitis) was greatest during the period of maximal oxygen consumption of the cells, were a prelude to more recent studies, some seeking the substrates and enzymes in cellular oxidations that may provide the energy for virus synthesis, others seeking the oxidative mechanism that may be diverted from normal processes to cellular synthesis of virus. W. F. McLimans and associates reported, 1949, 1950, results of measurements of oxygen utilization in individual hen's eggs after infection with Newcastle disease virus as tending "to support the hypothesis that the rates of virus multiplication within a host cell may be regulated by the over-all respiratory quotient of that system", reduced respiratory quotient being accompanied by reduced rate of virus proliferation. D. J. Bauer (Wellcome Laboratories, London), 1951, from comparison of the enzyme activity of normal mouse brain and of the same tissue after infection with viruses capable of multiplying in it (yellow fever, lymphocytic choriomeningitis, lymphogranuloma inguinale), concluded that increase in host-cell enzyme activity associated with nucleoprotein metabolism during virus infection indicated that the virus may upset "a balance between inhibition and activation of the host enzymes", and may actually organize the host-cell metabolism in favor of virus synthesis. Investigations under way in the University of Michigan virus laboratory, including studies by Ackermann and associates (Brown, Ainslie, Johnson) since 1950, indicated that proper functioning of the Krebs cycle in the cell is intimately related to growth of virus in the initial stages of infection. Other studies reported 1952 and 1953 by Ackermann and Johnson led to the conclusion that the energy required for viral synthesis derives from oxidative phosphorylative activity of the host tissue. Studies from the same source directed to the cellular site of virus synthesis suggested that certain of the oxidative reactions of the Krebs cycle essential for propagation of influenza virus are localized in mitochondria. In related studies, effects of analogues of various amino acids and other antimetabolites on the growth of virus (influenza, by Ackermann, 1951; poliomyelitis, by Brown, 1952) in tissue culture and reversal of these effects by specific metabolites were reported as an approach to learning host-cell metabolic mechanisms essential for virus synthesis. Other investigators have recognized with Ackermann that one value in these experiments may be in "pointing up one site of the host metabolism where some drug might act usefully". Referring to these and his own experiments, Horsfall observed, 1952, "if the objective of interrupting viral multiplication by chemical means is to be attained, present evidence supports the idea that this will come about through substances which act on intracellular components, possibly on enzyme systems of susceptible host cells, rather than on the virus *per se*". S. S. Kalter and associates, 1951, suggested a correlation between protein metabolism and virus multiplication in the host. Testosterone increased both protein synthesis and proliferation of influenza virus while relative lack of the hormone (in castrate mice) was associated with diminished rate of virus growth. Administration of ACTH and cortisone, known to increase protein catabolism (or possibly to prevent protein synthesis), was followed by decreased virus growth.

Craigie, 1947, applied the term "cryptic" infection to a hypothetical state in which the virus has lost its cytoclastic properties and multiplies inside the host cell "at just the tempo that will insure there being enough virus to maintain infection when the cell divides", with a resulting infection that would not be detected by the usual methods. Although, according to Craigie, cryptic infection in the case of viruses affecting man and animals was at that time still in the realm of hypothesis, recent studies (bacteriophage experiments reported by Lwoff and Gutmann, from the Pasteur Institute, 1950) of the "latent" or "dark" period following infection of cells by certain bacterial and animal viruses have added substance to his hypothesis. Lwoff observed, 1952, "whether a noninfectious phase is present in all viruses is not known, but one can say that it has been found in every case in which it has been carefully looked for". It has been reported thus far for influenza (Hoyle, 1948; Henle, 1949), for pneumonia virus of mice and for mumps (Horsfall, 1950), for vaccina virus (Briody and Stannard, (1951), Theiler's mouse encephalomyelitis (F. K. Sanders, 1953).

As to what happens to the virus immediately after entry into the cell, one hypothesis, first advanced by Luria, 1946, on the basis of work with bacteriophage, suggested that when the virus has penetrated the cell it may split into a number of units which become foci of self-replication by using substrates and energy sources from the host. Confirming the hypothesis, Hoyle, 1948, Henle and Henle, 1949, suggested, on the basis of evidence from influenza virus injected into the chick embryo, that multiplication of influenza virus occurs in a stepwise fashion; an "incomplete" particle, considered to be an "immature" virus without infectivity, emerges as the fully infectious virus only in the final stages of the growth cycle. Hoyle suggested that during the latent phase, the injected virus is in a soluble state; others consider that it becomes so closely bound to host substance that it cannot be detected as a separate entity. One approach to the question as to what degree the original virus and to what degree the host cell contribute the substance that forms "new" virus employs radioactive tags attached to invading phage, to host-cell substances, and to substances in the nutritive medium employed by the host cell for synthesis of its own protoplasm. Another uses different naturally occurring mutant strains of bacteriophage that can be distinguished by their different effects on the host; on infecting certain bacterial strains with two or more such different "genetic markers" the final effects of "recombination" within the host cell may be gathered from the mutants ultimately liberated, some of which combine, in one new mutant, characters known to belong to two or more of the original phages used.

According to a view emerging from bacteriophage work, the substance of the new virus is apparently derived from the host, not from large preformed host elements but from the smaller elements in the "metabolic pool" from which the cell draws for synthesis of its own protoplasm. In the same direction is the observation of Meneghini and Delwiche, 1951, on the basis of radioisotopic study of the materials transferred during infection with tobacco mosaic virus, that a considerable portion of the fresh virus is synthesized from the small molecular weight compounds available to the plant for the normal process of cellular growth. In bacterial cells, three fourths of the nucleic acids contained in newly synthesized bacteriophage were shown by Cohen, 1946, to be derived from those synthesized by the host after virus invasion. Such nucleic acids, however, were not of the ribose type dominant in the bacterial host cell before virus invasion but of the viral desoxyribose type. Summarizing the picture as outlined by experimental work with bacteriophage, Evans observed, 1952, that on entrance into the host cell the infecting virus apparently breaks up; "it appears that the actual process of viral synthesis is not initiated by the virus particle as we know it, but only by a portion of it. Further, since the actual materials of this surviving fragment are handed on to the progeny in a random fashion, the role of the effective fraction of the virus is apparently to initiate a distortion or transformation of the normal metabolic activities of the cell into those associated with the manufacture of new virus particles." In short, "it would appear that it is a case of the normal machinery of the cell being converted to the synthesis of virus particles." Whether the same mechanisms will explain what happens when mammalian viruses invade the cells of animals and man has yet to be established.

In addition to the work cited above on bacteriophage, and, to a degree, on influenza, work on poliomyelitis in Howe's and in other laboratories is also concerned with metabolic mechanisms in the virus-infected cells, possibly bearing on virus multiplication. Howe referred to this work in 1950 as suggesting the possible importance of "some characteristic protein" in the synthesis of virus.

The principal question, according to Delbrück, 1952, is whether the replica is formed directly from the pattern, or indirectly (by the cell's first making a "mold" and then casting the replicas from the mold). "Furthermore, how much molecular turnover takes place in the original particle from which replicas are made?" On the answer to the question whether viruses multiply by division through the intervention of zygotes, as in sexual reproduction, or through some one of the numerous possibilities of nonsexual reproduction, Delbrück considered, hinges "the whole question of the standing of viruses within the system of biology, whether they are degenerate or primitive microorganisms or whether they are cellular constituents evolutionarily on the march toward greater independence from the parent cell".

## VIRUS STRAINS AND VARIATION

Strain differences in viruses are recognized to account for various phenomena including notable differences in clinical manifestation, differences in duration of immunity. Antigenic differences between strains within the same type may be sufficiently great to hamper seriously practicable attempts at vaccination, as in influenza; on the other hand, the close immunologic relationship between vaccinia and variola accounts for the efficacy of smallpox vaccination. Knowledge concerning the number and nature of strains in various viruses has accumulated unevenly, intensively for some viruses, sparsely for others. According to Kunkel, 400 different strains of tobacco mosaic virus had been recognized by 1947. More than thirty strains of yellow fever virus had been studied by 1939, leading to effective methods of vaccination. Some eight hundred strains of the three known serological types of poliomyelitis virus had been reported as the result of typing work in all parts of the world by September, 1954 (A. J. Rhodes). Intensive study of bacteriophage strains since 1944 has been one of few systematic approaches to the biological bases of strain variation.

Current concepts of the origin and nature of strain variation (in both virology and bacteriology) derive largely from genetic work, especially the basic concept that mutation in higher forms represents a sudden alteration in chromosomal or genic substances as the result of which a new character appears, sufficiently stable to be passed on to subsequent generations. Burnet, 1945, considered valid the working hypothesis that "heritable variations in bacteria and viruses arise by a process of discontinuous mutation essentially similar to gene mutation in higher forms and that the mass transformation of a strain, as observed in practice, is the result of selective survival and overgrowth of one or more mutant types".

Of the genetic character of strain variation, two recent lines of research (with reference to both bacteria and viruses) offer suggestive evidence: identification in bacteria of desoxyribonucleic acid-containing bodies and their chemical similarity to chromosomes, and identification of desoxyribonucleic acid in viruses, notably in bacteriophage. A second line of work, developed in 1946 in both bacteriology and virology, concerns the phenomenon of "genetic recombination" in which two strains that infect the same host may be shown to yield a third possessing known, separate, genetic properties of the first two. Genetic recombination, observed in 1946 in bacteriophage, by Delbrück and Bailey, up to 1952 had been observed only in several closely related larger phages. Especial significance therefore attaches to the 1951 report of Burnet and Lind that genetic recombination can be demonstrated in at least one animal virus, influenza, in which one host inoculated with two different strains yielded a third strain combining known qualities of the first two. They postulated a mechanism similar to that suggested by work with bacteriophage: that during initial stages of infection the original viruses break up into subunits which multiply independently and that some of these from each strain recombine to produce the "hybrid" third strain. The biologic significance of genetic recombination has been pointed out by various workers, Burnet, Delbrück, Hershey and Bronfenbrenner. The latter team observed, 1952, that solution of the mechanism of genetic recombination may yield a clue to the fundamental problem of virus origin. On the practical level, these and other investigators have recognized the relevance of genetic recombination to rise and fall of viral epidemics and to the unsolved problem of survival of disease in interepidemic periods.

The varying capacity for adaptation of different strains (of a single type of virus) has significance for research, for explaining epidemic character, for control of virus infection by vaccines. Whether or not a strain will become well established with epidemic characteristics depends (Francis, 1952) on its ability to adapt itself to a host. Changes in virus properties in the course of adaptation to new host species or to new tissues, in some cases resulting in attenuation of virulence, have been an important factor in development of vaccines. Illustrative are: modification of neurotropism in a pantropic strain of yellow fever virus yielding, after serial passage through tissue cultures, the strain now used in vaccination against yellow fever; modification of the paralyzing canine "street virus" of rabies to the milder "fixed virus" resulting from continuous passage through rabbits. Variations in the other direction — enhancing virulence — may also occur: change in a strain of herpes simplex virus through adaptation to different tissues (by serial passage in rabbits) resulted in enhancing its virulence, finally rendering it capable of producing encephalitis.

During recent years new strains of viruses causing encephalitis have progressively been "discovered", although some of these have later been considered to be the same virus in widely separate areas. Resemblances and differences — in eastern, western, Venezuelan encephalomyelitis, St. Louis, Japanese B, Russian spring-summer encephalitis — are definitely a matter of current interest and study. Hammon, 1948, presented the common ancestry hypothesis for the encephalitides, or certain of them, postulating a "stem virus" for at least St. Louis and western equine viruses.

While there can be no finality in establishing the number of poliomyelitis types, Salk considered, 1952, that development of a procedure for control of poliomyelitis needed to be concerned with only the three types, Brunhilde, Lansing, Leon. On the basis of the typing committee's studies, observations are being assembled on the differing geographic and temporal distribution of the three types, on differences in the clinical diseases they respectively cause (asymptomatic, nonparalytic or abortive, spinal, bulbar), on the different sources (feces, blood, central nervous system) from which each type is most frequently isolated. Salk characterized data so far collected on the first hundred strains, classified according to the three currently known types, as "only a beginning". Evidence, however, indicated that all three types were world-wide in distribution. Bodian, 1952, pointed out that earlier studies had shown that strains of the same antigenic type manifested differences in virulence, in capacity to invade and destroy nerve cells, in capacity to reach nerve cells from peripheral portals of entry.

The marked capacity of influenza viruses for variation has been stressed consistently (Hirst, Francis, Burnet, Horsfall, Andrewes, Wilson Smith). The continuing antigenic variation of influenza A is significant not only in regard to control through vaccination but also in regard to concepts concerning origin of variant strains or factors influencing dominance of one variant over others. In addition to the two distinct immunologically unrelated serologic types of influenza — A, isolated in 1933 in England, B, isolated in the United States in 1940 — a third immunologically distinct type, C, was suggested by Taylor, 1949, 1951, by Francis and his associates, 1950. Horsfall noted, 1952, that immunological differences between individual strains within one influenza type may be so great as to cause difficulty in identification and classification. Andrewes (directing the World Influenza Center, London) noted, 1950, that strains antigenically related to the first A virus (strain WS) isolated in 1933 appeared up to 1935 but not thereafter for fifteen years; A viruses recovered between 1936 and 1945 were all more or less closely related to the 1934 standard A type, another strain, PR8. Since 1946, however, those resembling the PR8 strain have been largely or wholly replaced (in Australia, America, Europe) by viruses related to FM1 strains of A, more commonly known, because of their wide differences from the original A type, as A-prime. "Such a replacement of one virus by another", Andrewes observed, "if it is indeed almost universal throughout the world, is a phenomenon of remarkable importance epidemiologically" since it may be paralleling replacement of a lethal type of virus by less vicious strains. World Health Organization reports in 1953 indicated that strains recovered from 1951–52 epidemics and from 1952–53 outbreaks in continental Europe, Britain, Pacific areas, South Africa, Australia, the United States were also related to the A-prime strains. Wilson Smith, 1952, noted as now "abundantly clear" the error in "our earlier conception of a few antigenic types developed possibly by the process of sudden chance mutations". Instead, he pointed out, "one now recognizes a constant evolution of new antigenic types which replace the old types from which they are derived". In the same direction is Burnet's observation, 1953, that the general experience of workers with influenza A is that there has been a continuing series of changes in serological characters of which WS, PR8, A-prime represent convenient examples picked from the "changing continuum". His group advanced the hypothesis that, since influenza has always to move through a partially immune population, it survives in its extensive and active movement all over the globe by serological adaptation to the host, that is, "by a process of continually emerging serological novelty". Wilson Smith, 1952, advanced the hypothesis that incorporation of host protein may account for the changed character of new strains by changing virus structure. In support of this hypothesis he cited the impossibility of entirely separating the purest available preparations of influenza from host protein (Knight, 1946); he suggested that far from being a "contaminant" the host protein might be an essential property of the new variant, accounting for its changed biological properties.

Horsfall and Archetti, 1950, presented experiments suggesting that human antibody (whether the result of natural infection or vaccination) may account for antigenic variation of influenza A viruses or of any other closely related group of influenza viruses. In experiments passing four closely related A strains through the chick embryo, they exposed these to immune serum from other antigenically related strains, the amounts of antiserum being sufficient to neutralize only partially the four strains, presumably with reference to the common antigenic property they shared with the strains for which the antiserum was specific. Their findings showed that "antigenic variants emerge regularly", that such variants are "predictable in terms of the immune serum used". They advanced the hypothesis that the emerging variant represents multiplication of those virus particles from the various strains that were most resistant to the antiserum employed, so that they possessed "a preferential advantage for multiplication". Referring to these experiments, 1952, Horsfall observed, "Thus, immunization against but one sector of the total antigenic spectrum of a virus . . . would provide a host environment which, in some cases, might be expected to favor selection of a new antigenic variant." Francis, 1952, considered "extremely doubtful" the hypothesis that "changes in influenza virus proceed with succeeding years as an orderly controlled variation based upon the antibody content earlier developed by the population". However, if it proves to be true that the antigens of older epidemic strains are progressively less available in the strains of succeeding years, the result should be eventually to force variation back in the direction of the original strain, thus creating the recurrent cycles of strains suggested in "classical notions of the periodicity of influenza". Francis inclined to attribute certain pessimistic conclusions regarding influenza vaccination to the fact that current vaccines reflect preoccupation with antigenic differences and dependence on serological reactions to only the dominant antigen, neglecting lesser antigenic components. Finer analysis of these components and tests of sera collected over recent years for evidence of immunity against them, were concerned, 1954, with the possibility of establishing shared antigenic principles for a sufficient number of strains to insure broad protection not only against existing strains but against future strains which might appear containing the same antigens, if in other combinations.

The biologist's dream that ultimately mutations can be directed beneficently animates certain work going forward in chemical laboratories. Earlier studies of Stanley and of Knight, 1947, of differences in amino acid composition among strains of tobacco mosaic virus suggested that the new strains that tend to appear or to become dominant when a virus is grown in an unnatural host may be attributable to the fact that the new host cells provide a somewhat different supply of amino acids and enzyme systems, and, in the effort to adhere to some basic pattern, amino acids that would not normally be used for synthesis of the virus are built into its structure. In his 1947 Gibbs medal address, Stanley said that the differences in content of glutamic acid and lysine between the ordinary and the killing strain of tobacco mosaic led to the belief that the killing type "arose from the ordinary strain by virtue of two successive mutations . . ." Demonstration of tobacco mosaic strains in which mutation was accompanied by only two differences, by introduction of new amino acids, or by elimination of one led him to speculate: "There is reason to believe that changes, such as those responsible for the conversion of virulent smallpox virus to cowpox or vaccinia virus, the formation of the mild 17D strain of yellow fever virus, or the sudden appearance of a killing strain of polio-myelitis virus are accompanied by similar changes in the structure of these viruses." Knight suggested that the significant differences he found between the PR8 strain of influenza A and the Lee strain of influenza B, with regard to five amino acids (and possibly also varia-tions in other constituents), might "provide at least in part a chemical explanation for some of the differing properties of the PR8 and Lee strains of influenza viruses".

## VIRUS INTERRELATIONS

Of investigative work bearing on similarities and interrelations in viruses, there is little that goes beyond observation and speculation; but, in the long, complicated and frustrating effort to arrive at under-standing of the nature of viruses, and to detect possible common de-nominators among so many and such disparate virus agents, so unlike in their effects, any accumulated incidental detail is not negligible. It is in this perspective that mention is made here of an uneven body of information on interrelations among viruses, including a few demon-strated findings and a greater number of mere inferences, the compari-sons resting sometimes upon such uncertain ground as clinical similari-ties; sometimes on epidemiologic data concerning simultaneous or consecutive outbreaks of two virus diseases; sometimes on evi-dence pointing to interference between two viruses; sometimes on serologic reactions with which cross immunity may or may not be correlated.

### THE VIRUSES OF THE PSITTACOSIS, LYMPHOGRANULOMA, PNEU-MONITIS GROUP AND OF PRIMARY ATYPICAL PNEUMONIA

Investigations of primary atypical pneumonia in man in which known bacteria could not be identified led, during the last decade, to studies that have resulted in identification of a rapidly increasing list of viruses causing pneumonia in animals and, according to Meyer, 1952, indistinguishable from those causing psittacosis (Baker's feline pneumonitis, 1944; spontaneous mouse pneumonitis, Gönnert, 1941,

Nigg and Eaton, 1944; opossum meningopneumonitis, 1949; others) and some that are considered probably infectious for man (San Francisco human pneumonitis virus isolated by Eaton, Beck and Pearson, 1941; Illinois pneumonitis virus, reported by Zichis and Shaughnessy, 1945; Louisiana pneumonitis virus, Larson and Olson, 1946). Resemblances commonly pointed out among some of these pneumonitis viruses, psittacosis of man and of birds, lymphogranuloma, include relatively large size (300 to 450 millimicrons); morphological and staining characteristics; intracellular inclusion bodies; capacity for propagation in the yolk sac of embryonated eggs; capacity to infect mice by the intranasal route; certain antigenic components in common on the basis of complement-fixation tests. Rake, who placed the psittacosis-lymphogranuloma group (confined to psittacosis, lymphogranuloma, murine and feline pneumonitis, the Louisiana and Illinois pneumonitis viruses) in Bergey's 1948 manual with rickettsia, noted, 1953, two opinions in the committee created by the Fifth International Congress of Microbiology to offer a tentative system of classification and nomenclature for this group, one assigning the group to viruses, the other to rickettsia. Andrewes, 1953, referred to the group as lying, as does rickettsia, between bacteria and the more typical viruses. Over a dozen years ago, Eaton and associates had made the familiar suggestion that the viruses of the group may be variants descended from the same parent strain which has become adapted to various tissues and species. The common ancestry hypothesis has been offered also with regard to inclusion conjunctivitis and trachoma, which some investigators (Thygeson, 1952) would also include in the psittacosis-lymphogranuloma group (in a separate category intermediate between virus and rickettsia) but which others (K. F. Meyer, 1952) would definitely exclude from it. Bedson suggested that differences might perhaps result from long residence in a particular host species: psittacosis in a variety of birds, lymphogranuloma venereum, trachoma and inclusion conjunctivitis in man.

Horsfall pointed out, 1952, that certain viral or rickettsial diseases of established etiology "may simulate atypical pneumonia very closely, as psittacosis or ornithosis, Q fever, occasionally influenza". The agent of atypical pneumonia has yet to be isolated. A 1948 study of fifty-eight cases of primary atypical pneumonia reported in the *Lancet* noted that the explosive outbreak of primary atypical pneumonia coincided with reduction to zero of incidence of hepatitis, suggesting that the same virus might be operating; fresh cases of hepatitis did not return until the pneumonia epidemic had subsided. According to this study, the possibility could not be ruled out that certain febrile cases described as anicteric hepatitis were really cases of primary atypical pneumonia.

## INFLUENZA IN RELATION TO OTHER VIRUSES

Since Francis and Magill commented fifteen years ago on the difficulty of differentiating influenza clinically from Rift Valley fever, various workers have pointed out how other viral infections (common cold, primary atypical pneumonia, abortive measles, dengue, lymphocytic choriomeningitis, Venezuelan equine encephalomyelitis) may simulate influenza. With the exception of swine influenza, however, no other virus had, up to 1952, been shown to possess common antigens with the human influenza group. Francis and Shope between 1934 and 1939 (and subsequently other workers in this country and England) suggested that swine influenza and the human influenza A, although immunologically distinct, share a common antigen which is present in greater quantity in the human virus. On the basis of virus hemagglutination behavior, Burnet, in 1945 and 1946 studies, associated mumps with Newcastle and a group of influenza viruses. In 1953, Burnet (as exponent of a committee on classification of influenza viruses) recommended that influenza (A, B, C), mumps, Newcastle disease of fowls, fowl plague be combined in a single group primarily because all agglutinate red cells of chickens, but also because the virus units are of approximately the same size and (except for mumps virus) of the same spherical shape, though they differ in tissue tropism.

## THE POX VIRUSES

The relation of variola, vaccinia, alastrim of man with pox diseases of animals has been the subject of considerable study, but F. B. Gordon, 1950, did not consider that recent work altered the theories prevalent since 1936 concerning the evolution of this family of viruses. Buddingh commented, 1953, on physical and/or biochemical features shared by members of the pox group. Use of new methods for testing immunological relations, or of the electron microscope for characterizing morphological properties continues to distinguish individual variations within broad resemblances in the group. Buddingh suggested adding to it tentatively molluscum contagiosum and rabbit myxomatosis; he did not include chickenpox, since recent studies with the electron microscope showed differences justifying its exclusion.

Burnet, 1945, described the relationship of vaccinia to smallpox as, historically, a matter of controversy. Although by modern work "it appears to be adequately proved that some strains of variola at least can be 'converted' into vaccinia by consecutive passage through monkeys to rabbits and calves, no thorough study seems to have been made of the processes by which the change takes place, and since the phenomenon is the classical example of virus variation this absence of knowledge is to be regretted". Findlay early suggested (1936) that perhaps vaccinia is a stable variant of variola (or alastrim) which appears when it is transferred to a new host. However, since J. B. Nelson, 1943, and North, 1944, showed that variola propagated on the chorio allantois of the developing chick did not develop properties of vaccinia but remained stable, explanations for the change have yet to be found. Early studies of cross immunity in animals suggested that vaccinia protects against variola more effectively than variola protects against vaccinia. Summarizing various explanations of this offered during the past twenty-five years, van Rooyen and Rhodes, 1948, referred to the view that variola contains a group (vaccinial) antigen as well as a highly specific (variolar) antigen, the group antigen being responsible for resistance, the specific antigen for virulence in man, and that on animal passage the specific antigen is lost and the variola virus degraded into vaccinia. Buddingh, however, thought, 1949, that this hypothesis had not been substantiated, and that in evaluating reports of transformation of variola to vaccinia by successive passage in one or more animal hosts the possibility of contamination could not be excluded. He noted, 1953, that while there is evidence (but not proof) that some of the strains in current use for vaccines represent strains originally isolated by Jenner, various empirical methods commercially employed to maintain vaccinia since Jenner's day have resulted in "what must be regarded as essentially artificial or, at least, laboratory strains" with presumably the one common attribute of capacity to induce human vaccinia that prevents smallpox. The need of "more adequate experimental study" (Burnet, 1945) of the relationship of classical smallpox and alastrim has been stressed. Findlay once suggested the possibility that classical smallpox represents the activity of virus plus a specifically associated hemolytic streptococcus, while alastrim represents the activity of the virus alone. However, the alternate view, that the difference lies essentially in the virus, is described as the more orthodox.

All of the animal pox viruses, whether of cattle, swine, mice, fowl, or birds, became of interest with the discovery that cowpox conferred a degree of immunity against smallpox in man. A number of studies by newly devised methods have been concerned recently with discovering immunological relations among them. McCarthy and Downie, for instance, noted, 1948, that the minor antigenic differences among the viruses of variola, vaccinia, cowpox, ectromelia, demonstrable by neutralization techniques, were not greater than those within influenza A viruses. Frank Fenner, 1948, described smallpox, alastrim, and generalized vaccinia as "the closest human analogues of mousepox".

## Herpes Zoster and Varicella

Periodic discussions as to whether herpes zoster (shingles) and varicella (chickenpox) may be two strains of the same virus or actually identical stress similarities: in the histology of the vesicles; in type of elementary and inclusion bodies extracted from the vesicles; in size; and (studies in the electron microscope) in shape. While earlier investigators considered the seasonal incidence of the two identical, Dahl, 1946, reported maximum incidence of varicella from January to March, of zoster in August, sometimes from October to December. Other differences noted include epidemic incidence of varicella, sporadic incidence of herpes zoster; difference in age incidence, varicella occurring commonly, zoster rarely, in the age group under twenty. Varicella in children (Stokes, 1952) more often induces zoster in exposed adults than it does in exposed children; zoster, whether in children or adults, is an apparent source of varicella in children (almost never in adults). Among several hypotheses advanced in ex-

planation is that of van Rooyen and Rhodes, 1948, that children coming in contact with zoster are susceptible, so that the virus general-
izes and causes an attack of varicella, whereas adults coming in contact
with varicella are relatively immune "and either the virus produces
no disease, or else an attack of zoster, which may be regarded as varicella occurring in a partially immune person". Neither virus has
been studied extensively, and the available evidence of relationship is,
according to Buddingh, 1949, "only circumstantial"; a critical
demonstration of relationship awaits the propagation of the viruses
under experimental conditions.

## YELLOW FEVER, RIFT VALLEY FEVER, DENGUE

Circumstantial evidence of interrelation consisting of clinical resemblances among diseases caused by the viruses of the dengue group,
yellow fever, Rift Valley fever of sheep, has been discussed repeatedly since Findlay, 1932, published objective data showing that
dengue and Rift Valley fever are separate entities. The International
Health Division considered, 1948, that although monkeys actively
immunized against dengue were at times found relatively less susceptible to yellow fever than normal animals, and although the converse
also seemed to be true, "the immunological overlap" might "not be of
sufficient account to play any part in the epidemiology of the two viruses." Reviewing part of the program of the Armed Forces Epidemiological Board, Sabin reported, 1950, a definite antigenic relationship
between the dengue viruses and those of yellow fever, Japanese B encephalitis and West Nile fever as demonstrated by the complement-fixation test. In 1952 he reported additional evidence that these viruses,
with St. Louis encephalitis, may constitute "a distinct, generically
related group" including discovery of a strain of mice exhibiting an
inherited resistance to this entire group of viruses but not to others
(western equine, herpes, rabies, Rift Valley fever, lymphocytic choriomeningitis) and the finding of an antiviral (nonantibody) factor
in human milk which neutralizes all members of the group but not
western equine, herpes, poliomyelitis viruses. Sabin noted, however,
that this group relationship between dengue and other viruses is not
associated with significant, active cross immunity since human volunteers immunized with the 17 D strain of yellow fever were not resistant

to small amounts of dengue virus although an interference phenomenon was observed between the two viruses both in these human and in earlier monkey experiments.

## INTERRELATIONS AMONG THE ENCEPHALITIDES

The lengthening list of recognized viruses causing encephalitis in animals and man includes a number of clinically distinguished entities placed in very tentative subgroups: eastern, western and Venezuelan equine encephalomyelitis viruses; St. Louis, Japanese B, Russian spring-summer encephalitis viruses, to which louping ill (a disease of sheep which induces a mild nonfatal encephalitis in man) and West Nile viruses have certain resemblances; a group of newer and less studied encephalitis viruses isolated from mosquitoes in Africa, Columbia, Brazil and San Joaquin Valley, California. The viruses of the first two groups have in common small size (between twenty and thirty millimicron), similar biological effects on the cells of the central nervous system, epidemiological characteristics including frequent occurrence in domestic and wild animals and transmission by insects; immunologically they have distinctive likenesses and differences (Hammon, 1948). Immunological evidence has shown that North American types of equine encephalomyelitis virus, western and eastern, and the Venezuelan type (which were at first regarded as occurring only in horses) are often associated with clinically unrecognizable infection in various domesticated and wild animals and numerous fowl and bird hosts; all of these viruses are believed to be transmitted by biting insects (Hammon, 1948). The eastern and western viruses, in spite of their biological similarities, have significant differences (shorter incubation period and swifter lethal course for the eastern virus) and are, according to Olitsky and Casals, 1952, serologically and immunologically so distinct as to be regarded as causing separate disease entities. As to members of the second tentative group: various reports (Lennette, 1943; Olitsky and Casals, 1952) have pointed out that Russian autumn encephalitis has now been identified as Japanese B encephalitis and, according to Olitsky and Casals, is "probably identical with Australian X disease". While Russian workers have regarded the Russian Far Eastern virus (and louping ill, which in Russia appears to be clinically indistinguishable from Far Eastern encephalitis) as closely related to the Japanese B, West Nile, St. Louis viruses, Casals, 1944, pointed out that these relationships had not been established. Geographic distribution, certain serologic overlapping, uniformity in size of the viruses, clinical resemblances have led to the familiar suggestion (Olitsky and Casals, 1952) that the arthropod-borne epidemic summer viral encephalitides (St. Louis, western, eastern, Japanese B and Russian Far Eastern) may have "a common ancestor which on dissemination over the world has been acted upon by environmental factors", assumed, by several Russian and American investigators, to be insect vectors and animal reservoirs in newly-invaded areas to which the virus became in time adapted. Lépine observed, 1953, that there exists around the world in the hot temperate zone a continuous belt of seasonal insect-transmitted encephalitides, a vast interlocked family "linked by variable degrees of antigenic power and, sometimes, by complete cross-immunity". Laboratory data supporting the "common stem" virus hypothesis for at least St. Louis encephalitis and western equine encephalomyelitis was reported, 1945, by Hammon and Reeves: both are transmitted by *Culex tarsalis;* both infect horses and produce inapparent infection in other animals; both viruses may be acquired by the mosquito from the blood of fowls in which they produce no visible signs of infection; both have been found in the central and western parts of the United States; both are diseases of summer; both have been found in mixed epidemics.

## Relation of Poliomyelitis to Other Viruses

The possibility of a connection between encephalitis (in animals and in man) and poliomyelitis has been suggested within the past fifteen years by: simultaneous outbreaks of western equine encephalomyelitis and poliomyelitis; simultaneous appearance of poliomyelitis and St. Louis encephalitis (noted in California, 1937, by Hooper Foundation workers). Rhodes, 1953, mentioned many references (Theiler, 1941; Gard, 1943; Burnet, 1945; van Rooyen and Rhodes, 1948; Jungeblut, 1951) to similarities in biologic properties of Theiler's mouse encephalomyelitis and poliomyelitis. Koprowski observed that these two viruses and the little-studied virus of Teschen's disease in swine seem to be within the same size range and are ether resistant.

Immunological relationships between mouse encephalomyelitis virus and the human and Lansing strains were reported by Dalldorf and Whitney, 1945. Melnick and Riordan pointed out, 1947, the confusion that can arise from natural occurrence of the mouse virus in albino mice used in the study of human poliomyelitis virus.

On possible relation between the Coxsackie group and poliomyelitis viruses isolated together from fatal paralytic cases, Melnick asked, 1950: "Is it possible that infection with poliomyelitis would have been a mild affair in these patients had not C virus infection been superimposed on poliomyelitis infection?" "Close similarities in clinical features" between the disease produced by the Coxsackie viruses and the minor illness frequently regarded in the past as "abortive" nonparalytic poliomyelitis suggested, Rhodes pointed out at the 1951 poliomyelitis conference, that much that had been written about abortive poliomyelitis "must now be accepted with reserve". Dalldorf had suggested that the decreased incidence shown in his studies of paralytic poliomyelitis in the presence of Coxsackie virus may suggest that the C virus has a "sparing" effect on poliomyelitis virus, and in 1951 he reported that Nancy and Conn-5 types of Coxsackie viruses interfere with the activity of Lansing poliomyelitis in mice. Other investigators have been unable to detect interference experimentally and demonstration (Rhodes and associates, 1950; Melnick and associates, 1951) that C and poliomyelitis infections can occur simultaneously in the same individual was regarded (Schlesinger, 1952; Melnick and Curnen, 1952) as evidence that interference between the two viruses does not occur in man.

## HERPES SIMPLEX IN RELATION TO OTHER VIRUSES

As indicating capacity of herpes simplex, commonly in the dermotropic list, to attack nerves on occasion, Burnet, 1945, mentioned three authenticated cases of invasion of the central nervous system during the course of a primary infection. The possibility that herpes simplex may attack the brain has been more closely studied since Armstrong, 1943, recovered the virus from a case of suspected lymphocytic choriomeningitis. Since then herpes, according to Scott, 1952, has been recognized as a cause of herpetic meningoencephalitis with symptoms that may range from an uncomplicated aseptic meningitis (usually resulting in recovery) to encephalitic signs such as somnolence, dizziness, aphasia and ocular palsies. Most of the proved cases of encephalitis have been established by isolation of the virus and by typical brain damage, in fatal cases.

As to the possibility that herpes simplex is the causal agent of von Economo's encephalitis (lethargica, sleeping sickness), various workers in this country have registered a negative view: Horsfall, 1947, who found the theory "not substantiated by the experimental facts"; Scott, 1952, who suggested that occasional isolation of herpes in epidemic encephalitis might be merely the "result of a coincidental latent infection"; Olitsky and Casals, 1948, who considered the encephalitides occasionally induced by herpes virus in man distinct from von Economo's encephalitis lethargica. The question first arose in the twenties when Doerr induced encephalitis in the rabbit with herpes simplex and when C. Levaditi and his associates reported isolation of an agent resembling herpes simplex from a fatal case of von Economo's encephalitis. The latter on occasion shows the same meningeal, ocular and encephalitic symptoms as herpetic encephalitis. Summarizing extensive French work and a few other studies, van Rooyen and Rhodes, 1948, observed, "on the whole, the evidence of the last few years has tended to strengthen the view that herpes virus is the cause of lethargic encephalitis". Failure to isolate the causative agent leaves the question without definitive answer.

## BEHAVIOR OF VIRUSES IN THE BIOLOGICAL CYCLE OF MAINTENANCE BY TRANSMISSION FROM HOST TO HOST

Theobald Smith's concept of infectious diseases as "incidents in a developing parasitism" is as applicable to diseases produced by viruses as it is to diseases produced by bacteria or other agents. Viruses also illustrate the continuous struggle of all parasites to find food, shelter and an environment favorable to propagation of their kind; they are one of the parties in the "truce between two living things, accompanied by predatory processes whenever opportunity is offered one or the other party". The more efficient parasites (Francis, 1952) live in comparative harmony with their hosts, the more predatory (virulent) injure the host cells and may, with the death of the host or through mobilization of the host's physiological resistance, lose in the struggle for survival unless transmission to a new host is already accomplished and the cycle begun again.

Transmission of viruses from one host to another (from man to man, or from man through intermediary hosts and vectors back to man) depends upon the virus's opportunity: to gain entrance to the host's tissues in spite of natural defenses at portals of entry; to adapt to the environment of the host's cells and use their components for self-multiplication; to achieve exit from the host and find effective means of transition to a new host. The portals of entry often, if not always, provide the means of exit, and the materials and agents through which the virus leaves the host body may serve as a means of transmission to fresh hosts. Direct methods of transmission by a chain from host to host include handling, inspiring or ingesting infected material or infected air. Indirect transmission may be accomplished through contaminated water, milk, food, or by insect intermediate hosts or vectors providing the mechanism for the virus's escape from one host and entrance into another. In many virus diseases combined or alternate methods of transmission have complicated study.

Baffling uncertainties about the means by which parasites are transmitted from host to host under natural conditions have often delayed control of infectious diseases. More is known of the transmission of viruses that cause clinical disease than of viruses that pass from host to host without doing so. Yet whether the parasite actually injures the host cell and thus produces infectious disease is only an accidental or incidental part of the complex host cell-virus struggle. The complexity, moreover, is increased by great individual variation in the host cells — some succumb in the struggle, some eliminate the parasite, some neutralize its disease-producing properties. In this last event, resulting in establishment of equilibrium, the host may become a carrier, a reservoir, a vector, all three of which are among the more elusive factors in the transmission, and in the epidemiology, of virus disease.

## METHODS OF VIRUS TRANSMISSION

### INTRODUCTORY

Of critical importance in control of virus diseases through understanding the methods by which they are transmitted is knowledge of man's biological role in the cycle of virus infection. Is man the sole source of a given virus, as John R. Neefe, 1949, suggested for hepatitis ("to the present time, no extra-human host for hepatitis has been recognized"), as Enders, 1952, suggested for mumps? Or is man merely suspected of being the ultimate source of the virus because negative results have thus far attended investigation of other possibilities, as in the case of the common cold? If man is the ultimate source of the poliomyelitis virus (since all known strains, even those now adapted to rodents, are of human origin), is maintenance of the virus dependent on multiplication in man? If so, does the virus multiply in nervous tissue only, or may it, as various workers have suggested, multiply in the intestines? If the virus does multiply in the intestines, how does it reach them — by virus inhaled through the nose or ingested? That the virus leaves man, at least during epidemic periods, by way of the alimentary tract has been amply demonstrated in recent years by studies of feces, sewage. Are these a source of further infection through flies and contaminated food? Or, since the virus is also "shed in the oropharyngeal secretions" (Howe, 1952) by asymptomatic carriers and in patients with abortive poliomyelitis, is the virus disseminated chiefly by this means and swallowed, thereby localizing in the intestines? These are some of the wider implications in the biological cycle of a virus that make important investigation of method of transmission not merely as a public health problem but also as a critical part of research on the nature and activity of viruses. If man is only an occasional, an accidental or incidental host in diseases primarily of lower animals, as in rabies and yellow fever, where is the ultimate reservoir? Are there intermediate hosts, and if so are they readily recognizable by frank infection or are they silent reservoirs related to infection in man merely as a source of the virus carried by insects from such animal reservoirs to man? Do the insect vectors perform merely a temporary mechanical function in transferring the virus for a limited period, or do they remain infected so long as they live?

These are questions that must be answered differently for different viruses and that have not been as yet answered conclusively for some. It is now generally recognized that for some viruses there may be multiple methods of transmission; a 1945 account of infectious hepatitis in the Army described three methods of spread, respiratory routes, blood-sucking insects, "unsanitary conditions". Howe, 1949, suggested that a "dual mechanism" in the spread of poliomyelitis (pharyngeal secretions, flies infected from fecal sources) might account for the "epidemiologic complexity which has eluded understanding". Burnet suggested, 1945, that in nonepidemic periods fecal contamination may be a chief method of transmitting the virus but that during epidemics it is more probably spread by droplets. Ward, Melnick and Horstmann, 1945, suggested that flies might initiate poliomyelitis transmission continued thereafter by person-to-person contact. In referring to evidence that poliomyelitis virus may escape by way of the mouth as well as by the fecal route, Bodian observed, 1953, "but there is no conclusive evidence as to which of these routes is of principal importance in transmission of infection from person to person". The transmission problem is not to be explained in terms of simple mechanics: Levaditi, 1946, is cited as visualizing a widespread dispersal of poliomyelitis virus at the outset of an epidemic, associated with an increasing neurotropism and a changed susceptibility in the population. In this concept, immune persons who become infected are believed to act as healthy carriers, while the fully susceptible develop paralysis, the partly susceptible, abortive infection. A method of transmission effective in laboratory experimentation may not be the natural method of transmission of a given virus: experimental infection of mice with different strains of psittacosis virus by intranasal, intraperitoneal, intracerebral, intravenous, subcutaneous, or alimentary routes throws no light on the contact method by which the virus is transmitted from man to man (Meyer, 1952). There remains the complicating theory that some viruses may be continuously present, an hypothesis advanced to explain herpes simplex infection as evoked only at intervals by "trigger mechanisms".

The complexity of the whole subject of virus transmission is due not only to the numerous possibilities involved, ranging from theoretically ever present virus to transmission by various direct and indirect contacts with skin, secretions, excretions, air-borne particles. Complicating the picture also is advancing knowledge of numerous temporary or ultimate animal reservoirs and intermediate hosts, wild and domestic birds and insect vectors.   Where animal hosts and man are both concerned, which is the ultimate reservoir (if there is one), which is carrier, which is host, which is intermediate, which is obligate host without which infection cannot take place?   That the maintenance of a virus may be the result not of chance but of an obligate biological cycle is suggested by the method of transmission of one plant virus disease, X-disease of peaches, which, according to a 1947 account in *Horticulture*, cannot spread from peach to peach but must go from peach to chokecherry, or from chokecherry to chokecherry, and from chokecherry to peach.

## TRANSMISSION BY CONTACT, DIRECT AND INDIRECT

While human contact is the accepted means of transmission of a number of virus infections, the nature of the contact, with regard to many viruses, remains undefined.   Studies since 1944 (Francis and associates; Paul, Melnick and associates; Bodian and associates) of "interpersonal contact" as the means of transmission of poliomyelitis have focused increasingly on the higher rate of infection found among family contacts, especially in families in which a clinical case appears. Francis, 1952, cited evidence that the virus is not uniformly disseminated throughout a community during an epidemic but occurs "in focal concentration of dense infection in families or intimate groups". On the basis of evidence in this direction, especial attempts have been made to determine whether selective use of gamma globulin with familial contacts would be more economical than widespread use.

One form of contact (direct or indirect) does not exclude another. Lymphogranuloma venereum may be spread not only by sexual intercourse but also by infected pus on the fingers.   Direct contact with secretions and excretions  does not necessarily exclude less direct contact with contaminated objects.   For all methods of transmission that involve secretions, excretions, dried tissue, the length of time in which the viruses in them remain viable and infectious is obviously important.   Duration of the period of communicability is not known for primary atypical pneumonia (Horsfall, 1952); for varicella (Stokes,

1952). For mumps, available evidence (Enders, 1952) suggests that it may extend from twenty-four to forty-eight hours before to at least six days after salivary gland enlargement is noted. Measles, according to Rake, 1952, is particularly infective during the catarrhal stage, but infectivity wanes rapidly after the rash appears. The infectivity of the smallpox virus, on the other hand, persists in contaminated articles and surroundings long after the patient has passed the acute phase. Crusts kept in the dark at room temperature yielded the virus after 417 days (Downie and Dumbell, 1947) and when kept in a vacuum were found to be infective after more than two years.

Transmission of virus by droplets has been considered a major possibility in smallpox, as in measles, in chickenpox. Infected secretions (nasal, oral, pharyngeal) and excretions (fecal, seminal, urinary) may be wet (as in droplets) or dry (as in dust), varying in infectivity according to their state. Studies of various forms of contact with secretions in individual virus diseases, while often not conclusive, have yielded data of a certain epidemiological importance. The National Office of Vital Statistics, 1951, attributed a recent outbreak of acute epidemic conjunctivitis in Hawaii (about 3,000 cases in school children; and from 5,000 to 6,000 on all of the islands) to "a primary spread by droplet infection in the schools with further family spread at home". Rubella, according to Rake, 1952, is transmitted by nasopharyngeal discharges of the patient, either directly or from freshly soiled clothes. Nasopharyngeal secretions, droplets inhaled within close distance to the infected person or borne on the air within enclosed, crowded spaces, or farther afield, have seemed a logical, if not demonstrated, means of transmission for pneumotropic and respiratory viruses. With a view to determining whether the concept that virus infections may be air-borne could be confirmed, three members of the department of veterinary science of the University of California, 1948, collected air from poultry houses containing birds infected with the pneumoencephalitic Newcastle disease virus, and, after drawing the air through a fluid, made cultures which they found contained sufficient concentrations of the virus to kill chick embryos. The possibility that psittacosis may be transmitted by air-borne dried droppings entering the respiratory tract was stressed by Bedson, 1940, by Cox, 1947, and, 1952, by Meyer, who, while considering direct contact (with feathers, excreta of sick or dead birds) chiefly responsible for transmission to man, mentioned the possibility of indirect transmission by inhalation of dried particles suspended in the air. Andrewes, of the common cold research unit of Britain's Medical Research Council, observed, 1949, that the old idea of droplet infection in the common cold "has in some quarters lost popularity in favour of the conception (Wells and Wells, 1936) of droplet-nucleus infection", according to which the many small particles leaving the nose or mouth evaporate instantaneously to a diameter of less than ten millimicrons, remain suspended in the air for an hour or more, and (since, in any case, probably only a minority of the nuclei carry microorganisms) are inhaled only in infinitesimal quantity. Since mice and human beings have been experimentally infected by inhalation, droplet transmission of influenza has been frequently mentioned. Francis observed, 1943, that there is little reason to regard influenza as air-borne "except when in crowded quarters the differentiation between direct transfer and impregnation of the air becomes academic". The Commission on Acute Respiratory Diseases reported, 1946, that approximately twenty-five per cent of human volunteers were experimentally infected with primary atypical pneumonia by nasal and oral discharges from the upper respiratory tract of patients. Olitsky and Casals, 1952, cited Armstrong's suggestion of a decade earlier that the virus of lymphocytic choriomeningitis may be transmitted from the house mouse to man by dust (containing dried nasal secretions, semen, urine, feces).

### TRANSMISSION THROUGH CONTAMINATED WATER, FOOD, MILK

It is a short step from demonstration of the presence of virus in feces and sewage to incrimination of water courses. So long ago as 1912, the possibility that poliomyelitis may be water-borne was raised by Kling, in Sweden. Gordon cited an unpublished statistical report by A. T. Dempster from the University of Michigan School of Public Health, 1948, that of 121 cities of over 25,000, cities with little or no treatment of their water supply had the highest incidence of poliomyelitis, cities treating water by filtration and chlorination or softening had the lowest case rates. A 1940 epidemiological study by Casey and Aymond implied that the increasing incidence of poliomyelitis in the past few decades might be related to the growing tendency of communities to liquefy excreta without making adequate provision for disposal of the accumulated fluids. For eighty-seven incorporated communities with water supply but without sewerage systems, according to this study, the poliomyelitis rate was 83.6 cases per 100,000 inhabitants, whereas for twenty-seven incorporated communities that had both water supply and sewerage systems the rate was 26.6 cases per 100,000 inhabitants. Maxcy, however, observed, 1943, "there is on record at present not a single instance of an explosive outbreak of this disease which has been attributed to simultaneous exposure of a group of people to a common source of water". Efforts have naturally been made to discover whether methods commonly employed in water purification plants (sand filtration, aeration, alteration of pH, storage, alum precipitation, ultraviolet radiation) would remove poliomyelitis. Farquhar, Stokes and Schrack described, 1952, an epidemic of viral hepatitis in rural Pennsylvania in which infection "was apparently spread both by drinking water and by contact".

Proof of transmission of poliomyelitis virus by food contaminated by flies carrying the virus from feces of patients or sewage rests upon proof of transmission of infection by the oral route. Ward, Melnick and Horstmann reported, 1945, that food exposed with fly bait in twenty rural homes of poliomyelitis patients was capable of inducing inapparent poliomyelitis in chimpanzees. Howe, 1952, noted that diligent search had failed to trace epidemics to contaminated food. Melnick and Penner, however, 1952, in studies of survival of poliomyelitis virus in flies and their excreta showed that the virus could be detected in flies for seventeen days and in their excreta for ten days. The virus present in human stools survived drying at room temperature for at least three days. When these samples were fed to flies the virus in the dried excreta of the insects could be recovered for from one day to two.

Incrimination of milk as a means of transmitting virus — based on the reported tracing of a poliomyelitis outbreak to milk in the classic instance of the 1926 Broadstairs epidemic in Great Britain, and in an outbreak (Goldstein, Hammon and Viets, 1946) among cadets at a naval training school — was described by Francis and associates, 1948, as "entirely without laboratory support" but not impossible. Howe, however, considered, 1952, the attributing of five small outbreaks to consumption of raw milk contaminated with poliomyelitis virus as rather complimenting the vigilance of epidemiologists than as indicating a dangerous route of transmission. W. J. Murphy, 1946, reported a milk-borne epidemic of viral hepatitis.

### LATENT AND SUBCLINICAL INFECTION, ABORTIVE ATTACKS, CARRIER STATES, RESERVOIRS

Howe estimated, 1952, that between one and two hundred nonparalytic or abortive cases of poliomyelitis occur for every paralytic case; the ratio of apparent to inapparent infection with this virus has varied from 1:100 to the 1:1000 of Turner's estimate. The late Paul Clark commented on the number of poliomyelitis cases that are never diagnosed at all. Buddingh, 1949, considered that persistence of immunity in measles might be accounted for by retention of the virus in a latent form. Enders, 1952, cited the finding of specific complement-fixing mumps antibody in the blood of approximately half the tested adults that denied having had the disease. Horsfall, 1948, regarded observations of his own (with Rickard, 1940), and of Francis earlier, as suggesting that subclinical influenza infection "may be as common as, or even more common than, manifest infections". Scott, 1948, considered the evidence that seventy to ninety per cent of adults have circulating antibodies against herpes simplex virus to imply numerous subclinical infections resulting in a widespread carrier state. An hypothesis (cited by Stokes, 1952) similar to that advanced for latent herpetic infection would explain herpes zoster in adults as a varicella-infection of nerves precipitated by cold, nervous pressure (or exposure or massive doses of varicella) in individuals who have had varicella in childhood and in whom the virus remains latent in nerve cells until evoked by a sufficiently powerful stimulus.

Latent or symptomless infections may result in lifelong immunity, in a carrier state, or a reservoir. Carriers have loomed large in studies of virus transmission. Maxcy defined, 1952, two classes of carriers: hosts that are about to have a clinical attack (incubatory), or that have had an attack (convalescent or chronic); and, secondly, hosts that have subclinical or inapparent infections. Francis, 1952, defined a carrier as one who maintains the virus, the state being always a subclinical infection. In this concept the frequently used term "healthy" carrier becomes a misnomer. Carriers are sometimes incriminated as transmitters because of dearth of other explanations for the presence of virus at a given time and place and because of inability to account in other ways for survival of viruses between epidemics. University of Michigan investigators (in a five-year study of the sources of infection for poliomyelitis outbreaks) observed, 1945, that current stress on carriers might be partly due to obvious difficulty in establishing a history of person-to-person contact. A not inconsiderable body of work, however, justifies stress on carriers in poliomyelitis. Howe, 1952, felt that the leisurely spread of the disease without known connection between recognized cases points to a major role for subclinical cases and carriers in transmission. The virus may be "carried" in pharyngeal secretions or in stools. Epidemiological studies (Francis and associates, 1945 to 1952) indicated "that subclinical infection not uncommonly persists in apparently healthy individuals for as long as five weeks or more".

Van Rooyen and Rhodes, 1948, cited the reference of Le Bourdelles, Lesaffre and Rogez, 1946, to the "highly modified, perhaps ambulant, case of smallpox occurring in the immune person" as "an important source of infection". Carriers of smallpox were designated, 1945, by the American Public Health Association as active cases without remaining constitutional symptoms, recent contacts with cases, and exposed vaccinated persons who may have unrecognized forms of the infection.

Experimental evidence of a "fecal carrier state" in viral hepatitis, lasting from five to fifteen months in adult volunteers, was reported by Capps and Stokes, 1952. Of transmission of serum hepatitis through human plasma, Barnett, Fox and Snavely observed, 1950: "No known method of excluding donors or treating whole blood is capable of eliminating this virus. Healthy carriers exist . . ." Havens and Paul observed, 1952, that serum hepatitis is definitely transmitted by blood or its products obtained from an apparently healthy carrier, as indicated by the tens of thousands of cases of hepatitis transmitted before and during the last war by injections of plasma or administration of yellow fever vaccine containing human serum. Such transmission of the virus was confirmed by transfusing blood from suspected asymptomatic carriers to human volunteers (Stokes and associates with workers at the National Microbiological Institute, 1954).

Meyer, 1952, summarized evidence that psittacosis is common among apparently healthy birds that spread the infection in aviaries where conditions contribute to virulence and high mortality. As to human carriers, a 1952 report (Meyer and Eddie) refers to the "unusual history of a patient known to be a psittacosis carrier for eight years without transmitting the disease". The case was not considered to indicate that chronic psittacosis in man is contagious.

Burnet's view, 1945, as to human carriers of influenza, was: "At the present time there is no visible alternative to the view that human influenza viruses survive between epidemic periods in the tissues of human carriers." But Francis, in the same year, although he had earlier reported recovery of influenza virus from "healthy" contacts, observed that there is no evidence for chronic human carriers of this virus. Horsfall, 1948, thought that unequivocal evidence for the "existence of (influenza) virus carriers among human beings" had not been obtained.

The role of animals in providing reservoirs that keep a virus going in nature is illustrated by forest animals in jungle yellow fever, mice in lymphocytic choriomeningitis, birds and animals in psittacosis, dogs and wild animals in rabies, by the steadily growing lists (cat, calf, mouse) of animals found to harbor pneumonitis viruses, and of wild birds, domestic fowl and animals incriminated in recent years in transmission of encephalitis viruses that attack both horses and man. An animal reservoir is a logical supposition since something besides human infection must keep certain viruses going. Possible rabies reservoirs mentioned in the past decade include, among domestic animals, besides the dog, cats, horses, cows, hogs, sheep, swine, goats; among wild animals (Johnson, 1947, 1948), wolves, squirrels, raccoons, skunks, foxes, coyotes, bobcats, mountain lions, mongooses, jackals, vampire and other bats.

Simmons and associates, studying dengue in the Philippines, 1931, suggested that certain members of the *Aedes* species by keeping the infection going among susceptible monkeys can give rise to a type of jungle dengue which may be as important in the epidemiology of human dengue as jungle yellow fever is in the epidemiology of human yellow fever (Sabin, 1952). Among more unusual possibilities with regard to virus reservoirs is the complex cycle suggested (1939) by Shope for the virus of swine influenza which he traced through a circuitous route involving the swine lungworm as actual reservoir and intermediate host of the virus, and the common earthworm as the intermediate host of the lungworm, which must spend three of its developmental stages in its earthworm host before it can parasitize swine. Swine acquire their lungworm parasites by eating earthworms found in the soil. If the third-stage lungworm larvae are laid by an adult lungworm inhabiting the lung of a pig with influenza they will be carriers of the masked virus. The "masking" of swine influenza virus in its lungworm intermediate host explains (Shope, 1950) the means by which the virus survives in nature from one outbreak to the next. Similar reservoirs may explain how "lots of other viruses" (Shope) survive from one periodic outbreak to the next (hog cholera, poliomyelitis, measles, cattle plague, foot-and-mouth disease). Stanley, commenting, 1946, on Shope's hypothesis, said that although the virus cannot be demonstrated directly when in the lungworm larvae within the earthworm, it appears to be present at the start of the sequence of events and at the end: "The situation may be likened to that of a train going through a tunnel — you may see the train as it enters and as it leaves the tunnel, but it is not apparent while in the tunnel." Burnet, 1945, thought it "quite possible . . . that the Shope cycle may represent the most ancient mode of life of the influenza viruses. But there is equally no valid evidence that it is not a mere biological accident, perhaps dating only from the human pandemic of 1918."

Expanding horizons characterize the search for reservoirs for various viruses obviously not limited to man-to-man transmission. The virus of equine encephalomyelitis, first isolated from horses and mules, is known from experimental studies, from observations in nature and in the clinic, to attack a wide variety of mammals (including man) and birds, apparently always through insect vectors. Infections in animals, both those occurring naturally and those artificially induced, frequently occur in clinically inapparent form. Experimental evidence (Ten Broeck, 1940) indicated that birds may carry the eastern virus in the blood without other signs of infection, and viremia in infections with the western and St. Louis viruses was demonstrated in horses, birds and fowl (Hammon and Reeves, 1941 to 1949). In studies by Hammon and Reeves in the state of Washington, 1948, specific antibodies against western equine or St. Louis viruses (or both) were reported in the blood of about fifty per cent of the domestic birds (chickens, ducks, geese, owls, pigeons and turkeys) examined; in about twenty per cent of the local wild birds (quail, robin, sparrow, dove, flicker, hawk). Epidemiologists of the communicable disease center of the Public Health Service, reporting from Colorado, 1951, isolation of western equine encephalomyelitis virus twice from redwing blackbirds and once from a magpie, noted this as the first time the role of birds "has been definitely proved" by isolation of the virus from wild birds under natural conditions. Of the regional domestic mammals tested, about fifty per cent were positive, the cat being consistently negative; of the wild mammals tested, however, only about eight per cent gave a positive result. Many mammals and birds, especially chickens, have been suspected as a reservoir for Japanese B virus because on inoculation they develop viremia without other signs of infection. Hodes, Thomas and Peck, however, in Okinawa, 1946, and Sabin, on the basis of serum neutralization tests for the Army in Japan, 1947, found the virus widespread among horses and other mammals at a time when it was only occasionally present in chickens. Suspicion has fallen most heavily on fowl because Hammon and Reeves (1939 to 1947) found that the mosquitoes, *Culex tarsalis*, which are carriers of western equine and St. Louis viruses, and *Culex pipiens* feed on fowl, the latter exclusively.

Found originally in mice in which the virus is maintained in a colony by apparently normal carriers (Traub, 1935), lymphocytic choriomeningitis is now known, according to Olitsky and Casals, 1952, to occur naturally in guinea pigs, monkeys, dogs. To the parrot, once considered the sole reservoir of psittacosis virus, were early added as possible reservoirs the chicken (young and adult), canary, seagull, Japanese rice bird, Java sparrow, Peking duck, fulmar petrel. Meyer, 1948, considered it "now evident that the epidemiologist must carefully investigate every known avian and mammalian source before inquiring into the human spreaders of this virus".

In noting that little evidence has thus far been produced pointing to any animal other than man as the main reservoir of the human poliomyelitis virus, Gear, 1952, referred to his own finding in Africa (among birds), those of Hammon and others in the United States, of neutralizing antibodies to Lansing poliomyelitis virus in a wide range of domestic and wild animals as requiring further detailed study. The presence of these antibodies in rodents has been frequently mentioned.

## INSECT VECTORS

Investigations of insect vectors are aimed at determining whether these are infected temporarily or permanently; whether the virus can multiply only in a particular part of the insect (or requires the insect's saliva in order to start multiplication); whether the infected insect can transmit the virus to its offspring. The discovery that a given insect harbours a particular virus falls far short of proving that the insect transmits the virus; it has been demonstrated, for instance, that the fly can carry the poliomyelitis virus, but not that the fly is commonly involved in normal transmission of the disease to human beings. In spite of many years of research on mosquito transmission of various encephalitides, much of the experimental evidence accumulated against a given mosquito species (*Aedes aegypti*, *Culex tarsalis*) for a given form of encephalitis remains circumstantial. Proof of mosquito transmission, moreover, does not exclude other vectors: experiments of Berry and Syverton, 1941, demonstrated that wood ticks to which western equine virus had been transmitted could pass it on to their offspring, and wood ticks have been suspected by Russian workers as vectors of Russian Far East encephalitis. Although insects other than the mosquito, including lice, may be capable of transmitting equine encephalomyelitis to horses, mules, or man, they may serve rather as reservoirs than as direct transmitters (Kelser, 1947).

Insect transmission represents only one step in a complex chain of events: is the mosquito the ultimate reservoir, or does it secure the virus from some other source, human, or animal? Does the mosquito transmit merely from man to man, or from animal to man? For many years man was believed to be the sole source of the virus by which yellow fever was spread to man, the mosquito conveying the blood meal taken from one infected human by biting a second human. The finding (Stokes, Bauer, Hudson, 1928) that monkeys indigenous to South America could be experimentally infected with yellow fever, and that mosquitoes other than the *Aedes* (including forest mosquitoes) could transmit yellow fever in the laboratory, suggested that the man-*Aedes*-man chain might not explain wholly the transmission of yellow fever. Soper had suggested, 1936, that yellow fever in man might be an accident occurring during the course of an epizootic among lower animals. The finding of yellow fever in jungle regions where man does not exist, the failure of wide campaigns of mosquito elimination and vaccination to wipe out the infection indicated that man is not a necessary link and that, in the jungle, the mosquito may take the virus from animal to animal. Although "jungle" and "urban" yellow fever are clinically, pathologically and immunologically identical, the man-*Aedes aegypti*-man chain of the urban disease differs from the vertebrate-invertebrate-vertebrate jungle cycle of infection. The International Health Division's finding (jungle yellow fever studies in Uganda) that monkeys possessed immunity in regions where no humans resided, and that the virus could be isolated from mosquitoes in such regions, provided further support for the probability that there exists "an endemic disease cycle involving forest animals and preferentially arboreal mosquitoes without the participation of the human host". Meyer and Eddie, 1947, observed of equine encephalomyelitis that contact with horses is without consequence to man; "mosquitoes in all probability acquire the viral agent by feeding on birds with subclinical virus infections". Isolation during a nonepidemic period, by Smith, Blattner and Heys, 1944, of St. Louis encephalitis virus from blood-sucking chicken mites found in three separate localities in St. Louis County, and demonstration, 1948, by Smith and her associates, of transovarian infection of the mite suggested the possibility that mites of fowl or other birds may be the means for carrying this virus over the nonepidemic period for man. S. E. Sulkin, 1945, reported that chicken mites presumably form for western equine encephalomyelitis virus a permanent depot from which hens may be directly infected, and man and horses infected indirectly by other insect vectors, such as mosquitoes. The virus of Murray Valley encephalitis was believed (French, 1951) to be spread by mosquitoes from a natural reservoir in birds.

Fleas, bedbugs and, as previously mentioned, flies have all been suggested at one time or another as possible insect vectors of poliomyelitis, the geographical and seasonal incidence of which (in epidemic outbreaks) have made insect participation seem logical. Francis and associates considered, 1948, that demonstration of virus in flies of one species had shown that the stool of a patient with poliomyelitis can serve as a source of virus for certain flies which thus become "potential vectors". Howe, 1952, considered it obvious that if flies have a role in transmission it is accessory, since while virus had been recovered from flies with access to human feces during epidemic periods, there have been reports (Gear, 1952) of epidemics running a full course during fly-control programs instituted for other reasons. On the whole, he considered it difficult to assess the role of the fly in the "usual" spread of poliomyelitis.

## SIGNIFICANCE OF PORTALS OF ENTRY

Experimentation has confirmed the observation that a given virus may enter by more than one portal. The complexity of the factors involved in determining the dominant portal (if there is one) is suggested by early preoccupation with the gastrointestinal tract in poliomyelitis, succeeded by concentration on the olfactory portal, then reverting to the gastrointestinal after wide demonstration of the virus in feces and sewage. Numerous variables have been shown to modify experimental results — species, strain of virus employed with a given portal, for a given species. Rabies virus of the natural or street strain is (Johnson, 1952) pathogenic for all mammals by injection into the skin, subcutaneous tissue, muscle, or nervous tissue; strains of so-called fixed virus, while highly pathogenic by intramuscular inoculation for all laboratory animals and for large domestic animals, are noninfectious for man and dogs when given subcutaneously. Contaminated dust from the patient's room may bring in the variola virus not only by the respiratory portal (Smadel, 1952; Downie, 1951; F. O. MacCallum and associates, 1950) but also by other portals. Herpes zoster may enter by the nose, according to early workers (spreading by olfactory perineural lymphatics to the meninges and eventually to the spinal ganglia), or it may enter by the tonsils, spreading *via* the blood to spinal ganglia. Epidemiological observations and experimental evidence (Paul and Havens, 1952) at least suggest that "the intestinal-oral route" may be one of the natural ways in which infectious hepatitis is spread. In poliomyelitis, as several times stressed, the concept of widely disseminated virus from human sources (in sewage), confirmed by isolation of the virus from asymptomatic carriers and patients with abortive infections, has strengthened the view (Howe, 1952) that the virus "probably" multiplies primarily in the gastrointestinal tract, although on the basis of chimpanzee experiments "it is difficult to say" that presence of the virus in intestinal contents in man indicates true infection leading to immunity, or that the virus reached the intestinal tract by feeding. While observing that "the exact mode of entry of virus into the host is not known", Bodian, 1953, added, "but there is widespread agreement that the virus probably enters by way of the mouth and begins to multiply at primary sites of implantation in the oropharynx and in the lower intestines".

The relation of the portal of entry to immunity has been emphasized in the work of several groups on epidemic influenza. Burnet and associates have been interested since 1939 in the possibility of local immunity resulting from virus-inactivating or neutralizing substances in nasal secretions (believed by some to derive from serum antibodies in the blood). Francis, fifteen years ago, related histological changes in the nasal mucosa after instillation of influenza virus in ferrets to immunity, associated with the reparative process. "The conclusion appears justifiable", he observed, 1943, ". . . that influenza represents in its pathogenesis a specific injury inflicted by a virus of sharply selective affinities upon a specialized type of cell lining the respiratory tract, and that to obtain resistance these cells representing the portal of entry must be afforded protection." He reported, 1947, experiments showing that a small amount of immune serum given intranasally protected mice against pulmonary disease from virus administered intraperitoneally. Moreover, immune serum given by the same route several hours after intranasal administration of virus protected some animals. Experiments conducted by several groups of workers on influenza, in this country, Australia and the U.S.S.R., with inhalation of influenza virus, have been aimed at development of effective immunization at the portal of entry.

## POSSIBLE PATHS OF VIRUS TRANSPORT TO SPECIFIC CELLS

The more usual paths of virus spread involve the blood stream, as in yellow fever; the lymphatics, as in lymphogranuloma inguinale; the skin or mucous surfaces, as in warts; the nerve fibers, as in poliomyelitis and rabies. Rigid classification of viruses according to route of infection and tissue specificity has not, as indicated earlier, proved satisfactory. A neurotropic virus (Olitsky and Casals, 1952) "may also affect other tissues" besides nerve tissue; "there are degrees of neurotropism". A decade ago, Howe and Bodian had queried what, if the pathway of poliomyelitis virus is exclusively neuronal, "is the meaning of the general lymphoid hyperplasia so frequently described and the presence of virus in nasopharyngeal secretions and stools? May the virus be a common inhabitant of the upper respiratory passages or the gastrointestinal tract and only an exceptional invader of the central nervous system?"

### THE LYMPHATIC CHANNELS

J. M. Yoffey pointed out, 1947, that in the case of such a virus as vaccinia (from which, however, he would not generalize), the lymph node "far from preventing the spread of infection actually encourages it". McMaster and Kidd were cited as having demonstrated, 1937, that vaccinia virus reaches the lymph node, multiplies there, "and then leaves it and is carried to the blood stream by the lymphocytes in the efferent lymph". Burrows suggested that, for a majority of cases of poliomyelitis, acute lymphatic hyperplasia might be a more accurate name than infantile paralysis. Some workers have suggested that the poliomyelitis virus enters by way of the gastrointestinal lymphatics and "spreads to contiguous lymphatic tissues in the body". Wenner and Rabe, who detected the poliomyelitis virus in lymph nodes from six of nine fatal cases, 1951, proposed that the virus travels from the gastrointestinal tract into lymphatic channels with outflow into the blood stream and interstitial tissue spaces, and that after the period of viremia the virus collects in the lymph nodes. Yoffey and Drinker, however, after studying cervical lymph from monkeys (infected by intranasal instillation and intracerebral injection) at all stages of the disease, reported (of the one strain that they studied): "Virus was not found in either cervical or thoracic duct lymph; and tests on centrifugalized specimens showed that it was not present in the lymphocytes, as was the case with vaccinia virus." Early work on herpes zoster (Low, 1919) referred to spread by olfactory perineural lymphatics, on the way to the meninges, spinal fluid and spinal ganglia. The pelvic lymphatics, according to various workers, are involved in the route of infection in lymphogranuloma inguinale.

## THE BLOOD STREAM

The length of time during which viruses can be detected in the blood stream determines the transmission of some virus diseases, governs in others the possibility of preventing or attenuating infection. Only when virus can be detected in the blood can yellow fever and dengue be transmitted by the blood-sucking mosquito vectors. Faber and associates considered, 1950, blood invasion by poliomyelitis rare, "not an important part of the disease process in man", and secondary to primary neural infection. Jungeblut, 1950, envisaged three possible stages in progress of the poliomyelitis virus, the first alimentary, the second stage escape of the virus transiently into the blood stream, the third neural. A far more hopeful view of preventing or ameliorating poliomyelitis by gamma globulin followed the 1952 reports by Horstmann of Yale and Bodian of Johns Hopkins that when cynamologous monkeys and chimpanzees were fed the virus it could be found in the blood from four to six days thereafter. Up to that time the virus had been isolated from human blood only twice because it was sought in man in the acute phases, whereas these two investigators had found it in animals before symptoms appeared. Study of blood from human contacts with evidence of the virus in throat or rectum (Horstmann, 1953) and from asymptomatic, abortive and nonparalytic cases (Bodian, 1953) revealed viremia or antibodies. That presence of antibodies in the blood indicated that the virus was present in the blood stream before rather than after central nervous system invasion was suggested by observations on monkeys which showed little rise in antibody following infection from virus injected directly into the nervous system. Bodian considered that these studies supported the hypothesis that poliomyelitis virus enters *via* the gastrointestinal tract, with viremia in early stages and subsequent invasion of the central nervous system. Mechanisms of invasion of the virus from the blood stream into the central nervous system have been suggested by a demonstrated differential permeability to dyes of capillaries in the medulla, penetration at different sites conceivably determining localization of paralysis. The question whether viremia is an essential and constant prelude to invasion of the central nervous system (not yet established) is associated with the also unanswered primary question of the source of virus in the blood stream (Horstmann, 1953).

Studies have not revealed virus in the blood in rabies, although dogs can be infected by intravenous injection of the virus (Johnson, 1952). In smallpox there is support (Downie and associates; MacCallum, McPherson and Johnstone, 1950) for an hypothesis that the inspired virus may be spread from the respiratory tract by way of local lymph tissues and the blood stream to the viscera where it multiplies during the incubation period; with release of the virus from the viscera, fever begins and the virus is carried by the blood to the skin, mucous membranes and viscera where focal lesions subsequently appear. Viremia has been found in fowl and other birds with no sign of St. Louis encephalitis infection after infection by mosquitoes that have fed upon the virus. In eastern and western equine encephalomyelitis (Olitsky and Casals) the virus has been found in the blood of horses during the early visceral stages. The virus of infectious hepatitis can be readily isolated from the blood of infected persons during acute preicteric or early icteric phases. Serum hepatitis can be distinguished from its clinically indistinguishable counterpart, infectious hepatitis, by the presence of the former virus in the circulating blood during the long incubation period (in Neefe's 1944 report for so long as eighty-seven days before symptoms appeared) as well as in acute stages; this explains why human blood products derived from persons without apparent infection may be a source of infection.

## NEURAL ROUTES

One of the unanswered questions concerning "neurotropic" viruses (rabies, poliomyelitis, Borna disease of horses, herpes zoster, the encephalitides) is whether the presence of the virus in a given site in man represents initial progress toward specific nerve tracts, or rather exit from them. Do lesions in peripheral nerves mark ascent of the virus to the central nervous system or descent from it? Does absence of lesions in certain areas of the central nervous system mean that the virus has not invaded such regions or merely that it has left no histo-pathologic evidence of invasion? Does the presence of a virus in extraneural locations mean that this is the portal of entry of the virus or merely that the virus has "spilled over" from the central nervous system to this site? Isolation of a highly neurotropic virus from non-neural sources (in rabies, saliva; in poliomyelitis, pharyngeal secretions, feces) does not necessarily mean "that such an agent multiplies elsewhere than in nervous structure *in vivo*" (Olitsky and Casals, 1952).

The numerous ways in which neurotropic viruses may reach the central nervous system from the periphery differ for different viruses in the same host and for the same virus in different hosts (Sabin, 1939). From a given peripheral site, some viruses may pass along the regional nerves, while others, especially some of those that can multiply in non-nervous tissues and can occur in the blood in relatively high concentration, may first localize in some other site (nasal mucosa) and then follow a neural pathway into the central nervous system, or in certain hosts apparently actually grow through or pass directly across the cerebral blood vessels. Different viruses, according to their tissue affinities, may select different neural pathways from the same site in the same host.

Rabies and encephalitis have been described by various investigators as spreading diffusely through the central nervous system, in contrast to the more discrete distribution of poliomyelitis, along closed neuronal tracts. Webster, 1942, referred to "direct evidence that the (rabies) virus is not transmitted by the blood stream and indirect evidence that it is transmitted in association with the regional nerves". Schultz, 1948, thought the view that in natural infections rabies virus spreads to the central nervous system by way of peripheral nerves "is supported by the fact that the incubation periods tend to be longer following bites on the lower extremities than in the areas closer to the central nervous system". Referring to the evidence supporting the theory of neuronal spread, van Rooyen and Rhodes, 1948, nevertheless added, "the question is in need of review, using more sensitive methods"; they suggested further investigation of the role of blood and lymph.

Absence of evidence for neural spread of the viruses of eastern and western equine encephalomyelitis in monkeys, confirmed in guinea pigs, led Hurst, 1936, to further search for the path by which they invade the central nervous system. His experimentation led him to the concept, still held in 1948 according to Schultz, of a two-stage process, first a visceral involvement which may not progress to the nervous system and secondly, in some cases, involvement of brain and cord. In man (fatal cases), the St. Louis virus has been consistently found only in the brain, several (but not all) other tissues proving negative. The quantitative studies of Peck and Sabin, 1947, showed that after ninety-six hours the concentration of St. Louis virus in the brain, apparently by "spilling over" into the blood, had reached all organs except the inguinal nodes and intestines. Whether the virus in naturally occurring human infection follows the paths suggested in experimental animals had not been proved. Noting that two-stage infection (first in circulating blood, then in nerve) certainly occurs in some of the human viral encephalitides, Olitsky and Casals observed, 1952, "whether the virus passes directly from the blood into the central nervous system, whether, after leaving the circulation, it is deposited on the nasal mucosa whence it progresses *via* neurons and their processes to the central nervous system, or whether it goes directly by way of nerves to the central nervous system from the point of introduction into the body is not as yet definitely known for most of the agents producing encephalitis in man".

Howe and Bodian, Sabin, Faber and others are agreed that the poliomyelitis virus, once established in the peripheral nerves, is restricted to the nervous system, its progress thereafter being along closed neuronal pathways. Whether certain spinal lesions are the result of primary centripetal invasion of sympathetics from the lower alimentary tract or whether they represent a secondary, centrifugal movement of the virus after invasion of the central nervous system remains an open question. Faber and associates reiterated their belief, 1950, that during the initial stage of infection, and throughout asymptomatic and mild cases, the virus is confined to peripheral nerves, making its exit by them through neural connections to the mucous membranes of the upper and lower portions of the alimentary tract. In their view, when the central nervous system is involved, it is secondary to invasion of the peripheral nervous system. Bodian, however, in the course of monkey experiments since 1946 on the genesis of muscle spasm, found that, when the virus was injected directly into the central nervous system, muscle spasm appeared before the virus had reached the peripheral nerves and while it was still heavily concentrated in medulla and brain stem. These are areas for which recent research (Magoun, since 1946) has suggested a role in the regulation of muscle tone and relaxation. As previously noted, Bodian suggested that the virus could pass directly from the blood into the medulla from which it could sweep downward into the cord. In this view, virus excreted through the alimentary canal (in asymptomatic and nonparalytic poliomyelitis) has never found its way into the central nervous system.

Investigative work on routes of poliomyelitis infection illustrates the increasing tendency to challenge fixations, and to stress the importance of multiple variable factors in the conditions of experiment (species, strain, site of inoculation, dosage). Bodian recognized, 1952, lack of "rigorous proof" from any source "pointing to the route of transmission of virus from portal of entry to the central nervous system *in man*". Clear also is the increasing tendency to place experimental work in better focus and to check it constantly by observations in man.

## NEURAL MANIFESTATIONS OF VIRUS DISEASES

### INTRODUCTORY

Viruses commonly listed in the dominantly neurotropic group include rabies, poliomyelitis, various viruses causing encephalitis in animals or in man (eastern and western equine, St. Louis, Japanese B, Venezuelan, Russian spring-summer, Australian X disease, West Nile and Bwamba fever viruses, various other viruses which have been isolated from mosquitoes in the tropics and which although not yet shown to cause encephalitis in man have produced it in laboratory animals, viruses responsible for herpetic encephalitis, pseudorabies and ascending myelitis or B virus infection). To these (eight of them distinguished as epidemic) Olitsky and Casals, 1952, added as viruses causing encephalitis but in nonepidemic form, lymphocytic chorio-meningitis, louping ill and a small group of viruses ordinarily consid-ered not encephalitogenic but observed at times to induce enceph-alitis: herpes simplex, mumps, measles, lymphogranuloma, infectious mononucleosis ("probably caused by a virus"). They referred also to the so-called postinfectious "or demyelinating encephalitides" (viral etiology of which "remains obscure"), which sometimes follow vaccination against smallpox and rabies and such infections as mea-sles, influenza, mumps, varicella, variola, hepatitis, dengue, yellow fever.

So late as 1940, Goodpasture referred to the neural aspects of virus diseases as practically a virgin field for speculation. Obstacles to advance have included: difficulty in getting material from the spinal fluid; difficulty involved in animal experimentation; danger in apply-ing experimental findings to man; difficulty of some of the techniques for histological study of nerves and absence of such skills in pa-thology and bacteriology departments (until twenty years ago major centers for virus research). Rivers once commented on the need for "neurobiologists" in this field; within recent years there has been a steady increase in studies by neuroanatomists, neurochemists, bio-chemists and physiologists working (notably in poliomyelitis) at the cellular level on the relation of the metabolism of nerve to virus growth and spread. Neural manifestations of virus diseases range from mortal forms of paralysis and encephalitis to minor "nervous" symptoms. Individual variation is wide, influenced by the degree of neural involvement characteristic of a given virus, by strain, species, portal of entry (or site of inoculation), previous exposure to the same (or another) strain of the virus, amount of virus that reaches the cen-tral nervous system. Further, there are sometimes difficulties in deter-mining how neural manifestations evoked by viruses differ from neural accompaniments or sequelae of nonviral infections or indeed of non-infectious disease.

Important in attempts to assess neural manifestations of viruses is the question whether a given virus depends primarily or exclusively on nerve tissue for multiplication. The finding of poliomyelitis in the intestines led Evans and Green, 1947, to suggest that assumption of obligate neurocytotropism of poliomyelitis virus in the human body is "premature and may well be wrong". Syverton, 1951, regarded the assumption as "no longer tenable" in view of reports since 1949 that poliomyelitis virus could be propagated in cultures of cells from various extraneural tissues (Enders and associates, 1949; Syverton's group, 1951; others). Enders, at the second international poliomyelitis conference, 1952, although stressing the need to exercise caution in applying *in vitro* findings *in vivo*, added, "but our observations would seem to afford additional support for the hypothesis of extraneural multiplication". In the view, 1951, of Faber, however, whose own attempts to prove multiplication of the virus in the intestinal mucosa of monkeys had all failed, the theory of extraneural multiplication "remains without factual proof and only serves to becloud the pathogenesis of the disease". Views of other leading workers are more generally either doubtful or in the other direction. Jungeblut, 1950, thought clinical and laboratory evidence pointed to pantropic rather than strictly neurotropic quality in poliomyelitis virus. Melnick, 1952, referring to Horstmann's recent work as supporting the view that virus multiplication "can occur outside the central nervous system", mentioned as other possible sites of virus multiplication, lymph glands, the epithelium of the intestinal wall or the nerve cells adjacent to the intestinal mucosa. Bodian suggested, 1952, that virus multiplication may proceed in at least three successive phases — alimentary, vascular, neural. The foregoing views indicate in current discussions a distinct trend away from characterizing dominantly neurotropic viruses as exclusively neurotropic.

## NEURAL MANIFESTATIONS IN THE MORE NEUROTROPIC GROUP

In one of the more neurotropic group, *poliomyelitis*, various investigators have pointed out that traditional clinical preoccupation with the anterior horn of the spinal cord has tended to obscure the clinical significance of involvement of other parts of the central nervous system and of parts of the brain other than the medulla. Bodian, 1952, noted that recent studies (his own, those of Faber, of Baker and associates) raised questions as to "whether some of the symptoms which have been interpreted by clinicians in the past on the basis of anterior horn cell lesions are not actually due to brain stem or cerebral lesions". Howe, 1948, suggested that each paralytic poliomyelitis patient presents "a melange of signs and symptoms indicating damage to various parts of the central nervous system". Baker, of Minnesota's poliomyelitis research commission (who, with Brown and McQuarrie, has been correlating effects of destruction of medullary areas in bulbar poliomyelitis with changes in respiratory and cardiovascular symptoms), observed, 1949, that advances in neuropathology and neurophysiology, distinguishing different types of neural involvement, made it possible to modify the traditional fatalistic attitude toward bulbar poliomyelitis. By correlating clinical symptoms with what has been discovered of the function of various cranial nerves and parts of the medulla, he thought it now possible to foresee in which cases of bulbar poliomyelitis a more favorable, in which a less favorable, outcome is expectable. Ability to distinguish between different types of neural involvement would also guide treatment: physical clearance of the airways would be the treatment if the symptoms of respiratory failure were referable to tenth cranial nerve involvement (controlling swallowing), whereas oxygen therapy would be indicated if symptoms were referable to autonomic centers of the medulla (controlling respiration).

In addition to the well-known lesions found in fatal cases in the spinal cord, lesions in the brain are "so characteristic", according to Howe, 1952, as to distinguish poliomyelitis from other neurotropic virus diseases "perhaps even more clearly than do the lesions in the cord". In contrast to the random lesions found in the brain in other neurotropic virus diseases, those in poliomyelitis are characteristically concentrated in the motor cells of the reticular formation of the medulla and pons, and in restricted areas of the motor cortex, in which, according to Bodian, 1952, lesions are usually mild. In contrast to the encephalitides, for instance, in which the entire cerebral cortex is involved, in poliomyelitis only the motor (and premotor) areas have been found to be characteristically involved. Bodian, 1949, referred to the added significance given involvement of the reticular formation in poliomyelitis (in clinical interpretations) by the complex functions of the brain stem that have in recent years been localized in the reticular formation — as respiratory, vasomotor, swallowing and motor inhibitory mechanisms. Frequent association of bulbar and encephalitic manifestations was observed in patients studied in the 1946 Minnesota epidemic. McQuarrie reported encephalitis, "in one guise or another" (hyperexcitability, mental confusion, personality disturbances, convulsions, coma), in seventy-eight, or one sixth, of 464 cases admitted to the pediatric service at Minnesota. Referring to greater cerebral involvement in poliomyelitis than is suspected on clinical grounds, three McGill investigators in the pediatrics and neurology departments (Goldbloom, Jasper, Brickman) attempted, 1948, an electroencephalographic study of a small series of poliomyelitis patients with a view to extending clinical criteria of encephalitic involvement. The abnormal changes they observed have not been consistently noted in other reports and, in general, studies are not sufficiently complete (Howe, 1952) to justify interpretation. Howe considered cortical hypoxia the most logical explanation of encephalitic manifestations.

Adequate and controlled studies are not available to support or to refute the theory that an attack of poliomyelitis, either at the time or subsequently, may depress the level of general intelligence (as estimated by the Stanford-Binet scale) and/or lead to disturbed behavior or personality changes. The McGill electroencephalographic study, mentioned above, did not answer the question whether disturbed behavior may have an organic basis in the neural damage caused by poliomyelitis. Indeed the investigators suggested as one explanation for "the disturbed behavior which has been known to occur as a late sequel of poliomyelitis" psychologic trauma resulting from crippling disabilities and prolonged hospitalization. "However, the possibility that some of those disturbances may have an organic basis . . . has by no means been excluded." Bodian commented, a few years ago, that personality changes in poliomyelitis could hardly be the result of damage to the cerebral cortex, "since lesions are conspicuously absent from most of the cortex. Severe lesions are present, however, in the hypothalamus and thalamus in some of our cases, and in these cases general involvement of the brain stem is severe. If injury to these centers can contribute to emotional disturbances, then perhaps one can account for a correlation of electroencephalographic abnormality with severe behavior disturbances."

The acute encephalitis due to *rabies* has, according to various authors, been diagnosed only at necropsy since routine tests for distinguishing it from the encephalitis of poliomyelitis are not available. Establishing the causal role of rabies entirely on the basis of pathology offers difficulties (Johnson, 1952, others) because there are no gross abnormalities which can be regarded as specific for rabies; the lesions are similar to those found in other viral encephalitides.

In contrast to the "highly neurotropic" poliomyelitis and rabies viruses (Olitsky and Casals, 1952), *encephalitis* viruses have been listed as "ordinary neurotropic viruses". Necrosis of neurons has been described as the outstanding lesion for St. Louis, Japanese B, western and Russian Far East encephalitis. Meningeal reactions (in man) have been described in St. Louis and Russian Far East encephalitis and (in animals) in western equine and louping ill encephalitis. Whereas the cord is frequently involved in St. Louis and in Russian Far East encephalitis, it may be spared in western and eastern encephalitis. Most striking in Japanese B encephalitis is destruction of the cerebellum, in which respect Japanese B resembles louping ill. Clinical evidence of mental impairment, personality changes or disturbed motor function was reported by Lewis, Taylor and associates, 1947, in about a third of a series of cases of Japanese B encephalitis in the native population of Okinawa. Olitsky and Casals noted, however, 1952, neurologic or psychotic changes in only 3.1 per cent of the survivors in 2,000 cases. More frequent and more severe residual impairment (in horses and men) has been noted in eastern as compared with western encephalomyelitis (Kelser and others). Clinical forms of the meningeal involvement in lymphocytic choriomeningitis, in both mice and men, may range (Smadel and associates, 1942) from aseptic meningitis to meningoencephalomyelitis.

Schultz, 1948, mentioned as evidence serving "to establish the fact" that herpes simplex "is at times responsible for encephalitis in man", four reports within a decade of isolation of herpes virus from encephalic lesions: Smith, Lennette and Reames, 1941; Armstrong, 1943; Smadel, Zarafonetis, Adams and Haymaker, 1944; Whitman, Wall and Warren, 1946. Until herpes simplex virus was isolated from a nonfatal case of meningoencephalitis in 1951 (by Afzelius-Alm) encephalitis due to this virus had been diagnosed only at necropsy. Florman and Mindlin, 1952, described a case of generalized herpes simplex in an eleven-day infant who developed meningoencephalitis and survived with neurological defects and chorioretinitis. Experimental work by Field, 1952, in England, demonstrated herpetic encephalitis following corneal inoculation of the virus. A view long held by certain French workers is that the herpes simplex viruses form a graded group, at one end of which are the dermotropic strains, at the other the neurotropic strains. The neurotropic and dermotropic properties of the virus are, in other views (Florman and Trader, 1947), however, considered to depend not on intrinsic properties of the virus but rather on the host.

From 1917, when von Economo's studies gave his name to this encephalitis (suspected of being of virus origin although the etiological agent has never been isolated), various workers have stressed microscopic lesions in the gray matter, especially in the mesencephalon and diencephalon. A five-year study initiated in 1936 at the University of Chicago on the relation of Parkinsonian symptoms to encephalitis began with induction of destructive lesions in thirteen monkeys, in ten of which the aim was to destroy the lenticular nucleus on both sides of the brain while in three the lesions were placed in the midbrain to destroy the substantia nigra as completely and as selectively as possible. The experiments were of especial interest "because of the similarity to the acute stage of human epidemic encephalitis in which the inflammation lies in the same part as that damaged mechanically in these monkeys".

## NEURAL MANIFESTATIONS IN VIRUSES NOT USUALLY CLASSIFIED AS NEUROTROPIC

Developing realization throughout the years that neural aspects are not limited to the foregoing virus conditions in which nervous tissue is predominantly involved has led to observations, of a generally speculative character, concerning neural manifestations (associations, complications, sequelae) in varicella, herpes zoster, mumps, influenza, canine distemper, dengue, lymphogranuloma inguinale, measles, German measles, primary atypical pneumonia, smallpox, submaxillary gland virus of guinea pigs, sandfly fever, yellow fever. According to Stokes, 1952, *varicella* is only occasionally complicated by encephalitis "from which most patients recover". Meningitis was mentioned by van Rooyen and Rhodes, 1948, as a possible if infrequent nervous complication of varicella along with encephalitis and myelitis. In *herpes zoster* in the (rare) cases in which inflammation of posterior nerve roots and ganglia spreads to the anterior horn, temporary or permanent paralysis may occur (Stokes, 1952). He found paralysis in approximately fifty per cent of cephalic cases of zoster. Various workers have mentioned aseptic meningitis as occasionally associated with it.

That *mumps* can directly cause central nervous system manifestations more severe than those of the aseptic meningitis syndrome was described by a group of virus workers (Sabin, Horsfall, Meyer, Scott, Snyder, discussing the diagnosis of neurotropic viruses), 1952, as "open to question". Among suggestive scattered reports is a 1951 note from the National Office of Vital Statistics of several cases of encephalitis without parotitis or with mild parotitis in local outbreaks of mumps in Seattle. Oldfelt, 1949, reported a study of seventy-five cases of mumps-meningoencephalitis which were preceded, accompanied, or followed by typical salivary gland involvement, treated at Stockholm Epidemic Hospital during 1942–1943 epidemics. Lasting ill effects from which fifteen were suffering from three to five years later included severe epilepsy, total unilateral deafness, vestibular dizziness, mild eye, ear, mental symptoms and obesity "possibly due to injury to the hypothalamus". In an outbreak of mumps in a boys' boarding school in England (reported by Henderson, 1952), eleven of fourteen patients had mild meningitis, four of them having no parotitis. In connection with California studies (of viral encephalitides in county hospitals) the International Health Division, 1948, commented on "increasing evidence that the mumps virus plays a rather significant role in the causation of central nervous system disturbances". A number of cases of encephalitis, or of meningoencephalitis, without clinical evidence of parotitis or orchitis, were shown, according to this report, "serologically to be due to mumps virus". The percentage of routine mumps cases that show clinical and subclinical involvement of the central nervous system is suggested by Army studies within the past ten years; one of these military studies (McGuinness and Gall, 1943) noted nervous system involvement (observed or suspected) in fifty-five of 1,378 mumps cases. In a Fort Benning study of 100 consecutive hospitalized cases of mumps, thirty-three showed clinical signs of meningoencephalitis and twenty-eight of these showed abnormal spinal fluid. No correlation could be made between central nervous system involvement and severity of salivary gland involvement or presence of orchitis. Greater use of recently developed serologic (especially complement-fixation) tests should, in the view of the Army workers, lead to more accurate diagnosis of mumps meningoencephalitis. Enders, 1952, noted that the white cell count of the spinal fluid has been an important aid in diagnosing the general syndrome of aseptic lymphocytic meningoencephalitis "of which mumps virus is only one of the known causes". He regarded as "debatable", however, any tendency to construe increase in spinal fluid lymphocytes, indicating latent encephalitis, as support for regarding mumps as a primary invasion of the central nervous system.

Nervous symptoms, some of them marked, have been noted in sporadic reports for *sand fly fever, dengue, infectious mononucleosis*. In describing a fatal case of *atypical pneumonia* with encephalitis, a 1943 United States Army study recalled the antigenic relation between viruses isolated from cases of primary atypical pneumonia and viruses of psittacosis, lymphocytic choriomeningitis and lymphogranuloma venereum, "all of which can produce meningitis as well as pneumonia, in man or animal . . ." Sabin and Aring in 1942, Zarafonetis in 1944, and Scott in 1945, reported meningoencephalitis in lymphogranuloma. At the 1939 Harvard symposium, Fothergill classified *vaccinia* among viscerotropic viruses causing meningeal reactions. Van Rooyen, 1948, cited workers in the early 1930's (including workers under the British Medical Research Council) describing involvement of the central nervous system in *smallpox*. Mental disturbances (with encephalographic evidence of damage to the brainstem and spinal cord) were reported in a case of *rubella*, in which serious neurological complications had been reported previously in the literature (Mitchell and Pampiglione, 1954).

A study of encephalomyelitis complicating *measles* at the Hospital for Infectious Diseases of Stockholm, 1949, led Jacobsson and Holmgren to conclude that the incidence and severity of measles encephalitis are increasing. While Hoyne and Slotkowski, 1947, estimated the incidence to be one to 642, Rake, 1952, estimated that about one in 10,000 cases of measles results in encephalitis but noted that the incidence may be higher in certain epidemics.

The traditional question whether *encephalitis following vaccination or infection* with various agents including viruses ordinarily not encephalitogenic (as measles, influenza, mumps, varicella, variola, infectious hepatitis, dengue, rubella, lymphocytic choriomeningitis, yellow fever, according to Olitsky and Casals, 1952) is due to the original virus or to another agent, or to a hypersensitive reaction, remains without conclusive answer. Malamud, 1939, favored the view that postinfectious encephalitis following measles is due to the measles virus itself. Shaffer, Rake and Holden, 1942, reported isolating the measles virus (in a monkey) from the brain of a fatal case. The concept of postinfectious and postvaccinal encephalitis as a manifestation of autosensitization to brain tissue was developed following the reports, 1948, of Jervis and Koprowski, and of Ferraro and Cazzullo, on production of "chronic experimental allergic encephalomyelitis" in guinea pigs and monkeys by injection of homologous brain tissue in an emulsion with paraffin oil, aquaphor and killed tubercle bacilli. Kabat, Wolf and Bezer reported, 1949, production of acute disseminated encephalomyelitis in monkeys by injection of a portion of their own individual brains with adjuvants, which they considered to provide additional evidence that the pathological changes now designated as postinfectious, postvaccinal encephalitis, and other diseases such as multiple sclerosis "may be a result of sensitization or antibody formation to an individual's own brain tissue". Olitsky and Yager, 1949, who produced the same condition in white mice by injections of normal mouse brain mixed with a modification of the adjuvant considered that these animals, in which signs indicative of marked involvement of the central nervous system and also of the respiratory mechanism occurred, may be the species of choice for study of the etiology of the demyelinating diseases. How such a sequence of events would occur clinically is, of course, completely unknown. Merritt, 1950, referring to failure of all attempts to isolate a virus from the brain and cord of persons who had died of postinfectious or postvaccinal encephalomyelitis reported that the character of the pathological changes in the nervous system of these patients was "unlike that which is seen in the nervous system of patients with fatal infections with the known viruses". He thought it likely that postinfectious and postvaccinal encephalomyelitis "are due to an allergic reaction".

## SUSCEPTIBILITY AND RESISTANCE TO VIRUS INFECTION

A great deal has been learned in recent years about the factors that govern immunity in various virus diseases, notably measles, small-pox, poliomyelitis, hepatitis, influenza, encephalitis, rabies. The knowledge achieved, however, also brings into high relief the valleys between the mountains, the gaps that must be filled before it will be possible to reckon concretely with all the factors that determine the epidemiology of virus diseases, the division of the population into susceptibles and nonsusceptibles in epidemics. In the meantime, epidemiological questions are, from time to time, posed in striking form by such phenomena as the appearance during the last war of poliomyelitis in English and American troops in the Far East, the Middle East and North Africa, although native populations of the same age appeared to be resistant to the disease; and the susceptibility to sandfly fever observed (Sabin and Philip, 1944) when troops or other people from areas where the disease is not prevalent move into endemic zones "where adult native populations are for the most part immune". The fact itself suggests the explanation but by no means supplies all the answers.

While the relation between the susceptibility of the mass and the susceptibility of the individual is appreciated, it is far from being understood. Involved are all the factors touched upon throughout the preceding discussion in the complex cycle of virus (or other) infection — the method by which a virus is transmitted in a population, the portal by which it gains entry into the host, its ability to spread in the host to a tissue where it is maintained or multiplied, its ability to leave the host (by secretions or excretions or through an intermediate insect vector) in a way that will insure infection of another individual and so continued maintenance of the virus. There are the further questions: whether man is the only or obligate host through which a virus may be maintained and multiplied, or an incidental host, or a host supplementary to the primary host or reservoir; what is the nature of the interaction of virus and host and what is the influence of environment on both. Answers to all of these are fundamental in understanding what determines survival of the virus, how individuals and populations become immune, in short, the epidemiology of virus disease. What is entirely clear is that knowledge of the epidemiology of virus disease, its occurrence in given host populations at given times in given environments awaits more certain knowledge of the factors that determine immunity of the individual. Critical among virus problems is the question (as once stated by Berry) why 998 people may be infected with poliomyelitis without ill effects while two succumb to the disease, and why one of those two develops paralysis and the other does not; or the question (as stated by Andrewes) why the common cold virus, constantly passing in a large community from one person to another, usually causes no or only abortive symptoms, developing into a real "cold" only in an individual rendered temporarily or permanently susceptible by conditions without and/or within.

Natural resistance or nonspecific immunity of the individual is resistance to infection not dependent upon a previous spontaneous or experimental contact with infectious agents or their antibodies. Acquired resistance or specific immunity is produced by the body's own reaction to a previous infection, to experimental or intentional production of the disease or a modification of it, or to injection of a vaccine containing antigens capable of stimulating production of protective antibodies. Mechanisms of immunity in bacterial infections are pertinent in virus study since, as many have pointed out, the problems of basic immunity are much the same, "related to the interplay of antibodies and the cells of the body, varying according to the mechanisms of infection and the characteristics of the agent" (Francis). The basic protective activity lies in the serum proteins (antibodies) preparing materials for disposal by digestion or excretion and serving in the maintenance of physiological repair. Both natural and acquired resistance are influenced by constitutional, physical and chemical factors (from without and within). Limited observations on certain of these factors may contribute moderately to clarification of both kinds of resistance, the mechanisms of which are still only partially understood.

## Factors that Influence Natural Susceptibility and Resistance to Virus Infections

It is, as will appear, convenient rather than accurate to attempt to discuss separately the multiple factors that influence natural susceptibility and resistance to viruses, such constitutional factors as age, sex, species, race, genetic background, endocrine influences (closely associated with such physiological states as maturation, pregnancy), nutritional states, other physiological variables, heightened susceptibility of different tissues, tracts, portals. The inaccuracy in discussing these influences separately lies in the fact that any one factor may be influential only in relation to another factor or factors. Furthermore, most of the available observations on these factors are at the descriptive level rather than at the level of fundamental mechanisms.

### Constitutional factors

Considerably more attention has been given by virus workers to lengthening the list of *species* found to be susceptible to particular viruses (since this both enlarges the possibilities of natural reservoirs and provides additional experimental animals for virus research) than to discovering the basis of species resistance. A vast amount of data, some of it still tentative, has been assembled on the characteristic species selectivity of viruses, both in nature and in the laboratory. Some (rabies, vaccinia) attack many species; others (Shope papilloma of rabbits, salivary-gland disease of guinea pigs) are highly species specific. Although occasional claims have been advanced to the contrary, the general opinion is that only man is susceptible to herpes zoster and chickenpox; Rous sarcoma virus has been considered virulent only for fowl. Human influenza, naturally infectious for man, may be induced experimentally in ferrets, mice, European hamsters; hedgehogs, cotton rats, white rats, guinea pigs, mink, squirrels, chipmunks, swine and monkeys have been described (Horsfall, 1952) as all "more or less susceptible" to inapparent infection upon intranasal inoculation. The natural susceptibility of ferrets to distemper has interfered with their use in influenza research. Rhesus monkeys will respond only to certain strains of St. Louis encephalitis virus by intracerebral inoculation, while cebus monkeys have been described (Olitsky and Casals, 1952) as wholly insusceptible. The susceptibility of mice to the St. Louis virus enabled Webster, 1937, to develop a strain of heightened susceptibility to this and several other encephalitogenic viruses, facilitating experimental work; chickens, doves, guinea pigs, rabbits and other vertebrates may harbor this virus, without evident signs of infection, in their blood from which it may be transmitted by blood-sucking insect vectors. Human beings, horses, mules are naturally susceptible to western equine encephalitis; it has been induced experimentally in a long list of animals but the degree to which these form a reservoir of the virus in nature is not yet clear.

Systematic investigation over thirty years in laboratory animals of susceptibility to yellow fever strains (pantropic, dominantly viscerotropic, neurotropic) is being extended to wild animals in the search for possible hosts of jungle yellow fever. Theiler's discovery over a score of years ago that mice are susceptible to yellow fever by intracerebral injection led to a protection test which has facilitated studies of the epidemiology of the disease; and the subsequent observation that the mouse-passaged strain while increasing in virulence for mice loses its capacity to produce fatal visceral yellow fever in rhesus monkeys led to employment of this mouse-adapted virus in vaccines by the French. Following the finding, more than twenty years ago, that the rhesus monkey was the most susceptible laboratory animal, various South American and African species of monkey were tested and found susceptible; it is possible that these monkeys act "as hosts for the preservation of the virus in nature" (Theiler, 1952).

Most strains of poliomyelitis virus are, according to various workers, pathogenic only for man and other primates. The search for a less expensive animal than the rhesus monkey for poliomyelitis research led to Armstrong's adaptation, 1939, of a human strain (Lansing) to the cotton rat and the Swiss mouse; the two other known types of human poliomyelitis virus (Leon and Brunhilde) were reported, 1953, adapted to Swiss mice by Public Health Service workers (Li, Habel, Schaeffer). Numerous investigators have reported infection of the cynomolgus monkey from Java and of several species from Africa and South America by application of recently isolated strains to the pharyngeal and tonsillar mucosa, or by feeding. The chimpanzee has been shown to be susceptible to oral inoculation by a wide range of

strains (Howe, 1952). In considering species as a factor in susceptibility it is necessary to take into account not only such variables as age
and differing routes of infection but also mysteriously varying susceptibility among individuals within the species, exemplified by resistance
of individual dogs and rabbits to rabies inoculation (Remlinger and
Bailly, 1937).

Available observations regarding *race* predilection in specific virus
diseases are scanty and not well documented. Burnet, 1945, characterized the reported relative insusceptibility of Negroes to yellow fever
as the only instance in which "a reasonably good case can be made for
the existence of inherent racial differences in resistance to a virus infection". Even in this case the apparently racial resistance might, he
thought, be associated with some other genetic factor. In a 1944–
1945 epidemic of poliomyelitis in South Africa (Gear at the Fourth
International Congress for Microbiology, 1947), the fact that Europeans were ten times more likely to contract the paralytic form of the
disease than the native Africans was described as possibly "due to an
inherent insusceptibility of the African or to dietetic factors, but the
most likely explanation appears to be that the Africans in their unsanitary surroundings have frequent contact with endemic strains of
the virus and so acquire an immunity not shared by the more hygienic
Europeans". This explanation has also been offered for the immunity of the native population to the poliomyelitis that attacked
members of the armed forces in Africa, the Near East, Japan.

Findings from plant and animal virus studies on *genetic* factors in
susceptibility include F. O. Holmes's report from the Rockefeller
Institute (1937) that local lesion response of pepper plants to tobacco
mosaic virus is transmitted as a single gene. Gowen, at Iowa, 1948,
described as the real pathogen the gene or group of genes that account for the "unfit" or susceptible individual. He demonstrated an
"entirely specific" genetic basis for disease resistance, describing as
independent the genes for resistance to typhoid and the genes for
resistance to the virus of pseudorabies. Webster suggested that, in
mice, resistance to the St. Louis virus is inherited on a single factor
basis with resistance dominant over susceptibility. Sabin, 1952, considered inherited resistance to the 17 D strain of yellow fever virus in
mice Mendelian in character, dependent on a single pair of genes

which depress the level of viral multiplication. Burnet, 1945, referred to "very little evidence" that heritable variations in resistance are operative in relation to human virus disease. Aycock, 1942, reported evidence of family susceptibility to the paralytic form of poliomyelitis; in the same year, Addair and Snyder expressed the view that twenty-nine cases of paralytic poliomyelitis in one family could be explained as an autosomal recessive of seventy per cent expression for susceptibility to paralytic poliomyelitis. Gates, 1946, considered this study striking evidence "of inherited susceptibility to a germ disease".

*Age* as a factor in virus susceptibility may have less reference to years than to degree of maturation, physiological change, endocrine development; perhaps all findings on age incidence should be regarded in this perspective. Dalldorf, 1950, commenting on the recognized susceptibility to the Coxsackie viruses of "suckling mice and hamsters, irrespective of the route of inoculation", added: "but we must remember that some viruses are dependent on the maturation of their hosts". Hudson with Woolpert, 1937 to 1940, found younger fetuses more susceptible to poliomyelitis than older and noted in guinea pigs during intrauterine development a gradually increasing resistance to infection with epidemic influenza with, at birth, a sudden loss of infectibility by other than intranasal routes. Insusceptibility of the newborn rabbit to respiratory infection has been studied (Kneeland, 1939) in the hope of throwing light on insusceptibility of the human newborn infant to the common cold. Equine encephalomyelitis, both eastern and western, occurs at the highest rates in children under five (Meyer and Eddie, 1947). In some of the human viral encephalitides (Japanese B, St. Louis), however, incidence is regularly higher in older persons. Sabin suggested, 1939, that resistance of older animals to some of the encephalitides might be due to involutional anatomic change in blood vessels, inhibiting the virus. He referred, 1952, resistance of rats to intracerebral injection of St. Louis and Japanese B encephalitis viruses (which at an earlier age had caused death) to a selective "maturation change" in the central nervous system.

The reasons why the age at which children are most susceptible to poliomyelitis has changed from 0–4 years thirty years ago to the present 5–9 years are not wholly clear (Howe, 1952). One theory is that improved sanitation may have so protected the youngest age group as to lessen its chances of acquiring immunity by contact with the virus and increase susceptibility at the later age (Sabin, 1949). Paul observed at the Fourth International Congress for Microbiology, 1949, that, in poliomyelitis, the shift in some countries, during the past sixty years, from an endemic to an epidemic disease has widened the host range to include older children and brought subclinical disease more and more to the surface. Data accumulated in recent years on poliomyelitis in various tropical regions in which it was once thought to be rare and in which epidemics among natives were unknown include a study of neutralizing antibodies in Cairo reported by Paul with Melnick, Barnett and Goldblum, 1952. More than half of the native children had acquired Lansing antibodies by the age of fourteen months: "The speedy acquisition of Lansing, Brunhilde and Leon antibodies in infants within some of these tropical areas suggests that young infants are heavily exposed there to poliomyelitis viruses" (Paul) so that the number of susceptibles seldom becomes large enough to give rise to an epidemic. Referring to studies (Lenhard, 1950; Olin, 1952; Longshore, Edwards and Hollister, 1951) reporting increase in fatality and in severe disability with increased age, Howe observed, 1952, "there is no longer doubt that age plays a role in determining the severity of paralysis". Paul, 1954, thought an answer to the question whether poliomyelitis "is really a much milder disease in infancy than it is later in life" was essential to understanding the epidemiology of the disease. He raised the question whether the infantile ratio of one case of apparent to about 200 cases of inapparent infection (as compared with a childhood ratio of one in a hundred) might be attributable to residual maternal antibody, that is "resistance inherited from the mother", which might equip the infant to sustain a modified attack of poliomyelitis "if he is fortunate enough to be heavily exposed in infancy".

Susceptibility of the young to measles needs no documentation. In a given population susceptibles effectively exposed to cases become cases, cases recovering from the infection become immunes (Maxcy, 1948). The susceptibles are continually replenished by birth and immigration.

Outstanding among the few available observations on *sex* as a factor in susceptibility to virus disease is the reported but not dramatic predilection of poliomyelitis for males (Draper, Toomey, Lacey and others). Of 2,432 cases in New York City reported in 1949 by the health department's bureau of preventable diseases, fifty-eight per cent were males and the mortality was greater among males. The obvious association between sex incidence and maturation and endocrine factors is taken into account.

In poliomyelitis, for instance, on the basis of both experimental and clinical observations, *endocrine* factors, associated with maturation and with the reproductive cycle, have been related to susceptibility. Aycock, fifteen years ago, suggested that body build of individuals characteristically susceptible to poliomyelitis pointed to "a subclinical endocrine difference". Gates, 1946, in citing the work of Draper and Dupertuis, observed that the period of second dentition (six to seven years) and the period of puberty (eleven to fifteen years), both critical periods in maturation, seem to be periods of heightened susceptibility to poliomyelitis. Aycock referred, 1939, to a "clinical impression of the frequent occurrence of poliomyelitis during pregnancy because of known changes in estrogens" and to experiments of his group indicating that "some hormonal factor associated with the economy of estrogenic substance is involved in autarcesiologic susceptibility to paralytic poliomyelitis". The thickening of the mucous membrane resulting from estrogens was considered to suggest that administration of the female hormone might produce a barrier against the poliomyelitis virus; forty-five of fifty-two castrate monkeys intranasally injected with poliomyelitis virus developed the disease while only twenty of forty castrate animals treated with estrogen became paralyzed. At about the same time (1938), administration of estrogen (and later injection of salt solution) was shown to increase resistance of rabbits to vaccinia infection. In 1950, Sprunt explained the phenomenon as due to limitation of spread of the virus in the skin by increased tissue fluids, which estrogens could maintain throughout the course of the infection. "The limitation in spread limits the number of susceptible cells exposed and thus decreases the chance of infection." Adrenal influence has also been invoked in study of susceptibility to poliomyelitis and other viruses. Gregory Shwartzman, 1950, found marked enhancement of poliomyelitis infection in mice and hamsters following administration of cortisone, or cortisone with ACTH. In two other 1951 sets of experiments (Ainslie, Francis and Brown; Foster, Sigel, Henle and Stokes), administration of ACTH to monkeys inoculated with poliomyelitis virus was reported to result in higher rates of paralysis. Adrenal steroid secretion was most marked at the time of paralysis in all affected animals, leading to the inference that pituitary-adrenal activity influences susceptibility. Commenting on recent experimental findings involving effects of cortisone on certain viruses, notably influenza, in the chick embryo and in mice (Kilbourne and Horsfall, 1951; Kalter and associates, 1951), Bauer observed, 1953, "Cortisone is evidently an important factor in controlling virus growth, but it remains to be seen whether its effect is specific, or whether it merely depends upon an over-all control of cell metabolism, or even on a facilitation of the spread of the virus from one cell to another." Six different hypotheses had been advanced by 1953 concerning the mechanism of action of ACTH and cortisone with reference to the general effect upon resistance to infection (whether by virus, bacterium, fungus, protozoon) with the suggestion that cortisone may have "the property of completely disorganizing the natural host-parasite relationship" (Lewis Thomas) with the outcome "overwhelmingly in favor" of the invading agent through enhancement of infection.

Among the *physiological states* (some but not all with endocrine bearing) that appear to influence susceptibility and resistance to virus infection, considerable attention has been given to pregnancy. Among thirty poliomyelitis victims of child-bearing age the percentage of pregnant women was more than four times that of prepregnant women among a corresponding group in the population at large (Baker and Baker, 1947). Taylor and Simmons considered, in a 1946 Colorado epidemic, the pregnant woman twice as vulnerable as the nonpregnant. These findings are relevant to developing work on the whole question of susceptibility and resistance to infections of all kinds during phases of the reproductive cycle. Associated with the virus infections during pregnancy is the question of passage of viruses across the placental barrier. There is increased investigative interest in the periods of pregnancy when this passage may take place, and in the viruses that may or may not pass the placental barrier.

No adequate explanation has been offered of the high rate (ranging from eighty-three per cent when rubella — German measles — occurs in the first month to sixty-one per cent when it occurs in the fourth) of congenital abnormalities in children born of mothers that have had the disease during the first four months of pregnancy. These effects were described in detail by Gregg and associates, by Swan and associates in Australia between 1941 and 1946, by Ober, Horton and Feemster, and Ingalls and Gordon, among others, in this country, 1947. The congenital malformations include microcephaly, deafness with secondary mutism, cardiac malformations, eye defects, especially cataract. The possibility that virus infections other than rubella may also cause congenital abnormalities led a group of workers at the Marquette University school of medicine, 1948, to analyze the Milwaukee health department's records for 1942–1945, interviewing married women who had had measles, mumps and chickenpox during pregnancy to learn the incidence of congenital anomalies among their offspring. Although the total percentage of anomalies resulting from these maternal infections did not, in this study, exceed the normal rate of 0.9 per cent of the 665 children born of these mothers, the Milwaukee workers stressed the need for further investigation. For poliomyelitis in pregnancy they reported twice the usual number of anomalies, and, if the poliomyelitis occurred in the first four months, nine times the normal rate. While the mechanism responsible for development of these congenital abnormalities of the fetus is now suggested to be an embryological rather than a virus problem, nevertheless, since the first line of control lies in preventing the maternal disease, increasing attention is being given to virus susceptibility and resistance in pregnancy.

An obvious physiological variable is the nutritional state of the host. Against the traditional belief that undernutrition provides excellent soil for any infection are cited observations suggesting that undernourished experimental animals and plants are more resistant to some virus infections than the well nourished. The effect of malnutrition has been interpreted as diminished capacity of the cells to support viral multiplication. Specific vitamin deficiencies investigated in relation to resistance of animals to various virus infections include: pyridoxine (vitamin $B_6$) deficiency reported to result in development of less pneumonia virus of mice than in mice fed adequate diets (Mirick and Leftwich, 1949); thiamin (vitamin $B_1$) deficiency reported to convert latent experimental psittacosis infection, without overt manifestations, to a fatal, necrotizing infection (Pinkerton and Swank, 1940), to reduce mortality from Theiler's virus infection, and to decrease (from eighty-one to fifteen per cent) incidence of paralysis in mice infected with Lansing type poliomyelitis virus (Elvehjem and associates, 1943, 1944). Henle and associates confirmed, 1944, the effects of thiamin deficiency on paralytic poliomyelitis but noted that mortality rates in the deficient and the control animals were the same. Study of protein factors in susceptibility and resistance followed naturally from concepts relating intracellular multiplication of viruses to intracellular host mechanisms of protein synthesis. In studies of plant viruses at the Rockefeller Institute, Spencer (1933–1942) found that tobacco plants kept on low nitrogen intake were more resistant to tobacco mosaic virus than plants on high nitrogen. Deficiencies of certain amino acids have been reported to diminish multiplication of bacteriophages (Cohen and Fowler, 1947; Price, 1950), and of influenza A and Lansing strain of poliomyelitis (Ackermann and associates, 1951). Reports that such effects are strictly intracellular, that they inhibit multiplication of the virus without inactivation of the virus itself have been interpreted as strengthening the hypothesis that virus multiplication (infection) and cellular metabolism are inextricably interwoven. Various theories are that possibly a specific intracellular mechanism may be required for growth of virus (Cohen and Fowler; Ackermann); or possibly that viral synthesis depends upon "the normal machinery of the cell being converted to the synthesis of virus particles" (E. A. Evans, Jr., 1952).

These studies are considered to provide evidence — contrary to accumulated clinical and experimental reports of the last decade that virus infections are generally unresponsive to chemotherapy — that (Horsfall, 1952) "some viruses are vulnerable to the influence of certain external factors even while occupying an intracellular position". The approach, however, must be through the influence on specific metabolites (amino acids, vitamins, hormones or, as Pinkerton put it, 1952, still undiscovered intracellular factors) or intracellular metabolic mechanisms (enzyme systems) without which a virus cannot multiply. While "amino acids seem to lead the field" at the moment, as intracellular requirements for virus multiplication, probably "other classes of substances also deserve investigation" (Horsfall, 1952).

The possibilities of physiologic variables are obviously infinite and the investigation of them casual. Among speculative possibilities is a relation between blood type and susceptibility to poliomyelitis, suggested, 1936, by Wilburt C. Davison of Duke, on the basis of clinical observations that few persons with group A B or group B blood seem to have poliomyelitis; "the titer of the neutralizing power of the serum of convalescent patients and normal adults is reported as lowest for persons who have group O blood". Francis, more than ten years ago (discussing influenza), observed, "the cause for the susceptibility of a certain portion of the population to respiratory diseases in general will be found in some anatomical or physiological alteration in the respiratory tracts of those individuals". Two years later, commenting on a British suggestion that the nasal substance capable of inactivating relatively large amounts of influenza virus may be an enzyme, Francis suggested that possession of this anti-influenza substance by some persons and lack of it in others "may explain" why some individuals contract influenza while others under the same conditions of exposure do not. Burnet, 1945, stressed individual variation in the liberation of antibody on the respiratory mucosa, as a possible factor in susceptibility and resistance to influenza: "A person with a capacity for rapid liberation, perhaps with an essentially allergic basis, might be better protected than another with an equal level of circulating antibody but with a less efficient mechanism for mobilizing it."

*Hypersensitivity* or "allergy" (mentioned earlier in connection with observations on experimental poliomyelitis in monkeys and also in connection with etiological hypotheses for postinfectious and post-vaccinal encephalitis) is a speculative factor in virus susceptibility and resistance generally, as it is in relation to all profound and not thoroughly understood biochemical and biophysical phenomena. The concept of the common cold as a hypersensitive reaction has now become a field of public speculation, somewhat influenced by promotion of antihistamines. Fox, Harned and Peluse reported, 1940, that a study of 1,200 cold-susceptible persons revealed that eighty per cent of them had various allergies or came from allergic families. Locke, 1949, citing Coca's work and concepts, thought that susceptibility to the common cold might derive in part from inability to maintain a continuously efficient defense in an interval of food-allergic reaction. The hypersensitivity hypothesis has been invoked also for primary atypical pneumonia. A favorable response of this "virus pneumonia" to ACTH was explained by Finland and associates, 1950, on the theory that ACTH probably inhibited allergic reactions to invading organisms. Fever that had resisted antibiotics subsided and symptoms were greatly ameliorated during administration of ACTH, but relapse occurred when treatment was discontinued.

## Acquired Resistance to Virus Infections

### Introductory

Immunity is not a fixed but a relative term, commonly used to describe both complete and partial resistance to infection. There are wide differences in duration of immunity in virus diseases: certain diseases with short, sharp courses of infection are followed by a solid "relatively permanent" immunity, as smallpox, measles, yellow fever (virus diseases in which blood invasion is essential). While second attacks have been reported in poliomyelitis, in mumps (Enders, 1948), in psittacosis (Cox, 1947), in herpes zoster, in varicella, in smallpox (the classic instance being the man that had been vaccinated by Jenner himself), they are rare. Illustrative of viruses in which the duration of immunity is described as not at all permanent are: influenza, the common cold, dengue, herpes simplex.

While immunological and serological phenomena in virus infections are similar to those in bacterial and other infections, since "the basic principles of immunology and serology are operative in all fields of biology" (Rivers, 1952), there are many conditioning factors, some of them more or less peculiar to viruses. There is, for instance, lack of response of viruses generally (with the possible exception of the psittacosis-lymphogranuloma group) to the "miracle drugs", in particular the antibiotics that have so greatly reduced mortality and morbidity in other infections (including the bacterial complications of virus diseases). The very swiftness and efficacy of this conquest of infection by such agents as antibiotics may, however (Francis), pose another problem. The "cure" may leave the patient without immunity; it is possible to envisage a population devoid of immunity, dependent upon drugs which might not be available. In contrast would be the strongly developed immunity against virus diseases of a population that had acquired active immunity from clinical or subclinical attack, from injection of vaccines, or that had acquired passive immunity through administration of serum containing neutralizing antibodies produced in the body of an actively immunized host. In the general acclaim of the undoubted usefulness of the antibiotics, here and there a voice has been raised suggesting that there is "something to be said" for permitting the individual to develop his own immunity.

Since the presence of neutralizing antibodies in an animal's serum "in most instances but not all" (Rivers, 1952) suggests that the animal is resistant to a given virus, studies of immunity in virus (and other) infections have stressed the sites and the mechanisms of antibody production. Of the sites "far too little is known" (Philip D. McMaster, Rockefeller Institute, summarizing, 1953, work from 1886 to his own current studies with Kruse using tagged antigens) and "even less about the mechanisms". McMaster emphasized absence of proof that any one type of cell is exclusively involved in antibody formation. "Numerous sites are involved", according to Treffers, 1952. Burnet and Fenner, 1949, in stressing the point that antibody production is not the function of a single cell type considered that it occurs wherever phagocytic cells of the reticulo-endothelial system are associated with lymphocytes and undifferentiated mesenchymal cells. Felix Haurowitz regarded antibody production as not restricted to the reticulo-endothelial system, the focus of most of the work over the years, or to the lymphatic system (focus of major studies since 1935 by McMaster and Kidd, 1937; Ehrich, Harris, and associates, 1940–1951; Dougherty, Chase and White, 1944; others) but as occurring "even in the nervous system or in the cornea". The mechanisms by which antibodies are produced to fit with remarkable specificity individual antigens have been explained by a general theory deriving from Paul Ehrlich's suggestion, 1896, that antigen and antibody particles are complementary. The hypothesis that "the globulins *are* the true antibodies and that their antibody function is due to the complementary adaptation of their shape to the shape of the determinant group of the antigen", offered by Breinl and Haurowitz, 1930, and an hypothesis independently advanced by J. Alexander (1931) and by S. Mudd (1932) formed the basis for Pauling's chemical studies leading to the theory, 1940, that although the sequence of amino acids in both normal globulins and antibodies is probably the same, the difference between them lies in the different mode of folding of their peptide chains. A certain support for this view was considered to be provided, 1950, by R. R. Porter's analyses of inactive gamma globulins of normal rabbit serum and of anti-ovalbumin from rabbit serum. Haurowitz (who has modified his original view) suggested, 1953, that antibodies are merely "a modification of the normal formation of proteins" caused by the presence of antigen. Burnet who has been the main opponent of the dominant view that antibody synthesis requires the continued presence of antigen, suggested with Fenner, 1949, that while antibody formation is started by antigen, it can continue after disappearance of the antigen from the organism. They considered it likely that certain proteinases in the antibody-forming cells are lastingly modified as they are engaged in destroying the original antigenic particles. Then these "trained" enzymes continue to synthesize the antibodies.

Theories regarding the necessity for the presence of antigen for formation of antibody are relevant to the revived controversy whether the infective agent must persist in the body after infection in order to elicit antibody and maintain immunity. Rivers, 1952, referred to the "sufficient instances" on record in which viruses have been recovered from immune hosts — as in salivary-gland disease of guinea pigs, psittacosis, infectious anemia of horses, lymphocytic choriomeningitis of mice. He thought it "not unlikely that in some instances there is a causal relation between the persistence of virus and enduring immunity", adding that failure to recover a virus from an immune host did not furnish positive evidence that it is not present since viruses in the intracellular stage may not be detectable. Melnick, 1952, considered the hypothesis that latent viruses explain persistence of antibodies and immunity in human populations "difficult to prove". In the same connection, Dalldorf, 1950, observed that Shope had shown that our tests for presence of virus may be inadequate and that persistence of immunity might be accounted for in other ways besides the constant stimulation of humoral antibodies: "union of virus with cells may be dependent on other immune mechanisms than those we have known so long". Among the other mechanisms was mentioned interference between the virus already within the cell and the virus freshly introduced. The already existent virus either by exhausting intracellular substances required for multiplication of the second or by competing with it for intracellular sites of multiplication, or metabolites (vitamins, amino acids) or metabolic mechanisms (enzyme systems) may exclude the second virus. Various workers have stressed the absence of proof that immunity depends on persistence of the virus, interference or other cellular mechanisms: Francis, 1952, described as "unlikely" the idea that continued production of specific antibody is contingent upon persistence of an antigenic stimulus. "Antibodies are effective in virus immunity according to the invasive mechanism involved, the type of parasitism and the availability of antibody at the portal at which virus makes its entrance into the body." He characterized the last, the amount of antibody available at the portal of entry, as the first line of defense against infection. Other workers, as Schlesinger, 1949, 1952, have raised the question, especially with reference to neurotropic viruses, whether immunity depends upon the formation or the concentration of antibodies at sites where the virus localizes or multiplies. McMaster, 1953, noted as still unanswered the question whether antibody merely accumulates in nerve tissue by seepage from the blood following its production elsewhere, is formed there by reticulo-endothelial elements such as microglia cells, astrocytes or other cells, or appears there because of infiltration of antibody-carrying lymphocytes or plasma cells. Morgan, 1949, reported finding in monkeys convalescent from paralytic poliomyelitis the highest antibody levels within the central nervous system, particularly in the areas most severely affected by the disease and associated with little or no circulating antibody either in serum or spinal fluid. The glial scar, the end product of the focal inflammatory process and the perivascular cuffing, still visible for a year after paralysis, may possibly, she considered, "represent the site of antibody formation". The hypothesis "that this antibody represents a local formation within the central nervous system produced by the abundant cells of the inflammatory process" was not confirmed by the mouse experiments of Sabin and Steigman, 1949. Schlesinger's 1949 studies of the possibility of active cerebral immunity to equine encephalomyelitis virus in mice led to development of a concept which includes local antibody production within the central nervous system, and which he believed applicable to the wide field of virus infections of the central nervous system.

On the whole question of relation of antibody level to resistance, it is in order to recall Francis's caution, 1950, against regarding antibodies as synonymous with immunity. Rivers, 1952, pointed out that some animals that have recovered from a virus infection "are resistant to reinfection without possessing demonstrable neutralizing antibodies". Webster, 1942, referred to studies of his group in which "certain dogs refractory to rabies have proved lacking in neutralizing antibodies and mice abundantly supplied with serum-neutralizing antibodies may not prove immune . . ." He would interpret demonstration of rabies-neutralizing antibodies as "an indication that virus has come into contact with tissues and incited a response but not necessarily that it has rendered the animals immune". Horsfall, 1943, referred to the "well-established" fact that most normal adult human beings possess in their serum significant concentrations of antibodies against influenza A virus; nevertheless individuals that possess serum antibodies against influenza A virus can, and frequently do, contract influenza A. He did not consider that there is a critical antibody level possession of which would completely prevent occurrence of influenza A; "and, conversely, the demonstration of a given level, however high, in the serum of a particular individual cannot be taken as evidence of existing immunity to the disease . . .". The evidence on influenza B virus points in the same direction.

The earlier mentioned finding of neutralizing antibodies against Lansing type poliomyelitis virus in the very young in the tropics (challenging the former belief that poliomyelitis was confined to the temperate zone) was interpreted as indicating early exposure and early immunization. Paul, 1952, thought that various surveys justified considering Lansing poliomyelitis as "a world-wide endemic disease", or, if we wish to be optimistic, as "an endemic immunizing agent".

Antibody surveys of the other types, Leon and Brunhilde, have only begun, but Bodian's 1949 report that a refined and concentrated sample from pooled human plasma contained neutralizing antibodies against all three antigenic types was regarded as pointing to the widespread existence of the three types throughout the United States. That strains of the Lansing type predominate generally, however, was indicated by reports from various parts of the world by 1954, showing that, of more than 800 strains collected and typed, about three fourths were of the Lansing type.

The two illustrations above, pointing to the apparently limited immunological significance of presence of neutralizing antibodies in one virus disease, influenza, and to the apparently great potential immunological significance of the presence of antibodies in another virus disease, poliomyelitis, are an index of the complexity of the whole problem of virus immunity and the widely differing factors, aside from differences among the viruses themselves, that determine it.

### ATTEMPTS TO INFLUENCE VIRUS RESISTANCE BY SERA AND VACCINES

#### SERA

The mechanism by which passive immunity in certain virus infections may be induced by parenteral administration of sera containing circulating antibodies from an actively immunized person or animal was described by Rivers, 1952, as "not known"; it has not been demonstrated whether the introduced antibodies protect susceptible cells against entry of the virus, whether they act directly on the virus in such a way as to prevent production of disease or whether they enhance destruction of virus by certain phagocytic cells. It is recognized that the efficacy of human serum and serum fractions (pooled "normal", pooled or individual convalescent serum, gamma globulin), in the few virus diseases in which they are believed to have a rational basis, depends upon administering the serum after exposure but before appearance of clinical signs and symptoms, since by the time these are evident the virus has probably reached the tissue cells, out of reach of the serum antibodies. In stressing the promptness and finality of the union that occurs when the virus reaches the cell Dalldorf, 1950, cited Andrewes "who showed that antiserum injected into the skin a few minutes before the inoculation of vaccinia virus prevented infection.   Five minutes after inoculation it did not — further evidence of the rapidity of the union of the two."

While not many years have elapsed since Bahlke and Perkins, 1945, expressed a somewhat general conclusion, that not only gamma globulin but also "serum in any form is for all practical purposes ineffective in the therapy of *poliomyelitis*", hope of prophylactic use of gamma globulin during epidemics to prevent attacks, attenuate their severity and reduce the number of paralytic cases brightened with the reports, previously described, that the virus appears briefly in the blood following infection of animals and man, including Bodian's 1951 demonstration that human gamma globulin protected monkeys if given early, before the symptomatic stage.   The hypothesis that antibodies administered just before or immediately after infection might be useful in preventing development of paralysis was tested by large-scale controlled trials of gamma globulin in 1951 and 1952 epidemics in various Iowa, Texas and Utah communities, under a committee directed by William McD. Hammon and including Lewis L. Coriell and Paul F. Wehrle, with Joseph Stokes, Jr., as consultant.   One half of 54,722 children between the ages of one and eleven received intramuscular injections of gamma globulin, the other half, gelatin. The results, according to the committee's moderate report summarized by the division of medical sciences of the National Research Council, 1953, indicated temporary protection, "significant" from the second to the fifth week, diminishing thereafter.   "No significant difference" was found between the number of cases of poliomyelitis that occurred in the treated and the control groups in the week following injection, "but there was evidence of mitigation of paralysis in the cases occurring in the children who had received gamma globulin".   In further trial of gamma globulin under the auspices of the communicable disease center of the Public Health Service, in collaboration with forty-five state and city health departments, provision was made for a study of 749 households in which 1,654 cases occurred.   The reasoning was that "household associates have an increased risk of developing poliomyelitis", and selective use of gamma globulin with family contacts, if shown to be effective, would be more economical than mass inoculations in preventing spread of infection.   The conclusion of the National Advisory Committee for Evaluation was, however, that administration of gamma globulin to familial associates of patient with poliomyelitis had "no significant influence on (1) the severity of paralysis development in subsequent cases; (2) the proportion of nonparalytic poliomyelitis occurring in subsequent cases in which gamma globulin was given before onset; (3) the classic pattern of familial aggregation of cases in the country at large". Sabin, 1954, considered gamma globulin "of practically no value," observing that "poliomyelitis behaves in a manner quite different from measles".

Attempts to stop *influenza* virus at the susceptible cells through which it makes its first attack are illustrated by trial of prophylactic serum in the U.S.S.R., reported at the 1939 International Congress for Microbiology by A. A. Smorodintseff, describing experiments in which only four of 650 men that received bi-weekly inhalations of vaporized influenza antiserum during the influenza epidemic of that year developed influenza as against 149 cases in 1,700 untreated controls. Horsfall, 1943, described the ninety per cent reduction in incidence claimed by the Russian workers as "in fact the most striking reduction in the incidence of influenza A in man so far achieved by any method of immunization" and expressed the hope that additional trials would be made. Francis, 1945, while referring to this experiment as the first attempt to secure passive immunization by antibodies applied directly to the respiratory tract in man, observed that the influenza commission's trials in human volunteers had not substantiated the Russian claims.

More than a decade ago, Lord Horder observed that the use of serum antibodies in *measles* had "passed the experimental stage". Convalescent serum, pooled adult serum, placental extracts, and gamma globulin all depend for their efficacy (Rake, 1952), "on the fact that most adults have suffered from measles and that pools of adult blood will therefore contain specific globulin antibodies". Globulin concentrates, he observed, given to children under six years, within seven days of exposure, result in complete protection of about fifty per cent of them and modification of the disease in the rest. In the case of a pregnant woman exposed to *rubella*, Rake thought that, while claims and reports appeared contradictory, "immune globulin in one form or another" could be tried "for lack of anything else".

The results of attempts dating back perhaps twenty-five years to use convalescent serum to prevent *mumps*, or, if too late for that, to prevent orchitis, have not been conclusive.  Enders, 1952, described the results obtained from serum treatment of a limited number of cases of established orchitis or meningitis as "equivocal", adding that limited data suggested that "concentrated convalescent gamma globulin is of some value in preventing the development of orchitis if given after the onset of parotitis".  Concentrated normal gamma globulin had been, 1945, reported to be of no value under the same circumstances, by Gellis and associates.  Enders, while not disparaging the temporary prophylactic value of unconcentrated convalescent serum administered soon after exposure, described the passive immunity so conferred as "lasting probably two or three weeks".  Commenting on the results of one 1944 trial (Stokes, Maris, Gellis) of highly concentrated preparations of immune globulin, Enders expressed the view that critical analysis of the available data left "some doubt as to whether the procedure is sufficiently dependable to be of value".

Maumenee, Hayes and Hartman thought that, in *epidemic keratoconjunctivitis*, the value of human convalescent serum used intravenously or instilled into the conjunctival sac had not, 1945, been generally proved.  Convalescent serum in a large series of patients seriously ill with *primary atypical pneumonia* was reported to be successful by R. V. Lee, 1944, but Horsfall, 1952, observed that convalescent human serum "has not produced an obvious effect".  Convalescent serum was described by Stokes, 1952, as of little, if any, prophylactic and of no therapeutic value in *chickenpox*.  Meyer, 1952, described human convalescent serum as without curative effect on experimentally infected animals, but antisera prepared by Hilleman, 1945, by inoculation of rabbits and chickens showed "protective effect on experimental infections".  The initial phase of viremia previously mentioned for the equine encephalitides early suggested to investigators the possibility of an approach to this virus.  Olitsky and associates demonstrated, 1943, that hyperimmune rabbit serum could prevent a lethal infection in guinea pigs if given after inoculation of *western equine encephalitis* virus but before symptoms appeared; later, however, fatal encephalitis occurred in some of the treated animals and it was believed that the antibody level had fallen before the incubation period (thirteen to forty-seven days) had ended. Specific antiserum for the *eastern* virus was described by Olitsky and Casals, 1948, as preventing the disease in experimental animals but "its use in man awaits further tests". Hyperimmune serum (prepared in horses) was described by Olitsky and Casals, 1952, as effective in experimental animals infected with *Japanese B encephalitis*. The same workers found no uniformity of opinion on Russian workers' use of hyperimmune goat serum as specific early in *Russian Far East encephalitis*. Havens and Paul, 1945, found human gamma globulin protective against *infectious hepatitis* if given during the incubation period. They with Stokes, Neefe and associates demonstrated that this passive immunity lasts from six to eight weeks or sufficiently long, in their view, to justify use of it restricted to persons involved in family outbreaks or exposed to epidemics in institutions or camps. In *serum hepatitis*, the variability of the protection offered by gamma globulin, in their view, "makes its use of questionable value".

### VACCINATION AGAINST VIRUS INFECTIONS

From accumulated knowledge of virus infection and from trials of vaccination, it has become clear: that active infection produces the most enduring immunity; that live viruses in vaccines are more effective than killed, but that fully virulent viruses may be dangerous; that attenuated viruses producing a degree of infection (which may be inapparent) can undoubtedly be useful; that killed viruses, while less useful since they do not stimulate infection, may retain sufficient antigenicity to stimulate antibodies. Some workers have felt that, in general, imitation of "nature's method of latent immunization" offers the best hope of successful control. Enders, 1948, referred to recent evidence (his own work on mumps, 1946, and that of the Pennsylvania group) that "clinically inapparent infections confer immunity as effectively as does an overt attack".

Current problems of virus vaccination include: difficulty of cultivating certain viruses at all or in sufficient quantity to provide antigens for vaccines; difficulty in sufficiently purifying and concentrating the virus while retaining sufficient antigenicity; difficulty in establishing amount of virus to be used; danger of toxic reactions; uncertainty as to duration of immunity conferred and possibility of bolstering it;

criteria for the comparative efficacy of live (fully virulent or attenuated) or killed viruses for vaccines. Living virus in a fully virulent
state is still used against some animal diseases, inoculated either by an
unnatural route or given under cover of a protective antiserum. The
disadvantages of this method have led to employment of attenuated
strains (occurring naturally or induced by passage through animals or
tissue cultures). By 1952, attenuated virus vaccines were in use
against yellow fever, rabies, smallpox, fowlpox, distemper, swine
fever, cattle plague, fowl plague, Newcastle disease, Rift Valley fever,
dengue, African horse-sickness. There is difficulty in producing just
the right degree of attenuation which if carried too far may fail to produce immunity (Beveridge, 1952); the opposite danger, that an attenuated strain may become suddenly virulent, is reflected in Stanley's
1945 observation on the need of constantly testing "active" vaccines
because of the tendency of viruses to change or mutate during reproduction.

A swift review of the present status of vaccination in various illustrative virus diseases furnishes, in a way, the basis for a synthetic current estimate of its potentialities. Horsfall fairly summed up the
current situation, 1950, when he described as "exceptional" the
"striking efficacy" of artificial procedures against smallpox and yellow
fever, "but in most cases effective control remains only a theoretical
possibility". It is, however, a possibility that is being pursued with
lively hope and, in connection with some viruses, with considerable
intensity. Since Jennerian vaccination against *smallpox*, introduced a
century and a half ago, contributed to the "virtual disappearance" of
classical smallpox from European civilization during the nineteenth
century there have been advances. Smadel, 1952, referred to the present methods of preparing and standardizing smallpox vaccine, made
from calf-lymph vaccinia virus, as carefully controlled by regulations
of the biologics control section of the National Institutes of Health in
this country. He thought that while, "in general", the vaccines (in
addition to the standard smallpox vaccine prepared in calves) made
from vaccinia virus grown in tissue cultures or in embryonated eggs
have not been widely accepted, the encouraging field trials in Texas
(Cook, Crain and Irons, 1948) of chick embryo vaccine over a number
of years "should assist in overcoming the prejudice against such

materials". Benenson, 1950, cited work (Hooker, 1929; Craigie and Wishart, 1933; Benenson, 1950) indicating that an immediate reaction can be obtained with inactive virus as well as with infectious material. However, while the immediate reaction probably indicates the immunity adequate for the usual exposures of American living, in the face of exposure to virulent variola strains, it "can be accepted as indicating immunity only if the vaccine used is known to be of high potency and has been applied by the proper vaccinating technic".

*Rabies* vaccination has been complicated by lack of statistical comparison of incidence of rabies in treated and in untreated persons similarly exposed; by the varying length of the incubation period (ranging from ten days to seven or more months); by the impossibility of knowing whether the rabid animal's bite transmitted a sufficient dose of virus to the victim; by the impossibility of knowing how much of the favorable result — when a vaccinated person is bitten but does not develop rabies — is to be attributed to a specifically immune response and how much to interference of the injected virus with the infectious virus (Francis, 1947). The percentage of people bitten by rabid dogs that actually develop rabies was placed by Kelser at twenty-five, by T. G. Hull, 1947, so low as sixteen per cent, by other estimates at from five to fifteen per cent. "Though relatively few people die of rabies each year" in this country (Johnson, 1947), "it is necessary to give the rabies vaccine treatment to about 30,000 persons each year", involving not only a time-consuming and expensive procedure but also a hazard of paralysis from the vaccine in a small proportion of those treated. While rabies vaccination is recommended by public health authorities throughout the world and while the mortality rate among treated persons is remarkably low, controlled clinical tests of the comparative efficacy of combined local treatment and vaccination and of local treatment alone have not been made (Johnson). It is generally accepted that if the incubation period is short, the disease cannot be prevented and is fatal; but that clinical evidence leaves "no doubt that rabies vaccine is effective in preventing the disease in the majority of the instances in which there is an expected incubation period of more than one month". Leading workers (Sellers, Johnson) unite in urging that vaccine treatment should not be given unless there is adequate evidence of exposure since "complications produced by the vaccine when given to persons only indirectly or remotely exposed have caused more deaths than has rabies" (Sellers, 1947).

After a half-century of debate and statistical analysis (on an international scale), Rivers, 1939, had to observe: "Fifty years after the introduction of antirabic vaccination, there is no agreement regarding the type of vaccine that should be used." McKendrick, summarizing, 1940, the results of over a million cases of dog-bite treated with vaccine (collected since the 1927 International Rabies Conference), concluded that no one vaccine was notably better than the others. Greenwood, in his analysis, 1945–46, of ten reviews made by the League of Nations, found no evidence of superiority in any one vaccine. Present rabies vaccines use the original strain and apply the principles of vaccination of Pasteur and his associates, 1882. In spite of improvements over the years in methods of harvesting and preserving the virus for vaccines, Habel described them, 1949, as still representing "the crudest type of biological material". Elimination of the allergenic factor held responsible for the paralysis following rabies vaccination (described by Johnson as "a specific sensitization to brain material") by "washing" the virus in chemicals (Habel, National Institutes of Health) and by other methods has been a recent objective of studies in public health and pharmaceutical laboratories.

Some workers on rabies vaccination would transfer emphasis from human vaccination to annual vaccination of dogs. On the basis of vaccination of almost two million dogs in 1946, the veterinary section of the Public Health Service concluded, 1947, that "rabies occurs ten times as often in an unvaccinated canine population as in one vaccinated"; the canine rabies vaccine proved ninety per cent effective when used in single doses, and "nearly one hundred per cent effective" with three doses at intervals of a week. Johnson has, however, emphasized that the effectiveness of vaccinating dogs depends on simultaneous use of control regulations, licensing, collection of unlicensed dogs, quarantine, attack on wild animal reservoirs.

Attempts through forty years to devise a vaccine for active immunization against *poliomyelitis* appear to be bearing fruit. Contributing factors included the successful large-scale propagation of the three types of poliomyelitis virus in non-neural tissues, experimental demonstration that strains of the three types when inactivated (by chemical or physical means) induced antibody in animals. The first decisive demonstration by Morgan, 1948, that monkeys inoculated parenterally with inactivated poliomyelitis virus produced serum antibodies and developed measurable resistance to challenge with virulent virus was followed by reports from several laboratories that the same method induced antibody in rodents, monkeys and man. In 1954, after three years of tests for safety and antigenicity (in 4,000 monkeys) and trials in 5,320 human persons, field tests were made of the experimental vaccine (containing strains of each of the three types, propagated in tissue culture, inactivated by formalin) developed by Salk at the University of Pittsburgh. The subjects were approximately 1,800,000 children in the first three grades of school, in 217 counties in forty-four states; 445,000 received the vaccine (in three injections, over a five-week interval), the rest acting as controls. The plan set up for the field trial and for its evaluation (after seven months, by a committee headed by Thomas Francis, Jr.) was designed to throw light on the nature and extent of the protection offered by vaccination against paralytic poliomyelitis under natural conditions of exposure. In continuing studies, especially of the duration of immunity, by the Salk group, especial concern has been with the question whether a killed-virus vaccine can produce as enduring immunity as infection.

For enduring immunity some workers (Sabin; Cox) look more hopefully to a vaccine employing living viruses of diminished virulence, preferably given by the oral route. Adaptation of various strains to the chick embryo, to mice, rats, passage through tissue cultures, combinations of these methods to develop strains that may eventually be used in a living virus vaccine have been reported from several laboratories (Li and Shaeffer, 1954; Sabin, Hennessen and Winsser, 1954; Melnick, 1954; others).

Some of the approximately fifteen years' work involved in development of *yellow fever* vaccine, in the International Health Division, has been touched upon, as has the accidental development in tissue culture, from the pantropic Asibi strain, of the 17D strain, in which both the viscerotropic and neurotropic properties were to a considerable extent lost. It is this live virus, now propagated in the chick embryo, that has been routinely, and in the general view effectively, employed in this country in manufacture of yellow fever vaccine. Theiler

(Nobel prize winner, 1951, for his work on yellow fever vaccine) cited, 1952, as "conclusive evidence" of the prophylactic efficacy of the vaccines the fact that since introduction of vaccination against yellow fever no accidental cases had occurred in laboratory workers. He described the results of mass vaccination, to date, as "satisfactory", citing especially the experience in South America where nearly 4.5 million persons were vaccinated in Brazil alone. The efficacy of 17D vaccine was tested under critical conditions when thousands of British and American troops later exposed to infection in Africa were vaccinated between 1939 and 1945. At least three complications (failure to produce antibody response; encephalitis; jaundice) that occurred before the present standardization of the yellow fever vaccine using the 17D strain have now been eliminated. The third complication, manifested in the first part of the last war in 28,585 cases of jaundice in Army camps following yellow fever vaccination, was considered (1943 report of the International Health Division) to have "probably been completely solved by the exclusion of human serum", and substitution of an aqueous-based vaccine.

Although efforts to develop successful vaccination against *influenza* have, within the last ten years, registered important gains (the culmination of studies in man conducted by groups of investigators in this and other countries since 1933), development of successful vaccines depends upon several objectives as yet not wholly attained. These include: sufficiently comprehensive knowledge of strains to insure inclusion of the particular strains responsible for the given outbreak ("listening posts" set up by the World Health Organization throughout the world should aid this situation); most importantly, development of methods not only of raising but also of sufficiently maintaining serum antibody levels (studies on adjuvants are directed toward this objective). Under the Army Epidemiological Board's commission on influenza, tests of existing vaccines under controlled conditions indicated that during 1943 and 1944 epidemics incidence of influenza A was from seventy to eighty per cent less among the vaccinated than among the unvaccinated, and that the attack rate of influenza B was ninety per cent lower in the vaccinated than in the unvaccinated.

The antibody response to vaccination has not precisely defined duration of the protection.  Commenting, 1952, on the variation in estimates (two to twelve months), Horsfall observed: "Numerous workers doubt that vaccination leads to definitely reduced susceptibility for more than a few months."  A member of the division of communicable disease services of the World Health Organization noted, 1953, that although in controlled trials (in various parts of the world) the unvaccinated have been attacked four times as often as the vaccinated, a number of the vaccinated still become ill.  Since, according to the World Health Organization, the immunity produced by vaccination is neither so lasting nor so complete as, for example, the immunity produced by vaccination against smallpox, and since it is clearly not practicable to vaccinate the whole population each year, the outstanding question in control of influenza is whom to vaccinate and when.  The rapidity of strain variation in epidemics of this "highly mutable virus" (influenza A) complicates the problem.  It has been suggested that effective vaccine against influenza A would have to contain the antigenic strain "prevalent in the *next* epidemic".  Francis, 1950, expressed a view that findings suggesting that a strain appearing in the southern hemisphere in one year is likely to appear the next year in the northern indicate rapid dissemination rather than simultaneous appearance throughout the globe.  In that case, there would be value in the international network of laboratories under the World Health Organization identifying strains, and there would be point in the "trial run" made in manufacturing a vaccine from a "new" strain in 1951, under the United States influenza study program, with A-prime strains isolated by Andrewes during the 1950 epidemic.  Of six American pharmaceutical houses that agreed to undertake rapid production and laboratory tests of the new vaccine, two produced 1,000 doses in twenty-two and twenty-three days respectively, and the longest time required for any of the six was sixty-three days as against the six months to a year previously required.  The demonstration was considered to indicate that a large number of commercial laboratories would be able to produce enough vaccine against a threatened epidemic initiated by a new and virulent type of influenza originating in this country or imported from abroad in time to minimize its effects in a large part of the population.  Smith, 1952, described as "obviously a gamble" the possibility of protecting against a devastating pandemic by international attempts "to catch up as it were with the antigenic vagaries of the influenza viruses" by obtaining sufficiently early information of the emergence of new types to incorporate them in a vaccine. He considered it, however, a gamble worth taking "in our present impotent state". Francis deplored, 1952, "a defeatist attitude" concerning results of trials of human vaccination, suggesting that large-scale influenza vaccination may be "capable of maintaining a more effective immunity of broad character than merely awaiting the influence of recurrent epidemics". He had previously pointed out that the preoccupation of many workers with the "minutiae of strain differences" led them to understress strain similarities, and to lose sight of the possibility that strain differences may be not qualitatively so great as to necessitate anticipating a completely new strain. Available evidence suggested to him that only a limited number of antigenic components have to be reckoned with. Analysis of antigenic components of strains that had appeared between 1943 and 1951 showed no completely new antigenic component in the later strains and none of the components present in the earlier years had completely disappeared in the later. A vaccine with the components found basic for the limited number of strains studied was under investigation, 1954, looking toward development of a practicable vaccine. Adjuvants might meet some of the difficulties "by stimulating much higher, broader, and more persistent responses to the different antigens". The mechanism by which adjuvants heighten and prolong the immune response beyond that which could be expected when inactivated virus vaccines are used has not yet been established; it has been intensively studied, however, in several laboratories in France and in this country, notably by Freund whose method of preparing adjuvants is employed by Salk. In 1953 Salk and associates reported persistence of antibody after more than two years in the first 200 (of a total of more than 20,000) individuals vaccinated with influenza virus vaccines emulsified in a mineral oil of low viscosity, with controls inoculated with an aqueous based vaccine. Since the adjuvant effect was not stimulated by oil-in-water emulsion, but only by water-in-oil emulsions, Salk explained it as "undoubtedly due to the direct contact of the oil with the tissues eliciting the gathering of phagocytes that not only attempt to carry off the oil but are also effective in antibody formation. The result is that there develops at the site of inoculation the equivalent of an 'antibody-forming' tissue or possibly an 'antibody-forming organ'. . . ." The fact that much smaller doses of virus were effective with emulsified than with aqueous preparations would "allow the incorporation of many strains in a vaccine, probably as many as may be required for inducing a uniform response to the total spectrum for each type".

The possibility of vaccinating man against influenza by spraying a mixture of attenuated strains directly into the nostrils has attracted major workers for more than a decade. Francis, who reported intranasal inoculation in 1940, said, 1945, that induction of mild infection without clinical injury might be expected to confer "a relatively durable resistance", and that, since in recovery from natural infection the protective capacity of the nasal secretions is enhanced, an unknown local mechanism might be involved. Burnet and his associates, after conducting extensive experiments with military personnel during the war, reported, 1943, "suggestive" results showing rises in antibody titers in twenty to thirty per cent of the vaccinated, although no epidemic had occurred to test the actual immunity. Others (Henle, Henle and Stokes, 1943) reported comparable success, but intranasal vaccination has not as yet passed the experimental stage.

Of vaccination against the *common cold*, Horsfall said, 1952, "vaccines have not been shown to decrease susceptibility to the disease".

Vigorous attempts have been made during the past fifteen years to develop effective vaccines against several of the *virus encephalitides* in horses and in man. The Department of Agriculture's vaccination campaign against equine encephalitis was reported, 1949, to have resulted in reducing the incidence among horses (in which the death rate is thirty-five per cent) to the lowest on record. A type of chick-embryo formaldehyde-inactivated vaccine of the *eastern and western equine viruses*, similar to that used with horses, refined so as to remove a large part of the foreign protein, has been developed for use in man; Beard's finding, 1940, that, after vaccination, several persons (on whom it had been tried experimentally) possessed demonstrable neutralizing antibody was confirmed by Morgan, Schlesinger and

Olitsky, 1942.  While this vaccine has been used to protect laboratory workers and those especially exposed, wider use of it in man, according to Olitsky and Casals, 1952, depends upon controlled field tests under epidemic conditions.  Randall, Maurer and Smadel reported, 1949, after the occurrence of infection with *Venezuelan equine encephalomyelitis* virus in two members of the Army medical center staff, injection of twenty persons with a formolized vaccine prepared from partially purified chick-embryo cultures.  These persons, subsequently engaged in large-scale manufacture of the vaccine, showed no signs of disease. A formalin-inactivated virus vaccine prepared by Sabin and collaborators, 1943, for *St. Louis encephalitis* was described by Casals and Olitsky, 1952, as having elicited neutralizing antibody in a small human series but as not available for general use.  A mouse brain vaccine against *Japanese B encephalitis*, prepared by Sabin and collaborators in 1943 and 1947, was effective in preventing experimental infection; and a chick-embryo type vaccine, prepared by the Army medical school, was used in immunization of laboratory personnel (Smadel, 1951).

Since cultivation of the *mumps* virus in the chick embryo has made available the larger quantities of virus necessary for inactivated vaccines, field trials have been made in man following Habel's demonstration, 1946, that monkeys could be protected from experimental infection by a virus cultivated in chick embryo and inactivated by ether and ultraviolet.  When tested, 1946, on groups of migrant workers imported from the West Indies to Florida, incidence of mumps was reported to be one third as great among 1,100 vaccinated as in the 700 unvaccinated controls.  Commenting on these trials in groups that totaled 2,825 (in whom 336 cases of mumps were observed), Enders noted, 1952, that these tests left little doubt of the protective value of inactivated virus vaccine, provided exposure occurs within four to six weeks after administration.

The outlook for producing immunity against *dengue* by vaccination has improved since, under the Army epidemiological board, Sabin and Schlesinger, 1945, reported cultivation in the chick embryo of a strain first passed intracerebrally through mice.  Sabin, 1952, observed that tests in human volunteers of the vaccine made from this strain showed it to be safe, stable, effective, and possibly useful in epidemics or for troops that are moved from nondengue into endemic areas.

Referring to the demonstration by Wagner, Meiklejohn, Kingsland and Hickish, 1946, that an inactivated (phenol-killed) chick-embryo *psittacosis* vaccine, if administered repeatedly in large amounts, stimulates production of antibodies in man, Meyer, 1952, described the degree of effectiveness of such measures in control of the disease in man as "not known".

### CHEMOTHERAPY AND CHEMOPROPHYLAXIS IN VIRUS DISEASES

#### CLINICAL AND EXPERIMENTAL EVIDENCE ON EFFECTS IN VIRUS INFECTIONS OF VARIOUS AGENTS, INCLUDING CURRENT ANTIBIOTICS

Horsfall, commenting on the possibility of some day finding chemicals that will so alter the metabolic environment of the cell as to inhibit virus multiplication, thought it "unlikely", 1949, that it would be possible by this means to immunize effectively large segments of a population against many viral diseases "in the foreseeable future". Chemotherapeutic aims envisaged for one virus, poliomyelitis, are suggestive: inactivation of the virus before it passes the portal of entry or after it has become established in excreta of patients or carriers; blocking of entrance of the virus into susceptible tissues such as those of the central nervous system; alteration of metabolic processes of susceptible cells before or after entrance of the virus, rendering them unsuitable for multiplication of the virus; restoration or improvement of damaged tissues, especially nervous tissues.

Eaton, 1950, emphasized the familiar view that the smaller neurotropic viruses are resistant to chemotherapy "not so much as a result of their intracellular site of multiplication, but because they lack vulnerable enzyme systems susceptible to direct chemical attack"; complete or partial enzyme systems in the larger viruses are inferred from indirect evidence. Among these larger viruses, Horsfall, 1949, named as three exceptions to the general truth (based on trial of approximately 4,000 specific chemicals) that "chemical agents have not been shown to exert a beneficial effect upon viral infections in man", lymphogranuloma venereum, trachoma, inclusion blennorrhea, which "appear to be favorably influenced by the sulfonamides and somewhat less so by penicillin". The action of sulfonamides was described by Andrewes and King, 1946, as an excellent example of interruption of viral multiplication by competitive metabolic blocking; p-aminobenzoic acid in the cell, apparently needed for reproduction of these viruses, is blocked by the structurally related sulfonamides. Thygeson, 1948, described the formerly hopeless outcome for trachoma patients as entirely changed by the advent of the sulfonamides, but he found penicillin without established value in this disease and in inclusion conjunctivitis. Reviewing ten years' experience (1941–51) in treating trachoma at the Missouri trachoma hospital, A. A. Siniscal expressed his agreement with various investigators (Thygeson, Sorsby, Wilson, Bietti, Richards, Forster, Poleff, Freyche, Loe, Cosgrove) that the sulfonamides have a specific effect on the virus. As to the specificity of antibiotic action on the virus, he observed: "I do not believe that trachoma *per se* is affected materially by aureomycin or any other antibiotic used in this work", but he (with others) did consider the antibiotics (penicillin, bacitracin, streptomycin, chloramphenicol, terramycin) useful in clearing up secondary infections.

Of another large virus, psittacosis, Early and Morgan, 1946, reported that sulfadiazine saved mice from death, but did not interfere with their becoming psittacosis carriers; the drug was found to inhibit growth of some strains in the chick embryo, both by these workers and by Meiklejohn, Wiseman and their coworkers, 1946, who reported that sulfadiazine and penicillin are effective against two classical strains of psittacosis in mice. Toomey and Lohrey, 1946, reported no benefit from sulfonamides given to human patients with psittacosis, but Rosebury and his associates, 1947, reported some improvement in patients from both sulfadiazine and penicillin. In reporting two cases of human psittacosis infection in which penicillin seemed to be effective, Meyer and Eddie, 1947, observed that only in the extracellular phase, when the virus is not actually multiplying, is it apparently susceptible to the bacteriolytic as well as bacteriostatic action of the antibiotic. The ultimate destruction of the virus when it has once penetrated the host cell depends on the enzyme action of the parasitized cell, *i.e.*, the immunity mechanism of the host.

Except for viruses of the psittacosis-lymphogranuloma group, experiments aimed at showing efficacy of the antibiotics against viruses "are either lacking or have given conclusively negative results" (Smadel, 1951). He warned against dependence upon clinical evaluations of infections of variable severity and irregular duration, often complicated by bacterial infection. "This part of the field is a quagmire which demands cautious treading." Numerous negative clinical observations or experimental reports on trials of particular drugs with particular viruses include: Reimann's 1950 statement that for virus pneumonia "that has been rightly diagnosed", penicillin and/or sulfadiazine are not effective; Bloomfield's 1950 statement that the "true cold" is not influenced by antihistamines or antibiotics; Horstmann's 1949 observation that "none of the antibiotics or sulfonamide derivatives which have been tried has had any effect in destroying the (poliomyelitis) virus"; the finding of Kramer, Geer and Szobel, 1944, that no one of numerous chemotherapeutic agents tested in mice against St. Louis encephalitis is effective; negative results of trial of sulfonamides, antibiotics, for herpes simplex in eggs, mice, rabbits; reports since 1943 from various workers that experimental influenza is not affected by such antibiotics as penicillin, tyrothricin, gramicidin, streptomycin. Experiments with various pneumonitis viruses in small experimental animals suggested the possibility that penicillin might be useful against nonbacterial pneumonias; varying opinions, none of them dealing with the action of the antibiotic on the virus itself, have thus far been expressed concerning the efficacy of penicillin against primary atypical pneumonia in man.

The excepted group again figure prominently, although not exclusively, in clinical trials of aureomycin: in lymphogranuloma venereum, by Wright, Sanders, Logan, Prigot and Hill, 1948; in inclusion conjunctivitis, trachoma, epidemic keratoconjunctivitis, lymphogranuloma by Braley and Sanders, 1948. Herrell, 1950, described the beneficial effects of aureomycin in experimental and clinical infections with lymphogranuloma-psittacosis viruses as yet to be established. In experimental infections of chick embryos with all viruses of the psittacosis-lymphogranuloma group (lymphogranuloma venereum, psittacosis, mouse, feline and human pneumonitis, and meningopneumonitis), Wong and Cox, 1948, reported that a single dose of 1 mg. of aureomycin injected thirty minutes prior to massive doses of infectious material afforded almost complete protection. Marked therapeutic activity orally was reported in mice infected intraperitoneally and intracerebrally with psittacosis or lymphogranuloma venereum viruses. Eaton noted, 1950, some evidence of clinical effectiveness of aureomycin in psittacosis, and abundant evidence of its "curative effect" in acute lymphogranuloma venereum. By 1950, various reports had claimed definite beneficial effects from aureomycin in primary atypical pneumonia. Eaton's experimental studies in chick embryos and cotton rats with a strain of virus isolated in 1942 from patients with atypical pneumonia were reported, 1950, to show definite activity of aureomycin. On the basis of "encouraging results" in a small series of cases treated with aureomycin, Schoenbach registered, 1949, a "feeling" that aureomycin is a "valuable chemotherapeutic agent" in primary atypical pneumonia. Meiklejohn and Shragg, 1949, with reference to an outbreak in an Army station hospital, compared efficacy of aureomycin in twenty-two patients with failure of penicillin in twenty others. Referring to these favorable reports and also to reports denying significant effect (Harvey and associates, 1949; Hirsch and associates, 1952), Horsfall, 1952, considered it "doubtful that there are adequate grounds for regarding aureomycin as an effective chemotherapeutic agent in this disease".

Studies of aureomycin in the virus field outside the excepted group include negative results of its use in early stages of human poliomyelitis (Appelbaum and Saigh, 1950); "rather convincing evidence" of its clinical effectiveness in herpes zoster, according to Herrell, citing clinical studies reported since 1948; little evidence, also according to Herrell, to support its clinical value in the common cold, influenza, poliomyelitis, encephalitis, variola, rubella; no therapeutic activity for it (Wong and Cox, 1948) in experimental influenza, rabies, Newcastle disease, Venezuelan equine encephalomyelitis, poliomyelitis.

Comparative trials of aureomycin and chloramphenicol in chick embryos infected with psittacosis, reported by Wells and Finland, 1949, showed that only one fourth as much chloramphenicol was required to produce the same effect. According to Eaton, 1950, results with chloramphenicol against intracerebral and intranasal infections with viruses of this group in mice were "not outstanding". Viruses of trachoma and inclusion blennorrhea, having certain resemblances to those of the psittacosis group, have been reported as show-ing high susceptibility to both aureomycin and chloramphenicol. Smadel, 1951, quoted Freyche's conclusion that on theoretical and practical grounds these antibiotics may be a specific therapy for these eye infections.    Chloramphenicol was reported by Eaton, 1950, to show "definite virustatic" action against atypical pneumonia virus infections in the chick embryo.    Smadel, 1951, expressed his feeling that in "virus" pneumonia (in which "it is almost impossible to di-vorce the viral and bacterial elements") a physician is justified in using for a few days, at least, aureomycin, chloramphenicol, terramycin, and also in virus infections with dermatological manifestations (herpes zoster, extensive herpes simplex, molluscum contagiosum).

Terramycin was reported to have no beneficial action on influenza A in chick embryos (Francis and his group, 1950) and in mice (Kass, Barnes and Finland, 1950).    Prompt favorable effects of terramycin were described (Kneeland and Melcher, 1950) as comparable to those of aureomycin on the course of primary atypical pneumonia in ten patients.    Ehrlichin, isolated from a nonstreptothricin-producing strain of *Streptomyces lavendulae*, was reported by Waksman and his associates, 1951, to have *in vitro* activity against pox viruses, bacterial viruses, influenza A and B; in mice, the anti-influenza activity was limited to B.

### HYPOTHESES ON THE RATIONALE AND MECHANISMS OF CHEMOTHERAPEUTIC AGENTS

"If the objective of interrupting viral multiplication by chemical means is to be attained, present evidence supports the idea that this will come about through substances which act on intracellular compo-nents, possibly on enzyme systems of susceptible host cells rather than on the virus *per se*" (Horsfall, 1952).    If it is true that viruses lack the complete enzyme systems for their multiplication, depending for them wholly or in part on the host cell, then chemotherapeutic substances can interfere with activity and multiplication of intracellular viruses only by action on the metabolic processes of the host cells by "chemi-cal blockade of cell metabolites" (Horsfall and Ginsberg, 1949).

Pursuing a theory that virus multiplication in an infected cell depends upon an altered or "abnormal sequence of some normal metabolic processes of the cell", Cohen and Fowler, 1947, reported that blocking the availability of the amino acid tryptophane, essential to bacterial metabolism, by addition of the analogue 5-methyltryptophane inhibited growth of both bacteria and the infecting bacteriophage. Ackermann, in Francis's laboratory, reported, 1951, that blocking availability of the amino acid methionine to mammalian cells growing in tissue culture, by addition of the analogues methoxinine and ethionine, inhibited growth of influenza A. That four amino acids appear to be needed by cells to support growth of vaccinia virus was suggested by reports of inhibition of virus growth by analogues of glycine, valine and methionine (Thompson, 1947), of phenylalanine (Thompson and Wilkin, 1948). Pertinent to a theory that some particular cellular metabolic cycle is involved in virus synthesis are Ackermann's experiments attributing inhibition of growth in tissue cultures of influenza A by addition of malonic acid, antimycin and sodium fluoroacetate to blockade of the cellular citric acid (Krebs) cycle. Since growth in general is associated with nucleic acid synthesis, and it is known that mammalian cells make their nucleic acids from precursors different from those used by bacterial cells in the process, the search for metabolic antagonists of parasitic nucleic acid synthesis is one approach to bacterial chemotherapy. Hitchings and his associates pointed out, 1950, that this argument "applies equally well to bacterial, viral, rickettsial and neoplastic diseases". Evans, 1952, pointed out that recent work at the Pasteur Institute on bacterial viruses indicated that the nucleic acid of the bacterial hosts seemed to be involved in bacteriophage synthesis. "As components of nucleoproteins the purines and pyrimidines are intimately involved in biological systems" (Brown, Craig and Kandel, 1953). Their analogues which interfere with the synthesis of nucleic acids are known to affect the metabolic activity of certain bacteria and viruses. Diminished multiplication in the presence of these analogues was reported for vaccinia virus in tissue cultures (Thompson and associates, 1950); for Russian spring-summer encephalitis virus in tissue culture and mouse brain (Moore and Friend, 1951). Derivatives of one of the analogues, benzimidazole, were reported to inhibit multiplication of influenza A and B in tissue cultures (Tamm, Folkers and Horsfall, 1952). Other reports noted activity of benzimidazole against tobacco mosaic, psittacosis and, more recently, poliomyelitis virus in tissue cultures. Tried by Brown, Craig and Kandel, 1953, in experimental poliomyelitis (Lansing) in mice and monkeys, benzimidazole was found, in mice, to prolong the incubation period and moderately reduce mortality; in monkeys the incubation period was slightly prolonged but mortality was not decreased. These workers, in view of the fact that "few components which show antiviral activity in tissue culture are similarly effective in animals" (probably because of inability to exhaust or replace completely a given metabolite in the tissues of the intact host), considered the result of their experimentation to have a certain significance for chemotherapy in virus disease. On the theory that altering the cell's nucleic acid metabolism might prevent nerve damage by neurotropic viruses a Minnesota group (Schaeffer, Silver, Chin Chao Pi), 1949, treated mice infected with MM virus with nucleic acids, two of which appeared to prevent paralysis or death in two thirds of the treated animals. Incubation of the virus with a mixture of nucleic acids before inoculation resulted in a high degree of protection. The workers thought the hypothetical action of the nucleic acids might circumvent the cellular injury leading to the severe pathologic damage in the central nervous system, or it might lead to changes in the characteristics of the virus so that it would no longer have a marked affinity for the nerve cells.

Approaches to chemotherapy of virus diseases opened up by studies of virus-cell relationships include, as pointed out by Woolley, 1949, applications of fundamental knowledge of antagonism between structurally related compounds which may operate at the cell surface to interfere with interaction between virus and cell as well as within the cell to interfere with virus multiplication. Most attempts to stop the virus before it enters the cell are, as the earlier account of work on the hemagglutinating property of viruses indicated, largely directed toward modification, destruction or blockade of the receptors on the cell surface to which an increasing number of viruses shown to possess the hemagglutinating property are believed to attach themselves. The adsorbing properties of red cells may be blocked or altered or destroyed, as by periodate (Horsfall and Hardy, 1948) and by certain bacterial enzymes which have been shown (Burnet and Stone, 1948) to remove cell receptors from allantoic membrane of the respiratory tract of the mouse, preventing adsorption of subsequently injected influenza virus, making infection more difficult. Schlesinger, however, suggested, 1949, that in the living animal cell receptor substances are regenerated making the cells again susceptible and it is not known conclusively whether attachment of viruses to cell receptors represents the initial act in penetrating the cell (Hirst's 1943 hypothesis) or whether attachment to cell receptors represents some other function in the infective process (Hirst, 1952).

Realization that substances that exert their effect before the virus penetrates the cell "have little or no effect upon viral infections which are already under way" (Horsfall, 1952) has led to search for substances effective at a later stage. The search has included trial of highly purified bacterial capsular polysaccharides (experiments of Horsfall, Ginsberg and associates since 1947), especially in pneumonia virus of mice and in mumps. It was demonstrated, in the case of both viruses, that polysaccharide administered before the end of the latent period (i.e., before the first cycle of virus multiplication has been completed) inhibited multiplication of the virus, supporting the concept that this substance "interrupts the intracellular process upon which multiplication depends". Additional evidence of specific action of the polysaccharide upon some intracellular mechanism of the host cell was the 1950 finding that polysaccharide had no effect upon the virus *per se*, upon its adsorption by susceptible cells, and could not inhibit a variant of the mumps virus, the Newcastle or several other viruses. In the case of pneumonia virus of mice, however, the chemotherapeutic efficacy of polysaccharide was demonstrated (Ginsberg, 1950) by giving it long after inoculation of the virus, when viral multiplication was proceeding at a maximal rate and gross pneumonia was already present; it interrupted progress of the pneumonia lesion "and converted an overwhelming infection, which killed the control animals, into a modified disease from which the animals recovered".

In reviewing his own work and that of others on the polysaccharides, Horsfall, 1949, referred to the "small beginning although no more than a beginning" that has been made. "A tiny chink in the armour protecting viruses has been uncovered and this provides a hint that more effective and more useful procedures may be developed if the validity of the underlying concepts is supported by further work." This further work, in his view, must take into account the probability that, in man, "maximal viral multiplication occurs some time before frank clinical symptoms are evident". The needed work must also be guided by the implication of the experiments cited above suggesting that inhibition of viral multiplication results from alterations induced in the metabolic activities of the host cells, unfitting them for maximal viral multiplication.   This view defines the basic problem not only in terms of the nature of viruses but also in terms of the metabolism of the host.

CHAPTER 9

# Alcoholism

*Stressing metabolic approaches to an outstanding
psychological and social problem*

# INTRODUCTORY

Fundamental research on alcoholism suffers from the disadvantage that attends research on any condition that cannot be produced experimentally: chronic alcoholism has not yet been produced in animals. A more fundamental reason why research on alcoholism has not achieved the degree of biological perspective available for research on tuberculosis, cancer, poliomyelitis is the slow development of the concept that alcoholism is a disease. While the concept is not new — Thomas Trotter, in a doctor's thesis submitted to the University of Edinburgh in 1778, described drunkenness as "a disease produced by a remote cause"; and so long ago as 1830 the medical society of Connecticut urged on the state legislature the need of especial hospitals for this "disease" — the fact that the concept is still far from prevalent partly explains delay in support of fundamental investigative work. An inquiry addressed by a Rutgers University group to doctors, community leaders, the general public (reported a few years ago to the American Association for the Advancement of Science) showed that only one in five of those questioned regarded an alcoholic as a sick person; fifty per cent believed an alcoholic could stop drinking if he wanted to; fifty-eight per cent saw no difference between an alcoholic and a person that gets drunk frequently. The new approaches to the problem that began about 1940 are still inhibited by distrust of research on the part of the two extremist groups, the "wets" (who maintain that there are no problems) and the "drys" (who maintain that the problems can be solved only by total abstinence). The ambivalence of alcohol — the fact that it can be used for either harmful or beneficial purposes — continues to be a confusing factor in the development of research. A further — important — impediment to research on alcoholism is the relative underdevelopment of the "behavioral sciences" and consequent lack of fundamental study of alcohol-affected behavior.

Year by year, there are, it is true, impressive evidences of change in the public conception of alcoholism as a psychic and physiologic disease. On the social side, it is rather more than a straw in the wind that four states with sickness disability laws now pay benefits to medically proved compulsive drinkers who are unable to work; and that the committee on alcoholism of the Health and Welfare Council of New York City recommended, 1953, that alcoholism be recognized by law as a disease rather than as a penal problem. On the scientific side, researches projected by the now defunct Research Council on Problems of Alcohol, taken over in the programs of other research-oriented organizations now active in the field, have progressively recognized the complexity of the problem, the metabolic, neural, psychic, social and economic factors involved. Realization that the cause and the form of alcoholic disease vary widely in individuals has made it less and less possible to generalize about alcoholics as a group and to characterize them according to any universal mental, physical, moral, educational, psychological or biochemical characteristics differentiating them from nonalcoholics. Inability to determine whether alcoholism is a disease entity or the expression of various types of disorder, to determine whether the classic symptoms of alcoholism are end results of the effects of alcohol on the organism or the key to the metabolic and psychologic mechanisms that condition the organism to dependence on alcohol still confuses both the goals and the methods of investigative work.

The heart of the investigative problem thus becomes search for the factors that determine degree of dependence, the criteria that distinguish the compulsive from the merely heavy drinker. The subcommittee on alcoholism of the World Health Organization, 1951, defined alcoholics as "those excessive drinkers whose dependence upon alcohol has attained such degree that it shows a noticeable mental disturbance, or an interference with their bodily or mental health, their interpersonal relations and their smooth social and economic functioning; or who show the prodromal signs of such developments". How far addiction is psychological and how far it is physiological remains a question of perpetual interest. A physiologic basis of addiction in terms of nutritional deficiency or inherent biochemical defect is a major implication in various recent studies and in such hypotheses (MacLeod in Britain) as that specific intermediary metabolic reactions or systems may become so adapted to the presence of alcohol that alcohol becomes necessary for maintenance of metabolic equilibrium. Exploration of the assumed physiological basis of addiction has not thus far, however, according to a 1952 summary of existing knowledge by David Lester and L. A. Greenberg (Yale Laboratory of Applied Physiology), brought us anywhere near an explanation in physiological terms of the genesis of alcohol addiction. The present trend in investigative work is away from the concept that causes are either exclusively psychologic or exclusively physiologic (biochemical) and toward efforts to find biochemical correlates of such psychologic states as tension, anxiety, suppressed resentment, frustration often operating in alcoholism. A certain unsoundness in any implication that there are two separate fronts is suggested by C. J. Virden's 1950 observation (in a British discussion of addiction), "the distinction between the biochemical and psychological is not permanent, for psychological phenomena are open to biochemical investigation".

Clearly, only fundamental and systematic research in all directions, basic and clinical, physiologic, psychologic, social can lift the problem of alcoholism into the scientific atmosphere. The practical index of the present situation is that, while an increasing number of medical men, of the general public, of guardians of the law and the public welfare are willing to call alcoholism a disease of multiple and complex causes, there is little provision for treating it as a disease. Nor is there a present "cure" that does not involve abstinence.

## EXTENT OF THE PROBLEM OF ALCOHOLISM

Statistics on the extent of the alcoholism problem of the country must be speculative so long as there are no criteria for classifying either kinds of drinkers or alcoholic states, and so long as surveys catch rather those alcoholics that have landed in jails, asylums, county and city hospitals, than those that, by virtue of the economic good fortune of themselves or their families, remain at large, "statistically sequestered". Studies from 1940 to 1948 (E. M. Jellinek, World Health Organization, and Mark Keller, Yale Center of Alcohol Studies) led to an estimate that of a drinking population of sixty-two million approximately 3,800,000 are alcoholics, of whom over 900,000 are alcoholics with complications that have developed after at least ten years' heavy drinking.

The cost of alcoholism in terms of money is at least suggested by an inclusive Department of Commerce estimate that in 1946 the annual expenditure of the people of the United States for alcoholic beverages represented 6.1 per cent of total consumer outlay for all purposes, although this percentage of course includes the cost of liquor not only for alcoholics but also for millions of moderate or occasional drinkers. Significant also are not only the millions spent annually by the liquor industry to persuade people to drink ($27,920,643 for advertising liquor in 1940, according to the Bureau of Advertising of the American Newspaper Publishers Association) but also the millions, not easily estimated, to persuade them to stop drinking. Available estimates of the financial cost of extreme results of alcoholism include: $13,000,000 annually for caring for alcoholic addicts in mental hospitals (estimate of the Research Council on Problems of Alcohol as of 1940); over $175,000,000 a year for police and court procedures and for maintaining alcoholics in prisons; a New York City Department of Welfare estimate, 1953, that the "average alcoholic" cost the city $3,000 a year in hospital, jail, welfare and police expenses.

*The Manchester Guardian* recently observed that the relation of alcohol to motor accidents has reached the stage of international conferences. One of every six fatal traffic accidents in the United States during 1946 (David Geeting Monroe, University of North Carolina) involved a driver that had been drinking, and one of every four fatal accidents involved a driver or pedestrian that had been drinking. Experiments in the department of pharmacology of the Karolinska Institutet in Stockholm (Kjell Bjerver and Leonard Goldberg) led to the conclusion, 1950, that the role of alcohol in traffic accidents is "probably considerably greater than appears from official statistics" and "begins at a lower alcohol value in the blood than has previously been considered". Because of questions of legal responsibility involved in traffic accidents, a certain amount of research, sometimes with the cooperative interest of the police, has aimed at determining blood alcohol concentration as an index of intoxication, the effect of alcohol on visual fields or color vision, muscle balance, etc. Such determinations are made difficult by the recognized individual variation, some persons (not a few) showing signs of intoxication when the alcohol content of the blood is .05 per cent, others appearing sober when the concentration is eight times that or .4 per cent.

Alcoholism is often an essential factor in social problems listed under other labels, such as narcotic addiction and suicide. The Public Health Service noted as "an interesting phenomenon" a few years ago that about half of the morphine addicts under its care had first been addicted to alcohol. A ten-year study (reported 1948) showed that in over forty per cent of five hundred unsuccessful suicide attempts referred to the Chicago Psychiatric Institute by judges of the Chicago Municipal Court alcoholism was a precipitating factor.

The cost of alcoholism to industry and to workers includes an estimated $432,000,000 annually in loss of wages through alcoholism (Benson Y. Landis, economist, 1945). Conservative estimates derived from spot studies (*Quarterly Journal of Studies on Alcohol*, 1949) placed at 2,060,000 the number of regularly employed alcoholics; at twenty-two the number of working days lost annually by each male alcoholic, a total of 29,700,000 working days; at 1,500 annually the number of industrial accidents for which alcoholics are responsible. Nor does the label of alcoholism tell the whole story of alcoholism in industry: the Consolidated Edison Company in accepting, 1947, chronic alcoholism as a legitimate basis for disability retirement with the usual modified pay recognized realistically that the cirrhosis, hypertension, peripheral neuritis and other ailments for which many employees had formerly been retired on disability pay "were little more than convenient symptoms written down to ignore the fundamental trouble, chronic alcoholism".

While adequate data on the extent of alcoholism as a military problem in wartime are not available, there is a degree of suggestion in

H. J. Lawn's 1946 study of the first 700 men admitted to the Fifth South Carolina Rehabilitation Center. Eleven per cent had no history of drinking, thirty-one per cent were classified as social drinkers, seven per cent as moderate drinkers; the remaining fifty-one per cent were classified as alcoholics on three levels. All had begun drinking from one to three years before entering the Army.

Various attempts to measure the problem of alcoholism in terms of its influence on mortality have been made following Raymond Pearl's 1926 study (Johns Hopkins school of hygiene and public health) of alcohol and longevity. Statistical analyses, 1952, by Gunnar Dahlberg of death rates among alcohol addicts and a control group of "normal" persons of the same age and sex from the general population of Stockholm indicated a higher death rate among alcoholics between thirty and fifty-five than among the controls and a comparatively high death rate due to suicide and tuberculosis among alcoholics.

The cost of alcoholism, in all the ways noted above, has been used to bulwark the argument that rehabilitation of inebriates would probably cost much less than arrests, court procedures, jailing, losses due to accidents and to absenteeism, state and municipal hospital care notably for alcoholic psychotics, public support of dependents. Certainly the billion estimated by Landis, 1945, as the amount of the social bill "paid annually by the people because of inebriety" is in sharp contrast to the less than $500,000 currently estimated as the annual expenditure for research on alcoholism. While public understanding of the problem steadily advances, it is not yet the kind of understanding that insures popular or legislative support of fundamental biological research along a broad front. In alcoholism, even more than in most of the outstanding unsolved problems of medicine, interest in control and "cure" outruns appreciation of the need of the basic research that will make control and cure possible.

## TRENDS TOWARD BASIC RESEARCH ON ALCOHOLISM, DERIVING LARGELY FROM INTEREST IN CONTROL

Since research on alcoholism still holds the general status of a desirable but somewhat luxurious addition to control programs, it follows that the present volume of basic research is not large and that much of it has a strong clinical slant. In the direction, for instance, of evaluating new therapies, there is general alertness and activity: only a few months after the promotion in Denmark in 1948 of one of the most recent therapeutic expedients, disulfiram (antabuse), it was under more or less critical examination in the United States by physicians in over a hundred jails, detention homes, general and mental hospitals, clinics, in university and medical school departments of biochemistry, physiology, pharmacology, psychiatry, neurology, internal medicine. It is of course true that this and every other recognition of alcoholism as a medical or public health problem must be included among the advances that will aid in ultimately securing more fundamental research. Such advances multiply. At the international level, the World Health Organization's expert committee on mental health in 1952 appointed a full-time consultant, E. M. Jellinek, for its subcommittee on alcoholism. In the United States, the American Medical Association, which in earlier years had relegated discussion of alcoholism at annual meetings to neuropsychiatry sections, established, 1951, a subcommittee on alcoholism under the association's committee on chronic disease. The National Institute of Mental Health, in 1954 described as "the focal point of the Public Health Service's activities relating to alcoholism", gives consultative service to national, state and local agencies, maintains connection with (1) the National Research Council's committee on problems of alcohol, (2) the National States' Conference on Alcoholism, and (3) the National Committee on Alcoholism, promotes and supports training institutes, professional conferences, and special research projects. There is as yet in the United States, however, nothing comparable to the Swedish governmental program established in 1946 under which the Council for Medical Research distributes sizable annual grants for research in the universities, notably in the Karolinska Institutet which has been conducting such research since 1938.

## State Programs

In the United States the shift from the moral and punitive to the medical approach to alcoholism, from the concept of alcoholism as a private vice to alcoholism as a social problem, has, especially within the past decade, given remarkable impetus to assumption of responsibility for alcoholism in state public health programs. Following the action of the Connecticut legislature in 1945 establishing the Connecticut Commission on Alcoholism concerned with treatment, education, research, thirty-eight states and the District of Columbia had, by 1952, created boards or commissions. Twenty-two states had established new agencies or divisions in existing agencies for programs; sixteen of these included research (three in cooperation with hospitals and medical schools) or plans for future studies. Most of the state agencies were cooperating in surveys, education, therapy with health and welfare organizations, some with state hospitals and prisons, some with voluntary associations, nearly all with Alcoholics Anonymous. Larger state appropriations included in some cases funds for outpatient clinics (occasionally for inpatient facilities): Connecticut, $300,000; Delaware, $612,825; North Carolina, $150,000; Virginia, $117,325. New York's appropriation of $45,000 for research, North Carolina's contract for research in the social sciences division of the state university, Virginia's subsidy of research at the Medical College of Virginia and Connecticut's studies, some of them in cooperation with the Yale center of alcohol studies, represented direct provision for research. Summer schools of alcohol studies, patterned on the first full-time summer school held at Yale every year since 1943, have been held since 1950 in Wisconsin, Oregon, Texas, Utah. In state rehabilitation programs, inpatient facilities, especially those attached to medical schools, are regarded as significant since availability of patients for a continuous period is necessary for adequate study by medical students, for establishment of interneships and residencies in this field, for long-term studies of metabolic changes in alcoholics.

Local programs increase. A progress report of the National Institute of Mental Health for December 1953–January 1954 notes a statement by the director of the National Committee on Alcoholism that there are seventy-nine alcoholism clinics in the United States as against none ten years ago. While these are not dominantly research centers, they look hopefully toward research. The clinical director of the District of Columbia's Alcoholic Rehabilitation Program (now in its fifth year) recently commented on the degree to which the collaboration of other voluntary and official agencies brightens the prospect for research.

## THE YALE LABORATORY OF APPLIED PHYSIOLOGY

Outstanding for scientific approach to problems of alcohol, for spearheading on a national basis the effort to have alcoholism dealt with as a medical problem requiring fundamental biological research, have been two groups, the older a university group of investigators working even before 1930 in the Yale laboratory of applied physiology, the more recent a group of scientists drawn largely from university centers to serve on the Research Council on Problems of Alcohol. The older group, at the Yale laboratory, has, under Howard W. Haggard's direction, played a major part not only in stimulating research on metabolic, physiological, medical and, more recently, psychological and sociological aspects of alcoholism, but also in educating the public and the medical profession in more rational approach to the problem. The laboratory has supplemented its research, which continues to be the core of its activities, with educational activities (summer schools in New Haven and other parts of the country), consultation (for industries and states desiring programs, for hospitals planning clinics, many of which have been modeled on the Yale Plan Clinic, the first public clinic established for alcoholics, 1944). Besides publishing the *Quarterly Journal of Studies on Alcohol*, founded, 1940, by Haggard and Jellinek, the laboratory publishes the bimonthly *Alcoholism Treatment Digest* and maintains the *Classified Abstract Archive of the Alcohol Literature*, available, 1952, in twenty-three libraries and research centers. In 1945 the educational, therapeutic, consultative, publishing activities were combined in the Yale center of alcohol studies (Selden D. Bacon, director) which is separate from the research activities of the laboratory. The Yale summer school of alcohol studies (eleventh annual session, 1953) was designed not only for instruction but also for integration of efforts on several levels (medical, psychological, sociological, religious). The 1,479 individuals that attended the first ten annual sessions from forty-seven states in the United States and fifteen other countries included physicians, psychologists, sociologists, educators, clergymen, nurses, public health and social workers, representatives of the liquor industry, of Alcoholics Anonymous, of various states considering programs for control of alcoholism. In 1949, the center sponsored the first of the summer schools in other states. Under the medical direction of Giorgio Lolli, the Yale plan clinic has published studies evaluating medical treatment, studies of group therapy, sociological studies on such subjects as drinking patterns among various occupational and racial groups. The laboratory established and for five years maintained the National Committee on Alcoholism, a voluntary association now operating independently from its New York offices, with, by 1952 (its seventh year), some sixty community affiliates. The heart of the scientific program at the Yale center of alcohol studies, however, continues to be the metabolic studies conducted in the laboratory from which originated the program described above. Investigations under way in the laboratory before 1930 by Yandell Henderson and the laboratory's present director, Haggard, on anesthetic (later toxicological) properties of alcohol were followed by a series of investigations on absorption, distribution and elimination of alcohol, carried on by Haggard, since 1933 with Leon A. Greenberg, since 1940 with David Lester.

### INFLUENCE OF THE RESEARCH COUNCIL ON PROBLEMS OF ALCOHOL

The idea of the Research Council on Problems of Alcohol (now disbanded) originated in the mid-thirties when Norman Jolliffe, then chief of the medical service of the New York University psychiatric division at Bellevue, worked out a detailed project including clinical, laboratory, social science research on alcoholism; the project was not carried out when expected financial aid did not become available. Later, 1937, through the efforts of Jolliffe, Bowman and other interested educators, the council was established "to deal with alcoholism in the same general fashion as other public health agencies combat tuberculosis, cancer, syphilis, heart disease, and other major threats to human health". The American Association for the Advancement of Science assumed a leading role in developing the council (a membership organization), accepting it, 1940, as an associated society financially independent but with the association's endorsement and general direction in carrying out its scientific program. The council's scientific committee of forty-eight, which carried out its research program independently of the council, included by 1944 representatives of university departments of psychiatry, neurology, physiology, applied physiology, pharmacology, biochemistry, medicine, preventive medicine, heads of public and private mental hospitals. The *Quarterly Journal of Studies on Alcohol*, established 1940 by Haggard and Jellinek as a project of the Yale laboratory of applied physiology, served for a time as official organ of the council; later, in accordance with the principle of separating scientific and promotional activities, the *Journal* reclaimed its status as a scientific periodical published by the Yale laboratory. However, the *Journal* continued to include reports of investigations for which the council appropriated grants from funds placed at its disposal by foundations (the Carnegie Corporation of New York, the Dazian Foundation), the liquor industry (Seagram Distillers, Frankfort Distillers, National Distillers Products) and other agencies (Research Corporation). The first study, supported by a grant of $25,000 (Carnegie Corporation) and begun in 1939 at New York University, was a critical survey of completed work on effects of alcohol on the individual. The first of a number of symposia on alcoholism was held at the 1940 meeting of the American Association for the Advancement of Science. Studies supported in part by funds administered by the council (grants from donors noted above of from one to seven thousand) included an experimental study of effects on the fetal cortex of alcohol ingestion by the mother and clinical studies of alcohol toxicity, liver cirrhosis, craving for alcohol. By 1942, development of a consultation and research clinic for chronic alcoholics had been undertaken under the auspices of New York University with grants from Research Corporation and Seagram Distillers. Grants (most of them from the liquor industry) continued to be small, but the research program, conforming with the scientific committee's initial purpose to stress interrelation of practical objectives and fundamental scientific attack, has influenced public health concepts in state or medical school programs subsequently established over the country. Among reasons given by the council's last president (Anton J. Carlson) for discontinuing it, 1949, was "too much overhead with too little money for research". Various uncompleted research projects and residual funds were turned over to the division of medical sciences of the National Research Council which entrusted them to a committee on problems of alcohol, which thus became, 1949, the successor of the Research Council on Problems of Alcohol.

## THE NATIONAL RESEARCH COUNCIL'S COMMITTEE ON PROBLEMS OF ALCOHOL

The stated purpose of the National Research Council's Committee on Problems of Alcohol was "to initiate and support research, to correlate data, to provide advisory and administrative service for agencies concerned with pathological effects of alcohol". The committee was not, according to published statements of policy (*Science*, 1950), to "be concerned with education or public information" but rather to "offer technical advice to persons and agencies", governmental and private. The committee's eleven members included, 1952, two physiologists, two pharmacologists, representatives of medicine, biophysics, psychiatry, biochemistry (several of them with a record of basic metabolic research in alcoholism), two liaison members from distilling corporations. Although the committee has recognized the need of broad and deep research on psychological and sociological problems involved in alcoholism, it has restricted itself thus far to making small grants for research on biological and pharmacological problems related to alcoholism. It plans, however, to request the aid of other National Research Council committees and agencies outside the council in undertaking and financing psychological and sociological studies. In 1950 the committee had received $100,000 to be used over three years from the Licensed Beverage Industries. For 1951–52 the committee allocated approximately $25,000 for six projects in five university centers.

## UNIVERSITY CENTERS OF RESEARCH ON ALCOHOLISM

Few university or medical school programs on alcoholism now have a history so long or so extensive as Yale's. The previously mentioned grant of $25,000 made by the Carnegie Corporation to New York University, 1940, however, represented recognition of basic studies of the preceding three years by members of the psychiatry department

(Karl Bowman), the neurology department (S. B. Wortis), the department of internal medicine (Norman Jolliffe's studies of metabolic diseases brought to bear on metabolic changes in delirium tremens, on neurological changes associated with vitamin B deficiencies in alcoholism) and collaborative studies of these three departments furthered by the clinical material available in the Bellevue alcoholic wards. The investigations of James J. Smith, director since 1947 of research on alcoholism at New York University-Bellevue Medical Center, have moved from psychiatric to endocrine factors in alcoholism. The center was engaged, 1952, in extending its private treatment facilities through a clinic especially designed to serve industry.

From Stanford's department of medicine, since 1936, have come H. W. Newman's reports on the metabolism of alcohol in various species, including man, on the relation of rate of metabolism to habituation, more recently, 1951, on the effect of disulfiram on metabolism of ethyl alcohol. The Harvard department of nervous and mental diseases has for years brought to bear on the problem of chronic alcoholism its long-term basic programs on cerebral circulation, on autonomic function, electroencephalography. Subjects of studies in other Harvard departments have included: effect of alcohol on certain intermediary steps in carbohydrate metabolism (biochemistry department since 1938); alcohol diuresis, alcoholic polyneuritis (department of medicine, 1950); relation of craving to nutritional status (F. J. Stare, school of public health). At the biochemical institute in the University of Texas, Roger J. Williams and his associates have, since 1947, been testing Williams's hypothesis that genetically determined metabolic defects raising the requirement for certain nutritional elements may account for addiction to alcohol. In the medical branch at Galveston, G. A. Emerson was engaged, 1952, in studies of metabolic and endocrine factors in alcoholism. Studies in Cornell's psychiatry department by Oskar Diethelm have included since 1948 attempts to correlate emotional and biochemical factors in alcoholic patients. Subjects of studies in other university centers since 1949–50 include: at California, alcohol metabolism (C. H. Hine); at Indiana, toxicity of alcohol (H. R. Hulpieu); at Johns Hopkins, enzymes involved in alcohol metabolism (V. A. Najjar), factors involved in experimental production and control of pathological appetite for alcohol (C. P.

Richter), effect of injected alcohol on the vascular system of the brain (E. A. Walker); at New York State College of Medicine in Syracuse, mechanism of action of disulfiram on metabolism of myocardial and other tissues by Jay Tepperman. Among state university or medical school programs associated with state activity, 1950 to 1952, are studies at the Medical College of Virginia, 1950–51 (J. C. Forbes and G. M. Duncan, biochemistry), of effect of alcohol on metabolism of liver lipids, heart glycogen, adrenal factors in alcoholism, drug therapy; at the medical college of South Carolina, studies of alcohol metabolism in dogs (William McCord, J. C. Aull, Jr., and F. W. Kinard, chemistry). To these more or less continuous programs are to be added numerous scattered studies from departments of psychiatry evaluating therapeutic approaches to alcoholism.

## INDUSTRIAL INTEREST IN RESEARCH ON ALCOHOLISM

Illustrative of industrial interest in rehabilitation of alcoholic workers was the contribution ($25,000) by the Consolidated Edison Company and several other industrial grants, 1952, toward the first year's expenses of a clinic for alcoholics (referred by New York industries) set up in the department of industrial medicine of the New York University postgraduate medical school under joint guidance of Anthony J. Lanza, department director, S. Bernard Wortis, chairman of the psychiatry and neurology department, A. Z. Pfeffer, physician in charge of the clinic's permanent staff of medical and psychiatric specialists. The DuPont Company, 1951, reported restoration of a hundred valued employees through remedial programs, and the Eastman Kodak Company contributed to a Rochester community program resulting in acceptance of cases of acute alcoholic intoxication by all Rochester hospitals. More generalized evidence of industrial interest is mentioned in the following section on sources of financial support for research on alcoholism.

## FINANCING OF RESEARCH ON ALCOHOLISM

Funds for research on fundamental aspects of alcoholism have never been large. The university's contribution to the Yale center, aside from the building, including the laboratory of applied physiology, was described, 1952, as small, the center depending chiefly on voluntary contributions. For ten new projects requiring approximately $390,000 in 1949–50, the National Research Council's committee on problems of alcohol had only $53,028, inherited (with certain projects) from the Research Council on Problems of Alcohol. The committee interested the Office of Naval Research in aiding research at the Scripps Metabolic Clinic, La Jolla, California, on alcohol metabolism employing radioactive ethyl alcohol, and at the Biochemical Institute at the University of Texas. Other sources of support for the Texas work include Research Corporation, the Nutrition Foundation, the Rockefeller Foundation. The Licensed Beverage Industries gave $100,000 for three years to the National Research Council's committee, in 1948 made a grant to the National Safety Council for developing legal standards of intoxication in persons involved in accidents, and gave $5,000 to Northwestern for training technicians to perform chemical tests of intoxication. The liquor industry is also the indirect source of funds (derived from licenses and other taxes) used in several states for programs of treatment, education, rehabilitation, occasionally for associated research. Illustrative of governmental liquor revenue so employed are: in Connecticut, $300,000 (1951–1952) representing nine per cent of permit fees; in the District of Columbia (since 1950), ten per cent of retail liquor license fees amounting to $100,000; in Oregon, $120,000 biennially from liquor revenues; smaller sums from state liquor taxes in New Mexico, Alabama, Louisiana, Vermont. Pertinent here is the view of the Licensed Beverage Industries (cited by Karl Bowman, 1952) that the cost of programs for alcoholics should be met "from general rather than special sources". Recent state appropriations for control programs besides those previously mentioned for Connecticut, Delaware, North Carolina, Virginia include: New York's $245,000 (earlier $55,000); $15,000 allocated, 1951, by the Vermont General Assembly for a two-year program. In 1952 the Georgia commission on alcoholism asked the state for $334,000. State appropriations, some providing specifically for research in state universities, mark, in their increasing number and size, progressive recognition of alcoholism as a public health problem calling for state recognition and for fundamental research.

## GRADUAL PROGRESS TOWARD METABOLIC
## APPROACHES IN RESEARCH ON ALCOHOLISM

Among the ancient fixations that have diverted research on alcoholism and delayed approach to fundamental metabolic work and attempts at psychological and biochemical correlations has been persistent preoccupation with toxic effects of alcohol on this or that separate organ. This preoccupation has favored partial and incomplete approach to the phenomena of intermediary metabolism, ignoring initial and fundamental metabolic processes in which alcohol merely plays a part, in the attempt to attribute directly to alcohol tissue lesions and localized disturbance of function. Yet pathologists have supplied no evidence (L. H. Berry) of unequivocal chronic gastritis due to alcohol; there is scant evidence (Haggard and Jellinek a decade ago) of particular intestinal action on and by alcohol; experimental cirrhosis of the liver produced in rats fed alcohol could have resulted from well-known disturbances of fat metabolism due to lack of lipotropic dietary factors (W. H. Sebrell, Jr., and associates at the National Institute of Health), a condition that may occur in total abstainers; against the old view that alcohol produces "Bright's disease", experimental work has suggested that while alcohol is diuretic its effect on the normal kidney is slight. As to heart effects: electrocardiographic records of 2,400 men of an average age of 47.8 years, reported over a decade ago by H. J. Johnson, indicated no correlation between cardiac abnormalities and use of alcohol, a finding perhaps not incompatible with electrocardiographic studies by Russek, Naegele and Regan, 1950, suggesting indirect effect of alcohol upon coronary accidents through sedative action upon the higher nervous centers, eliminating the protective effects of pain and lessening caution. Direct effect of alcohol on the reproductive organs and system is not, according to a pamphlet based upon studies at the Yale laboratory of applied physiology, supported by the available evidence. Some years ago Jellinek observed to the scientific committee of the Research Council on Problems of Alcohol: "At present it does not seem justified to support researches on germ damage unless some investigator of great originality should place these researches on an entirely new basis." In general, investigative interest in the manifestations of alcoholism in particular organs and tissues has now departed from outmoded concepts of gross organ function and yielded to the larger perspective envisaging mechanisms of intermediary metabolism at the cellular level.

## METABOLIC IMPLICATIONS IN CONCEPTS OF ALCOHOL AS A FOOD

"Any discussion of the effects of alcohol on metabolism" (Harold E. Himwich, research director, Galesburg State Research Hospital, Illinois, discussing brain metabolism, 1951) "must be considered in at least two aspects: alcohol as a food and alcohol as a narcotic." The two are hardly, however, to be regarded as sharply separate. Because alcohol does not require digestion but is absorbed directly from the stomach and small intestine by simple diffusion, it is a readily available source of energy. Oxidation of one gram of ethyl alcohol yields approximately seven calories (Himwich, 1954) and on this basis one ounce of alcohol would produce approximately 200 calories. Alcohol cannot, however, supply what an equivalent amount of ordinary food would provide in minerals, proteins, or in the vitamins that form the prosthetic groups of various enzymes. There is, moreover, an upper limit beyond which alcohol cannot supply the caloric needs of the body. It can supply the energy needed for ordinary metabolic functioning but not the energy needed for unusual physical or mental work. Its power to mobilize energy seems to be counteracted by its narcotic effect. "There is a low limit upon the amount of alcohol that body cells can handle at one time. When this limit is reached, alcohol can become a poison to the cells; it slows them down, narcotizes or anesthetizes" (Yale pamphlet). The success that has attended supplying many known vitamin deficiencies to combat the lessened intake of food, recognized as a major problem in chronic alcoholism, should not obscure more recent data on the ten amino acids, the numerous fatty acids and components of phosphatides which are dietary essentials (*i.e.*, cannot be synthesized by the human body), each of which has a specific and indispensable part to play in the cycle of intermediary metabolism which can be blocked at almost any point by lack of an intermediary compound. All discussions of alcohol as a food point to need of fundamental understanding of the complex mechanisms of intermediary metabolism, but ancient and oversimple concepts of alcohol as a direct food, a direct toxin, or a direct stimulant still cloud the picture.

## METABOLIC IMPLICATIONS IN CONCEPTS OF ALCOHOL AS A MEDICINE

Outstanding among therapeutic properties claimed for alcohol in various forms and dilutions (aside from its toxic action on bacteria, leading to many practical uses) are its anesthetic and analgesic capacity, its power to stimulate or depress respiration, circulation, brain metabolism. "Alcohol is in fact an anesthetic like ether or chloroform. In deep intoxication surgery could be carried out painlessly" (Greenberg, 1953). It is impracticable as a general anesthetic only because of its effect on vasomotor and circulatory mechanisms, and because "the anesthetic doses are too close to the lethal" for safety (Himwich, 1954). On the analgesic powers of alcohol, opinions, according to Himwich, 1954, have changed. It is possible that alcohol may work by changing the reaction of the individual to pain rather than by raising the pain threshold. Random illustrative reports of clinical trial of alcohol's analgesic properties include: a 1951 report (M. Karp and J. K. Sokol) on alcohol as a useful drug in angina pectoris, in other cardiac conditions, in cancer (on the basis of nine years' use of intravenous infusions for sedation of 2,000 surgical patients); a 1951 report (E. R. Chapman and P. Williams, Jr.) on use of alcohol for obstetrical analgesia (on the basis of clinical trials of intravenous injections of 7.5 per cent ethyl alcohol in five per cent glucose in a hundred unselected obstetrical patients).

The apparent stimulation (of heart rate, blood pressure, respiration) that follows minute doses of alcohol has been interpreted as essentially depressant, the result of the depressing effect of alcohol on higher cortical centers, the function of which is to inhibit the activity of nerves playing a part in normal cardiovascular activity. Thus, Dodge and Benedict ascribed the more rapid heart rate after drinking alcohol to removal of the inhibitory influence on heart rate usually exerted by the brain through nerves to the heart. Through the nervous system, alcohol "turns the heart loose", or stimulates the cerebral circulation. Arthur Grollman (carrying on his studies of circulatory dynamics at

Bowman Gray, 1942) likened the apparently stimulating effect of alcohol in transient heart failure, syncope or shock to the effect of "other irritants such as smelling salts", or to reflex stimulation induced in the mucous membranes of the gastrointestinal tract. Experimental studies, in his view, had demonstrated that alcohol affects the circulation only slightly, and indirectly, by sedative action. While observing that "the narcotic effects of alcohol may emanate from other avenues also", Himwich regarded depression of brain metabolism as the significant phenomenon. Admitting that the "complete explanation of the narcotic process is not at hand" for any drug or for alcohol, he mentioned two views designed to explain the mechanism of the narcotic process. One of these views postulates as of primary importance interference with cellular oxidation. Another view casts doubt on the primary importance of interference with oxidation as explaining the narcotic process and stresses rather the view that depression within synaptic transmission of the nerve impulse, regarded as the basis of the narcotic action of alcohol, depends upon a metabolic block, interference with the turnover of energy-rich phosphate. "Thus the impairment of the cerebral metabolic rate observed in alcoholic stupor may be secondary to the failure in the formation and breakdown of organic phosphates." Understanding of the mechanisms by which alcohol exercises its narcotic effects clearly involves full understanding, not yet achieved, of the mechanisms of narcosis generally. So long as this fundamental knowledge is not available, there is slim scientific basis for attempts to use alcohol as a stimulant or a sedative. In present perspectives, the regulation in the first world war requiring Army doctors to use whiskey in pneumonia (skeptics among medical officers had to choose between violating their scientific conscience and facing court-martial) seems curiously archaic. Nor does scientific evidence support the power of alcohol to increase muscular output or to sharpen intellectual function. MacLeod, 1950, found no reason for thinking that alcohol can be used directly to further performance of muscular work, although "as a readily oxidized substance it can furnish heat and also probably spares carbohydrate and fat". As to its ultimate effect on intellectual function, initial stimulus from alcohol appears to be overbalanced by impairment in fine coordination and in reaction time; pertinent in this regard is one physician's pragmatic summary: "Alcohol can never make you do a thing better; it can only make you less ashamed of your mistakes."

## METABOLIC IMPLICATIONS IN OBSERVATIONS ON SO-CALLED ALCOHOLIC DISEASES

The net effect of a brief survey of some of the fairly numerous conditions popularly and clinically associated with alcoholism is to deprive alcohol of a direct causal role and to focus attention on the general malnutrition, specific nutritional deficiencies, the metabolic derangements in psychoses, neuropathies, pellagra, liver cirrhosis and other pathological conditions frequently found in alcoholics — but not peculiar to them.

It has been recognized for many years that *delirium tremens*, although it accounts for approximately thirty-seven per cent of all cases of alcoholic psychosis (Yale pamphlet, 1952), "befalls only a fraction of chronic alcoholics" (Bowman and Jellinek, 1941), cannot be attributed to alcohol directly but grows "on the ground of metabolic disturbances". These disturbances may involve metabolism of carbohydrate, lipid, protein, water, loss of the detoxicating function of the liver, acidosis, depressed oxidation in the brain and other evidences of disturbed metabolism "in complex interaction". This concept of multiple metabolic disturbance is reflected in treatment of delirium tremens with many substances, including intravenous glucose, insulin, vitamin B complex, ascorbic acid, liver extract. Commenting on the idea that delirium tremens may be, in part at least, a withdrawal syndrome, Himwich mentioned recent studies of addiction (in this case to the barbiturates) at the federal drug addiction hospital in Lexington, Kentucky, revealing a picture "strikingly similar to delirium tremens".

*Wernicke's syndrome*, an encephalitic syndrome which can occur in nonalcoholic conditions, has been referred to thiamine deficiency. All of a Bellevue series of twenty-seven cases of Wernicke's syndrome (twenty-four of them alcoholics) responded to thiamine therapy. In a Japanese prison camp, Wernicke's encephalopathy (attributed in this case to malnutrition, not to alcohol) was reported by de Wardener and B. Lennox, 1947, to be rapidly and completely cured by thiamine

therapy.   The deficiency of thiamine chloride attributable to alcoholism and other factors has been described by various workers as "the
important etiological factor" underlying the histopathologic processes
in the brain in Wernicke's syndrome (F. W. Bailey, 1946).   Although
various vitamins of the B group are known to be involved in tissue
metabolism as parts of coenzymes, "it is only in thiamine deficiency
that an obvious defect in the brain tissue metabolism has been detected" (Elliott, 1952).   This statement is based on the work of
R. A. Peters and his associates (Banga and Ochoa) at Oxford, 1936
and thereafter, showing that deprivation of thiamine beyond a critical
level reduced the oxidation of carbohydrates in the brain (of pigeons
and of rats) and that this resulted from lack of diphosphathiamine
which is synthesized (in the brain and other tissues) from thiamine
(known since 1937 to act as a coenzyme in carbohydrate oxidations)
by phosphorylation.   Summarizing certain observations made earlier
at the Mayo Clinic, and more recent studies at the Elgin State Hospital, 1943–1946, under the auspices of the food and nutrition board
of the National Research Council, Russell M. Wilder observed, 1952,
that thiamine deficiency, when moderate, "leads to disturbances of
attitudes and behavior" and, when severe, "to serious disorders of the
central nervous system".

*Korsakoff's psychosis* is known to be more common among nonalcoholics, and to occur (Haggard and Jellinek) in lead poisoning, arteriosclerosis, syphilis, occasionally as a complication of pregnancy.   In
the Bellevue series of Wernicke's syndrome mentioned above in which
all responded to thiamine therapy, the Korsakoff's psychosis that
followed reversal of Wernicke's syndrome in several of the alcoholic
patients did not respond to thiamine.

About ten per cent of chronic alcoholics, it is estimated, suffer from
*pellagra*.   Of 241 cases of pellagra in Ohio hospitals reported, 1942, by
Bean, Spies and Blankenhorn, 169, or 70.1 per cent, described as
"primarily alcoholic", were attributed to dietary deficiencies or unsatisfied vitamin wants.   So-called alcoholic pellagra was defined by
Robinson, 1951, as one of the pseudo pellagras in which psychic disturbances precede by weeks or months the recognizable tissue lesions
(dermatitis, stomatitis, glossitis, ulceration) of classical pellagra which
are quickly cured by nicotinamide.   Advanced psychic and neural

symptoms are not relieved by nicotinamide, probably because cerebral neurons are actually destroyed, but less advanced symptoms are relieved by multiple vitamin therapy, including especially thiamine and riboflavin. Since nicotinic acid is an essential component of two coenzymes (diphosphopyridine nucleotide, coenzyme I, and triphosphopyridine nucleotide, coenzyme II) active in the hydrogen transport system in which energy is produced by intracellular oxidation of carbohydrate, the neuropsychiatric changes (memory gaps, changes of mood, stupor, coma) were described (Jolliffe, Wortis, Stein) as probably directly related to metabolic disturbances in the brain. Observations on two different species have yielded diverse results. Elvehjem (1939) was unable to detect in dogs a decrease in the coenzyme activity of the brain in acute deficiency of nicotinic acid. On the other hand, rats on a diet deficient in nicotinic acid exhibited subnormal levels of that substance in the brain (S. A. Singal, V. P. Sydenstricker, G. M. Littlejohn, 1948).

Blankenhorn and his associates, 1946, considered the "direct cause" of *beriberi* heart disease in twelve alcoholics seen at the Cincinnati General Hospital between 1940 and 1944 to be not alcohol but rather diet deficient not only in thiamine but also in other water-soluble vitamins, particularly niacin, riboflavin, ascorbic acid.

A Research Council's statement of a few years ago pointed out that the *various peripheral neuropathies* to which fifty per cent of chronic alcoholics are subject can be avoided by vitamin B administration.

R. S. Boles and coworkers, on the basis of autopsies performed on alcoholics at the Philadelphia General Hospital between 1942 and 1946, while regarding alcohol as a contributing or predisposing factor in some cases, recommended abandoning, as unscientific, reference to any type of *liver cirrhosis* as "alcoholic". Early experimental work in the National Institute of Health, in producing liver cirrhosis in rats by dietary means, without alcohol, had led Lowry, Daft, Sebrell to observe, 1942, that the participation of alcohol in liver cirrhosis is probably in acting "as a toxic substance on a liver already damaged as a result of dietary deficiency". The relation between hepatic damage and the metabolism of alcohol has been the subject of investigations by Sirnes (Oslo), who studied, 1952, the influence of different types of liver injury on the rate of alcohol oxidation, which occurs essentially

in the liver.  His work indicated that alcohol oxidation is profoundly
affected by lesions in the peripheral parts of the liver lobes, the chief
site of alcohol oxidation.  According to Beams, 1946, enlargement
(probably fatty) of the liver in an early stage in alcoholism responds
to treatment with high protein, low fat diets supplemented with
choline and cystine.  Impairment of the liver's handling of fat was
described by Greenberg, 1953, as probably responsible for development of liver cirrhosis "which occurs with particularly high incidence
among alcoholics".  Rouleau and Nadeau in France, 1951, found that
lipotropic substances and vitamins brought about improvement in
liver function in thirty-eight alcoholics without resort to total abstinence.  Some light on the relation of degree of habituation to fatty
liver was contributed by Texon's 1950 study of five hundred patients
admitted to the alcoholic pavilion of the Knickerbocker Hospital,
New York: after five years of excessive drinking, incidence of fatty and
of normal livers was equal but after ten or more years nine out of ten
alcoholics had liver disease.  Aside from the demonstrable role of malnutrition in liver cirrhosis in chronic alcoholics, there is still investigative interest in the question whether metabolic disturbance more
directly attributable to alcohol may also be operative.

## INVESTIGATIVE INTEREST IN RELATION OF HABITUATION TO RATE OF ALCOHOL METABOLISM

Around the question whether habituation to alcohol might increase the capacity of the organism for its oxidation has grown up a
voluminous literature, and a divided opinion.  Jacobsen, however,
cited, 1952, as a majority opinion the view that the metabolic rate of
alcohol is independent of concentration, and that habituation has no
effect on the metabolic rate.  Experimental findings (in rats, with C14
labeled alcohol, Bartlett and Barnet, 1949; in dogs, Newman, 1947,
Loomis, 1950) have supplied neither uniform nor conclusive answers
to the question whether higher concentrations of alcohol "condition"
the organism to a higher oxidation rate.  Lester and Greenberg
thought, 1952, that the whole controversy might be referable to "inaccurate analyses for alcohol in the blood".  Studies of the Yale center
of alcohol studies showed that the effects of a moderate amount of

alcohol were less in the group of habitual heavy drinkers, greater in the group of occasional light drinkers. But the heavy drinkers "turned out to be fully as much below par as the inexperienced drinkers in tests of speed of motor response, auditory and visual discrimination, tactile perception, digital dexterity and other faculties. They merely had their 'sea legs'." According to Greenberg, 1953, "the experienced drinker's 'habituation' to alcohol may be largely, if not entirely, psychological". Himwich (1954), citing the experiments of Fleming and Stotz, noted that "absorption of alcohol was most rapid in the heavy drinkers, slowest in the abstainers, and intermediate in the moderate drinkers". The position of the three curves was reversed, however, after the first hour and then absorption became slowest in the heavy drinkers.

### KNOWN AND ASSUMED STEPS IN THE METABOLISM OF ALCOHOL

Oxidation of alcohol (as tentatively outlined by Himwich, 1954) occurs in five major steps: formation of acetaldehyde accomplished with the aid of alcohol dehydrogenase; production of acetic acid which may be catalyzed by several enzymes including xanthine oxidase, aldehyde oxidase and aldehyde dehydrogenase. The first two steps take place chiefly in the liver but not exclusively since the brain also is capable of initiating oxidation of alcohol though at a slower rate. The three subsequent steps, formation of acetyl CoA, condensation of the latter with oxalacetic acid to yield citric acid, and finally oxidation of citric acid to $CO_2$ and $H_2O$ are not located chiefly in the liver but are widespread throughout the body, including the brain; also they apply not to alcohol alone but to carbohydrate, fat and protein.

There is not clear agreement as to which enzyme systems are involved in the first step, formation of acetaldehyde. The question whether the major role is played by alcohol dehydrogenase, an enzyme localized mainly in the liver (studied in partially purified form by C. Lutwak-Mann, 1938, and, since 1950, in crystalline form obtained from horse liver by Bonnichsen in Hugo Theorell's laboratory), or whether catalase participates in the physiological oxidation of ethyl alcohol (through reaction with hydrogen peroxide) has not yet been answered in the laboratories that have been working on oxidation of alcohols (D. Keilin and E. F. Hartree, 1936, 1945, at Cambridge; Hugo Theorell, 1950–51, at the Karolinska Institutet, Stockholm; Britton Chance, 1947–1951, at the Johnson Foundation, University of Pennsylvania) and among workers that have more recently come to this question through interest in the human problem of alcoholism (Erik Jacobsen, 1952, at the University of Copenhagen; Grant R. Bartlett, 1952, at the Scripps Metabolic Clinic, California). Solution of this problem will affect views concerning the relation of the rate of alcohol oxidation to alcohol concentration in the blood since (as Jacobsen pointed out, 1952) if alcohol dehydrogenase is responsible for all of the oxidation of alcohol, the rate of alcohol oxidation would be constant without regard to blood concentration of alcohol.

While the acetaldehyde resulting from the first step is "much more toxic than alcohol itself", the acetic acid to which it is further oxidized in the second step in all the tissues of the body is "a harmless substance" (Greenberg, 1953). Acetic acid is the normal intermediary by which all fats, carbohydrates, proteins are broken down and enter the metabolic pool *via* the tricarboxylic acid (Krebs) cycle (Konrad Bloch, 1947). This fact explains (Jacobsen, 1952) why alcohol can replace the calorie-producing factors of normal nutrition. Oxidation of acetic acid through the Krebs cycle requires vitamin $B_1$.

From considerations of the metabolism of alcohol emerge two points that could be of practical importance in control of alcoholism. One of these is the determining influence of food, notably protein and fat, in prolonging the emptying time of the stomach, thus delaying intestinal absorption of alcohol and reducing its effects. The other is the search for procedures and substances calculated to hasten oxidation and for that reason potentially useful in treatment of acute alcoholic intoxication. The influence of insulin in this regard is mentioned later. Himwich, mindful of the complex processes of intermediary metabolism, reviewed (1954) some of the substances tried with reference to their indirect as well as their direct effects, and subscribed to belief that the power of certain amino acids to accelerate the oxidation of alcohol is well substantiated. "Apparently the experimental methods holding most therapeutic promise for the oxidation of alcohol are those which employ pyruvate as an intermediary metabolite." From a more pragmatic point of view, Greenberg, 1953, found successful "none of the attempts thus far made to increase the rate of alcohol oxidation and thus to shorten the period of intoxication".

MacLeod, 1950, referred to "the strikingly uncomplicated character of the main route of alcohol metabolism" as leaving little scope for investigation of the basic problem in alcoholism, the possible metabolic basis for addiction. His own experiments since 1947 have been motivated by the working hypothesis that some metabolic mechanism — perhaps that of acetate metabolism or perhaps some reaction system in the tricarboxylic acid cycle into which alcohol would enter through acetate — becomes so conditioned to the presence of alcohol that alcohol becomes necessary for maintenance of equilibrium; as alcohol is rapidly oxidized in the liver, this metabolic requirement must be met by additional alcohol. Since the effects of alcohol are best known on the nervous system, he suggested that the reaction systems conditioned to alcohol for their maintenance be sought in the intracellular mechanisms of nerve cells rather than in other tissues in which the same mechanisms operate.

## TISSUE SITES OF ALCOHOL METABOLISM IN TERMS OF LOCALIZATION OF ENZYMES

From the earliest days of study of enzyme reactions in terms of units of activity in minced or homogenized tissues, variations in content or concentration of specific enzymes in various tissues have been recognized. Studies in specific tissues of enzyme-activated reactions in alcohol oxidation have been largely concerned with the liver, generally accepted as the primary site of continuous removal and oxidation of alcohol by enzymes. Studies *in vitro*, indicating that the liver carries out eighty per cent of the first oxidative step, the formation of acetaldehyde, are in harmony with correlations of the over-all rate of alcohol oxidation with the amount of liver tissue in the body: a number of workers have reported experiments showing that hepatectomy reduces markedly ability to metabolize alcohol. As indicated above, after the formation of acetaldehyde and its oxidation to acetic acid in the liver, study of the steps and the sites from which acetic acid is distributed by the blood stream to other tissues for further metabolism has been pursued in less detail.

Of these other tissues, kidney and brain have come in for more frequent speculation; heart and diaphragm were mentioned by Bartlett and Barnet as having "a slight ability to oxidize alcohol, although insufficient to contribute appreciable energy to their own metabolism or to the organism as a whole". Finding in their own rat experiments a high rate of oxidation in kidney slices, these workers felt that while it was not possible definitely to "exclude the kidney as a factor in primary activation of alcohol oxidation", the rat might possibly be "an exceptional species in this regard". In pointing out that metabolic processes of the brain (dependent largely on oxidation of glucose) probably cannot be supported adequately by oxidation of alcohol, Himwich, 1951, nevertheless recalled the few findings providing "reliable evidence" that the brain can oxidize alcohol: as Dewan's isolation, 1943, from beef brain, of an oxidase capable of oxidizing alcohol to acetaldehyde; also evidence implicating, in oxidation of alcohol to acetaldehyde, flavoprotein, a large class of respiratory enzymes found in the brain. The possibility that the brain may be capable of only the first step, oxidation of alcohol to acetaldehyde, and that it cannot complete the oxidation of alcohol to $CO_2$ and water was suggested as a possible explanation of negative findings with isolated brain tissue by Bartlett and Barnet, 1949. Support for the view that in man alcohol cannot substitute for glucose in supplying food necessary for the energetic processes of the brain was found in the 1941 report of Wortis and Goldfarb that patients in hypoglycemic coma could not be returned to consciousness when alcohol was substituted for glucose.

### RELATION OF ALCOHOL TO MECHANISMS OF CARBOHYDRATE, LIPID, PROTEIN, WATER METABOLISM

The developing concept of metabolism as a largely reversible reaction continuum (Fritz Lipmann, 1946), with two major accompaniments, transformation of potential energy of foodstuffs into utilizable energy and synthesis of needed compounds from the breakdown products of energy-yielding oxidation, makes it possible to appreciate the measurable value of alcohol in energy production and its limited value in supplying building blocks for metabolic needs. Hopkins once remarked, "The body ... is in general able to deal only with what is customary to it." An excess of energy-producing material such as alcohol which provides few of the radicals needed for synthesis of proteins, enzymes and other vital body constituents must, it appears, disturb the dynamic metabolic continuum and may at specific points disrupt it. John P. Peters (Yale, medicine), discussing the interrelations of foodstuffs, 1952, pointed out that the reversible glucose-glycogen cycle is no longer to be viewed as simply as in time past, but that each alternate step depends upon the tissue cells involved and their specific complement of enzymes. Metabolic blocks, in the light of the peculiar orientation of enzyme systems in liver, muscle, may possibly be overcome or circumvented by "introduction of appropriate intermediary products at strategic points". The relevance of these fundamental ideas to the scarcely touched problems of the role of alcohol in relation to metabolic equilibrium is to point the relative futility of attempts to discover specific interrelationships between alcohol and separate foodstuffs on the level of reaction rates or concentrations. MacLeod reported, 1947, experiments designed to test the possibility that interference by alcohol with the normal processes of intermediary metabolism may result in alterations responsible for the "physiological drive" leading to addiction. In liver slices, oxidation of acetate "was greatly reduced when ethyl alcohol was present at concentrations occurring physiologically after alcohol administration". Results of rabbit experiments, in which rise of blood acetate after administration of alcohol indicated a temporary disturbance of the normal mechanisms which prevent accumulation of acetate, and of a few other scattered experiments on effects of alcohol on the tricarboxylic acid cycle of reactions were in harmony with MacLeod's concept that alcohol exerts its effects on certain features of oxidative metabolism to which carbohydrate is a chief contributor.

Although there is no doubt that at the level of acetic acid or acetate the breakdown products of alcohol and of *carbohydrate* would be indistinguishable, the question whether alcohol interferes specifically with some step in the reversible reactions between glucose and glycogen (the storage form of sugar in the body) has not been answered. Pyruvate was established more than twenty years ago as the route through which lactic acid is oxidized in one of the independent pathways of sugar oxidation. MacLeod referred to some kind of interaction "that recurs *in vivo* between pyruvate and ethyl alcohol, either of which is able to accelerate the disappearance of the other from the blood stream". However, the hypothesis that pyruvate accelerates the metabolism of alcohol (Westerfeld, Stotz and Berg, 1942; Himwich, 1954) has been disputed by Gregory and associates, 1943; on the basis of experiments with dogs, 1951, by McCord, Aull, and Kinard. One line of reasoning (Haggard and Jellinek, 1942) as to the way in which alcohol may disturb storage and mobilization of sugar by the liver is that, during emotional excitement, the rate of breakdown of glycogen into glucose rises with consequent rise in level of blood glucose. In a study of glucose tolerance (rate of glucose utilization measured by the time required for the blood glucose curve to return to normal after ingestion of glucose) in 303 cases, reported in 1943, Voegtlin, with the O'Hollarens at Shadel Sanatorium, found that "the carbohydrate metabolism of the alcoholic patient was severely deranged in over half of the cases studied". Glucose tolerance tests on fifty chronic alcoholics, reported, 1946, by Karlan and Cohn, showed increase of rate of utilization in twenty-two (forty-four per cent), decrease in five (ten per cent) and normal rate in twenty-three (forty-six per cent). Control tests of a hundred nonalcoholic psychoneurotics showed only seven with longer glucose tolerance curves. These workers registered their view that hypoglycemia does not lead to alcoholism, but that the resulting faintness, restlessness and hunger, accompanied by mental states, do increase the desire for alcohol. Delirium tremens and the alcoholic psychoses generally have been largely attributed by some workers to toxic intermediate products from disturbed carbohydrate metabolism. In trying fructose in alcoholism, A. Pletscher and associates reported, 1952, rapid disappearance of alcohol from the blood following intravenous administration of fructose (which is converted to glucose in the intestines). Whether or not this finding, and similar effects from intravenous levulose, reported by F. Heim and associates, 1953, confirm the generally accepted disturbance of carbohydrate metabolism in alcoholism or have therapeutic implication remains to be seen.

Acetic acid or some closely related compound was for more than forty years postulated as a principal intermediary in *lipid metabolism* before use of isotopes made possible its identification. Curran and

Rittenberg, 1951, in discussing the possibility that ethyl alcohol or acetaldehyde may be an intermediate in the utilization of acetate for cholesterol synthesis, concluded (after testing the hypothesis by *in vivo* and *in vitro* experiments with alpha-deuterioethyl alcohol) that "ethyl alcohol is not an immediate precursor of cholesterol, but that it undergoes biological conversion to either acetic acid or an active acetyl radical before utilization in cholesterol synthesis". Lester and Greenberg observed, 1952, that low incidence of arteriosclerosis in alcoholics "suggests the merits of experimental investigation of the effects of alcohol on cholesterol deposition". J. C. Forbes and G. M. Duncan (chemistry, Medical College of Virginia), on the basis of experiments undertaken to determine whether animals receiving alcohol showed a distinctly higher level of neutral fat and cholesterol in their livers than those fed the same diet without alcohol, reported, 1950, that chronic alcoholization did not increase the tendency toward development of nutritional fatty liver, a finding not entirely in agreement with the previously mentioned rat experiments of Sebrell, Lowry and associates, who found in the alcoholized group a "somewhat greater" degree of cirrhosis. The presence in the diet of lipotropic substances in amounts proportionate to caloric intake was considered to be the chief factor in prevention of fatty livers in pair-fed rats studied by C. H. Best, W. S. Hartroft, C. C. Lucas, J. H. Ridout (Banting Best Institute, Toronto), 1949. The control rats given sucrose in amounts equivalent to three-fourths of the caloric value of the alcohol consumed by the alcohol-fed rats had an incidence of liver fibrosis and average fat content in the liver "actually slightly greater than the corresponding values in the alcoholic group". Administration of choline prevented both the fatty infiltration and the cirrhotic changes in each group. The hepatic changes in both groups were attributed to choline deficiency induced either by alcohol or sugar, which, when taken in excess, "supplants choline-containing foodstuffs and at the same time, by increasing caloric intake, augments the demand for the lipotropic agents". On the basis of a series of experiments paralleling those of the Toronto group, Klatskin, Gewin and Krehl of Yale reached the conclusion, 1951, that alcohol increases the demand for choline not by raising the caloric intake but in some other way, possibly by blocking its action in the liver, by altering its absorption from the intestinal tract, or by altering its rate of endogenous synthesis.

*Protein metabolism* enters the alcohol picture notably in its relation to lipid metabolism. Knowledge of factors that control fat deposition in the liver dates from 1932 when Best's experiments on depancreatized insulin-treated dogs suffering from massive infiltration of fat into the liver led to the discovery of the lipotropic action of choline. Tucker and Eckstein demonstrated (1937) that the amino acid, methionine, is also lipotropically active and the relations between choline and methionine, elucidated by du Vigneaud and his associates (1939), rounded out the nutritional concept of fatty livers produced by a deficiency in the diet of labile methyl groups which are used for synthesis of choline. Both choline and methionine are supplied in the diet in lean meat, liver, casein and other protein foods. Proteins ingested above the amounts needed to supply amino acids for specific purposes and for replacement of body proteins, including enzymes, are broken down into nitrogen and materials that are oxidized through the channels of either carbohydrate or fat. Earlier mention was made of the suggestion of Himwich (citing work on dogs, by Westerfeld, Stotz and Berg, on cats, by Eggleton, on rabbits, by LeBreton and on excised hepatic tissues, by Leloir and Munoz) that amino acids derived from protein food probably accelerate alcohol combustion in the liver by passing through a pyruvate stage as proteins are converted to carbohydrate in the liver. That indirect and direct effects on lipid and protein metabolism may result from the well-known vitamin deficiencies associated with alcoholism is suggested by recent studies on the role of vitamin $B_{12}$ in metabolism. Schaefer and his colleagues reported, 1949, that vitamin $B_{12}$ reduces the requirement of the body for choline and further studies on transmethylation (transfer of methyl groups), Fields and Hoff, 1952, indicated that folic acid, ascorbic acid and other substances such as desoxyribosides and glutathione participate in these reactions. More direct influence of vitamin $B_{12}$ on protein metabolism was suggested, 1950, by reports (Charkey and coworkers) that $B_{12}$ enhanced utilization of amino acids in protein synthesis.

Rat experiments bearing on the relation of alcohol to *water metabolism* have indicated that increase in extracellular fluid in alcoholism could be accounted for only by loss of intracellular water. A series of studies comparing diuresis following drinking of water and of alcohol by M. Grace Eggleton (physiology, University College, London), 1942–1946, suggested that alcohol diuresis is of the same nature as water diuresis mediated by the posterior pituitary. Measurements of urine components in seven subjects, 1946, showed after alcohol an initial drop in acidity followed by a rise consistently higher than that following water. One property of water and alcohol diuresis (Eggleton and Smith, 1946) distinguishing it from all other types of diuresis is a unique response of the kidney accompanying increased flow of urine; in general, increased urine flow includes also increased excretion of chloride, but in water and alcohol diuresis chloride output is decreased. Results of experiments with dogs (five normal and three with surgically interrupted supraoptico-hypophyseal tracts) were, 1951, considered by H. B. Van Dyke and R. G. Ames (pharmacology, Columbia) to be in agreement with the hypothesis that alcohol interferes with release of antidiuretic hormone from the neurohypophysis. They found no evidence that diuretic doses of alcohol alter renal function directly; they considered that an increasing level of alcohol in the blood is necessary, but not alone sufficient, to inhibit secretion of antidiuretic hormone and that an adequate secretion of the hormone can appear and continue in the presence of a high concentration of alcohol in the blood. Silkworth and Texon at the Knickerbocker Hospital, 1950, interpreted their finding of low blood chlorides in nineteen of twenty-five patients who had been drinking heavily before admission to the alcoholic pavilion as possibly contributing to the craving for alcohol. Lester and Greenberg stressed, 1952, the need of a great deal of further work on the problem as to how and why alcohol "exercises an effect on water balance and on electrolyte excretion and shift" (as manifested in edema seen at autopsy in acutely intoxicated individuals, in thirst after heavy drinking and perhaps in a part of the hangover reaction).

## Endocrine Influences in Metabolism of Alcohol

Workers currently interested in endocrine factors in alcoholism have stressed the need of distinguishing between endocrine dysfunction that might result from chronic toxic effects of alcohol and constitutional endocrine imbalance assumed to predispose to habituation. The recurring difficulty of precisely allocating responsibility relatively to cause and to effect is again obvious here. Lester and Greenberg, 1952, summed up one view: "If endocrine malfunction is present in an alcoholic, it is probably a complication rather than the cause of the alcohol addiction." The route by which a worker might be led to approach the possible relation between endocrine dysfunction and alcoholism is suggested by the testimony of James J. Smith, director of research on alcoholism at the New York University-Bellevue Medical Center, that when he began his investigations he inclined to the belief that alcoholism is a personality problem, an "escape" from emotional immaturity. But "the more I saw of alcoholics at Bellevue Hospital, the more clearly were metabolic factors in the disease evident". Under the guidance of this perception, his group proceeded to its work on the relation between alcohol and pituitary-adrenal-gonad functioning in rats and men. The approach was not new: endocrine dysfunction, chiefly hypofunction of pituitary, adrenals, thyroid, had been mentioned by workers in the thirties as part of the mechanism of delirium tremens. The conclusion of the Smith group that alcohol stimulated and exhausted the adrenals through the pituitary derived in part from observation of biochemical and clinical similarities between delirium tremens and Addisonian crisis (an acute episode in adrenal cortical insufficiency), and from finding effective the addition of adrenal cortical extract, used in Addisonian crisis, to routine therapy for delirium tremens (saline and glucose infusions, vitamin C). To test the theory that adrenal insufficiency, possibly not primary but referable to pituitary insufficiency, is associated with chronic alcoholism, Smith used the eosinophile index in the circulating blood, one of several indices of adrenal cortical response to stimulation. Counts were made in a series of seventy-three alcoholics after test doses of ACTH and of epinephrine; results (reported at the second clinical ACTH conference, 1951) were interpreted as indicating defects in the pituitary-adrenal responses of twenty-five per cent and defects at the hypothalamic level in seventy-five per cent. These interpretations of the tests were criticized by Kark, who, from studies of 284 persons, 1952, favored abandoning as of little value the epinephrine test in diagnosis of adrenal, hypothalamic or pituitary function. Involvement of the hypothalamus in alcoholism was suggested by Smith, 1950, on the basis of its relation to pituitary disturbance generally and on the basis of such "forcible" clinical implications as profound disturbances in the alcoholic of sleep and appetite which, in part at least, are considered to be regulated by the hypothalamus.

The adequacy of the evidence so far presented in support of theories of either primary pituitary-adrenal insufficiency associated with alcoholism or of secondary insufficiency resulting from alcoholic intoxication has been challenged. Karl Bowman (psychiatry, University of California and Langley Porter Clinic) observed, 1952, that the work classifying alcoholism as a metabolic disease associated with some degree of adrenal cortical insufficiency "has not as yet produced any important contributions tending to prove or disprove this theory". The Lester and Greenberg 1952 summary noted "no evidence at present for exhaustion of the adrenal as a result of its hyperactivity, even if this is, or can be, induced by alcohol". These authors described as requiring confirmation reports of acute effect of toxic amounts of alcohol in lowering the ascorbic acid and cholesterol content of the adrenals. This finding was reported, 1951, by Forbes and Duncan, from rat and guinea pig experiments based on tests of adrenal cortical secretion developed by C. N. H. Long, in which reduction of the ascorbic acid and cholesterol content of the adrenals was correlated with increased synthesis and release of hormones. Among those testing the possible relationships in clinical studies, Norman M. Mann (Blue Hills Clinic, Hartford), 1952, suggested that available evidence should be a deterrent to the "over-enthusiastic" in routine use of cortical hormones in alcoholism.

Insulin (mentioned in the earlier reference to rate of alcohol metabolism), in the presence of adequate carbohydrate, evokes rapid formation of pyruvate, believed (Himwich) under certain conditions to accelerate alcohol metabolism. However, Himwich considered, 1954, that results of current work indicate that "it is not insulin *per se* but some indirect effect of insulin on carbohydrate metabolism that may be the important factor". D. J. Feldman and Howard D. Zucker found, 1953, "as yet no clinical evidence that the use of insulin hastens the metabolism of alcohol in the body". Newman, 1947, emphasized the need of repeating experiments of the twenties and thirties that had yielded conflicting results, as, in one direction, that administration of insulin with alcohol (to animals) resulted in accelerating metabolism of alcohol and in another direction, that insulin had no effect on metabolism of alcohol in man. Investigation of the insulin-alcohol relation, which H. Pullar-Strecker, 1945, thought may at least suggest a common denominator in metabolic disturbances of alcoholism, involves the whole sweep of intermediary metabolism.

## METABOLIC APPROACH TO NEURAL AND PSYCHIC FACTORS IN ALCOHOLISM

The mechanisms accounting for the effect of alcohol on the central nervous system are far from being understood in metabolic terms. Understanding of its dominant narcotic effect involves, as previously mentioned, understanding the mechanisms of narcosis generally, hypothetical explanations of which have been discussed for fifty years. They range from concepts related to observations of the physical behavior of protoplasm to concepts relating narcosis to mechanisms of cellular permeability involving the lipoidal layer of the cell membrane in certain physical phenomena at the cell surface, to concepts of changes that occur within a cell in response to stimulation at the surface. To these have been added more recently biochemical concepts related to specific intracellular reactions in systems regarded as necessary for the metabolic equilibrium of the cell. As to the precise location of the cells through which alcohol exerts its narcotic effects it is to be remembered that even those (Himwich, 1951; MacLeod, 1947–1952) who regard brain tissue as the most likely site of the narcotic action of alcohol (on the scanty metabolic evidence thus far available) consider that investigation has not as yet been sufficient to rule out other tissues.

It is probable that for a long time there will continue to be a division of emphasis among a number of groups, dominantly interested, respectively, in physiological, or in biochemical, or in neurophysiological, or in psychological approaches to the problem, and especially between the two large groups roughly comprising those that see alcoholism as a metabolic disease of which behavior is merely a symptom and those that see it primarily as a psychic disturbance. The division of emphasis does not greatly matter so long as research proceeds along all these fronts, or, more accurately, has in view all these approaches. Investigation of alcoholism should profit by the present general trend toward including in investigation of all mental and behavioral changes (and not only those associated with alcoholism) metabolic pathways and metabolic techniques. On the other hand, the "metabolists" are likely more and more to be forced to take into account evidence indicating that while many causes may be operative in alcoholism, addiction, as one commentator puts it, usually "begins with an anxiety state of some sort".

## BRAIN METABOLISM IN ALCOHOLISM

Attempts to arrive at some understanding of brain mechanisms in chronic alcoholism have involved pathological (and a degree of histo-chemical) study. Neither of these has been significantly rewarding as a basis for deducing what actually takes place in the brain of the alcoholic. Post mortem studies of alcoholics over a score of years have described both gross and microscopic central nervous system lesions (Harvard, Boston City Hospital, Washingtonian Hospital) considered to be degenerative rather than inflammatory. G. H. Stevenson, who, in 1940 autopsy studies, attributed brain changes in forty-four patients to vitamin deficiency (chiefly $B_1$ and $B_2$), thought that "pathologic changes in the nervous system in chronic alcoholism demonstrated in this presentation were relatively slight as compared with the profound and fatal illness of the patients". However, he felt that the changes responsible for the clinical picture "cannot be demonstrated under the microscope by methods now available". On the possibility that neuropathological changes found in alcoholics may be the basis for psychoses found in only a proportion, Walter L. Bruetsch's observation, 1952, made in the course of a discussion of mental disorders arising from organic disease, may be pertinent: "In psychoses due to intoxication, particularly alcohol, the changes in the brain are mostly of a transitory physicochemical nature."

That efforts to associate alcoholism with a specific biochemical brain "lesion" are not likely to yield an early return is suggested by the bare beginnings that have been made in histochemical study of the brain. Lowry (in the course of describing development of necessary micromethods for quantitative measurement of ten different enzymes, four lipid fractions, four phosphorus fractions, riboflavin, chloride) observed, 1952, "the structural complexity of the brain is such that interpretation of gross biochemical data seems almost hopeless".

Since analysis of pathological and histochemical data as yet justifies few conclusions as to the nature of the metabolic mechanisms in the brain involved in chronic alcoholism, informative sources also include the findings, the speculations and hypotheses of certain workers who have for years been concerned with oxygen consumption by the brain, with only occasional reference to alcoholism. Among such is Seymour S. Kety (National Institutes of Health), who, in 1950, observed that while the view that alcohol (as other narcotics, various anesthetic drugs and poisons) produces central nervous depression by intracellular block of vital enzyme systems is widely held, the exact site of the metabolic depression in narcosis is "not as yet well defined". Himwich suggested that alcohol may inhibit cerebral oxidations by inhibiting enzymes necessary for the catalytic effect of the four-carbon dicarboxylic acids on respiration (and so affecting the tricarboxylic acid cycle). Pronounced increase in cerebral blood flow and equally significant reduction in cerebral oxygen uptake were shown (Louis L. Battey, Albert Heyman, John L. Patterson, 1953) to be associated with severe alcoholic intoxication. A point consistently stressed by Himwich is that alcohol acts first upon the highest centers, the parts of the brain required for the most highly integrated activities, the functions with the largest cortical components. "The deeper depression of the more highly integrated functions is, however, not necessarily due to the presumably larger number of synapses involved in their activities but rather to the location of the synapses in cerebral areas with greater metabolic requirements." These higher areas (more susceptible perhaps because of their higher metabolic rate) can no longer exert their inhibitory control, "thus permitting the release of the anatomically lower structures". As a possible series of three events during narcosis, Himwich outlined, 1954: depression of energy-rich phosphate bond formation; a slackening of function for want of energy; diminution of oxygen uptake because of the lower metabolic requirements of the inhibited tissues. "We cannot conclude, however, that this rationalization of the narcotic process is correct, but must rather wait for further experimental results to test this explanation of the synaptic block caused by alcohol."

L. D. MacLeod, who also held the view that craving for alcohol could conceivably take place in tissue outside the nervous system, considered that "the most obvious and immediate effects of alcohol are exerted" in the nervous system and should be sought there. One clue to the peculiar susceptibility of the central nervous system to derangements, he suggested, lies in its "very high energy turnover", from which derived his view (or working hypothesis) that the process of alcoholic intoxication involves "primarily certain features of the oxidative metabolism". Because the Krebs cycle "is believed at the present moment to represent a generally valid scheme of oxidative and energy-yielding reactions occurring in a wide variety of types of cell and tissue", MacLeod studied the effects of alcohol on specific reaction systems in that cycle in cells, including especially brain tissue taken from rats intoxicated with alcohol or acetaldehyde. The working hypothesis orienting these studies was outlined as follows: "If it is believed that at least in a proportion of alcoholic addicts, there is a metabolic basis for the abnormality, then the craving for alcohol is presumably related to a need for the presence of alcohol in certain systems which have become adapted to its presence. Removal of the alcohol by the normal process of oxidation then apparently leaves the metabolism maladjusted so that more alcohol must be taken to restore the disturbed equilibria." In 1948 he had noted that a moderate amount of adaptation appeared to be part of the normal physiological response to ingestion of alcohol, leading to the suggestion that "a loss of flexibility in this mechanism could theoretically furnish a basis for the abnormal features of addiction".

MacLeod suggested as the most likely explanation (not yet demonstrated) of narcosis a highly differential action affecting some enzyme systems and leaving others unaltered. Assuming that impairment of oxidative efficiency in the central nervous system is primary, he planned experiments to explore other systems known to be active in nervous tissue, and possibly dependent on the efficiency of oxidative metabolism. For these experiments he chose the intact animal, pointing out that *in vitro* study of metabolic reactions in brain tissue must take into account the severe damage to an organ "which has lost not only the power to function as a nervous tissue but has also lost two-thirds of its power to turn over energy in chemical reactions". The only reliable guide is to obtain from study of the intact animal information about the intoxication process and extend it by reasonable hypothesis and testing to the human addict. In these 1952 experiments the degree of intoxication was assessed by performance tests. The finding that intoxication occurred in response to substances affecting not the sympathetic but the parasympathetic nervous system led to the view that in the intoxication process "some interaction occurs between alcohol and certain systems involving acetylcholine" (transient appearance of which is believed by many to be involved in transmission of nervous impulses at the ganglion). Instead of the unstable acetylcholine, a stable drug, carbachol, was used because its actions resemble those of acetylcholine; carbachol (carbamyl choline chloride) and alcohol showed a mutual potentiation or synergism. Explanation of the relation of (primary) impairment by alcohol of oxidative efficiency of the central nervous system to the apparent (secondary) disturbance of acetylcholine systems by alcohol was proposed; high levels of glycolytic and oxidative activity may be necessary to insure a large and flexible supply of acetyl groups for synthesis of choline, a part of the molecule of the phospholipid, lecithin, which occurs plentifully in brain tissue. This suggested interrelation between oxidative metabolism and acetylcholine (the brain has a high concentration of the enzyme cholesterase) may explain why the brain is so sensitive to narcotics and anoxia. The examination of such an hypothesis depends upon neurophysiologists' overcoming technical difficulties in studying formation and destruction of acetylcholine, which has so transitory an existence, and study of its effects on the properties of an organized structure such as the cell membrane. Further experiments with carbachol, MacLeod thought, might furnish further clues, as, for example, study of the effects of the drugs in alcoholics in whom intense craving for alcohol has suggested a physical need.

## ENCEPHALOGRAPHIC FINDINGS IN CHRONIC ALCOHOLISM

William G. Lennox (neurology, Harvard) once suggested that in some individuals (who display a cortical dysrhythmia that is inherent and not simply a result of alcoholism) alcoholism like epilepsy may be "a physicochemical disturbance of brain metabolism". Encephalographic studies designed to show whether chronic alcoholism is associated with abnormal encephalograms include those of M. Greenblatt, S. Levin, F. di Cori, 1944, who, on finding electroencephalographic abnormalities in only five per cent of fifty-five patients with uncomplicated alcoholism but in ten per cent of 240 normal controls, concluded that the electroencephalogram showed nothing of significance in chronic alcoholics without psychosis. In alcoholics with psychosis, encephalographic differences have been considered significant: a study of forty-seven psychotic alcoholics (delirium tremens) by a New York University and Western Reserve group, 1945 (Kennard, Bueding, Wortis), showed significant electroencephalographic changes compared with the encephalographic records of twelve nonpsychotic chronic alcoholics and a normal group. The use of encephalographic evidence to establish alcoholic psychosis and thus fix criminal responsibility was noted, 1943, in a foreign study concerned with a twenty-year-old student, who murdered his mother after having drunk four pints of beer. The encephalogram showed that the impulses from his brain were erratic and definitely abnormal. The jury found him guilty of murder but insane at the time of the crime. Such precise use of encephalographic evidence to establish alcoholic psychosis does not seem to be generally regarded as practicable in the present lack of more fundamental knowledge.

One focus of investigative interest is the difficulty in defining the significance of the lower alpha index noted in nonpsychotic alcoholics. Davis and Gibbs found, 1941, in fifteen nonpsychotic chronic alcoholics only two that had well developed alpha activity. Faure and Bannel (reporting from Paris, 1951), while noting no correlation between the clinical state of the alcoholic and his electroencephalogram in any one of twelve patients studied, added that the least intoxicated of them showed abnormal (low) alpha activity. Little and McAvoy, 1952 (neurology, University of Alabama), in their study of thirty-four confirmed alcoholics (with fifty-five normal controls) without manifestations of structural brain change or major psychosis, found that, while "the electroencephalograms of the alcoholics revealed no more abnormality than those of normal controls" (according to present routine standards of clectroencephalogram interpretation), the alcoholics showed a lower alpha index and less pronounced amplitude modulation. In raising the question whether depressed alpha waves mean tension as a cause or as a result of alcoholism, they observed that their experience confirmed the impression in a 1949 study by other workers that in patients in whom alcoholism appeared to be the primary difficulty, the alpha index tended to be low, while those in whom alcoholism is a secondary problem tended to show normal alpha activity; this impression, together with other findings, seemed to support the suggestion that the poor alpha type of record in alcoholics may be the result of the cerebral condition predisposing to alcoholism and not the result of alcoholism itself. "The testing of this hypothesis would require long-term follow-up studies of presumably normal controls to determine whether those showing low alpha indices in their EEG are more prone to become alcoholics than those with normal alpha indices."

## METABOLIC APPROACH TO PSYCHIC FACTORS IN ALCOHOL HABITUATION

Metabolic approaches are necessarily few and tentative in a field in which definition is so lacking as it is in the field of psychic factors in alcoholism. Informed workers sidestep attempts to define in psychological terms a unitary alcoholic personality. There is still admitted difficulty, moreover, in a majority of cases of chronic alcoholism, in deciding whether underlying psychosis was pre-existent or whether years of alcoholic excess have radically changed personality.

Alcoholics themselves, as certain psychiatrists have pointed out, incline to account for their addiction by psychic patterns — inferiority complex, resentment deriving from lack of affection in childhood, and all the other clichés, which, according to Abraham Myerson, 1944, the prevailing *mores* have presented to the drinker for convenient rationalization of his addiction. Current psychiatric reflections on alcoholism suggest that while no composite is justified, it can be said that many alcoholics show various combinations of some of the following traits: failure to adjust to social environment; a sense of inferiority and of frustration; overweening ambition without the energy or constancy to work; intense anxiety; emotional immaturity; terrified avoidance of adult situations; obsessive desire to be considered "normal" (as in captious unwillingness to admit inability to drink), and greater satisfaction with their own way of dealing with their difficulties than nonalcoholic neurotics usually show with their solutions. "Emotional vacuum" was the term Freyhan, 1946, used to describe a "sociopathological factor" he discerned in an increasing number of drinkers, a mass rather than an individual phenomenon, pointing toward a cultural crisis, lack of a philosophy of living and consequent lack of a sense of personal and social responsibility. More important than the intellectual impairment, according to a member of Bellevue's psychiatric division, summarizing, 1941, his experience, is the "deleterious effect on the individual's affective reactions and personality structure as a whole. More serious than the alcoholic's loss of memory is his loss of goal; long before he shows measurable signs of mental deterioration, he gives ample evidence of being less efficient socially. As to precisely what makes him so we are still in the dark."

Often stressed among psychic factors that account for the alcoholic's original urge to drink is the desire to escape neurotic anxiety, to brace himself for some dreaded *tour de force*, to blunt some devouring fear. The drinker's discovery that alcohol can, apparently, both brace and blunt then results in a pattern of drinking. Throwing a certain light on efforts of humans to use alcohol as a "cushioning" device, some 1945 experiments of Masserman, Jacques and Nicholson described administering alcohol to nine cats and then observing their response to shock stimuli (physically harmless air blasts or electric shock). Only three of the nine cats given alcohol developed neuroses (mild) whereas eight of the controls (to which alcohol was not given) showed some neurotic effect, in three cases severe.

Attempts to relate varying patterns of drinking to certain emotions were reported by Fleetwood and Diethelm, 1952. Certain biochemical factors in the blood of twenty-six alcoholic patients (observed during more than two years in from two to twenty-six psychiatric interviews) were demonstrated through their effects on contraction of rodent intestines and rabbit uterus: tension and resentment were correlated with the presence of two distinct cholinergic substances, anxiety with an adrenergic (nor-epinephrine-like) substance. Eleven of the patients after drinking six ounces of whiskey showed a reduction in the resentment factor "directly proportional to the amount of alcohol ingested". Alcohol, it was suggested, abolished the tension factor, decreased or abolished the resentment factor but only slightly decreased the anxiety factor. The inference was that if resentment is the cause of desire to drink it can be abolished by alcohol and drinking may proceed at a leisurely pace; but if anxiety, guilt or depression leads to drinking the drinker does not obtain relief so easily and drinks more heavily and more constantly in order to deaden emotions. Diethelm reporting, 1953, on his and Fleetwood's ten-year studies, declared the existence of "a close relationship between the psychiatric and biologic evaluations of the emotions . . . there is close correlation between what we call emotions of anxiety, tension, and resentment and the findings in the blood". They found, however, no special type of psychoneurosis in chronic alcoholism. "In about one-third of our patients psychoneurotic manifestations were expressed in immature and dependent or rigid behavior." Lester and Greenberg said, of the Fleetwood and Diethelm experiments: "aside from the question whether the emotions increase the titers of the factors, or vice versa", this type of study may open the way to "objective analysis and categorization of different types of alcoholics".

Whether emphasis is on mental disorientation or "ethical deterioration" or psychosis, it is quite clear that, except in acute alcoholic intoxication, correlation of these "symptoms" with metabolic values is still in its infancy. When such correlation is achieved in alcoholism, the general disciplines of psychiatry and psychology may be measurably advanced. Beadle suggested that study of the relation of metabolic derangements occurring in alcoholic intoxication to marked changes in mental function might offer a better approach (than study of normal metabolism) to understanding the chemistry of rational thinking. He recalled that study of one metabolic defect, phenylketonuria, led to the finding that persons who are unable to oxidize phenylpyruvic acid and who therefore secrete the acid in the urine are invariably idiots or imbeciles. He thought that study of normal metabolism would not have been so likely to clarify the importance of the phenyl-pyruvic acid transformation in relation to mental function.

## ATTEMPTS TO INFLUENCE SUSCEPTIBILITY AND RESISTANCE TO ALCOHOLISM

On the factors, constitutional and environmental, that may possibly influence susceptibility to alcoholism — age, sex, race, nutrition, weight, previous infection, intercurrent disease, psychologic and biochemical individuality, hereditary endowment, occupation, economic status, altitude (this does not exhaust the list) — there have been extended discussions but few conclusive findings of general application. Not only does a high degree of individual variation defeat attempts at generalization, but also the interaction of widely differing factors, the influence of one upon the other, makes suspect intensive stress upon any one. Students intrigued by apparent racial difference in susceptibility to alcoholism, for instance, have in more intensive study discerned how frequently cultural, religious, climatic, physiological, sociological, psychological influences rather than race have determined the drinking pattern. On the moot question of hereditary liability to alcoholic habituation, high estimates apparently bulwarking the possibility have been attributed to the fact that the records used were those of psychotic or criminal alcoholics. A constitutional hypersensitivity to alcohol was invoked years ago as possibly explaining alcoholic addiction. Advanced so early as 1903, the theory that addiction constitutes "an immunological response or allergy to alcohol" had a slender base in unconfirmed animal experiments reported from Germany in 1914, others from France, 1947 and 1948. In 1952, Margaret W. Robinson and Walter L. Voegtlin (physiology and biophysics, University of Washington) repeated the experiments in animals (rabbits) and also conducted them with serum from human abstainers, normal drinkers and addicts. Their negative results were described, 1952, by Lester and Greenberg as conclusively "laying to rest" hope of an experimental foundation for the hypersensitivity explanation of alcohol addiction.

The rationale of certain of the attempts to influence habituation reveals a metabolic aim, and the experimentation that has accompanied some of the therapies confirms more fundamental metabolic findings. Classified roughly (the classes are not always mutually exclusive), the therapeutic expedients aimed at habituation include: substitution therapy based on the assumed practicability of supplying vitamin deficiencies and compensating for endocrine dysfunction associated with alcoholism and considered to have a role in habituation; substances and procedures aimed at creating aversion; tetraethylthiuram disulfide (TETD, disulfiram, antabuse), for which is claimed a definite role in metabolism of alcohol; psychotherapy which ideally must be directed toward all the causes of alcoholism and take account of all the factors that influence susceptibility to it. Pertinent, with reference to the last in this list, is the general conviction among informed workers that whatever physiological or biochemical or physical methods are used must be accompanied by psychotherapy. Indeed the avowed aim in some treatments is simply to achieve abstinence for a sufficient period to make it possible to reach the patient with some form of psychotherapy.

## Vitamin Therapy

The basis of vitamin therapy in diseases and conditions associated with alcoholism, touched upon earlier, is not only multiple dietary deficiencies (appetite being satisfied by the high caloric value of alcohol) but also deficiencies conditioned by decreased utilization, increased requirements induced by the caloric burden of alcohol, and possibly by "a still unascertained specific destructive chemical effect of alcohol and fusel oils on ingested vitamins" (Alexander and other authors). Apparent absence of neuropathological evidence in behavior disturbances, psychoses, encephalopathies associated with chronic alcoholism has led to suggestions that the lesions are biochemical, disturbances of cellular function without morphological alteration of the cells (Jolliffe and associates). The precise ways in which vitamin deficiency may be related to habituation are still to be clarified.

Illustrative of work focused on the relation of vitamins to alcoholic habituation are experimental studies of R. A. Brady, and W. W.

Westerfeld (biochemistry, Syracuse), 1947, indicating that rats on a diet deficient in all vitamin B factors increased their intake of alcohol; addition of six vitamin B factors to the deficient diet did not prevent increased alcohol intake, but the supplement led to temporary interruption of alcohol intake after it had begun. Experiments with rats were the basis of Williams's explanation of alcoholism (and other conditions) in terms of genetically conditioned individual biochemical differences that produce a relatively heightened need for vitamins or other elements and lead to a craving for alcohol. He considered, 1951, that in rats the relation between vitamin deficiencies and desire for alcohol was shown to be "clear cut and unequivocal"; and that individual human variations leading to alcohol addiction might be requirements not only for vitamins but also for minerals and unknown or unrecognized substances. With the finding of the Williams group that rats and mice on vitamin deficient diets develop a craving for alcohol and choose drinks containing it, Jorge Mardones of the institute for investigation of alcoholism in the University of Chile expressed, 1951, substantial agreement (on the basis of rat experiments antedating Williams's); he favored a deficiency of an unknown substance, referring to his 1941 finding that rats appeared to lack "a thermolabile element of the vitamin B complex", designated $N_1$.

Criticisms of the concept of a nutritional or conditioned nutritional etiology of habituation have been leveled at the adequacy of the rat experiments and also at extension of conclusions from rat experiments to human alcoholism. Lester and Greenberg considered that the results of their studies in rats of nutrition in relation to alcoholism (the first report of which was published, 1952) challenged both the published data and the interpretation of them. A "choice" between water and alcohol solution (the latter the only additional source of calories offered to animals presumably unable to utilize other dietary caloric sources because of vitamin deficiencies) was, in their view, no choice at all. When a sucrose solution and other caloric foods were made available and the vitamin-deficient rats chose these in preference to alcohol, no "craving" for sucrose was suggested. The experimental results were also considered to be incompatible with "any narrow concept of human alcoholism as due to nutritional or genetotrophic defect as proposed by Williams"; the human alcoholic seeks intoxication but the rat's consumption of alcohol as a caloric source was spread over the day and never produced intoxication. Diethelm, 1953, described Williams's theory as attractive but not applicable to "the intricate problem of human alcoholism without a great many further fundamental investigations". Effects of vitamin "supplements" (used to test the presence of either vitamin deficiency or increased need) have been tried in a few alcoholic patients. "A diminished craving for alcohol" was reported, 1951, "in many patients receiving vitamin supplements" by Stare and his associates at the Harvard school of public health in a study of fifty chronic alcoholic patients, half of whom received massive doses of most of the known vitamins, the other half, placebos. Although J. A. Smith and his coworkers, also in 1951, drew no conclusions from a small series of six treated with vitamin B supplements in excess of maximum daily requirements (without other treatment or psychotherapy) they noted alteration in the drinking pattern of the patients (while under treatment) in decreased desire for alcohol, decreased tension, hostility, insomnia; they recommended further study.

## HORMONE THERAPY DESIGNED TO COMPENSATE FOR ASSUMED ENDOCRINE INSUFFICIENCY

There are reports of the use of ACTH directed toward metabolic defects in alcoholics attributed to pituitary insufficiency with consequent adrenal cortical and gonadal hypofunctioning. Reporting on treatment of twenty-five chronic alcoholics for over eight months with small doses (twenty-five mg. three times a week) of ACTH, J. J. Smith noted, 1951, benefit to all of the seventeen that tolerated the hormone without unfavorable side reaction. In view of the limited period of study and the lack of definite criteria, Smith considered the reduced incidence of alcoholism and the briefer duration of drinking episodes (when they occurred) to justify further investigation. Feldman and Zucker considered, 1953, that clinical management of acute alcoholic intoxication had been "radically changed" by introduction of the adrenal steroid hormones. "Although the exact relationship of adrenal function to alcoholism has by no means been conclusively demonstrated, it is evident that the use of these steroids in the acute alcoholic patient may result in striking and rapid improvement." Williams, in admitting that periodic and continued injection of the proper hormones might perhaps keep alcoholism in abeyance, also urged keeping in mind that it "is a definite function of the body to produce hormones" but not to produce vitamins. If vitamins and "materials needed in the nutritional treatment are completely available", in his view, hormones will be produced within the body "in normal fashion".

The metabolic mechanisms involved in three ways of using insulin in chronic alcoholism (in massive doses designed to produce shock; in subconvulsive doses, aiming at a mild degree of hypoglycemia not amounting to coma; in small doses, aiming at detoxicant action) are not well understood; nor has influence of insulin upon habituation been demonstrated. Voegtlin and Lemere (Shadel Sanitarium, Seattle) found, 1942, no competent evidence that either insulin or metrazol, whether in convulsive or subconvulsive dosage, affects alcohol addiction. Shock therapy in alcoholism has been recommended on the nonspecific ground that, as one British practitioner put it a few years ago, it provides a knockout that leaves the alcoholic patient "helpless and completely dependent physically and mentally on those around him" — *i.e.*, deprived of all defenses. Demonstrations that small doses of insulin shorten the withdrawal period (Vassaf and Hall, Ring Sanatorium and Hospital, Arlington, Massachusetts, 1946; Thimann and Peltason, Washingtonian Hospital, 1947) are not directed to habituation. Of interest in the whole discussion of hormone therapy in alcoholism is the philosophy expressed, 1951, by K. R. Beutner, "psychotherapy produces the desirable changes in endocrine imbalance more permanently than the administration of hormones can".

## SUBSTANCES AND PROCEDURES AIMED AT CREATING AVERSION

So long ago as 1785, Benjamin Rush observed that therapeutic use of the psychological principle of association was as old as the attempt of Moses to compel the children of Israel to drink a water solution of the Golden Calf which they had idolized. From this it is not a very far cry to the device of putting tartar emetic in a drinker's rum.

Myerson, 1944, described as logical and feasible creation of "a conditioned distaste for any chemical habit with a view to reversing it", but he added that the most successful method of carrying out the idea, sound in itself, may not have been achieved. Many hospitals, clinics, sanitariums now administer such substances as emetine hydrochloride, apomorphine, on the theory that the marked vomiting and nausea that follow intake of alcohol create a conditioned aversion to the sight, smell and especially to the taste of alcohol. The treatment breaks the alcoholic cycle and helps "through the first difficult period of surrendering drink as a way of life". The induced loathing wears off in time and the treatment may have to be repeated. Thimann, 1949, noted that, as in any other therapy, "but more so", the conditioned-reflex procedure should be supplemented by dynamic psychotherapy to reduce feelings of inadequacy and guilt. A report, by Lemere and Voegtlin, 1950, covering a follow-up of 4,096 patients treated (emetine) in the fourteen years from 1936 to 1950 showed that forty per cent remained totally abstinent; of those that relapsed 878 were retreated and of these thirty-nine per cent remained sober — an over-all abstinence rate of fifty-one per cent for thirteen years. Psychological factors considered to play a large part in the success of the treatment included: the understanding attitude of a staff encouraged to take into account the psychology of alcoholics; the cooperative attitude of patients who had voluntarily accepted the treatment, and who, in free and natural discussion of their common problems, influenced one another.

While little stress has been laid and little work done on metabolic mechanisms involved in "conditioning", more than an aversion reaction is claimed for apomorphine in a 1951 book by Harry Feldmann evaluating treatment of 150 patients (fifty-four per cent of whom relapsed). He suggested that apomorphine (as contrasted with emetine) acts directly on the "cause" of craving, exerts a profound effect on cerebral centers, specifically on the hypothalamus, and rapidly corrects the biochemical disturbances present in alcoholics. Biochemical data indicating toward the end of apomorphine treatment changes toward normal in blood (levels of urea, cholesterol, sugar, proteins, chloride, sodium), in urinary pH, in liver and kidney functions were considered evidence of central biochemical action.

TETRAETHYLTHIURAM DISULFIDE (TETD, DISULFIRAM, ANTABUSE)
FOR WHICH A METABOLIC ROLE IS CLAIMED

The Danish workers, Hald, Jacobsen and Larsen observed, 1948, that intake of alcohol after administration of tetraethylthiuram disulfide produced unpleasant and sometimes alarming symptoms (which might include, besides the usual nausea of conditioning drugs, vasomotor and cardiovascular effects resembling shock). These workers conceived the idea that some of the reactions between alcohol and disulfiram might be made to serve a therapeutic purpose in alcoholism. Clinical trial followed, accompanied by chemical and pharmacological studies on the symptoms expected to serve therapeutically, on unexpected side reactions and the dangers of some of these. By 1950 some 20,000 patients had been treated throughout Scandinavia, 11,000 in Denmark alone. Introduced into the United States at the suggestion of Glud in 1949, the drug was named disulfiram, 1952, by the Committee on International Pharmacopoeia of the World Health Organization to avoid confusion arising from differing proprietary names (antabus, antabuse, abstinyl, aversan, esperal, refusal) in various countries. Although in April, 1951, Oskar Diethelm described the use of disulfiram as "still in an experimental stage", in October of that year disulfiram was approved by the United States government for sale on a physician's prescription.

The complete mechanism of the metabolic interaction of disulfiram and alcohol is still unknown and still under study in various places. In 1949 Jacobsen and associates corrected their original conclusion that disulfiram caused increased formation of acetaldehyde from alcohol and suggested that accumulation of acetaldehyde in the blood of disulfiram-treated animals and man results from inhibition of the oxidation of acetaldehyde to acetic acid. Himwich referred, 1954, to additional evidence of the possibility that TETD attacks the enzyme concerned with oxidation of acetaldehyde to acetic acid. That oxidation may proceed by several alternate paths — involving one or more of various enzymes, xanthine oxidase, acetaldehyde oxidase, the carboxylase mechanism. In normal metabolism, the first step concerned with formation of acetaldehyde is slowest. But TETD renders slowest the second step of alcohol metabolism, oxidation of acetaldehyde to acetic acid. Disappearance of acetaldehyde was shown to be activated by acetaldehyde oxidases, one of which was purified by S. Black, 1950. Jacobsen, 1950, and Graham, 1951, reported *in vitro* experiments in which disulfiram inhibited acetaldehyde oxidases. Other evidence of the inhibiting action of disulfiram on oxidizing enzymes includes a 1949 report from T. P. Edwards of the Texas biochemical institute (studying the metabolism of the drug in liver homogenates) that its breakdown releases cyanide groups from the thiuram nucleus which act as inhibitors of oxidizing enzymes. In the liver preparation disulfiram inhibited the oxygen uptake by eighty-five per cent. Edwards concluded that, since only twenty per cent of the drug is excreted from the body unchanged, toxic breakdown products must interfere with cellular respiration, an effect observed *in vivo* without ingestion of alcohol and without increase of acetaldehyde. Suppression of this inhibition *in vitro* by ascorbic acid was reported by Niblo, Nowinski and Roark, 1951 (neuropsychiatry department and tissue culture laboratory, University of Texas, and the state psychopathic hospital), and intravenous ascorbic acid was found to exert a favorable effect upon the subjective symptoms of the disulfiram-alcohol reaction in patients (headache, palpitation, apprehension, weakness), possibly related to tissue anoxia. That the activity of ascorbic acid in these reactions may possibly be related to the observation of Forbes and Duncan, 1952, that alcohol in intoxicating doses rapidly depletes the ascorbic acid and cholesterol content of the guinea pig adrenal was suggested by G. P. Child (pharmacology, Albany), 1952.

Clinical observations have contributed to the present trend away from attributing the disulfiram-alcohol reaction exclusively to concentration of acetaldehyde in the blood. Bowman and his associates found, 1951, the intensity of the reaction and the time of its development not always related to concentration of acetaldehyde in the blood. Progressive increase in intensity of the reaction after repeated test doses of disulfiram and alcohol, observed by a number of clinical workers, has suggested also that the reaction is more complex than simple accumulation of acetaldehyde and is possibly a toxic reaction to the drug.

A hypothetical mechanism in the disulfiram-alcohol reaction was outlined by Jens A. Christensen (pharmacology department, Hahne-mann), 1951. Recalling earlier experiments by Nelson, 1943, and Koppanyi, 1945, indicating that acetaldehyde is a potent sympathomi-metic drug, he concluded from his experiments that disulfiram alters "the response of specific sympathomimetic receptor cells" to the action of acetaldehyde. There are other speculations as to the mechanism of the alcohol-disulfiram reaction.

Discussion of dangers and complications in disulfiram treatment suggests that the gravest are possible cardiovascular effects and psychosis. The danger of disulfiram treatment in patients with signs of myocardial deficiency or coronary disease has been stressed. That the cardiovascular hazard may not be limited to patients with dis-cernible cardiovascular defect is indicated by a 1951 report from Mack-lin, Sokolow, Simon and Schottstaedt, describing cardiovascular com-plications in sixteen of eighty-two patients under disulfiram treatment, all relatively young and all with "apparently normal cardiovascular systems prior to treatment". Feldman and Zucker, who considered the whole matter of contraindications to disulfiram treatment "over-inflated", observed, 1953: "Coronary artery disease and severe hyper-tension, as mentioned, are contraindications to test reactions, but experience shows they are not contraindications to treatment in a person stable enough to be informed of the dangers of possible reac-tions." Himwich considered, 1954, the profound effects of disulfiram on the cardiovascular system "a contraindication against its use in patients with coronary disease and with hypertension".

Since Martensen-Larsen reported, 1951, six cases suggesting that disulfiram (possibly because of unnecessarily high dosage) might prove a psychosis-provoking agent, other reports on this point have been published. Feldman and Zucker, 1953, regarded psychosis as the only real danger, finding "no absolute contraindications except a personality clearly on the borderline of overt psychosis". Bowman and associates attributed, 1951, "definite psychotic reactions in ten patients" in a series of a hundred "to withdrawal of the crutch alcohol and not to toxic effects" of the drug. Strecker and Lathbury, 1952, attributed complete personality disintegration in two cases to the un-controllable conflict that followed inability to tolerate the accustomed sedation. Inability to handle mounting anxiety that occurs with withdrawal of alcohol was cited by Gottesfeld and his coworkers, 1951, as possibly explaining psychotic sequelae in eight out of forty-two cases treated with disulfiram.   Dale and Ebaugh, 1951, considered that patients in whom alcoholism is a symptom of an underlying major psychosis do poorly under disulfiram.   Bennett, McKeever and Turk, 1951, in reporting transient psychotic reactions (which subsided with cessation of treatment), posed the question whether the drug might interfere with oxygen consumption in nervous tissue.   They also suggested that disulfiram might release pre-existing personality difficulties that had led to alcoholism.   The psychotic reactions following disulfiram therapy did not, however, seem to them to resemble the psychopathology of alcoholism.   Himwich's view, 1954, was that "with small daily doses of disulfiram psychotic reactions are rare".

Present evaluations of disulfiram and the extent of danger in its use are tentative.   Commenting on reports of deaths resulting from treatment, Jacobsen, 1952, observed that no one of the seventeen fatal cases among the eleven thousand alcoholics treated in Denmark between September, 1948, and June, 1951, "could with certainty be attributed to the effect of disulfiram alone".   Martin C. Becker and Gilbert Sugarman, commenting, 1952, on a death (apparently the first reported in this country) following intake of alcohol after disulfiram, suggested that while short-term studies of disulfiram treatment appear promising, complications of so grave a nature made long-term studies essential.   Meanwhile, "it seems timely to temper the current trend of enthusiasm".   As in the case of other therapies, the success of disulfiram is referable in part to psychiatric adjuvants.   Bowman, 1952, while conceding "a definite place for antabuse in treatment of chronic alcoholism", expressed the view that securing lasting results from it would require also individualized psychotherapy, a point stressed in the earliest statements of the Danish workers.

## PSYCHOTHERAPY IN ALCOHOLISM

All the resources and techniques of psychiatry are implicated in the psychotherapy of chronic alcoholics, and all the devices that have ever been developed for dealing with mental illness and disturbed behavior. In noting that "altered behavior" is the essence of the problem of alcoholism, Selden D. Bacon, of the Yale center, in a ten-year review of research on various aspects of alcoholism, observed, 1952, "the outstanding characteristic of psychological studies concerning alcohol or alcoholics is their relative absence in a field otherwise marked by prolific publication". Giorgio Lolli, medical director of the Yale Plan Clinic, pointed out that besides being an addict the chronic alcoholic "usually suffers from other neurotic or psychotic reaction patterns", and interruption of the drinking pattern is achieved only when the emotional energies tied to these conditions are liberated and mobilized to keep in check the addictive urge to drink. Even when total and permanent abstinence, the stated goal of almost every therapist in the field of alcoholism, is achieved, "the condition is not cured but only arrested". The neurotic or psychoneurotic complications, the personality, emotional, behavioral, social maladjustments of the alcoholic (factors only indirectly related to addiction) must also be dealt with; the alcoholic can remain abstinent only as the outcome of favorable readjustments of these.

Programs of treatment and re-education range from lectures and talks to all the resources of individual psychotherapy; they are contributed by hospitals and clinics, churches and religious agencies, various voluntary social agencies, by psychiatrically oriented social workers, nurses, physicians, by clinical psychologists and trained psychiatrists. Leaders among these stress the point that success of treatment depends upon the patient's inner understanding of the need for help and some desire to obtain it.

Many hold, as Lolli does, that while orthodox psychoanalytic techniques are not adapted to treatment of alcoholism, "psychoanalytically oriented abridged forms of therapy" are useful. Orthodox psychoanalysis besides being expensive (in time and money) is often not applicable to alcoholics, he pointed out, because of their constitutional instability and low tolerance of stress, which become acute when painful subconscious material is brought to the surface, resulting in relapse. He considered psychoanalytically oriented approaches as "offering the greatest promise of success". The approach and successes of Alcoholics Anonymous are, in his view, to be "interpreted on the basis of widely accepted psychodynamic principles".

PSYCHIATRIC USE OF THE GROUP PRINCIPLE OR SOCIAL APPROACH

The need to provide therapy for alcoholics outside the hospital and outside the boundaries of traditional psychotherapy, the prohibitive cost of individual psychotherapeutic treatment and the limited number of competent psychiatrists have all been factors in attempts to apply to alcoholism the principle of group psychotherapy. Identification with a social group is regarded as one approach to personality adjustment and social communication. The application to alcoholism of group therapy grew out of group psychotherapy techniques developed for other purposes by the armed forces during the second world war. By 1953, some form of group therapy was being employed in most of the more than twenty state-supported treatment programs and in many private facilities for treating alcoholics. According to Raymond McCarthy (director, alcoholism research, Mental Health Commission of New York State), who applied group therapy for a number of years in the Yale Plan Clinics, it is designed, under the leadership of a therapist who serves as a key figure and catalyst, to release emotional blocking and to induce in alcoholics a certain emotional shift, particularly in regard to interpersonal relationships. A 1946 report noted that in the preceding two years four different groups of male alcoholics from thirty-five to fifty years of age had met weekly at the clinic for spirited informal discussion of a topic presented by the group leader. In these meetings, emphasis seemed to be on intellectualization of the common problem of alcoholism and development of a more objective attitude toward it. However, group therapy that remains at the level of intellectualization is relatively ineffective since at this level "it is unlikely that any deep emotional shift among patients can be anticipated" (McCarthy, 1953). Group therapy is described as "not a substitute for individual therapy" but rather a supplement to it. Its techniques are still in the experimental stage: up to 1953 no systematic research had determined exactly what happens in group therapy sessions; "when such data becomes available it may be possible to refine the technique so that it will reach more patients".

A less formal application of the principles of group therapy inspires the program of Alcoholics Anonymous. Through it many alcoholics apparently achieve reduction of their difficulties through sharing of

guilt, through objective acceptance. In aiming at objective understanding of the problem, Alcoholics Anonymous relies for grace to
persevere not only on an extrahuman Power but also on the support,
spiritual and practical, of fellow members. It is true that one of the
organization's stated principles, "the socializing impact of group
participation", may not (McCarthy) be effective with those individuals who for any of a dozen possible reasons may have especial
difficulty in merging with the group pattern.

OTHER ASPECTS OF ALCOHOLICS ANONYMOUS

First formed in 1935 and by 1939 numbering only a hundred members, Alcoholics Anonymous claimed by 1950 a total of 3,500 groups
comprising 100,000 well-recovered members, a rate of about 2,000 additions each month, branches in thirty foreign countries. The key
principle of Alcoholics Anonymous, that the organization can be useful
only to those that genuinely want to stop drinking, explains both
the success and the limitation of the therapy. Of those that want its
help, according to a 1949 report, fifty per cent become sober at once,
twenty-five per cent have relapses but improve. The degree of deterioration, physical, neurological or psychic, is naturally an important
factor in the individual's capacity to be helped, and in the amount of
time required to help him. One of the twelve principles that constitute the A.A.'s tradition or "program of recovery" prescribes that
A.A. groups should be supported not by dues but by the members'
voluntary contributions. Among the other eleven principles of this
"tradition" are a provision that A.A. groups should never go into business, should remain "forever nonprofessional", should have a
minimum of organization, should maintain personal anonymity, etc.
The principle of anonymity is considered to have "immense spiritual
significance".

Groups of Alcoholics Anonymous have arrangements with local
hospitals for accepting promising patients. In 1945, the first year of a
cooperative arrangement, a thousand patients were referred by Alcoholics Anonymous for care to the Knickerbocker Hospital in New York.
The patient is placed under the care of two physicians, one of whom
takes over the medical treatment, the other of whom "looks after the

alcoholic and psychological aspects of the case". The minimum stay is five days. Alcoholics Anonymous secures the hospital against loss by guaranteeing the use of a certain number of beds at a nominal fee. A.A. makes the request for admission, signs out the patient, provides the hospital with regular shifts of nontechnical help (A.A. members). Certain classes of alcoholics ("good material") are sent to Rockland State Hospital with a court certification for a period of sixty days. "In many instances substantial results are accomplished during the brief period . . ."

To the frequently raised question as to whether the animating impulse of the organization is religious, representatives of the organization have replied: "If admitting that neither we ourselves nor any human relationship nor agency has been able to help us so far as the drinking problem is concerned and that we are desperately in need of help from somewhere, and are willing to accept it, if it can be found — if that is religion — the answer is, yes." The A.A., as C. Nelson Davis once expressed it, utilizes "spiritual power freed from the restrictions of organized religion, urging the acceptance of God (or a higher Power) and leaving the individual to form his own conception of that God or Power". Tiebout expressed the view that attempts to use the Alcoholics Anonymous program "without the God angle" have failed.

CHAPTER 10

# The Biology of Schizophrenia

*Illustrating interaction of physiological,
psychological and social factors*

It should be said at the outset that any objective and comprehensive picture of investigative work in schizophrenia is bound to suggest, at this time, a state of disorganization. Schizophrenia (as will appear hereafter) is still far from being a uniformly defined entity. Investigative approaches to it (neurophysiological, electrophysiological, biochemical, psychological, social) are still so disparate, so far from correlations, that work in any of them must be discussed rather with reference to ultimate objectives than to present achievements. In this period of transition, psychiatry itself is, as Ralph Gerard once put it, "unhappily schizophrenic, rooted in biological science and the body, and fruiting in social science and the nuances of human interaction". The aim in this brief review is simply to suggest the breadth and depth of the investigative field involved in study of schizophrenia, and the main disciplines concerned in reaching — ultimately — correlations between mind and brain, nervous function and behavior, between physiologic, electrical and metabolic activity, and the psychological manifestations of mental illness.

Among all the uncertainties, it seems to be entirely clear that schizophrenia is a number one riddle among mental illnesses and that there are many reasons for including it in the illustrative group of medicine's outstanding unsolved problems discussed in this volume. It is freely admitted that schizophrenia accounts for nearly half of all mental hospital patients, although hospital data, as will appear hereafter, convey only incompletely even the statistical story of schizophrenia.

## ADVANCING PUBLIC CONCERN WITH MENTAL ILLNESS GENERALLY

A necessary backdrop in considering the present outlook for research on schizophrenia is a changing public and governmental attitude toward mental illness and toward research aimed at discovering means of curing and preventing it. Few miracles have been wrought and it will take many years and much work to perfect and extend even the therapeutic goals now conservatively envisaged. The national mental health week of 1955 was ushered in by ringing a great bell cast from chains once used to restrain mental patients. The physical chains are gone; but hundreds of thousands of mental patients are still enchained by inertia and deterioration in institutions equipped for custody (and overcrowded even for that) but not for therapy (even the simplest occupational therapy).

It is something — it is a great deal — that the problem is under national review. In 1955, on the basis of Senate and House committee reports advocating the end of "mental pest houses where patients are confined indefinitely with slight hope of cure", Congress, without a dissenting vote, passed a mental health study act providing for a three-year survey to inform the government and the country on all aspects of mental illness. The act authorized an appropriation of $1,250,000 for the three years; $250,000 has been appropriated for the first year. In some enlightened quarters at least, the whole concept of the mental hospital as the main dependence for dealing with the mentally ill is under challenge. At hearings on the joint resolution, the chairman of the American Medical Association's Council on Mental Health expressed the view that there is "good reason to question fundamentally the concept of a mental hospital as the primary tool for treating the mentally ill". The American Psychiatric Association's medical director described the mental hospital as merely part of a network of community services designed to prevent hospitalization or at least to shorten it. The superintendent of St. Elizabeth's Hospital, certainly not an inexperienced witness, expressed, 1955, the view that in the first year in a mental hospital patients have a fifty-fifty chance of release; in two years, the odds against being released alive rise to sixteen to one and by the time a patient has been hospitalized for eight years the odds are more than ninety-nine to one.

Behind these governmental and professional recognitions is a public increasingly conscious of the degree to which mental illness enters into the social and economic problems of the day. On the one hand there is steadily advancing interest in the neuroses and psychoses of childhood. On the other hand the increased span of life (in one sense a medical triumph) has meant more mental illness among the higher age groups, whether in the form of cerebral arterial degeneration or of the psychological depression and aberration that result from the extreme loneliness and isolation which is the lot of many of the aged. It will avail us little, a Hoover commission task force pointed out, 1955, to increase the life span by the miracles of modern medicine "if we are to end ingloriously with the senile psychoses".

Accelerated public interest in the mental field is reflected in many other ways: in the trend toward establishing mental health clinics in general hospitals; in according new status to psychiatry in the medical schools, converting what was once relegated to Saturday afternoon sessions in the fourth year to a discipline given place in each of the four years; in increasingly numerous organizations — international, national and local — reflecting the public concern. Expressions of it at the international level include the World Federation for Mental Health, with thirty-seven member nations which sponsored the international congress on mental health in Toronto in 1954; the World Medical Association which stressed psychological medicine at its conference on undergraduate education in London in 1953; a mental health section in the World Health Organization although its activities are, as yet, planned on a modest scale and involve less than one per cent of the total annual income available to the organization from all sources. "Thirty times as much", the *London Times* commented, "is spent on the control of communicable diseases."

In this country, the federal government recognized the dimensions of the problem by the National Mental Health Act of 1946, providing for the establishment, 1949, of the National Institute of Mental Health, with a comprehensive program including federal research grants to investigators in the universities. Since its establishment, according to the federal secretary of health, education and welfare, 1954, twenty-nine states and territories have initiated mental health programs and twenty-four states have extended their programs; local and state funds for mental health activities increased from 2.5 millions in 1948 to 12.4 millions in 1954. Some states are establishing research programs and building new research institutes with funds provided by patients' families. In Illinois alone, current funds for these purposes are reported to be about $5,000,000. At the governors' conference in 1954, administration of mental hospitals was described as the greatest single problem of the states, often representing the largest item in the annual expenditure.

Among voluntary organizations, the National Association for Mental Health was established in 1950, merging the National Committee for Mental Hygiene (established 1904), the National Mental Health Foundation and the Psychiatric Foundation. In May, 1955, there were forty-four state mental health associations (twenty-nine of them associated with the national) and 425 local associations. The association's 1954 campaign raised about $1,000,000, seventy-five per cent of which was retained by the state and local associations. Most of the association's research expenditures to date have been in the field of schizophrenia; its largest grant was from the Masons' organization which during the past twenty-one years has given the association more than a million for this purpose.

Other national organizations with particular interest in mental health include the American Psychiatric Association, which with the American Medical Association has formed a joint commission on mental illness and health, including representatives of sixteen organizations. Other organizations included in the commission's planning are the American Association of Psychiatric Clinics for Children, the American Hospital Association, the American Psychological Association, the Social Science Research Council, the Group for the Advancement of Psychiatry, the American Orthopsychiatric Society, the American Group Therapy Association, the American Association of Psychiatric Social Workers, the Commission on Religion and Health of the Federal Council of Churches of Christ in America; also certain national organizations dealing with especial aspects of the mental health problem as the American Association on Mental Deficiency; the National Epilepsy League and the American branch of the International League Against Epilepsy; the National Committee on Alcohol Hygiene, the National Committee on Alcoholism, the National States' Conference on Alcoholism and Alcoholics Anonymous.

Foundation interest in behavioral problems is illustrated by the Rockefeller Foundation's concentration of interest in the field over many years, and by activity, in this area, of the Commonwealth Fund, the Milbank Memorial Fund and, more recently, the Ford Foundation which in 1955 allocated $15,000,000 to strengthen and extend research in mental health over the next five to ten years. The foundation had reached the conclusion that at present the most effective opportunity for service in this field lay in emphasizing research aimed at determining the causes of mental illness and developing and testing effective methods of treatment and prevention.

In spite of the organization of public sentiment, present accomplishment in control and prevention of mental illness, and in research into its causes and its therapy shows up dimly against the picture of present needs. A summary, 1954, by Kenneth E. Appel, president of the American Psychiatric Association, showed that 37,000 patients in twenty-nine public mental hospitals had no psychiatric treatment whatever, that twenty to thirty per cent overcrowding in seventy per cent of the country's hospitals left little opportunity for constructive treatment programs, and that, if hospitals were to include treatment and not merely custody, 15,000 more psychiatrists would be needed. Federal figures for 1953 indicated that the average state hospital still spends no more than about $2.50 a day to cover maintenance and treatment for each patient. Quite aside from the fundamental questions (for the future) as to whether mental hospitals are to be the main dependence in dealing with the mentally ill, and aside also from the question whether current therapies (various forms of shock, "psychosurgery", experimental drugs) are the best present hope, it remains true that these procedures — since they involve certain hazards — require hospitalization and that hospital facilities presently available do not permit wide application of even remedies considered by some to have possibilities. Not a single state mental hospital meets, as yet, the personnel standards defined by the American Psychiatric Association: the average state mental hospital is understaffed about forty per cent in physicians, seventy-six per cent in clinical psychologists; it is also understaffed in registered nurses, hospital attendants, psychiatric social workers. These figures do not take into account the additional personnel that would be required to provide intensive individual or group psychotherapy, generally regarded as an imperative concomitant for all other forms of therapy.

## THE EXTENT OF THE PARTICULAR PROBLEM OF SCHIZOPHRENIA

Statistics on the extent of schizophrenia should certainly be prefaced by admission that all figures on a condition that is far from being a uniformly defined clinical entity, diagnosable by definite criteria, must remain, in a degree, suspect. Profound workers in the field have repeatedly stressed the multiple nature of both the causes and the manifestations of schizophrenia. In some views, the usefulness of the term schizophrenia as a diagnostic label "has reached a nearly farcical stage". Hudson Hoagland (director, Worcester Foundation for Experimental Biology) once observed, in recommending removal of schizophrenia to the symptom class: "I do not consider schizophrenia a more specific term than headache." It lacks (Nathan S. Kline, director of research, Rockland State Hospital, 1953) "even one operationally discriminating attribute".

This perspective is needed for the statement, previously cited, from the National Institute of Mental Health, 1954, that approximately fifty per cent of the half million patients resident in the state hospitals of the country suffer from schizophrenia; some of these are admitted in early youth and "stay in for the rest of their lives". The total picture, moreover, is not, as previously suggested, conveyed by hospital data. Such figures do not take into account the schizophrenic private patients of psychiatrists (a limited group); or the undefinable (but not limited) group on the list of practically every general practitioner, patients whose schizophrenic-like reactions continually impair response to treatment for other conditions; or the completely unregistered and undiagnosed schizophrenics not in any institution and under no psychiatric or medical care; or the borderline and mild cases, the "schizoids", more or less identifiable in any group of the population at any level. In sum, as William Malamud once observed, schizophrenia far from being limited to hospitals is "actually more prevalent outside of them".

## TRADITIONAL AND PRESENT CONCEPTS
## OF SCHIZOPHRENIA

If any conclusion emerges from the not too well founded arguments as to whether schizophrenia is dominantly attributable to disordered psyche or disordered soma, it is probably that, whether causes are primarily psychogenic or primarily somatic, "they are always both" (Bellak). The fact that definitions of schizophrenia tend to be in terms of psychology easily arises from the fact that whatever physiological, neurological, electrical and chemical mechanisms may be involved, the manifestations of schizophrenia are certainly psychological.

Just what the "split personality", etymologically conveyed in the term schizophrenia, is now meant to include may be dubious, but the stress upon fission is not too far out of line with current definitions emphasizing the schizophrenic's dissociation of emotion from experience, withdrawal from the world around him, break with reality. The battling over definitions of schizophrenia has been going on since the concept was created by Kraepelin in 1898. Of possible causal factors, forty separate categories have been mentioned — variously assigned to genetic, anatomical, neurophysiological, biochemical, endocrine, infectious, psychological, social and other areas.

One way of reconciling the competing etiological influences has been to envisage not one schizophrenia but a number (*die schizo-phrenien*, Eugen Bleuler, 1911), connoting multiple causes and multiple manifestations, in curious and confusing combinations. Bleuler himself described subdivision of the *"schizophrenien"* as "a task for the future". It is still so relegated: F. C. Redlich (psychiatry, Yale) expressed, 1952, merely the hope that as more is known of the etiology of schizophrenia, more specific classifications of the different conditions now thus inclusively grouped under that name may be possible. One current view, expressed by L. J. Meduna (Neuropsychiatric Institute, University of Illinois), 1953, to the American Foundation, considered it possible now to "hypothetically differentiate" other forms of schizophrenia from "true schizophrenia produced by heredity". Some would reserve dementia praecox, still often used as synonymous with schizophrenia, for the more constitutionally determined cases, leaving schizophrenia to describe "presumably psychogenic cases whose course is often more benign" (Robert P. Knight, psychiatry, Yale, 1952).

Manfred Sakel stressed, 1954, the importance of distinguishing between "badly moulded" people with a psychological personality distortion and people whose deformation is the result of a biochemical and organic dysfunction. So long as the nature of the structural damage and the origin of the biochemical and organic dysfunction assumed to characterize schizophrenia are not clear, some workers find it difficult to postulate the clear distinction described by Sakel. Even on the psychological level, definitive differentiation between schizophrenia and the neuroses has been a knotty problem for clinicians. Some of the efforts to point out essential differences between the conditions seem to end by stressing likenesses, or by citing the possibility of neuroses that "border on" schizophrenia or of coexistence of neurosis and schizophrenia in the same person. Otto Fenichel, while observing, 1945, "it certainly is not true that psychoses represent a kind of higher degree of neuroses", nevertheless envisaged "certain neurotic persons who without developing a complete psychosis . . . have a readiness to employ certain schizophrenic mechanisms whenever frustrations occur". They have not broken with reality but they give signs of breaking.

## ROLE OF HEREDITY IN CONCEPTS OF SCHIZOPHRENIA

That the tendency to schizophrenia is inborn was referred to by Winfred Overholser of St. Elizabeth's Hospital (at the 1954 annual meeting of the National Association for Mental Health) as now definitely known. Many workers without regard to whether they are dominantly committed to a physiological or to a psychological or a social and environmental approach (L. J. Meduna, I. A. Mirsky, Franz Alexander, Karl M. Bowman, W. C. Menninger, F. C. Redlich, Edwin F. Gildea, Frieda Fromm-Reichmann, L. S. Penrose, E. T. O. Slater, Derek Richter and others) have expressed agreement on the role of heredity in schizophrenia postulated by Bleuler in 1911.

The genetic vulnerability of schizophrenics could, in the view of Franz J. Kallmann (New York State Psychiatric Institute), be described "psychodynamically" as the individual's inability to be a part of the *milieu* in which he lives. Kallmann pointed out, 1952, that "no analysis of a statistically representative group of blood relatives of schizophrenic or manic-depressive patients has so far been completed in any country without showing a significant increase in the expectancy rate for either psychosis". While the expectancy of schizophrenia in the general population is not lower than 0.7 and not higher than 0.9 per cent, the expectancy rate for relatives of schizophrenics, by Kallmann's findings, varies from 7.1 per cent for half-sibs, through about fourteen per cent for full sibs and two-egg co-twins, to 86.2 per cent for one-egg twin partners. Between 1938, the date of his volume on the genetics of schizophrenia, and 1952, Kallmann had studied 1,250 twin family units with four types of psychoses, including 953 schizophrenic twin index families. The twin studies made by him and by Rosanoff in the United States and also by various workers in Germany showed, as a universal finding, that from sixty to eighty per cent or more of the uniovular twins of schizophrenics themselves become schizophrenic.  E. T. O. Slater (Institute of Psychiatry, Maudsley Hospital, 1953) observed: "That is very nearly conclusive about the significance of the hereditary factor."

Less conclusive have been various opinions on the nature of the gene factors involved.  Differences of opinion have been concerned not with the existence of vulnerability which is widely accepted but rather with just what it is that is inherited.  According to Julian Huxley, 1951, the genetic mechanism cannot transmit mental experience nor any result of mental experience, but merely the capacity for having a certain kind of experience, including in some animals the capacity for learning by experience.  It is a purely material mechanism and accordingly "cannot be either operated or transformed except by the tedious, difficult and often wasteful material process of selection, natural or artificial".  Kallmann considered, 1954, that the basic dysfunction in the etiology of schizophrenia, the "diverse inadequacies in the adaptive capacity of potentially vulnerable persons", could be best explained by "a recessive unit factor which produces the specific potentials of disordered behavior patterns by a metabolic disturbance in the enzymatic range".  Referring to Kallmann's work, Slater regarded as "still much in dispute" the question whether there are "many different genes responsible for schizophrenic psychoses, or perhaps only one and whether recessivity or dominance is the rule".

The possibility of establishing the nature of the constitutional vulnerability (in schizophrenia) eventually in terms of biochemistry has been of increasing investigative concern.  The present evidence seems to Gerard to "speak strongly for heavy weighting of an inherited biochemical aberration as a dominant factor in the causation of schizophrenia.  Indeed, it deserves thought that the psychoses — notably schizophrenia and cyclothymia — may be primarily disturbances of the units of the nervous system, biochemical in nature and genetically carried; while the neuroses may be primarily disturbances in the patterns of function and interconnections of the neurone units, weighted on the physiological rather than the chemical, and resulting more from unfortunate relations of the individual to his environment than to his ancestors".  Mention was made just above of Kallmann's reference to the possible genetic significance of "metabolic disturbance in the enzymatic range".  In a communication to the American

Foundation, 1953, he described "biochemical identification of the basic disturbance produced by the mutant schizophrenia gene and of the alternative integrative function depending on the action of its normal allele" as a "prerequisite" to further progress in genetic research on schizophrenia. Richter, referring to biochemical tests that have now been found for detecting a number of the genes in man, stressed the prophylactic importance of "identifying heterozygotic and unexpressed homozygotic carriers of the genes predisposing to schizophrenia". The work on phenylketonuria, he thought, illustrated the way in which the genetic approach could be aided by development of a simple chemical test. He conceded that in the schizophrenias we have probably to deal with something a good deal more complex than phenylketonuria but added that R. Gjessing's observation of nitrogen retention as a metabolic defect in periodic catatonia encouraged the belief that biochemical methods might some day be useful in the genetic approach to schizophrenia and hence in prophylaxis of it. He did not underestimate the difficulty of identifying predisposing and inhibiting chemical factors.

On the practical question whether emphasis on genetic predisposition invalidates psychological concepts of schizophrenia and is incompatible with belief in its curability, there are differing views. Slater, 1950, attributed lack of adequate appreciation of the heredity concept in general psychiatry partly to the fact that this concept "has run counter to psychodynamic trends derived from the advancement and increasing popularity of psychoanalysis". Jan A. Böök (medical genetics, University of Lund), 1952, found "no conflict between a genetic theory and the idea that psychologic and other factors may precipitate or impair the symptomatology of psychoses, appearing in persons having a specific genotype". Malamud stressed the power of environment to modify the "aggregate of hereditary characteristics" in schizophrenia. Ralph W. Gerard (Neuropsychiatric Institute, University of Illinois) deplored, 1952, the "artificial dichotomy" between heredity and environment.

Discussing the "heredity-environment fallacy" before the American Society of Human Genetics, its president, Laurence H. Snyder, commented, 1950, on the fear of the psychologist or sociologist that attitudes could not be changed "if there were any genetic basis for the original development of individual differences in behavior". According to Snyder, while science does not prove that differences in knowledge, customs and personality are not transmitted biologically, "there is little scientific evidence either way on the possible genetic basis for personality". In his view, certainly "the genes and their accompanying cytoplasm do not alone make a man or woman. There is always an environment in which the individual develops, although the relative effects of differences in gene substitutions and differences in environmental forces will vary from trait to trait . . . If the anthropologist, the psychologist, the sociologist and the geneticist are to join forces in the genetic analysis of racial traits which are significant in the level of intelligence, personality and social behavior, the implications of multifactorial inheritance must be carefully studied."

## The Age Factor in Concepts of Schizophrenia

Those whose view is oriented by genetic concepts of schizophrenia think the importance of the age factor inheres in the time at which trigger mechanisms become operative. While various workers have pointed out that the characteristic schizophrenic symptoms are by no means always manifest at an early age, schizophrenia has been traditionally regarded as a particular problem of adolescence, and the young schizophrenic as "stranded on the rock of puberty". Physiologists emphasize the stresses and strains of physiologic development at that time and the possibility of pathological maturation. Psychodynamists are less concerned with the physiologic changes than with adolescence as, psychologically, a crucial period of development. Schizophrenic breakdown at that time is attributed to "failure of personality organization under the increasing demands of society for independence and productive functioning" associated with early adult years (Knight, 1952).

Stress on adolescence is less significant in the concepts of some schools than stress on much earlier experience, whether of soma or of psyche. Some of the hypotheses stressing the significance of early years go back to prenatal influence. Current research in the United States, testing the hypothesis that prenatal influence in terms of obstetrical complications is correlated with a child's postnatal behavior, was mentioned, 1954, at the fifth international congress on mental health at the University of Toronto (Paul V. Lemkau, Johns Hopkins). The significance of developmental influences in neurophysiological functioning was touched upon in studies described, 1952, to the conference on biological aspects of mental health and disease, illustrated by embryological studies of the fetal cerebral cortex conducted since 1941 at the Carnegie Institution of Washington (J. B. Flexner, V. B. Peters, L. B. Flexner). Brosin referred to the importance attached by Lashley and Thorndike to chemical embryological factors in efforts to elucidate the characteristics of the immature brain. "After fifty years of investigation", Brosin observed, "we know that we must get back more and more to the earliest years of the patient's life. The potentiality for schizophrenia . . . seems to be established at that time . . ." Less literal acceptance of the determining effect of early childhood experience was suggested, in one of the 1953 Salmon lectures, by the late Ralph Linton (anthropology, Yale): "Recent research seems to indicate that the predominant role assigned to infantile experiences by certain schools of psychoanalysis is not supported by the evidence." Nursing patterns, toilet training, etc., seem to be much less significant as personality determinants than was formerly supposed.

Donald O. Hebb (psychology, McGill University) and his group have given particular attention to the way in which early experience provides thinking animals with the mechanisms which are later integrated into perception, concepts and general intelligence. Most of the outstanding psychological manifestations of the schizophrenic — his lack of capacity for abstraction, his break with reality, his loss of faculty for communication, his emotional withdrawal, disintegration of his ego — have been, by various workers, quite directly related to childhood. Kurt Goldstein (1953) attributed lack of capacity for abstraction in schizophrenia to "development of anxiety in the early period of childhood". To emotional deprivation during infancy has been attributed incapacity to achieve full maturity, forcing the individual under the traumata of life to "regress to an infantile or partially infantile emotional level" (Malcolm L. Hayward, Institute of the Pennsylvania Hospital, 1953). The breakdown in faculty for communication which characterizes the schizophrenic has been attributed (Jurgen Ruesch, psychiatry, University of California, 1953) to inability to learn in early childhood the necessary means of efficient communication with others.

## ASSOCIATION OF PSYCHOLOGICAL, PHYSIOLOGICAL AND SOCIAL FACTORS IN CONCEPTS OF SCHIZOPHRENIA

Realization that a collection of symptoms, however enlightening, is a less and less satisfactory way of defining any illness is likely to follow any review of current definitions and concepts of schizophrenia such as those touched upon above. Certainly the congeries of psychological manifestations which bulk largest in attempted definitions of schizophrenia do not comprehensively define it. Even within the confines of psychology, these manifestations result rather in a mosaic than in an integrated psychological picture. Of the single stones in the mosaic some are of the greatest importance: Freud's recognition of the significance of unconscious processes, his emphasis on withdrawal from the world to a state of narcissism, and on sexual motivation; rejection of overemphasis on this motivation by Jung and Adler; Jung's stress on buried complexes; Kraepelin's theory concerning the schizophrenic's capacity to bring his intellect — which may remain intact for years — fully to bear upon a fantastic universe of his own; the theory stressed by a number of workers that the odd psychological characteristics of schizophrenia may be associated with "a relatively clear sensorium, a good memory and clear conception" (Bellak); Fenichel's observation that schizophrenic thinking is comparable to that found "in the unconscious of neurotics, in some children, in normal persons under conditions of fatigue and in primitive man".

The degree to which reliance has been placed upon psychological as contrasted with neurophysiological and biochemical definition of schizophrenia is easily explicable by the conventional trend — in academic as well as in lay circles — toward comprehending the whole field of mental health and illness in the term "psychiatry", the literal limited meaning of which is therapy for the (disordered) psyche. It does not connote neurophysiological and biochemical mechanisms, nor does it connote the mechanisms of normal psychology. It connotes, rather, therapeutically oriented studies of the abnormal psyche, of abnormal human behavior. Study of the abnormal psyche has been responsible for a vast amount of deduction, for many suggestive revelations and for even more hunches. It nevertheless represents an empirical working backward, the starting point being mental disease rather than the principles, mechanisms and organization of mental health. That study of the process in reverse sheds some light is not to be denied; but it can never be a substitute for approach through normal psychology and physiology. Psychiatry, moreover, has not yet developed a firm core of generally accepted basic knowledge because of the nature of its materials, which do not easily lend themselves to demonstrable verifiable experiment of the kind that has contributed to the advancement of physiology and chemistry.

Social factors have been well recognized in traditional definitions of schizophrenia though in fairly general terms: Adolf Meyer's "psychobiological" concept presented schizophrenic reactions as the outcome of maladaptation of the individual to his environment; J. C. Whitehorn (psychiatry, Johns Hopkins) stressed the schizophrenic's distrust of "the social facade so meticulously maintained by ordinary mortals". Recognition of the environment, the "society", upon which the individual organism is dependent takes the study of schizophrenia and of psychosis generally not only into the more or less charted fields of conventional sociology but also, inevitably, into anthropology, into the physical sciences that account for soil and climate, and for other factors in human ecology, into economics, history and other fields in the attempt to assess cultural influences and, indeed, the whole "civilization" which the individual organism reflects, and to which it must adjust.

The schizophrenic, in most definitions, is a dislocated unit who has withdrawn from the world around him, has suffered a breakdown of communication between him and the life of his day. Reducing the social aspects of the problem of psychosis to ultimate simplicity, William G. Lennox suggested, 1951, why "the study of the brain more than the study of any other organ of the body carries the student into the wide field of human relations". A disordered heart or kidney impairs the productivity of the individual, but "a disordered brain can disrupt a whole community or nation".

The breadth and complexity of the areas in which the causes of schizophrenia may lie sufficiently explain the lack of competent definitions of it. Among efforts to achieve more accurate definition by taking a "fresh look" at schizophrenia and to describe objectively characteristic traits — psychological, physiological, biochemical, sociological, etc. — are a ten-year project conducted at the Worcester State Hospital, Massachusetts, a program established, 1951, in a special research facility of the Rockland State Hospital, New York, a study just completed in the Michael Reese Hospital, under the direction of Samuel J. Beck (psychology laboratory) with a five-year grant from the National Institutes of Health. Participants in the last-named study, disclaiming, 1954, any intention either to confirm or to refute any existing concept of schizophrenia, proceeded to "describe the schizophrenic person, by operational trait data . . ." on reaction patterns. Any pattern emerging from this description was regarded as an hypothesis of schizophrenic behavior. "Six such patterns have so emerged which are therefore that many hypotheses . . ." One hundred and twenty "operational traits" were tabulated by these workers, according to frequency of appearance in their six schizophrenias.

## SOME OF THE OUTSTANDING CURRENT NEEDS IN RESEARCH ON SCHIZOPHRENIA

In projecting this chapter the American Foundation asked representative investigators of differing "schools" to suggest the current lines of work from which, in their view, light on schizophrenia could most hopefully be expected. The more profound of the replies, while freely admitting a given worker's preference for physiological (biochemical or neurophysiological) or for psychological emphasis, stressed the critical need of converging work from all these directions including the little-explored social influences in the current "civilization" that determine and/or modify the behavior of the individual. Those that had worked longest and delved most deeply in any one of the above fields tended most to stress the fundamental danger inherent in disconnected consideration of any one approach or exclusive preoccupation with emphasis upon any one of the three, physiological, psychological, social. The present reviewers feel that, in spite of the present gaps in knowledge and absence of correlations, leaders representing all these approaches do definitely look and work toward the day when, conjointly, they may arrive at more precise definitions of schizophrenia, better correlation of the interacting physiological, psychological and social factors involved in it, and development of less empirical methods of treating it.

Lack of ideas, of a fresh approach, rather than lack of money in schizophrenia research was stressed in many of the communications to the American Foundation. This is not to say that research funds in this field are adequate; high grade personnel and the finely devised techniques increasingly being developed for work on the nervous system are costly. The comparative lack of funds for research in mental illness has been well publicized: as in the 1953 statement of the National Association for Mental Health that they amount to only about $4.15 per patient as compared with $28.20 for poliomyelitis, $26.80 for tuberculosis, and $27.70 for cancer; as in the Magnuson report's note, 1951, that over the five-year period, 1946–1951, the nation's grants for mental health research were less than five per cent of grants and contracts for all types of medical research; as in the estimate at the first National Governors' Conference on Mental Health, 1954, that less than one per cent of total state mental health budgets is expended for research — four millions out of a total expenditure of about 560 millions.

A more hopeful financial note, so far as schizophrenia is concerned, was struck at the end of 1954 in a communication to the American Foundation from the National Institute of Mental Health that in the preceding seven and one-half years its research grants and fellowship branch had supported fifty-seven schizophrenia projects at a total cost of $1,965,176. In order to spur mental health research and assist in opening research careers to qualified young psychiatrists and scientists in related disciplines, the institute had announced, 1954, a new series of research grants designed to enable a limited number of qualified workers to devote from two to five years to full-time research.

It remains true that a dominant need is explicit formulation of problems in the field in order to determine where money could most productively be spent. A decade ago the National Research Council, in view of "intensified awareness of a need for better understanding of human behavior", requested a committee on "neurobiology" to survey the status of needs in all areas concerned with research on the nervous system. These areas included physiology, psychology, anatomy, histology, embryology, clinical neurology, psychiatry, neurosurgery and comparative biology. A report of the work of the committee was published (under Paul Weiss's chairmanship) in 1952. While this report, and much of the work discussed in the rest of this chapter, have no specific reference to schizophrenia, the present reviewers believe that any logical discussion of research bearing upon an entity so ill-defined as schizophrenia involves basic work in the whole field of neurobiology, comprehending the disciplines mentioned above. The orienting conviction of the National Research Council's committee was that research in all these disciplines related to the nervous system and ultimately to behavior had become highly departmentalized, reflecting lack of cross correlation and reflecting also reliance upon excessive superstructures of speculation, built upon narrow and often shaky foundations of fact. "Inconsistencies and incompatibilities within each field and among the various fields have provided us with a confused rather than unified concept of the nervous system, its construction, function, development and diseases."

The existing deficiencies, as the committee recognized at the beginning of its work, were of two kinds. The first of these was deficiency in fundamental knowledge. While in most of the disciplines, modern and promising methods and techniques were available, they were not, in the committee's view, being used to the best advantage. Only rudimentary knowledge was available of the finer structural anatomy, cytology, physical chemistry, chemical composition, physical structure, functional organization, developmental mechanisms and regenerative and adjustive powers of the nervous system. Almost unexplored "at least so far as systematic fundamental approach is concerned" were the mechanisms of drug action on the nervous system; differential chemical properties in relation to brain function; analysis of the development of behavior. While important advances were noted for each of these fields, these isolated achievements were described as "pathetically small islands in a vast sea of ignorance". During the past decade, more islands, sometimes chains of islands, have appeared on the face of the deep, but more content is needed in all the directions noted, more islands — and more connections with the mainland. With reference to the second present deficiency, lack of proper evaluation, correlation and integration of knowledge that is already available, the National Research Council's committee noted a more or less recent "healthy change for the better".

The American Foundation's recent correspondents in various divisions of the neurobiological field consistently stressed the need of integration and correlation — and the difficulty of achieving it. The very workers that have this goal most clearly in mind are also those that see most clearly the length and the turns in the road winding toward it. "I can't find any way", wrote George H. Bishop, 1953, "to correlate cortical physiology either with neurochemistry or with psychology. So far, these things just come in different packages; they don't dovetail. Somebody will have to do some repackaging. What kind of 'idea' can you relate to the electrical discharge pattern of cortex or to the oxidative or lipoid metabolism of the nerve cell?" Bishop himself put his finger on one of the many reasons for lack of progress in correlation of physiological and psychological phenomena, i.e. the rapid development, through new techniques, of present knowledge of physiologic mechanisms, swiftly making ancient good uncouth: "Four-fifths of the physiology postulated as the basis for behavior is likely to be soon revised" by rapid advances in knowledge, necessarily followed by revised perspectives and new hypotheses.

In spite of the undoubted fact that lines of physiological and psychological research seem to be at present parallel rather than converging, it is something that profound workers of differing predilection do orient their research philosophy on what seems to them the scientific necessity that the lines must converge. This philosophy animated such statements as that of Gerard, 1953, that it is "neither hopeless nor premature" to attempt to establish the link between neurophysiology and psychology; of Whitehorn, 1952, stressing the absolute necessity to work out "some mutually comprehensible *modus vivendi* between dynamic psychiatry and 'organic psychiatry' "; of Hebb, whose book aimed "to present a theory of behavior for the consideration of psychologists" and at the same time to show anatomists, physiologists and neurologists "how psychological theory relates to their problems" and how they may contribute to that theory. In happily pragmatic vein, a member of the psychoanalytic school observed, attributing the sentiment to Freud, "let the biologists go as far as they can and let us go as far as we can. Some day the two will meet." The error of positivism on either side was stressed, in a communication to the American Foundation, by I. Arthur Mirsky (director, department of clinical science, University of Pittsburgh School of Medicine, 1953): "The biochemist who insists that only a biochemical derangement initiates the syndrome is as biased as the psychoanalyst who insists that only some derangement in psychosexual development initiates the syndrome." The hopeful view that "the days of disparate schools and conflicting opinions dogmatically held are over" was set forth, 1953, by the chairman of the Mental Health Research Fund at its Oxford conference; he thought he discerned an overriding desire on the part of the specialist to "absorb as much of the other man's vision as he can".

One obvious obstacle to correlation is the insularity that results from highly specialized training. The limitation of an investigator's particular training may also limit his research field — and sometimes his point of view. Kurt Goldstein, 1953, (writing to the American Foundation) attributed his own dominant concern with psychological aspects not to belief that progress is to be expected from psychological rather than from chemical research but rather to his own lack of training in chemistry. There are lively comments from both directions — on the average psychiatrist's ignorance of physics and chemistry; on the biochemist's and the neurophysiologist's lack of appreciation of the psychological area to which his own work does not reach.

Realization that many disciplines are involved in research on schizophrenia has resulted in a few examples of multidisciplinary approach to study of a considerable number of the same patients over long periods ("a thousand tests on one rat rather than one test on a thousand rats"). One illustration is the previously mentioned project at the research facility of the Rockland State Hospital described by its director, Nathan S. Kline, 1953, as including simultaneous and continuous studies of the same patients for an extended period, aiming "to develop an integrated interdisciplinary framework for the description of personality organization". The project utilizes "the knowledge, interest, skills of neurophysiologists, sociologists, psychologists, physiologists, endocrinologists, biometricians, biochemists, geneticists, anthropologists, statisticians, nurses, attendants, and an electrical engineer and a mathematical logician". Other examples include the Columbia Greystone project in which the same group of patients (those subjected to psychosurgery and a number of controls) were studied for more than three years by a group of neurologists, anatomists, psychiatrists, psychologists; a similar study in the Boston State Hospital by members of the Harvard psychiatry department with the cooperation of biochemists, psychologists, neuropathologists, physiologists, sociologists; a Tulane study, reported 1954, in which the behavior of patients subjected to a new surgical procedure was studied by a group including psychiatrists, psychologists, physiologists, neurologists, neurosurgeons, biochemists. These projects reflect increasing realization that the attack must be at once multiple, involving both the basic and clinical sciences, and concentrated: "The problem of schizophrenia is not going to be settled by one or two men working here and there" (Donald W. Hastings, psychiatry and neurology, Minnesota Medical School, 1953). Instances of the increasing institutionalization of "behavioral science" include the new center for advanced study on the Stanford campus and the University of Michigan's new mental health research institute, created to accommodate the behavioral science committee long active at the University of Chicago, under the chairmanship of James G. Miller.

The important thing, as more than a few workers have pointed out, is that the investigator of schizophrenia, whatever his especial preoccupation, shall consistently have in mind the total picture. This is the only thing that will ever unite some of the extremists in the most widely disparate of the fields. The psychodynamists charged with using "methods of low precision to the exclusion of others" tend to separate themselves from the point of view as well as the procedures of the neurophysiologists, electrophysiologists, chemists. On the other hand the high-precision methods of the latter group may narrow perspective. "A highly precise method may be applicable to only so small a segment of the phenomenon being studied as to afford little information about the phenomenon as a whole" (Altschule, 1953). Richter and others have commented that the limited amount of fresh

brain biopsy material (secured directly and during prefrontal leucotomy) limits the amount of information available from analysis of
it. There is considerable margin for error in examining only small
fragments of the brain without a concomitant histologic study of the
whole brain as well as of other organs or tissues. The fragmentary
material, together with the fact that not all submicroscopic changes
are as yet objectively demonstrable, tend to invalidate many of the
conclusions drawn from biopsy and postmortem material.

Increasingly conscious of the limitations of the interpretations based
on the unavoidable piecemeal approach, leading investigators, notably in recent years, have stressed the need of greater concern everywhere with the whole picture, with those integrating and coordinating
mechanisms that alone can give meaning to specific and limited findings. Weiss observed, 1953, that while there have been remarkable
advances in knowledge of enzymatic, metabolic and electrical properties of single neurons, there is still "virtually complete" ignorance of
what makes them operate in *harmonious coordination*. A coherent neurophysiological explanation of how single nerves act in coordinated
groups was described by Hebb, 1949, as the outstanding need in
psychology in attempts to work out a neurophysiological basis for
behavior. Kline observed, 1952, that only when the total pattern of
organization is understood will it be possible really to understand the
disorganization of personality that characterizes schizophrenia.

## Need of More Extensive Work In Comparative Biology

F. M. Burnet of Australia said, 1953, that "as a biologist" he fancied
that the effective generalizations needed "may eventually be found
more readily from the study of animal behavior than from too undivided attention to the human being". It has not been possible to
produce schizophrenia in animals although, by drugs and other
means, certain schizophrenia-like reactions have been produced
experimentally in them as in man. Considerable experimental work
bearing on various aspects of neurophysiology, neuroanatomy and
neuropsychology has been done in some species, practically no work
in other species. Many investigators have stressed the need of con-
structing a wider biological framework by extending experimental
work to a wider range of animals, including wild species.

Philip Bard (physiology, Johns Hopkins), 1952, found reason to believe that "information that cannot be obtained in any other way" could be reached through systematic study of, for instance, specific aspects of cerebral organization in a series of mammals from marsupial to monkey. It is true that species differences are important and sometimes insufficiently taken into account, but in systematic study right down — or up — the line, these differences become less striking, a fairly smooth curve can be plotted and "an 'extrapolation' to man is likely to yield a good working hypothesis". The leads from comparative biology that have given direction to work on the human nervous system could be illustrated in many directions — as in orientation of more intensive work on the human rhinencephalon by observation that in some animals, at least, the rhinencephalon does much more than mediate the sense of smell; as in the fact (once noted by W. E. LeGros Clark) that certain basic mechanisms in the cerebral cortex — obscured in man by other processes — are more accessible to study in the reptilian brain.

Further animal ablations might, in Bard's view, throw light on the neural bases of both stereotyped and learned modes of behavior, be useful in analysis of complex central mechanisms, and help to explain the imperfectly understood therapeutic mechanisms of lobotomy and topectomy in man. Bard recognized the considerable gradation in animal experimentation, in that it is one thing to decerebrate a cat or dog and study the preparation briefly and "quite a different matter to decerebrate an animal and keep it alive and in good condition for five months", as can now be done.

The significance of many cortical areas has been established or suggested by experimental work. Woolsey's group mapped the sensory areas of the cortex in a small number of diverse species by the method of recording evoked potentials. It was then possible to make correct prediction as to the loci of the areas in the brains of intermediate and "higher" forms and to test these predictions during surgery in man. The results also established for the first time homologies between the widely differing fissures of the different species. The mapping of the fundamental units of structure for man's nervous system was described by Sam L. Clark (neuroanatomy, Vanderbilt), 1952, as "not even near completion", pointing to the need of extensive and systematic work on many species. As yet, not all the details of the nervous system of even the best known animal, the earthworm, are clear. While considerable work has been done on the nervous system of various invertebrates and fishes, amphibians, reptiles, birds and mammals, not all the needed details in any one animal species have been established. When experimental embryology has provided approaches to basic principles of development in the salamanders and chicks, the same kind of work in other species is indicated — and often lacking. Gross anatomical observations by Frederick Tilney and O. Larsell supporting localization of representation of different body parts in the cerebellum call for further comparative studies and correlation of findings in gross anatomy with physiological studies of living animals. The work of George E. Coghill's group with amblystoma, and of W. F. Windle's group with cat and rat (correlating developmental changes in the nervous system with appearance of behavior patterns) call for extension to other species.

In these behavior patterns, in the correlation of the neuroanatomy and neurophysiology of animals with their behavior, there is dominant interest if little work. According to Karl S. Lashley (neuropsychology, Harvard, and director, Yerkes laboratories of primate biology) there were, in 1952, not more than five institutions in this country conducting definitely organized experimental research combining neurological and behavior studies. "And even these are heavily weighted toward one side or the other." He pointed out that comparative psychology is as greatly needed as comparative anatomy. "There are comprehensive studies of the behavior of the rat, of the chimpanzee and of man, but little is known of any other species." S. L. Clark once pointed out that since, superficially, the brains of bees and ants seem entirely inadequate to account for their complicated and well-organized behavior, experiments correlating the structure of their brains and their behavior could be of great importance. In most medical school psychiatry departments, experimental institutes and laboratories, as pointed out in 1948 by James G. Miller (chairman, psychology department, University of Chicago, and at that time chief clinical psychologist in the Veterans Administration), were "almost unheard of".

One comparative study directed toward defining genetic rather than neurophysiological factors that may play a part in the determination of normal variations in behavior has been going forward for some years in the cross-breeding program at the Roscoe B. Jackson Memorial Laboratory, Bar Harbor, Maine, designed to bring to light underlying variations in canine behavior from strain to strain, by measurements of the speed of learning, the intensity of emotional reactions to a given stimulus, the degree of dependency, in various pure strains.

Efforts to identify the areas, tracts and interconnections involved in intellectual and emotional functions motivated some of the work, over many years, of John F. Fulton and associates (physiology, Yale) concerned with ablation of various parts of the brains of primates. Primate investigation has been greatly furthered by the above-mentioned Yerkes laboratories of primate biology.  Lashley observed, 1955, that the laboratories' main investigations have been in the fields of cerebral function, comparative intelligence, sex physiology in chimpanzees.  As the most important contribution from the laboratories, Lashley named Carlyle Jacobsen's reduction of temper tantrums in chimpanzees by brain lesions, the discovery that led Moniz to the operation of prefrontal lobotomy in man.

That something about mental illness might be learned from animals by "experimental" observation was suggested by a Canadian governmental investigation into the cause of "madness" in Nova Scotia moose.  The working hypothesis, 1954, was that the brain disease from which the moose were suffering was caused by a dietary deficiency of certain minerals and vitamins.  The Provincial Lands and Forestry Department of Canada, on the basis of incomplete research, offered the hypothesis that the madness was to be attributed fundamentally to climatic changes that have taken place in Canada during the last few hundred years.  As the climate has grown warmer, certain types of plant food on which the moose depended for a balanced diet have disappeared.  The moose would normally move north in search of cooler temperatures and essential foods, but since Nova Scotia is a peninsula with a narrow land-bridge to the mainland they could not do this.  Instead, "slowly dying of malnutrition, scrawny and tick-infested, they lope around the countryside, their motor and sensory nerves out of order.  Half blind, they crash into fences or get entangled in bushes or trees until they die." The report noted that biologists are attempting to treat the moose by feeding them the minerals believed to be lacking in the food at present available to them, "in much the way Nova Scotia farmers give their cattle supplemental cobalt to keep them well". The analogy is considered at least to point toward currently publicized possibilities of curing or alleviating human mental disturbances, including schizophrenia, by biochemical means.

In capacity to develop such means, man with his frontal lobe has the advantage over animals. That the advantage is sometimes with the animals, that animals may have developed better ways of solving the problems of their world than man has developed for solving the problems of his was suggested by one philosophic observer of animal behavior (Edward C. Tolman, psychology, University of California) in a discussion at McGill University, 1954. Much of our human inability to solve critical political and social problems arises, according to Tolman, from lack of belief in the soundness of our own way of life, and a consequent paralyzing fear. To justify the fear we seek a scapegoat, and find it in, for instance, "Communism", envisaged as a "threat to our own way of life". This, according to Tolman, is a psychological mechanism which afflicts man in our current civilization but from which animals are free. "The lower animals do not, to my knowledge, go in for scapegoating . . ." They are not driven to it by any doubt as to the sanity of their own society, by any fear that they will be either nazified or communized.

## Need of Orienting Schizophrenia Research by Normal Mechanisms

The harm that has resulted from primary, exclusive or uncontrolled preoccupation with abnormal or interrupted physiological and/or psychological mechanisms and manifestations has been stressed by some workers in all schools. Psychiatry has been charged with being less interested in the music from normal violins than in the sour notes that come from *some* violins. Neurophysiology, neuroanatomy and biochemistry as disciplines are naturally focused on the normal, but, even so, approaches through them to study of schizophrenia and other forms of mental illness are often confined to pathological phenomena.

In investigation of all mental illness, the need of studies of not only normal but also of "superior" people as the necessary background for studies of the abnormal was stressed at the Oxford conference. In this connection, R. N. Sanford (psychology, University of California), commenting on a previous speaker's plea for examining the brains of people after leucotomy, recommended "the same sort of examination of brains of people who never got sick". Commenting on study of the anatomy and physiology of the frontal cortex from material that has suffered post-mortem change, one worker observed: "so little normal material has been available that our criteria of what is normal requires serious reinvestigation". Study of the biochemistry of schizophrenia justifies conclusions only when it is conducted against the framework of biochemical study of normal organisms; otherwise there is no basis of comparison and no justification for inference. Knowledge of normal physiologic responses to environmental changes in cells is requisite for understanding the abnormal physiologic responses of schizophrenics.

Orienting the social approach to schizophrenia by study of the normal offers peculiar difficulty. Defining the social norm would be a severe challenge to the present sum of human knowledge. The environment is connoted in all descriptions of schizophrenia and one of its leading characteristics, the breakdown in communication between the individual and his environment, can be understood (Jurgen Ruesch, 1953) only on the basis of understanding *normal* interpersonal relations on all levels, ranging from the relation between individuals to relations involved in the family and in larger social, political, economic, cultural organization. In this field, as in others bearing on schizophrenia, stress has been laid on the need of reinvestigating certain current values and perhaps of adopting new criteria. Trigant Burrow (when scientific director of the Lifwynn Foundation) questioned whether the fact that certain behavior is socially accredited insures its social normality. This question stretches to far horizons the fields calling for reinvestigation.

It is in the psychological area that need for orientation by the normal is greatest — and perhaps least existent. Understanding of one of the traditional psychological "aberrations" of schizophrenics, lack of capacity for abstraction, can be achieved (Goldstein, 1953) only if study of it is based on knowledge of normal capacity for abstraction. Without the balance and the check of work upon the normal, psychological theory even more readily than physiological or biochemical outruns facts. That psychological theory had done just that was pointed out, 1951, by Hebb. Reviewing some of the psychological theories badly in need of substantiation of some kind, Hebb inquired: "Do we have any evidence that the child learns because he needs affection? Or that because the very young infant is biologically dependent upon the mother he 'wants' to do anything?" Until we learn how far such theories agree with fact "we are arguing in circles".

The psychological "fact" referred to goes far beyond the usual implications of a psychiatry aimed at therapy of the mentally ill. "Neglect of psychology in medicine — or rather its displacement by rigid symbolic formulations not amenable to validation by controlled observation and experiment — deprives psychiatry of an opportunity to participate in the processes that have enriched other branches of medicine in the past half century" (Altschule, 1953). The spectacularly increased attention to psychiatry in medical schools, previously noted, has not been paralleled by a developing relation of psychology to the psychiatric field. Rarely, as James G. Miller pointed out, do medical schools offer, for the training of psychiatrists, "the wide field of experimentation and investigation which at present forms the systematic science of psychology". In his view, "the average well-trained clinical psychologist knows more about the psychology of the mind, the normal functioning of the personality and related topics than does the average well-trained psychiatrist". Little more than a beginning had been made in his judgment, 1948, in applying clinically the findings available from psychology on such subjects as maturation, perception, learning, memory, motivation, group behavior and many forms of functioning involved in mental illness. Psychology, in brief, has much more to contribute to psychiatry than psychiatry has yet accepted, or solicited. However greatly the research field on schizophrenia would be extended by involving the field of normal as well as abnormal psychology, it remains true that recognition of the dimensions of the whole field may best orient limited investigation of any part of it.

In summary, the outstanding research needs in schizophrenia

include more study of comparative biology; more use of fundamental work in psychology correcting psychiatric theory and bringing it into focus by relating it to the principles that govern normal as well as abnormal behavior; more attention to social and cultural factors which all schools of thought admit to be powerful influences; pursuit of neurophysiological and biochemical correlations with psychological manifestations.

## PHYSIOLOGICAL EMPHASIS IN RESEARCH BEARING ON SCHIZOPHRENIA

Belief that the phenomena of behavior and of mind are ultimately describable in concepts of the mathematical and physical sciences is (Lashley) "the faith to which we all subscribe", while admittedly still awaiting the works that will "ultimately" support it. The faith covers certainty that the brain is the organ of "mind", that whenever the brain functions there is organic change — in the caliber of blood vessels, in alteration of heart beats, in more subtle changes in glands or viscera, that "there can be no twisted thought without a twisted molecule" (Gerard). This belief would appear to leave little room for a mysterious agent that is not physical and yet has physical effects. "One cannot", Hebb once observed, "be logically a determinist in physics, chemistry and biology and a mystic in psychology." We cannot say that "because we have not yet found out how to reduce behavior to the control of the brain no one in the future will be able to do so".

Failure in the search over decades to find structural defects or organic lesions specific for schizophrenia has added to the prestige of the psychological as contrasted with the physicochemical approach to mental illness, including schizophrenia. "At the very time" (Frederic A. Gibbs, 1953) "when our electronic techniques have advanced to the point where we can make electron pictures of the brain . . . and when, with radioactive tracers, we can study the intimate chemistry of the brain, the physicochemical approach to the understanding of mental illness is being largely abandoned in favor of the psychological approach." "Largely abandoned" must be interpreted conservatively, in view of the support that exists for the concept that psychiatry "is a biologic science (Bruetsch, neuropathologist,

1952) dealing with biochemical and pathological processes in the cerebral tissue, which may affect mental health". Some of the investigators whose work is definitely slanted toward psychological emphasis join with neuroanatomists, electrophysiologists, biochemists in urging this biological perspective for the present research on schizophrenia. Harry C. Solomon (psychiatry, Harvard, 1953) in a letter to the American Foundation stressed "going to the basic facts" in research on schizophrenia. Among the sources of the "basic facts" he included experimental stimulation and ablation of parts of the brain (as in the work of Bard, Magoun); experimental production of schizomimetic symptoms by such drugs as lysergic acid, mescaline; search for the neurophysiological and biochemical mechanisms by which certain physical therapies as convulsive shock, insulin coma, etc., apparently affect the thinking, feeling and behavior of the schizophrenic patient. Concern with neurophysiological and biochemical factors has been a tradition for years in some psychiatric centers, as the Elgin State Hospital in Illinois. Currently, centers of psychiatric work in which biological perspective is apparent include the Langley Porter Clinic at the University of California (Bowman); the psychiatry department of Washington University (Gildea); the Rockland Hospital Research Facility (Kline); the New York State Psychiatric Institute; the Worcester State Hospital; the Neuropsychiatric Institute of the University of Illinois; the newly established Mental Health Research Institute at the University of Michigan; Harvard's psychiatry department, contributing work in physiology, psychiatry, chemistry and biochemistry, through staff members at the Boston State Hospital and at the McLean Hospital in which Altschule's physiological studies, Folch-Pi's chemical analyses of the brain have been conducted for many years.

On the other side of the picture, there are still in the ranks a good many psychiatrists whose vision is limited to the possibilities of psychotherapy, with or without shock therapy, possibly with a hopeful eye also toward chlorpromazine and reserpine in empirical use. If these psychiatrists rather than those mentioned above prevail, psychiatry will never feel the impact of the physiology, chemistry and modern physics that have revolutionized other branches of medicine. Between the psychiatrists and the physiologists there must be a greater meeting of minds — and also an extension in the training of both. In which connection Altschule recommended more "expert physiologists and chemists with some knowledge of psychiatry rather than psychiatrists with fragmentary knowledge of physiology".

Clearly there is still imbalance between the psychological and the physiological approaches and there is present need for wider support of neurophysiological, neuroanatomical, electrophysiological and neuropsychological work. Various workers, citing the physical findings of an earlier age that believed in an organic basis for insanity but made little headway in physiological investigation of it, have stressed the present need of reinvestigation of some of the unproductive work of the past, making use of the immensely improved tools of the present, radioisotopes, finer electronic, microscopic and electrographic devices, better staining techniques, new morphological approaches and new structural concepts. The earlier physiological work was done under different conditions but there was a not inconsiderable amount of it. It included attempts to find out whether hyperactivity or hypoactivity of some function might be a distinguishing physiological mark of schizophrenia; it reflected preoccupation with quantitative physiological variations (Yale workers recalled a 1911 article in which forty-three pages were devoted to variations in serum lipids, proteins, non-protein nitrogen in schizophrenics), in oxygen saturation, carbon dioxide content in arterial blood, in hemoglobin concentration, erythrocyte sedimentation, leukocyte and lymphocyte counts; it included numerous functional studies on circulatory factors (measurement of cardiac rate, peripheral blood flow, arterial pressure in schizophrenics), on pituitary-adrenal function, with somewhat less attention to the thyroid and the sex steroids.

The present dominance of psychological over physiological motivation in research has a rational evolutionary history: at the very time when physiological work on mental illness in this country was at low ebb so far as results were concerned, Freud's work stimulated investigative imagination by apparently offering a new and hopeful approach. Perhaps Freud suffered the fate of many other discoverers — *i.e.*, over-exploitation of only part of his original concept. E. D. Adrian told the British Association, 1954, that "Freud would have liked to build up a system based on the physiology of the brain, but he was soon too deeply committed to the psychological side". Pavlov's conception of human behavior, on the other hand, although based on brain physiology, had unhappily become perhaps "more disturbing than Freud's because Pavlov's notion of the conditioned reflex has come to dominate one side of the world" but "we must not think the less of it because it has been used to justify political system foreign to ours". Referring to both Freud and Pavlov as scientists of surprising originality and influence on research, Adrian added, "but the fields they explored are still waiting for the next advance to show how much they will yield".

Very recently, 1955, Pavlov's disciples among psychiatrists in this country organized a new national psychiatric society in dissent from the traditional Freudian school and in support of the Pavlovian principle that subjective findings are not dependable unless confirmed by measurement of physiological processes. Those associated with the chief organizer of the new society, W. Horsley Gantt (Johns Hopkins) included John C. Whitehorn (psychiatry, Johns Hopkins), Ernst Gellhorn (neurophysiology, University of Minnesota), Howard S. Liddell (animal psychology, Cornell), William G. Reese (psychiatry, University of Arkansas) and David McK. Rioch (neuropsychiatric division, Army Medical Center).

In discussing presently neglected areas in research on mental illness, the Magnuson report pointed out that one of the chief lags was in physiological basic research. The "basic" is important. The range of work comprehended in research on the nervous system in " total perspective" represents, Weiss observed, 1953, "problems of molecular organization, histological structure, geometry of connections, biochemistry of metabolism, chemical and electrical correlates of conduction and transmission, pharmacological response to drugs; problems of coordination, specificity, of integrative, regulatory and interpretative functions and their derangement, as well as the whole problem of the developmental mechanisms through which all of this has come about". While admitting that work from these many directions had resulted in many conflicting versions of the brain, Weiss seemed not to question the possibility that clinician and anatomist, psychologist and physiologist, cytologist and biochemist would be able ultimately to clarify their common objectives. Indeed, he envisaged the nervous system as the field *par excellence* for combined effort, as "perhaps one of the most heartening examples of active resistance to specialist isolation".

## CURRENT TRENDS IN NEUROPHYSIOLOGICAL (AND NEUROANATOMICAL) WORK IN RELATION TO ULTIMATE EXPLANATION OF BEHAVIOR

### INTRODUCTORY: THE POSSIBILITY OF PSYCHOLOGICAL CORRELATES ORIENTING NEUROPHYSIOLOGICAL RESEARCH

Neurophysiology aims, as Lashley once put it, at "ultimate synthesis of neurology and psychology", at definition of behavior in terms of neural mechanisms. Thinking, wishing and dreaming are just as much functions of the organism as are breathing, running and digesting. "They are merely more complex, and less understood" (Cobb, 1952). That all human behavior is a function of the activity of the nervous system and other physiological systems was described by Hoagland, 1952, as a "hardly debatable premise". Such disturbances of brain function as schizophrenia, however, evidently occur at a molecular level, "too subtle to yield directly to present-day analysis by neuroanatomists and neurophysiologists". Schizophrenia is no less an "organic" disease than any other, "but science is not as yet sufficiently advanced to analyze the brain mechanisms involved in either normal or abnormal behavior at the level necessary for understanding so complex a problem".

That, nevertheless, efforts at neuroanatomic and neurophysiologic analysis should be prosecuted vigorously has had significant confirmation: from H. W. Magoun (chairman, anatomy department, University of California at Los Angeles), who observed, 1953, to the American Foundation that the most valuable contributions to understanding of schizophrenia are likely to come from long-time studies on the neurophysiological correlates of behavior; from Frederic Gibbs (chief, division of electroencephalography, neuropsychiatric institute, University of Illinois), who observed, 1951, that "until an understanding of brain function underlies psychology, psychiatry, and sociology, these sciences will necessarily remain superficial and weak in their powers to predict and control". He described the science of brain "engineering" as now, however, at about "the same stage of development as were electrical science and engineering in 1892". While explanation of behavior in terms of neural mechanisms seems, even to some of the most diligent workers in fundamental neuroanatomy and neurophysiology, almost too remote to justify hope, others feel with Adrian, 1954, that we are at least "beginning to trace a closer connection between what is going on in the different parts of the brain and what we happen to be doing from moment to moment. For what it is worth, we can see a physical reason for our restless lives and our insatiable curiosity."

Some of the most significant advances in neurophysiology in the last twenty years — concerning patterns of interrelated activity of nerves, concerning neural centers of "emotion" and their representation in lower and higher cerebral structures — are only now beginning to percolate to psychiatry. Hebb commented that psychology has not yet fully assimilated such fundamental neurophysiological contributions (most of them since 1928) as those of H. Berger on the electrical activity of the brain, of J. G. Dusser de Barenne on the physiology of the cerebral cortex and subcortical influences, and of R. Lorente de Nó on "internuncial" neurons, all of which have broadened the concept of cerebral interconnections and mechanisms. Those interested in the dimensions of the present research field in schizophrenia would do well to bear in mind that a great deal of the ultimately — and presumably — pertinent neurophysiological work is being done by workers not in the least concerned with mental illness: there are men who have been working on the single axon for years whose interest continues to be — not schizophrenia but axons.

One of the reasons why validated correlation of even the simplest psychological concepts with neurophysiological mechanisms is still remote is the rapidity with which neurophysiological theories are superseded through advancing knowledge. The "toppling" of current theories (not yet superseded by entirely stable substitutes) was commented upon by George H. Bishop (neurophysiology, Washington University), 1953. He estimated that at least ten years might be required for present changing concepts to crystallize. "This crystallization is the next important step. One aspect of it will be to coordinate cell physiology and cell chemistry into an integrated understanding of neural mechanism." Favorite hypotheses of the past have been, or are being, demolished by new findings, new prominence for hitherto neglected brain areas, new hypotheses related to interconnections between them, to the manner in which sensations are relayed, to the primary importance of integrating principles, to a newer theory of the electrical activity of the nervous system, postulating continuous rhythmic activity of the brain cells, rather than activity in response only to stimulus, new stress upon not only the immediate reactions of the nervous system but also "those more persistent changes which alter its habits and give us our memories" (Adrian). Even without reference to the far goal of psychological correlates for neurophysiological findings, the infinite reach of the problems involved in study of the development, structure, chemistry and function of the nervous system might well (as phrased by one participant in a recent conference on some aspects of the nervous system) make a nuclear physicist shudder.

## PROBLEMS WITH A NEUROANATOMICAL SLANT

If the "biological value of a brain" (Julian Huxley, 1951) lies in its being "an organ for general coordination of all information about significant changes in the outer environment and the animal's own organism, then all available facts about the structure, chemistry and function of the nervous system are essential to solving the problem of mental illness, including schizophrenia". The need of considering *together* the "structure, chemical composition and function of an excitatory tissue" was stressed, 1954, by George Wald (biology, Harvard): "Only at grosser levels of analysis can anatomy, chemistry, and physiology be dealt with separately. At the molecular level they are one and must be so regarded." This is the conviction that underlies modern "anatomical" work on the nervous system and its structural units from the individual neuron to the cerebral cortex. Increasingly, study of the particular unit, area or pathway is oriented by recognition of the integrating mechanisms which the unit serves.

There is a difference in emphasis (rather than in substance) among groups of workers as to how far hopes are still to be tied to detailed study of the structure and function of particular areas of the brain in the ultimate effort to explain behavior. Virtual abandonment of the old, almost phrenological, concept attributing distinctive functions to distinctive areas has by no means meant abandonment of interest in the detailed structure of these different areas and the particular way in which they contribute to the sought-for integrating pattern. The question upon which leading workers differ is more or less procedural. F. O. Schmitt (biology, Massachusetts Institute of Technology) somewhat deplored the tendency among neurophysiologists to bypass detailed analysis of structure and chemical composition of neuron components in favor of concentrated work on the nerve impulse. He favored, rather, concentrating on the vast amount of detailed work on structural and chemical composition of neuronal components that must be done "before we shall be in a position to state what is really there".

There may be no real incompatibility between certain workers' emphasis on the need of intensive work on separate units and the stress of other workers on the importance of orienting work by concern with integrating mechanisms. W. E. LeGros Clark, who cited, 1950, the scorn some investigators have expressed concerning "the extent to which the anatomist may go in his cytoarchitectual parcellations", nevertheless regarded tedious cytoarchitectural surveys as a necessary preliminary to tracing fiber connections and as thus having direct reference to experimental investigation of functional localization. Clark thought that many instances could be adduced in support of the anatomists' thesis that "functional localization is in most cases reflected in structural localization".

Lashley did not attack the premise. "Please do not take it", he observed, "that I deny the functional value of the precise anatomic arrangements of the nervous system. On the contrary, I believe that the secret of cerebral, perhaps of all neural integration lies in the nature of the topological representation of the sensory surfaces and of the motor apparatus. What I wish to emphasize is the need to examine the possible integrative mechanisms which are provided by the mosaic projection in the sensory and the motor systems, and the need to give adequate consideration to such topological relations in any theory of neural organization . . ." Lashley urged the need of investigating the finer details of internal cortical structure, both the nature of the network within functional areas and the modes of interconnections between areas, in order to clarify the nature of patterns of neural activity which they can mediate. The psychological data must be analyzed "not in terms of formal logic, which has been the customary procedure, but with reference to the patterns of activity which they represent . . ."

The form and function of the nervous system are so intricately interwoven (Sam L. Clark, 1952) that the investigator of function finds it necessary to unravel details of morphology. "From the way the nervous system is constructed for conduction it is frequently possible to interpret the function of a pathway or 'center' by determining its connection." Various neuroanatomical problems bear upon outstanding current problems of neurophysiology, as, for instance, the importance of the synapse in the conduction of the nerve impulse. Neuroanatomically speaking, why, asks Sam L. Clark, are synapses variously formed as they are? What is the exact relationship of two neurons at synapses? How is the morphology of synapses related to the production of humoral substances which are related to transmission of the nerve impulse? These and many other questions are raised, including those requiring answer on a microscopic plane.

At some levels, morphological details call for study in terms of chemistry and physics. In this connection such methods as use of radioactive substances and of micro-incineration have not been completely exploited as a means of studying the distribution of various elements in the nervous system. Much needed is more intensive study of alterations as a result of pathological processes both in the chemistry of neurons and their morphology. The moot question of how and why, in the evolution of the vertebrate nervous system, the gray matter increases in volume and complexity must be answered in part by morphological studies. Within different animal forms, the general distribution of the masses of gray matter raises anatomical questions. "Even the reasons for segregation of the large mass of gray matter into separate suprasegmental structures, cerebellum, tectum and cerebrum are not at hand; and within these the localized distribution of representation in specific areas offers opportunity for fruitful investigation . . ."

As to the study of nervous pathways, quite aside from the facts that can be gleaned from blunt dissection of major bundles of white matter in the brain, understanding of almost every pathway that has been described depends upon further investigation. There is need of further knowledge of the intricate interconnections of parts of the gray masses within the cerebrum, *i.e.*, basal ganglia, and thalamic, subthalamic and hypothalamic nuclei. This need is emphasized by the now recognized relation of the reticular system to the general problems of inhibition and excitation.

Studies of single units and of immediate responses of single sensory and motor fibers are essential to broader, integrated approaches. "It should be borne in mind that recent work on cerebral mechanisms has been guided and interpreted in terms of results obtained by analyses of units in peripheral nerves and in autonomic ganglia" (Bard, 1952). There are obvious difficulties in anatomical and physiological correlations. Many neuroanatomical facts, for instance, are devoid of functional significance. "For example there are conspicuous fiber tracts within the central nervous system to which no function can be assigned." On the other hand, physiological studies have revealed the existence of functional connections for which there appears to be no anatomical basis. The problems can best be solved and advances best be made, according to Bard, by cooperation between neuroanatomists and neurophysiologists. One suggested direction for this cooperation was a fresh attack on the relation of cytoarchitectural fields of the cerebral cortex to functionally defined areas and to the thalamic nuclei.

## CHANGING CONCEPTS OF BRAIN FUNCTION THAT HAVE RESULTED FROM CONCERN WITH PARTICULAR AREAS

### INCREASING INTEREST IN LOWER AREAS AND IN THEIR CORTICAL CONNECTIONS

Over-preoccupation with the cortex and neglect of more primitive areas, notably the *rhinencephalon*, has been widely stressed in recent years. Bard and other leading investigators found no valid evidence for the old idea that these structures subserve olfactory functions and, on the contrary, good reasons for supposing that they are not parts of the "smell brain". LeGros Clark, 1953, envisaged the cerebral cortex as an organ which, broadly speaking, refines the behavior mediated by these more primitive structures. J. A. Bates at the Oxford conference noted considerable agreement among workers with this idea that the cortex acts as a sort of super-computing-machine "which puts frills on something more fundamental that is going on beneath it".

Nearly two decades ago, Bard observed: "The more closely one examines the operation of the brain, the more unsound appears the practice of distinguishing sharply between cortical and subcortical functions." Alfred Meyer (Institute of Psychiatry, University of London) thought it, 1953, "not inconceivable" that a pathological change in subcortical rhinencephalic regions "has been overlooked in schizophrenic brains". In the newer thinking, interest has measurably shifted from the frontal lobe to the temporal lobe, and from the temporal lobe downwards through the thalamus to the reticular substance of the brain stem.

Heinrich Klüver (experimental psychology, Chicago), at the 1952 Macy conference on cybernetics, observed that later experimental work has lent support to the hypothesis advanced fifteen years ago that the rhinencephalic structures constitute an anatomical substrate of emotions. The rhinencephalon, according to LeGros Clark, probably serves some quite important function, linking the activities of the hypothalamus and cerebral cortex. "Much of it forms a complex mechanism whose activities are predominantly related to emotional processes, and, if this is so, it may prove to be of the highest importance among those factors which determine abnormalities of affect, and, indirectly, disorganization of normal cortical activity." Wilder Penfield (Montreal Neurological Institute), 1954, in making the point that no area of the cortex is independent and that none is capable of function without its corresponding portion of the old brain, observed: "Indeed, it seems to be through the brainstem that the new capacities of each area of the cortex are utilized." In this concept, the sensory areas of the cerebral cortex are simply way stations in the several currents that carry different forms of sensation into the centrencephalic (Penfield's term) integrating system, and the cortical areas are way stations in the stream of out-flowing impulses that produce motor activity. Penfield and Jasper described the continuous electrical rhythms of the brain as apparently "under the separate, independent control of the brainstem reticular system". In the reticular system is included the adjacent thalamus.

Study of interrelations between several structures of the rhinencephalon and the higher cerebral centers furnished experimental basis for the belief that many structures in the rhinencephalon are associated with the emotional "background" of higher intellectual functions. Describing a complex circuit between one of the component structures, the hippocampus, and the hypothalamus (parts of which had also once been relegated to the rhinencephalon) and the frontal lobes, Clark referred to reported "dramatic changes in affective behavior" in animals, resulting from ablations involving the hippocampus. On the basis of Bard's animal experiments (cats) Cobb observed, 1953, that it would seem that "when different parts of the archicortex . . . are released from higher control, exaggerated emotional reactions take place".

Various workers over a period of twenty years have suggested that the *thalamus* holds the secret of much that goes on within the cerebral cortex. Penfield and Jasper noted, 1954, that earlier electrophysiological studies in their laboratories had shown important projections from the sensory receiving areas of the cortex (particularly auditory and visual) back into the thalamus. LeGros Clark more than fifteen years before this had described the cortex as "a dependency of the thalamus and not *vice versa*". Several earlier workers (Dempsey and Morison; Dusser de Barenne) had, in the thirties, reported suggestive evidence that the thalamus is the "pacemaker" for cortical electrical rhythms.

The *reticular system of various nuclei*, regarded until recently as merely "background" for thalamus and brainstem, may, according to Clark, actually be "the primary physical basis of the background of conscious awareness". The reticular system of nuclei is "an exceedingly primitive component of the vertebrate brain. On the other hand, the cerebral cortex is a comparatively late development which in the course of evolution (it is suggested) has been elaborated to form a sort of scanning mechanism utilized by this primitive system as an instrument which makes possible a high degree of sensory discrimination, but not constituting *by itself* the ultimate basis of conscious experience . . ." If these concepts are well founded, then it becomes "of great importance that we should know something about the structural organization and connections of the reticular nuclei". Actually, "we know very little".

Work on the *hypothalamus* over the last twenty-five years has contributed to breaking down the rigid concept relegating intellectual reactions to the frontal lobes of the cerebral cortex, emotional reactions to the autonomic system. Between the two and linking them lies the hypothalamus which may not only regulate autonomic function but also be regulated in turn by higher centers in the frontal lobes. Cobb, 1950, pointed to "much new evidence from the studies of electroencephalograms" that the hypothalamus "has an influence upon the electrical activity of the cerebral cortex". He favored regarding the hypothalamus not as the "sleep center" of the traditional concept but rather as a "wakefulness center", the activity of which tends to keep the cortex alert.

Although up to 1950 no direct anatomic pathways had been established from the frontal lobes to the hypothalamus, LeGros Clark referred, 1953, to "functional evidence" (1945 demonstration of electroencephalographic changes indicating cortical discharges following electrical stimulation of the hypothalamus of animals) that the hypothalamic nuclei "are under direct cortical influence", the nature of which "can presently only be conjectured". According to Meyer, 1950, "Clark has gone so far as to regard the frontal lobe as the projection area of the hypothalamus".

An important gap in knowledge concerns the significance of the relation between the hypothalamus and the anterior pituitary (which has no direct innervation) and the possibility of "neurosecretion", suggested by the fact that the two are joined during early embryonic development. In calling attention to this, 1953, Clark suggested that the mode of interaction between the hypothalamus and the pituitary, still not fully understood, may be found to have some quite fundamental part in cerebral activity as a whole.

In the view of Gellhorn (concerned with the integration of the autonomic nervous system), 1953, we reach *"per exclusionem* the hypothalamus as the structure in which functional reactivity seems to be altered" in the functional psychoses — including schizophrenia. Information bearing on central representation for autonomic function has been developing over the past twenty-five years. Experiments, notably by Ranson and associates (anatomy, Institute of Neurology, Northwestern University), in the late twenties and early thirties, on the role of the hypothalamus in such discrete autonomic functions as cardiovascular reflexes, visceromotor functions, water metabolism, sleep, strengthened developing concepts of central representation of autonomic function and were described, 1953, by Clark as showing that "the so-called autonomic functions of the body are not so autonomic" in the sense of being independent of cerebral mechanisms. The higher levels of integration of the autonomic nervous system, according to Penfield and Jasper, 1954, have been regarded as located in the brainstem centers, in the hypothalamus and, in some views, in the cerebral cortex.

Schizophrenic patients were divided (by Funkenstein, Greenblatt and Solomon), 1952, into several groups according to their autonomic reactions to autonomic drugs. Those that showed the poorest prognosis in terms of autonomic pattern also showed, in psychological tests, the most marked impairment in abstract thinking and the greatest clinical deterioration. Schizophrenic lack of capacity for abstract thinking was interpreted as a "release" of the autonomic nervous system from higher controls. Comparison of the autonomic reaction (as gauged by the reaction to the drugs used) before and after shock therapy in a hundred patients suggested that autonomic function may have prognostic value as to whether electroshock will or will not be effective in given cases of schizophrenia. This is in line with the view (Gellhorn) that electroshock therapy operates by stimulating the hypothalamic sympathetic-adrenal systems.

"To relate mental disease to a dysfunction of the autonomic nervous system", probably at the diencephalic level, was stated by Gellhorn as the purpose of the last two chapters of his 1953 volume devoted to physiological foundations of neurology and psychiatry. "Is it possible to measure central autonomic reactivity in the human being and thereby to obtain objective evidence of an interdependence between mental behavior and the reactivity of autonomic centers?" As a result of testing the reactivity of autonomic centers (by means of blood pressure response to mecholyl) in patients afflicted with neuroses and functional psychoses, and of correlating these responses with changes resulting from shock therapy, Gellhorn noted correlation between improved autonomic response and psychological improvement in response to shock therapy. Where such experiments seemed to indicate that the diencephalon is not at fault, Gellhorn felt that such physiologic therapies as electroshock, insulin coma, and high concentrations of carbon dioxide which act on the diencephalon and alter autonomic balance should not be applied. "Perhaps psychotherapy, whose point of attack must be quite different, should be tried."

There are those that fear that advancing preoccupation, in neurophysiological research, with subcortical regions and mechanisms may go too far: O. L. Zangwill (experimental psychology, Cambridge University), at the Oxford conference, observed, "however much our interest may be drawn to the importance of subcortical mechanisms in connection with the bare facts of wakefulness and sleep", we cannot lose sight of "the relevance of cortical mechanisms to the aspects of consciousness that are responsible for effective intellectual adaptation". There is little real danger, however, that increased attention to subcortical areas, about which much remains to be learned, will inhibit research on the cerebral cortex; work on it has become so greatly intensified within recent decades that periodic reviews, to cite one commentator, are out of date before they can be printed. Only a small part of this large investigative field is touched upon below.

### THE TEMPORAL LOBES

The temporal cortex was described by Penfield, 1954, as "an area of the brain to which no certain function has been previously ascribed". He observed that during the preceding twenty years, in the course of operations on the human brain, he had discovered from time to time that stimulation of the temporal lobe cortex occasionally produced a psychic response. The patient might exclaim in sudden surprise that he heard music or that he saw something he had seen before (the *déja vu* phenomenon) but the patient remained aware of his present environment. In other words, the electrode, applied to the temporal cortex, recalls a specific action or event. It is as though the temporal cortex contained a continuous strip of cinematographic film, a strip that includes the waking record from childhood onward. The functions of the temporal cortex thus suggested were described by Penfield and Jasper as, first, to provide a storehouse of potential recollections and, secondly, to play some role in the comparison of present with past experience.

Connections between the temporal lobe and the cerebral cortex have in recent years been traced electrophysiologically by Gibbs. Clark, stressing comparative neglect of the temporal lobe, had observed that although its anatomical connections are still obscure, it "occupies a strategic position". Through it the cerebral cortex "may exert an important control over regions of the brain not known to influence cerebral activity as a whole". He described the temporal lobe of the cerebrum as a far more distinctive feature of the primate brain than the frontal lobe: "its progressive enlargement was a very early manifestation of the evolutionary development of the primates". He mentioned, 1953, indirect evidence suggesting that the temporal lobe may be functionally connected with "basic mechanisms" such as the hypothalamus, the reticular nuclei of the thalamus, and other regions. One piece of evidence suggesting connections with the hypothalamus was a 1950 report from workers in the Harvard psychiatry department (Chapman, Livingston, Poppen) that electrical stimulation of the tips of the temporal lobes in patients during surgery had an effect upon blood pressure.

### THE FRONTAL LOBES

The frontal lobes, long regarded as the silent areas, because they give no discernible response to stimulation, were described nearly a decade ago by Ward Halstead (experimental psychology, Chicago) as "the portion of the brain most essential to biological intelligence", the organs of civilization, "the basis of man's despair and of his hope". Penfield described enlargement of these lobes in man as without doubt "associated with man's supremacy in the intellectual field". When both frontal lobes are amputated "the luckless individual forfeits capacity for planned initiative. He may have gained peace of mind but he has lost a type of insight that is difficult to define." These lobes account for the conclusion that the sensory and motor elaborations of function are not the only uses of the cerebral cortex. The controversial point has been whether the seat of intelligence could be localized, as it was in older concepts, in the frontal lobes, or whether it is, as in newer concepts, throughout the cortex.

No real antithesis is involved in this argument, according to Clark; the essential fact is that the cerebral cortex provides a mechanism which effectively combines the concepts of functional localization and functional integration. J. LeRoy Conel (research associate, Childrens Hospital, Boston) 1952, on the basis of work on the human cortex at various stages of development, thought the minute parcelling of the cortex into subdivisions "not justified by any significant differences in microscopical structure". Percival Bailey (neurology, University of Illinois College of Medicine) 1952, on the basis of years of neurosurgical work felt "certain" that differences in function between areas of the cortex depend on the external connections rather than upon the intrinsic structure.

Cobb, observing, 1952, that recent experiments (involving cutting association fibers in animals and sectioning the corpus callosum in man) had thrown doubt on the early doctrine that intelligence is physiologically based on associative or long-circuiting mechanisms in the cortex, cited K. U. Smith's view, 1951, of the cerebral cortex as not essentially an organ for association of received and remembered perceptions, but rather a reaction system. Cobb interpreted "modern thinking" (admitting some vagueness in it) concerning the functions of the cerebral cortex as getting away from the idea of local storage and as "approaching a theory of neurons which react in certain combinations, perhaps in patterns of reverberating circuits", the concept supported anatomically by Raymón y Cajal, physiologically by Lorente de Nó. The supporting anatomical data challenged the concept of the brain as a simple, central telephone exchange connecting sensory input with motor output. The reverberating circuit picture envisaged series of small nerve cells besides the main tracts, with short collateral axons "forming many synapses, circuits and nets" which "cause varied delays of the nerve impulses and comprise a mechanism for summation, facilitation, after discharge and inhibition" of nerve impulses. This theory of cerebral mechanisms, according to some electrophysiologists and some psychologists, may some day completely reorient psychological theory of behavior in relation to neurophysiological mechanisms.

Whether finally correct or not, according to Gerard, 1955, "it will be useful to explore further some of the behavioral consequences that can flow from reverberating neurone circuits. It was early pointed out that such circuits free behavior from being time bound to the stimulus. . . . Consciousness and creative behavior are both evoked by the reverberation of circuits, while routine unattended behavior is presumably handled by messages running quickly and with no or minimal repetition through well-grooved 'reflex' channels. Along the same lines, dreams might result from unresolved pressures left from the day or generated from the environment and would represent such continuing reverberation and irradiation in brain neurones. If dreams represent maintained brain activity — as borborygmi accompany a maintained digestive activity — their presence with unresolved situations is physiologically reasonable." Much the same considerations would apply to hallucinations . . . When neural activity is maintained, more and more neurone loops will be activated to that level which is associated with conscious awareness and with focussing of attention. Such a neurophysiological picture is obviously congruent with the psychodynamic one of drives or pressures which are unsatisfied, with the accumulation of something — unfortunately called energy — which finally overflows in healthy or unhealthy ways. On the possible connections between neurophysiological and psychological activity (consciousness, etc.), Gerard observed, it is at least now possible for neurophysiologists to make "informed guesses".

Indeed, the concept of reverberating circuits is beginning to appear as a possible explanation of schizophrenic behavior and even as an approach to therapy, in studies psychological and physiological (at McGill) and in new surgical experiments on the brain of psychotic man (as at Tulane). Some of these have envisaged the schizophrenic as caught in a closed reverberating circuit imprisoning him in his own ideas or hallucinatory world, and excluding the external world, impulses from which were not sufficiently powerful to overcome the reverberating circuits. By another hypothesis, the schizophrenic is imprisoned in lower reverberatory circuits through some improper firing of these from higher areas. Interruption of the lower circuit by electrical stimulation of the higher area presumed to influence it has been tried as an experimental research project on a small series of human schizophrenic subjects (the Tulane project).

Much neurophysiological and neurosurgical work has in the past been concerned with testing the hypothesis that the frontal lobes of the cortex are the particular center for consciousness, for capacity for abstraction (lack of which is frequently cited as an outstanding characteristic of schizophrenics), for intellectual function generally, and for certain aspects of behavior and personality. Unequivocal knowledge is still lacking, however, of specialized functions for the frontal lobes. Referring, 1951, to the status of present knowledge of the functioning of the cerebral cortex, Samuel Beck (at the third research conference on psychosurgery) observed: "I am not saying 'frontal lobes' because we do not know their function." Cobb considered, 1950, that the admittedly "great fund of information concerning the function of the frontal areas" accumulated, for instance, through frontal leucotomy and its recent variations does not "justify localization of special frontal function". Hans Lucas Teuber, describing, 1952, work with M. B. Bender (psychophysiology laboratory, New York University College of Medicine), observed that current studies had singularly failed to prove the point that frontal lesions produce the most marked disturbances in the higher intellectual functions in man. ". . . In contrast to the data available for the macaque, we have yet to find any one deficit characteristic of losses of frontal lobe tissue in man . . ." Admitting that those in their own group with frontal lobe lesions due to gunshot wounds also showed deficits in intellectual function, Teuber added "but the deficits are not specific for frontal lobe lesions, since they appear in equal fashion, and often more markedly, after involvement of the posterior lobe substance . . ."

A University of Wisconsin group (Harlow, experimental psychology) stressed, 1952, their finding that "the different cortical areas play markedly unequal roles in the mediation of our diverse intellectual processes". Hebb registered the support of his group for this general conclusion concerning differential contributions of parts of the cortex to problem-solving. Lashley, 1952, thought that differences in cytoarchitecture suggested that various areas may have fundamentally different types of circuits and hence may differ in the kinds of integration they mediate "but there is no more direct evidence of this". Lashley had "come to believe" that almost every cell in the cerebral cortex may be excited in every activity, that behavior does not depend upon any localized conducting pathways within the cortex, that habits are not stored in any limited area. Such facts point to "the conclusion that there is multiple representation of every function . . ."

Modern concepts of cortical functioning thus stressing the differential contribution of different areas, the significance of connecting tracts, and above all the concept that the cerebral cortex functions as a reaction system, alterations in the components of which constitute the physiological basis of learning, represent, in sum, broadened emphasis on reaction patterns rather than on structural areas.

## Contributions of Electrophysiology to Concepts of the Integrated Activity of the Nervous System

"It has now become almost a complaint", Bates observed at the 1952 Oxford research conference, "that people cannot become neurophysiologists until they have acquired a working knowledge of electronics, and to acquire this is a far more formidable task than it was in the days when the measuring instruments were the kymograph and galvanometer . . ." The concept that the brain is electrically active, not merely when stimulated but also constantly, has been progressively substantiated by electrophysiological work, and in this sense (Hebb, 1949) electrophysiology has been much more than a method and a technique and may be the imminent means of working toward "the ultimate psychological problem, the meaning of behavior and perhaps a new neurophysiological basis for explaining it".

Some physiologists still regard with reserve the electrical techniques as an ultimate dependence. Most physiologists, Burnet commented a few years ago, are now electrophysiologists. He described the recently available gadgets of infinite adaptability for measurement of electrical changes in nervous tissues, the electronic brains and the cybernetics now figuring in research on the nervous system, as "magnificent" but as having "no bearing whatever on the pressing problems of insanity, behavior disorders, and feeblemindedness". He could not escape the feeling that the electrophysiological trend lay also in the direction of infinite and futile elaboration. "I am afraid I feel that way about electrophysiology; but I must also admit that from the president of the Royal Society downwards electrophysiologists have the highest status today in the scientific world." Even some of those whose work has significantly employed electrical techniques in exploring some of the areas and pathways with apparently discernible relation to memory, consciousness and thinking stress rather the hopes than the certainties inhering in electrophysiology. Penfield and Jasper pointed out in their 1954 volume that although it was known seventy-five years ago that electrical currents are generated within the brain "during its activity", the "basic elementary mechanisms underlying the electrical activity of the brain are still poorly understood".

The appeal of electrophysiology is that it is one way of recording what is going on *at the time it is going on*. In the domain of neurophysiology are: the properties of synaptic connections, the structure and reverberating characters of nerve nets and loops; the shape, intensity, and spread of electric and of chemical fields and the associated synchronization of electrical rhythms and discharges (Gerard, 1955). Application of electrophysiological method has made possible such achievements as mapping in detail major sensory areas of the cerebral cortex, as demonstrating that several sensory modalities have specific representations in the cerebellar cortex, as showing that tactile sensibility has a detailed topographical pattern of representation in the thalamus and the dorsal column nuclei. There is a peculiar interdependence in knowledge of electrical effects in the nervous system and structural knowledge of the separate units and areas. Adrian pointed out almost a decade ago (1947) that it is from records of electrical changes in nerve fiber that "we have most of our information about the events which take place in the nerves and the brain". At present, he admitted, we are quite a distance even from understanding the molecular changes which give rise to the difference of electric potential between an active and an inactive part of the cell surface.

On the over-all question of the origin of the brain's electrical activity, many speculations have been offered. Brazier, 1951, referred to it as clearly an aggregation of many components. The Belgian investigator Bremer rested the case on a postulated inherent rhythmicity of all nerve tissue. Lorente de Nó's concept of self-exciting chains of nerves in closed circuits sharply revised the earlier concept of the nervous system as a mere reflex organ.

As yet, however, electrophysiology has not provided an adequate picture of the pattern of electrical activity of even a large group of cells. Bishop observed, 1952, that he did not expect to see in his day "the recording of a large enough complex from the whole brain to represent even the simplest type of mental behavior". Nevertheless, Bates noted that less than fifteen years after the neglected report on the spontaneous electrical rhythm of the brain by Berger, a psychiatrist, had been validated by Adrian, a physiologist, he had seen in Jung's laboratory in Freiburg the record of activity of a single cortical nerve cell in a conscious human subject.

Some micromethods, now intensively applied (in animals) in a few laboratories scattered over the globe, are expected to provide, ultimately, a coherent picture of the coordinated electrical activity of the brain as well as of its unit of activity, the single cell. Microelectrodes, fractions of a thousandth of a millimeter in diameter, inserted into a cell or fiber, are being used (in the laboratory of neurophysiology, Washington University, by Tasaki and associates; in Yale's physiology laboratory by Chang; by Gerard and associates, University of Illinois; at the University of Washington, Seattle, by Amassian and Woodbury; in Australia, by Eccles; in Paris, by Fessard; in the National Institute of Mental Health, by Frank) to study the nature of the nerve cell and of its parts, the action of synaptic structures, the mechanism of transmission of the nerve impulse from cell to cell. Larger electrodes, placed close to units but outside them, to record some one unit preferentially in order to detect the presence or absence of activity of the given unit, are being employed in other laboratories (by Jasper, at McGill; by Lloyd, at the Rockefeller Institute; by Marshall and Frank, at the National Institutes of Health; by Hartline and Kuffler, in the biophysics department of Johns Hopkins). The hope is that, by constantly enlarging the number of electrodes and multiplying the number of simultaneously active zones, the television techniques of electrophysiology may make it possible to distinguish patterns of activity for whole areas. The ultimate objective (John C. Lilly, Johnson foundation for medical physics, University of Pennsylvania, 1952) is "to see and record enough of the electrical action of the brain concurrently with bodily behavior to begin to offer evidence useful in psychiatric research". Then, "pushing this *fantasy* a little further than is cautious", Lilly envisioned the day when it might be possible to "look" into the brain electrically and discover, without interposition of speech or hearing, what needs to be learned. The remoteness of present research from this ultimate objective is indicated by Lilly's observation that at present not even so many as 100 electrodes have been simultaneously activated.

The possibility that new electrophysiological techniques and knowledge may be clinically valuable in approach to problems not now accessible by other techniques and disciplines was suggested by Chang in a 1952 report of his own studies. The result of his work with implanted microelectrodes to discover the electrical response of parts of the single cell led to his observation that "identification of cortical dendritic potential seems to point to a possibility of utilizing the dendritic potential as a means to diagnose certain kinds of nervous disease such as schizophrenia", since impairment of the cortical dendrites can now be demonstrated by ordinary technological techniques.

One illustration of new types of study facilitated by electrophysiological techniques is the recent multidisciplinary study in Tulane's pyschiatry department (Robert G. Heath and associates). The orienting hypothesis of this five-year study was that schizophrenia is a disorder of the "lower levels" of integration; that the septal region, which they defined as embracing connections with the hypothalamus, hippocampus, etc., is probably "a correlating structure interposed between the higher neocortical level and the diencephalic and midbrain structures"; and that while localization of schizophrenia in the septal region is not implied, the septal region is "a key area in which the dynamic process is reflected".

The concrete objective was to demonstrate that the lack of awareness (outstanding in a hundred traits studied intensively in twenty-six schizophrenics, and commonly considered characteristic of the condition) may be related to the septal region. Following a series of experiments in cats and monkeys, the findings were tested in man: craniotomy permitted implanting electrodes in the septal region of twenty-three patients, twenty of whom were schizophrenics and three of whom were victims of intractable pain. Study was made of the results of psychological tests of the patients before and after stimulation of the implanted electrodes. The electrical records, in Heath's view, appeared to offer some confirmation of "our basic hypothesis — that is, that schizophrenia is associated with abnormalities in the septal region of the forebrain".

The report of the Tulane experiments led a conference of leading investigators (neuroanatomists, psychologists, psychiatrists, neurophysiologists, electrophysiologists) to present a considerable number of challenging questions, bearing on many of the conditions of the experiment, on the methods used, on the adequacy of the controls, etc. One of the questions challenged the exclusive specificity of the implanted electrodes to stimulate the specific areas aimed at. The unphysiologic strength of the currents employed (greater than in shock therapy), it was further suggested, might have been destructive rather than stimulating. After all the challenges had been aired, one of the conferees suggested that the surprising feature was not that shortcomings should be found in the work but that it should have been attempted at all.

That electrophysiology may throw light on the cerebral mechanisms presumed to operate in some of the empiric therapies currently employed in mental illness was suggested in the 1952 annual report of the National Institute of Mental Health. Some of the studies noted as under grants from the institute (for example, studies of George A. Ulett, Washington University) were concerned with quantitative recording of changes in brain waves produced during convulsive therapy. Such recordings "may increase understanding of neurophysiological mechanisms related to the therapeutic effects of shock treatment". They should help also in illumining the chemical phenomena resulting from or accompanying shock therapy. Bishop at one time referred to electrophysiology as an essential link between the biochemists and the psychiatrists.

RATIONALE OF ATTEMPTS TO APPLY NEUROPHYSIOLOGICAL PRIN-
CIPLES IN VARIOUS FORMS OF BRAIN SURGERY

Various brain operations (ablation, severing of associative fibers) represent attempts at therapeutic application of present neurophysiological knowledge. Whether these attempts are premature and neurophysiological knowledge is at present inadequate for such direct and practical application is one of the burning questions in this field.

The psychological effects claimed for these operations are briefly mentioned in a later section of this chapter, concerned with psychological emphasis in approaches to schizophrenia. Concern in this section is with the neurophysiological stimulus that has prompted development of these operations and the neurophysiological aims of the procedures. As to the exact neurophysiological objectives, it must be said at once that these surgical procedures do not, in general, rest upon comprehensive and exact knowledge of the tissue that is being ablated or the pathway that is being severed. The extent to which these surgical procedures (grouped under the somewhat unfortunate term, psychosurgery) have, nevertheless, been widely used, in a variety of modifications, for certain forms of mental illness is indicated by the report at the third psychosurgery research conference, 1951, of 18,600 psychosurgical operations for various forms of mental illness in the United States during the fifteen preceding years. Of these, 6,490 were done in state, city or county mental hospitals, ten per cent in general hospitals with psychiatric wards, ten per cent in Veterans Administration hospitals, four per cent in private mental hospitals, twelve per cent in other hospitals included in the survey. As of 1955, the estimated total was reported to be at least 20,000. The operation is used in schizophrenia although a leader in the psychosurgical field, Walter Freeman (neurology, George Washington) in a communication to the American Foundation, 1953, described lobotomy as "less successful with schizophrenics than with other types of functional mental disorder of equal duration. It is frequently successful in early cases, say with disability under six months".

This is not the place to evaluate psychosurgery generally or any of the many forms of it (prefrontal lobotomy, transorbital lobotomy, leucotomy, topectomy, thalamotomy, gyrectomy and variations of some of these). In addition to several comprehensive studies of various procedures in limited series (projects of the Boston Psychopathic Hospital, and of the Columbia Greystone Associates), there are numerous reports of the results of particular operations on particular series and of conclusions drawn from these results. Illustrative is Walter Freeman's 1954 statement that "transorbital lobotomy in the state hospitals of West Virginia has been performed on 602 patients with the result that a substantial number of patients (thirty-eight per cent) are able to live at home". Freeman added that lobotomy is a prime factor in abolishing violent wards, that in a state hospital a lobotomy project accomplishes notable savings in the maintenance of patients; and that discharged patients earn more in a year than the total cost of such a project.

The neurophysiological observations and theories that seem to have led to therapeutic psychosurgery may go back so far as 1928 in which year (as reported by E. Jefferson Browder at the 1951 psychosurgical research conference) a surgeon severed association fibers between the frontal and parietal lobes in three patients in an attempt (not markedly successful) to relieve psychosis. In 1935, Fulton and Jacobsen reported, as earlier mentioned, favorable behavioral changes in chimpanzees following ablation of the frontal association areas. These experimental results were applied to humans by Moniz, and the Moniz technique was used by Freeman and Watts, 1936, in prefrontal leucotomies in patients suffering frequent relapses into the psychotic state.

There have been many modifications of the Moniz technique. "At least four major types of psychosurgery" were mentioned at the 1951 conference: the lateral transcranial operation, the less drastic procedures such as transorbital lobotomy, topectomy, thalamostereotomy. The many changes in procedure and in locus of the operation have reflected developing neurophysiological knowledge. Fulton, for instance, observed in 1951 that "two notable developments" during the preceding three years — first, the use of a more restricted operation; and secondly, adaptation of the operation to the particular mental illness — in his judgment had reduced the empirical nature of the operation and brought it into greater accord with "basic physiology". A part of the development in type of operation, locus and procedure has naturally resulted from psychosurgical experience — from such neurosurgical observations as, for instance, that the closer to the motor cortex the operations of lobotomy were carried out, the greater was the incidence of convulsive seizures.

The development of psychosurgical procedures has paralleled changing concepts of cerebral areas and cerebral functioning. Hypotheses increasingly stressing the related importance of all parts of the brain, and stressing brain functioning as a total phenomenon could not help changing somewhat, in psychosurgery as in other directions, exclusive preoccupation with prefrontal areas, with little reference to the influence upon these of other areas and other pathways. In the 1930's, in the very year of the Fulton-Jacobsen observations on chimpanzees, Penfield and Evans had concluded after extensive removals of the frontal lobe that maximum amputation of the right or left frontal lobe has "for its most important detectable sequel, impairment of those mental processes which are prerequisite to planned initiative". In 1948, Penfield (reporting a short series of bilateral frontal gyrectomies, designed as a hopeful substitute for lobotomy) concluded that the "farther the bilateral excision extended back into the superior portion of the intermediate frontal cortex, the more severe was the intellectual deficit". In later observations Penfield pointed out that while one frontal lobe could be removed with little or no detectable deficit, large removal of one lobe extending back into the superior intermediate frontal area would damage those conscious intellectual processes essential to well-planned initiative and to understanding of future consequences of present action. Denny-Brown, 1951, had described the damage to the frontal lobes through leucotomy as resulting in "peculiar indifference to the seriousness or indeed painful consequences of any situation".

A sound neurological basis for psychosurgery would require (in addition to more precise and better standardized methods) comprehensive, detailed and differentiated neurophysiological data. Lack of this inclines the objective observer to balance against reports of "dramatically" beneficial effects of psychosurgery and against the favorable implication of such a study as that at the Boston Psychopathic Hospital, such conclusions as that of Kenneth E. Livingston, resulting from intensive experimental work (especially concerned with representation of autonomic function in the back part of the frontal lobe): "In spite of extensive experiments with modified forms of the lobotomy procedure, the minimal effective anatomical lesion has not been defined and the physiological basis for the operation has not yet been clearly established."

Also to be taken into account is the view of some workers in the mental field that the amount of neurophysiological information available is not yet sufficient to justify the hazards. There is a somewhat ominous implication in the usual recommendation that psychosurgery be used only "after everything else has been tried", and even then only if the degree of the patient's suffering and/or the difficulties in managing him seem to justify a therapeutic step so serious and so irreversible. Making frenetic patients institutionally manageable is, it is pointed out, an objective quite different from the cure of the individual. Analysis of the effects has not progressed to the point of making possible even a clear definition of the hazards. A rough and ready estimate of the hazards by Francis C. Grant (neurosurgery, University of Pennsylvania), at the 1951 research conference, outlining "what a standard lobotomy may be expected to do for a patient with intractable pain and an inoperable lesion", gave such a patient a ninety-two per cent chance of surviving, an eighty per cent chance of complete relief from pain, a forty per cent chance of change in personality.

Some — apparently not few — neurologists and psychiatrists consider the risk too great. Until neurophysiological knowledge is more adequate, they are repelled by the idea of applying any surgical, anatomical and physiological procedure to functioning so integrated and so complex as that of the human brain in intelligence and in behavior. So powerful and so radical an expedient, they reason, is not adapted to empirical use. Brain operations were described, 1953, by L. J. Meduna, in a communication to the American Foundation, as a straight admission of our ignorance: "We do not know what schizophrenia is; we cannot cure it; and therefore we cut out that part of the brain which enables the patient to mind his own condition. From that point on, the patient loses his capacity to 'mind' and therefore he is satisfied."

As a research tool Fulton described psychosurgery as having

opened new horizons in the "fundamental sphere of the functions of the central nervous system in relation to emotional expression and also to the integration of intellectual function".

NEUROPHYSIOLOGICAL WORK ON THE NERVE IMPULSE AS<br>RELATED TO EFFORTS TO EXPLAIN BEHAVIOR

The nerve impulse, according to Eccles, 1953, is to be regarded as the universal currency of the nervous system. While much of the neurophysiological work dealing with the origin and transmission of nerve impulses may seem indeed remote from the objective of explaining behavior, it is considered by many to be a necessary precedent to defining the gap that certainly still exists between sensory and motor mechanisms and behavior. Even in mammals so low as the rat, Hebb pointed out in 1949, it has not been found possible to describe behavior as an interaction directly between sensory and motor processes: "Something like *thinking* . . . intervenes" and it is clear that behavior (even in the rat) is not completely controlled by immediate sensory events: "There are central processes operating also."

Neurophysiologists generally would agree that further advances in understanding cerebral function (and certainly in understanding schizophrenia) depend primarily on testing hypotheses that envisage central activity in terms of nerve fiber conduction and synaptic transmission. Bard pointed out, 1952, that the present day neurophysiologist has the same regard for his knowledge of nerve conduction that William Harvey's followers had for the demonstration that blood circulates because of the motions of the heart. Work on the mechanism of conduction of the nerve impulse developed largely in the 1920's, including the work of Erlanger and Gasser. Many questions concerned with the mechanisms of propagation of the nerve impulse along the neuron and across the synapses remain unanswered and there are many hypotheses designed to explain the nerve impulse whether in relation to resting nerve or to active nerve during excitation. Outstanding is the membrane or ionic hypothesis, postulating selective permeability of a neuronal membrane to potassium and sodium ions. Eccles described the ionic hypothesis, 1953, as still "in an early stage of development" but as providing an essential basis for further work. Modifications of the ionic hypothesis have resulted from work of

Lorente de Nó, Ralph Gerard and British workers, A. L. Hodgkin, A. S. Huxley. Regarded as a classical theory, it has nevertheless not been conclusively established. Since the neuronal membrane itself has not been seen directly but merely inferred from biochemical and physicochemical evidence, there are those who question its existence.

The importance of synaptic transmission of the nerve impulse lies in the fact that the synapse is the site at which delay and inhibition of the impulse takes place. The physiology of the synapse includes transmission of excitation at the neuromuscular junction as well as at synapses in autonomic ganglia and in the central nervous system. In the view of some investigators, the building up of "neuronic reaction-complexes" to form the continuous thought of the individual — memory, learning, capacity to draw upon old experience, to form judgments when faced with new experience — may depend upon what happens at the synapse perhaps in terms of organic, chemical or electrical change. The premises are as yet unproved but various workers consider the role of synapse as a key problem ultimately linking mind and brain.

Referring to present intensive study of transmission at the synapse, Bard observed, 1952, that while the problem has been well outlined and while much useful information has been obtained by recording potential changes, both slow and rapid, from gross electrodes on or in the cord and on spinal roots, interpretation of some of the results has been both difficult and varied. In his view, some of Eccles's studies, recording potential changes within the somata of individual spinal neurons, are likely to "reshape some of our thinking about the intimate character of synaptic processes". Bard thought it likely that further testing, "at the subcellular level", of the hypothesis that basically both excitation and inhibition are mediated by chemical transmitters, will lead to a substantial breakthrough in neurophysiology.

In spite of all the unsolved problems connected with the purely neurophysiological aspects of transmission of the nerve impulse, Bard expressed the view that recent fundamental work by Hodgkin, Curtis and Cole, by Lorente de Nó and others suggests that the remaining mysteries may be greatly reduced in the near future. He mentioned, as perhaps the least understood aspect, the way in which energy is made available for conduction, particularly for restitution of the resting potential. While the techniques of enzyme chemists have not yet been able fully to determine the specific chemical changes involved, significant advances toward this knowledge were, in Bard's view, being made.

Recognizing the vastness of the gap still existing between demonstrable physical and chemical fact on the one hand and learning, consciousness, intelligence on the other, H. J. Muller observed, 1955: "As, through association and analysis, an increasingly coherent and serviceable formulation or representation of the world outside becomes built up out of the neuronic reaction-complexes, we become justified in speaking of intelligence". Something of what happens in that mysterious process by which "the nerve impulse is somehow converted into thought and thought converted into nerve impulses" (Penfield) was simply set forth by Adrian, 1951: "The sensory inflow brings information about the events taking place outside" but before the response is made (at any but the immediate reflex level) "the great central mass of nerve cells has to fabricate a radically different pattern of messages to send out to the muscles". That pattern depends on "what happened to us a year ago as well as on what is happening now", *i.e.*, on stored memories, previously learned information and reactions, making it possible to "interpret" incoming sensory messages in the light of past experience, involving "learning", cognition, choice, behavior.

The reason why defense of the old idea that the input shapes the structure of the output is "a losing fight" (Weiss, 1951) is that without the aid of, and prior to the appearance of a sensory input from the outside world, basic behavior patterns are developed within the nervous system "by virtue of the laws of its own embryonic differentiation". The basic configuration of these motor patterns "cannot possibly be a direct product of the patterns of the sensory input". The sensory input is required for release, facilitation and modification but not for the primary shaping of the output. The nervous system is not a network of monotonic elements, but rather "a hierarchical system in which groups of neuronal complexes of different kinds are acting as units, the properties of which determine the configuration of the output pattern. Some of these higher units are rigidly fixed in their functions, others are modifiable by experience." Even the simplest nervous system, Weiss summarized, has three primary attributes — autonomy of pattern, rhythmic automatism and hierarchical organization — "and this, I think, unifies our view of the nervous system".

The problem of pattern, structural and functional, was described (Bishop, 1946) as the central problem of neurophysiology. And the patterns are those not of a static but rather of a dynamic, constantly active system or a composite of many interacting systems. It is "practically certain" (Lashley, 1951) "that all the cells of the cerebrospinal axis are being continually bombarded by nerve impulses from various sources and are firing regularly probably even during sleep". The input, according to this premise, is never into a static system, but rather into a system that is already actively excited and organized. "In the intact organism, behavior is the result of interaction of this background of excitation with input from any designated stimulus." It is determined not by the activation of isolated paths through an otherwise resting system but by momentary patterns of synchronous firing involving large areas.

Commenting on the expectation that such patterns may ultimately provide the missing link between mind and brain, Russell Brain, 1951, soberly emphasized the immensity and complexity of the task involved: "Not only are there twelve thousand million nerve cells out of which the patterns can be made, but nervous patterns exist in time, like a melody, as well as in space. If you look at a tapestry through a magnifying glass you will see the individual threads, not the pattern; if you stand away from it you will see the pattern but not the threads. My guess is that in the nervous system we are looking at the threads, while in the mind we perceive the patterns, and that one day we shall discover how the patterns are made of the threads." The psychologist as well as the neurophysiologist is thus concerned with patterns (Lashley, 1952), "but the patterns of behavior differ in a fundamental way from those of structure. The structure is fixed like the keys of a piano but the behavior patterns play over the structure, as the fingers of a musician play over the keys, producing the characteristic chords . . . throughout the range of the keyboard. The ultimate task of neurophysiology is to discover the relation between the fixed structural patterns and the evanescent functional ones . . ."

## TRENDS IN DOMINANTLY BIOCHEMICAL WORK

### INTRODUCTORY: CURRENT HYPOTHESES CONCERNING CHEMICAL FACTORS

While conceding that the biochemical approach to schizophrenia is "not more basic than any other approach" (Mirsky), many workers concerned with other approaches have an increasingly chemistry-conscious outlook. Some of the biochemical work pertinent to schizophrenia is related to physiological systems other than the nervous, and has been going on for many years. For it has long been recognized that the metabolic changes found in patients with psychoses "are either cause or effect of the psychoses, or both; they cannot be regarded as neither". The biochemical work briefly reviewed in this section is confined to the nervous system; all other systems (*e.g.*, circulatory, endocrine), as Eccles pointed out, 1953, "produce their effects on the 'mind' or 'self' secondarily to their direct or indirect action on the brain". Recognition of the importance of biochemical factors in mental illness has been responsible for establishment of particular laboratories for study of cerebral metabolism in a few mental hospitals (most of them associated with medical schools) as at the University of California, 1953, the McLean Hospital, 1944, and at the National Institute of Mental Health. The staffs of these laboratories, concentrating on the chemistry and metabolism of the brain, are progressively carrying their work to deeper levels, obviously subscribing to Hoagland's observation that all behavior depends upon physiological events determined basically at the molecular level.

As yet it cannot be maintained that biochemical work directed toward mental illness has in great degree penetrated to the molecular level. Nor have chemical correlates of behavior been as yet either fundamental or persuasive. Describing present attempts at unraveling the chemical pathology of mental disease as "little more than shots in the dark", Derek Richter added, 1950, that in schizophrenia, "which is perhaps the biggest single problem in the whole of medicine", we still have practically no quantitative data on the biochemical composition of the brain, on the distribution of the lipids, nucleoproteins, or most other substances of biochemical interest. The biochemical problems that will need to be solved if psychiatry is to be provided with a firm biochemical basis have been described as sufficient to keep generations of investigators productively employed.

Weiss, 1951, in stressing subtle chemical relations as "instrumentalities in biological relations in general", urged more intensive study of these relations in the nervous system. Here, there is clear evidence that different types of nerve cells have distinctive characteristics "decisive in the making and breaking of functional connections and that conformance or nonconformance between elements may decide whether a synaptic junction will be passable or impassable". The fact that correlations between these subtle chemical reactions and nerve excitability and response are not significantly demonstrable, and that correlations between these subtle chemical reactions and behavior are even less demonstrable, does not alter, as many workers have pointed out, the necessity of working toward them.

Belief in the goal, however remote, gives significance to even the most highly limited studies of the chemistry and metabolism of the brain and the nervous system; to study of chemical phenomena in nerve excitation and transmission; to study of the key processes of shock therapy on the theory that the biochemical phenomena induced by shock should throw light on schizophrenic processes. It supplies perspective for wide study of drugs and chemical substances which, used empirically, seem to have therapeutic value in schizophrenia or which appear to produce, in animals or man, psychological effects comparable to characteristic symptoms of schizophrenia.

With reference to the nerve impulse briefly discussed in the preceding section, there has been a "welcome decline" in the "dichotomizing approach" which at one time tended to force a choice between *either* electrical *or* chemical (acetylcholine) factors in transmission of nerve impulses. The pluralistic view is not new; it was stressed by Bronk so early as 1939, by Gerard, and by others. Almost a decade ago Bishop observed: "Emphasis in work on the excitatory process seems to be shifting from concern with electrical versus chemical transmission to the question of the relation of chemical and electrical phenomena in the institution of the impulse. That excitation in general has an electrical sign, and that the chemical environment may affect both the intensity of response and the ability of the adjacent tissue to be excited in propagation, has been obvious enough.

The question is, can one or another chemical phenomenon be considered the one essential of excitation, say of the change in the membrane's resistance, viewing other agents as modifiers of this process." At the third Macy conference on the nerve impulse, F. O. Schmitt expressed the view that current knowledge did not justify exclusive concentration on acetylcholine to the exclusion of other possible elements: "As in the case of muscle, much biochemistry of intermediary metabolism, of enzymes, of proteins and of other components will probably have to be done before nerve mechanisms can be viewed except as through a glass darkly . . ."

Different concepts of the role of acetylcholine are now to be considered as differences in emphasis rather than as sharp antitheses. Dale's suggestion in 1914 that acetylcholine was the substance whose action was most suggestive of mediation of nerve impulses was described, 1955, by A. S. V. Burgen and F. C. MacIntosh, (physiology, McGill) as "brilliantly justified". These investigators, after summarizing the evidence in favor of the chief proposals concerning roles of acetylcholine in nerve activity, pointed out that, while most physiologists would probably agree on a number of these proposals, "there would be no unanimous assent to any one proposition". The vigor of some of the objections to Dale's proposal (1936) that acetylcholine is the mediator, probably the sole mediator, for transmission of excitation from the motor nerve endings to skeletal muscle has diminished in the face of the recently summarized "very strong" evidence referred to above. As for the role of acetylcholine in transmission of excitation at synapses of autonomic ganglia, Burgen and MacIntosh considered the evidence also very strong, although here also dissenters favor the evidence for electrical transmission. The role of acetylcholine in transmission at autonomic postganglionic nerve endings has been studied chiefly in terms of vagal endings impinging upon heart and stomach muscle and on sweat glands. In 1921 Otto Loewi isolated a chemical agent, which he identified, 1926, as acetylcholine, at the junction between vagus nerve endings and heart muscle. Burgen and MacIntosh found no opposing evidence over the intervening years but also no direct evidence that acetylcholine is the sole transmitter of excitation at these autonomic neuromuscular junctions. Within recent years, acetylcholine has been postulated as not only the junctional transmitter but also as playing an essential part in conducting the impulse along the axon. Proposed by von Muralt in 1937 this hypothesis has been extended since 1946 by Nachmansohn and his associates at Columbia whose work has emphasized the unity in activity of nerve cells with all other cells and has pointed to the need for integration of energy-producing metabolism with electrical manifestations of nerve activity. The evidence so far appears to satisfy many physiologists, but critics of Nachmansohn's concept of acetylcholine as an essential part of the metabolic cycles that result in alteration of the permeability of the nerve membrane and consequent production of the electric potential (which probably transmits the impulse) appear to regard it as not established although possible.

With accumulating evidence that acetylcholine acts as the transmitter of excitation at the synapses of autonomic (cholinergic) ganglia, the question has become more insistent whether acetylcholine transmits excitation at the synapses of the central nervous system. On the basis of work in England (Feldberg, Gaddum, Young) and Australia (Eccles), Burgen and MacIntosh observed that even if it is not the universal central synaptic transmitter, the acetylcholine theory, alone, accounts convincingly and satisfactorily for many observations although there is no direct evidence for any one synapse. Some progress can be expected from knowledge of acetylcholine synthesis, shown by work in Nachmansohn's and Lipmann's laboratories since 1945 to require energy from adenosinetriphosphate and acetylcoenzyme A, and thus to be linked with intermediary processes in all cells. That the tricarboxylic acid cycle through which oxidative energy is produced and made available for the activities of all cells exists in brain cells was considered by R. A. Peters (biochemistry, Oxford) proved "beyond further doubt" by work in his laboratory, 1953. Work since 1939 (J. H. Quastel, biochemistry, McGill; others) has resulted in significant findings: acetylcholine and its enzymes are found in large amounts in the central nervous system, some neurons in which are highly sensitive to acetylcholine; anticholinesterase drugs affect the activity of the central nervous system; changes in central nervous system activity are associated with transient changes in concentration of acetylcholine, which appears to be released with physiological activity, especially of the cerebral cortex. Some studies of acetylcholine in the brain have been directed to the possible significance of it in mental disorders, including schizophrenia.

In man, the psychotic nature of the reactions resulting from administration of an antagonist of acetylcholine, diisopropyl fluorophosphate (used as are mescaline and lysergic acid for "experimental" induction of psychotic reactions) was attributed to "partial inactivation of brain cholinesterase" by some (as noted by Pope, 1952, in reviewing the field) but by others (as noted by Lilienthal, 1952) to interference with cellular respiratory mechanisms not involving acetylcholine. In a study of cholinesterase activity in human cortical biopsies (twelve deteriorated schizophrenic patients and nonpsychotic controls), Pope found, 1952, that five of the twelve showed an over-all cholinesterase activity in excess of the range in the nonpsychotic controls, suggesting exhaustion of acetylcholine supplies. While he considered the series too small to justify conclusions, Pope thought his findings did at least "suggest a chronic increase in the rate of neuronal discharge in the cortex" of the schizophrenic patients. Hemphill and Reiss observed, 1950: "If all the statements concerning acetylcholine production and nerve transmission are true, it is reasonable to expect that abnormalities in the production or destruction of acetylcholine should produce deviations from normal mental activity . . ."

## OXIDATIVE METABOLISM OF THE BRAIN — ESPECIALLY CARBOHYDRATE UTILIZATION — IN SCHIZOPHRENIA

Knowledge of the metabolic mechanisms involved in providing the energy for the brain's work has come, over the past twenty years, from some of the major biochemical laboratories of the world (those of Warburg, Meyerhof, the Coris, Krebs, Lipmann) concerned not with schizophrenia nor indeed with any aspect of the relation of neural function to behavior, normal or abnormal, but rather with the mechanisms involved in the production, transformation and utilization of energy in all tissues.

Interest in carbohydrate metabolism in schizophrenia although largely concerned with nervous tissue has not been restricted to it. There have been more generalized, but not broadly productive, approaches concerned, for instance, with comparisons of more or less accepted indices of carbohydrate metabolism in normal and in schizophrenic patients. Meduna, whose concern with carbohydrate metabolism, 1953, was associated with his hope of ultimately developing a chemical or biological treatment to replace shock therapies in schizophrenia, noted disturbed carbohydrate metabolism in certain groups of schizophrenic patients. His studies over many years suggested to him the presence of an abnormal anti-insulin factor in blood and urine of patients diagnosed as schizophrenic. Gerard, who assigned "a large role to metabolic factors in schizophrenia, with emphasis on carbohydrate metabolism and endocrine factors", described work at the Neuropsychiatric Institute, Illinois, by I. Boszormenyi-Nagy, as suggesting "a general cellular difference in carbohydrate metabolism in schizophrenics as compared to normals", *i.e.*, breakdown of glycogen in erythrocytes from a group of schizophrenics followed a qualitatively different path than that in erythrocytes from normal persons. The more intensive and progressive biochemical work directed toward mental illness, however, has been concerned with carbohydrate metabolism in the brain, oriented by the conviction that the metabolic basis of the electrical activity of the brain inheres (Gibbs) in its close relation to oxidation of glucose by the brain's nerve cells.

Broadly speaking, it is considered that the functioning of brain tissue *in vivo* depends "in the main" upon oxidation of the sugar carried to it by the blood, the small store of glycogen present serving only temporarily as a reserve (R. A. Peters, 1955). It has been calculated, for instance, that between eighty and ninety per cent of that functioning is sustained by metabolism of the blood glucose reaching the brain. When the blood glucose is depleted, as in hypoglycemia, it has been found that oxidation of noncarbohydrate substances, ordinarily suppressed by the presence of glucose, begins, but at a relatively low rate. There is no evidence of oxidation of fat (K. A. C. Elliott, Montreal Neurological Institute, 1955). That only glucose serves to restore the function of brain cells after insulin-induced hypoglycemia may be explained (Meyerhof, biochemistry, Pennsylvania, 1952) by findings in Cori's laboratory that, whereas liver and muscle have several hexokinases (enzymes activating the first step in glucose utilization), brain tissue contains only one. "Why", Cori asked, 1952, "is glucose essential when pyruvate could, from an energy standpoint, be just as effective as glucose, although it is not equivalent to glucose? We know, of course, all the steps that occur between glucose and pyruvate. Their function is one of the mysteries, I believe."

As to oxygen: the suggestive finding is that cells of the cerebral cortex, if deprived of oxygen for more than five to ten minutes, will not completely recover (other parts of the brain and spinal cord may recover if the period of oxygen deprivation has not exceeded twenty to thirty minutes).

Studies of the mechanisms involved in the above findings are of first importance in attempts to establish the relation of oxidation of glucose to schizophrenia, and in confirming or refuting the view of various workers (as Meduna, 1953) that undue acceleration or retardation of oxidation of glucose in the brain must result in "alterations of the thresholds of cells and consequently in relation to their activity of external stimulation". A step toward investigating oxygen supply to the brain, dependent upon cerebral circulation, was described by Kety, 1953, in work in the laboratory of cerebral metabolism at the National Institute of Mental Health concerned with developing a technique for studying the blood supply to every portion of the brain during life. "Previously the only method of studying the brain was by autopsy when the condition and functions of the living brain could not be observed." There were, as yet, no generally applicable techniques for studying the localized metabolism of the brain *in vivo*, with a minimum of disturbance of function and relations. No method had as yet been devised for measuring glucose consumption in the brain of living subjects even to the degree that oxygen consumption could be measured.

On the level of physiological and psychological effects of interruption or diminution of glucose oxidation in the brain through oxygen lack, there is a body of data, originating largely from wartime work in aviation medicine. Disturbances of sensation, memory, visual function, behavior in atmospheric conditions of high altitudes have confirmed the dependence of the brain on blood-borne oxygen. Other studies of oxygen consumption of brain tissue, possibly ultimately relevant to hypotheses invoking cerebral metabolism, especially inhibition of oxygen consumption, as a cause or approach to cure of schizophrenia, have been oriented toward analysis of the mechanism of action on nerve tissue of anesthetics, analgesics, narcotics, convulsants, nutritional deficiencies, drugs and chemicals studied experimentally or clinically in modification of nervous activity. To a lesser degree, data have accumulated from studies of the physiological effects of lowered blood sugar as a means of diminishing the energy-producing metabolism of the brain in connection with insulin shock as a hazard of insulin therapy of diabetes, and with the physiological and psychological effects of insulin shock therapy used empirically since 1927 in treatment of schizophrenia.

Theories directly implicating abnormalities in the oxidative metabolism of the brain in schizophrenia, whether expressed in terms of oxygen lack or carbohydrate lack, serve chiefly at present to indicate possible directions of approach to study of brain metabolism in the living subject. While the theories are highly speculative and may be wrong, "if we didn't have some hypotheses, we could hardly find experiments we wanted to do" (Gerard, 1952). McFarland, 1952, referred to numerous early studies, including his own in 1938, suggesting oxygen deficiency in certain forms of schizophrenia but he also thought that conclusive evidence was yet to be obtained that impaired oxidation is of *primary* importance in schizophrenia. Of its significance, however, he had no doubt; he cited his own and other experiments over many years on animals and man, indicating sensory and mental deterioration in normal subjects "and even loss of insight" resulting from anoxia. These findings confirmed his belief that "the so-called 'psychic' functions appear to be related to velocities of certain chemical processes in the tissues" and that these, rather than "repression or regression influenced by emotional mechanisms", provide the basis for mental disease. Nathaniel Kleitman (physiology, University of Chicago, 1952) correlated "greater degrees of awareness" with "greater oxygen consumption". While the extent to which central neurones are caused to "fire" by changes in their immediate chemical environment, rather than by nerve impulses, is not known, it "may be very large" (Gerard, 1955).

Kety, referring, 1953, in a communication to the American Foundation, to an earlier study of a group of young male schizophrenics considered sufficiently large to justify a conclusion, found that total cerebral blood flow and cerebral oxygen consumption in patients with schizophrenia was not markedly different from those values in normal young men. He suggested, however, that normal cerebral metabolism in schizophrenia might simply mean that it takes just as much oxygen to think an irrational thought as to think a rational thought. He also pointed out that over-all metabolic rate may not adequately measure the metabolism of local areas of the brain. From this conviction followed his study, mentioned earlier, at the National Institute of Mental Health, of blood supply to local areas. The attempt to relate the oxygen consumption of the brain to its more abstruse functions was described by him at the 1952 meeting of the Association for Research in Nervous and Mental Diseases, as an effort to "bridge a very large gap". While there is "a great deal of reason at the present time to think that the oxygen consumption of the brain is a necessary and a vital constituent of cerebral metabolism and mental activity", he observed, it is "analogous to the energy which is needed to keep the filaments of the electronic tubes in a radio hot, and what the tubes do with their heated filaments may be a question of an entirely different order". Trying to find differences in over-all cerebral oxygen consumption associated with changes in mental activity or function might, he thought, be "something like trying to tell the differences between the Philadelphia Orchestra and a high school band on the basis of the caloric intake of the players".

In view of developing concepts of oxidative or energy-producing cellular metabolism (in all organisms from yeast cells to man) as carried out in its final stages through the uninterrupted turning of the oxidative mill (the citric acid or Krebs cycle), utilizing all foodstuffs, whether carbohydrate, fat or protein, the apparent dependence of brain cells upon glucose for fuel has puzzling aspects. It would be difficult to envisage brain metabolism as operating outside the principles of the "metabolic pool" of Schoenheimer or the energy transfer system of Lipmann, involving utilization of all foodstuffs and not merely carbohydrates. Concepts of the biological unity of all living cells in terms of energy-producing metabolism give a certain significance, therefore, to more or less isolated observations or proposed studies of alterations in brain metabolism outside the carbohydrate pathways.

One of these observations, suggesting a possible role for amino acids in oxidative metabolism of the brain, is that glutamic acid, an amino acid of increasing biochemical interest, is oxidized, after several intervening steps, *via* the citric acid cycle (S. Ratner, pharmacology, New York University, 1954). Glutamic acid has been described as "the most important of noncarbohydrate materials oxidizable by the brain" *in vitro* and the "only amino acid which has been found to be oxidizable in this tissue", although not so readily oxidizable as glucose and not capable of replacing glucose *in vivo* (Elliott, 1952). The observation that glutamic acid seemed to increase mental activity in feebleminded children led to a few studies of glutamic acid in relation to schizophrenia. Studies with microquantitative techniques have shown that glutamine, the amide of glutamic acid, penetrates the blood-brain barrier more easily than its parent substance. Restoration following intravenous glutamic acid of animals in insulin coma, which was accompanied by increase in blood sugar insufficient to restore consciousness, may have been due to a catalytic stimulation of the central nervous system rather than to oxidation of the amino acid in the brain (Heinrich B. Waelsch, New York State Psychiatric Institute, 1955).

Knowledge of complexes of proteins with nucleic acids (nucleoproteins) and with lipids (lipoproteins) is recognized as essential to understanding the structure and activities of all living cells. Studies of changes in nucleoprotein metabolism in the brain cells of schizophrenics were reported, 1948, by the cell physiologists, Holger Hyden and Hans Hartelius (Karolinska Institutet, Stockholm), who had long been concerned with the role of nucleic acids in vital processes. Work since the early thirties in Caspersson's laboratory at the institute had resulted in development of methods for determining the chemical, especially protein, composition of individual cellular structures. Hyden and Hartelius, using chemicals to stimulate nucleoprotein formation in the cell, found that administration of malononitrile was followed in rabbits by functional stimulation of nerve cells, and in schizophrenics by evidence of mental stimulation. They also reported cytochemical studies indicating decreased nucleoproteins in nerve cells removed during frontal lobotomy from the pyramidal area of seven schizophrenics.

Attention to influences associated with lipid metabolism has at least opened up new vistas in mental research, as it has, increasingly, in many other fields. A pattern can be discerned suggesting that most, if not all, of brain lipids, which constitute half of its solids (Hemphill and Reiss, 1950), are lipoproteins (Folch-Pi, 1952). In pointing out that modern techniques have opened this field to "all comers", Folch-Pi suggested that knowledge of this type "holds promise of throwing light on the physiology of brain, both in health and in disease". Further study of brain lipids and lipid compounds might, he thought, have especial relevance to development and maturity. Research on brain metabolism is obviously at the stage of finding not the right answers but the right questions.

## BIOCHEMICAL PHENOMENA IN SHOCK THERAPY AS POSSIBLY ILLUMINATING SCHIZOPHRENIC PROCESSES

On the theory that the key processes involved in insulin shock therapy are reduction of oxidation of glucose or of energy-producing metabolism in the brain, considerable attention has been given to shock therapy as a means of throwing light on schizophrenia. "Unfortunately", as pointed out by Henry W. Brosin (psychiatry, University of Pittsburgh, 1952), "there has been no comprehensive study linking this clinical work with the large amount of research on hypoxia on airmen and the high altitude studies which were stimulated by the war." Kety pointed out, 1950, that in schizophrenics receiving insulin shock, "cerebral oxygen consumption was reduced to fifty per cent of the normal figure while the utilization of glucose in the blood was practically negligible". By Kety's calculation, "the glycogen of the brain will support cerebral metabolism for about ninety minutes at the low level present in coma. This period is roughly equivalent to the time in which the patient may remain in deep hypoglycemic coma without irreversible damage to the brain . . ." That sympathetic centers are stimulated by lack of blood sugar for normal oxidative mechanisms in the brain was suggested by Gellhorn (1938) who considered that the central nervous system mechanisms operate at the diencephalic level as a regulator of autonomic activity.

Himwich considered that the common denominator in all shock therapies, either hypoglycemic or convulsive, is deprivation of energy:

"oxidative metabolism is inadequate to support cerebral function, and anaerobic breakdown of energy deposits is called upon to maintain the brain". In the hypoglycemia of insulin shock, he considered, the brain is deprived of glucose and cerebral metabolic rate is depressed below normal levels; in electroshock or metrazol convulsions, "brain activity is raised to such a high pitch that it cannot be sustained by the oxygen and sugar coming to the brain in the blood . . ." He considered that "the longer and more gradual assault made by hypoglycemia" yielded better results for some types of schizophrenia, the shorter and more intense convulsive attack better results for the affective psychoses. The consecutive group of signs or symptoms appearing as the reaction to insulin progresses in hypoglycemia was interpreted by Himwich, 1953, as gradual changes in function in areas of the brain, beginning with the higher cerebral areas and finally reaching the medulla. He thought this gradual progression might mean that utilization of sugar varies in different parts of the brain.

Another theory (cited by Elliott, 1952) as to what happens in the brain cells deprived of glucose because insulin has lowered the blood sugar is that in the absence of glucose the cells may use "non-carbohydrate material", presumably from the cell structure, and this "would be expected to alter the functional condition of the tissue". Sakel's hypothesis, 1950, of the mechanism of reduced blood sugar levels by insulin administration included the proposal that the altered metabolism forces the dormant cells of the brain to function actively and to take over the functioning of the "psychotically acting cells" which are suppressed by the "many component factors" of the insulin treatment. By the Sakel concept, the brain, the main organ for performing and processing mental and emotional activities, operates with only a fraction of its specific nerve cells assigned to a given function, most of the brain cells being dormant, in reserve, but under normal circumstances not always on call. If part of the nerve cell group of the brain is diseased, the processing of thought and associations performed by this employed fraction will naturally produce distorted thoughts and psychotic reactions. The dormant reserve cells of the brain are not automatically called upon to compensate or substitute for the malfunctioning cells as in other vital organs, and therefore do not automatically take over to carry on the normal function. Permanent "cure" in schizophrenia, according to Sakel's hypothesis, would depend upon the ability of the reserve cells to take over permanently the functions of "distorted and therapeutically eliminated brain cells" that were responsible for malfunctioning in psychosis.

The light that study of shock therapy throws on brain metabolism and on metabolic approaches to cure of mental illness is subject to varying evaluations. Discussing Himwich's views of the effects of lack of blood sugar on brain metabolism presented at the symposium of the Association for Research in Nervous and Mental Diseases, C. F. Terrence (director, Rochester State Hospital) — on the basis of hypoglycemic treatment of over 1,000 schizophrenic patients, 500 of whom had been followed up for more than ten years — found, 1953, "no facts to present that by this treatment any permanent change occurs that alters the pathways or does anything to alter the metabolism of an individual cell or groups of cells or a part of the brain". Meduna, endorsing, 1953, the necessity that therapy must be physiological, included insulin coma in his observation that all the present treatments in schizophrenia involving shock and brain operations "are to say the least stupid and barbaric treatments". What should be sought, in his view, is "a treatment that will do away completely with the coma and the shock and produce the biological and biochemical changes necesssary to cure schizophrenia".

This brief review is concerned only with the metabolic mechanisms predicated for insulin shock and not with present evaluation of shock as therapy. Such evaluation would offer present difficulties. On the one hand, there is considerable testimony similar to a recent report from the New York State Department of Mental Hygiene that, as a result of the development of the various shock therapies, the recovery rate for schizophrenia has tripled over the last forty years. On the other hand, there are statements such as that of Meduna above and those of other workers who regard all forms of shock as still at best "very crudely guided procedures". Summarizing opinion in 1949, Leopold Bellak wrote, "it may well be that no one of the shock treatments brings about a long-range improvement or recovery or even an over-all decrease of the length of hospitalization". In some recognition of what has been added to present knowledge, Kety observed that whether or not we accept insulin therapy as important in treatment of schizophrenia, "we can certainly agree that insulin therapy has led to a considerable increase in our understanding of carbohydrate metabolism in the brain".

### INCRIMINATION OF TOXIC WASTE PRODUCTS IN SCHIZOPHRENIA

Metabolic changes appear to be fundamentally associated with mental disorders and psychoses resulting from or accompanying such conditions as infection, intoxication, trauma, circulatory disturbance, convulsive disorders, nutritional deficiencies, endocrine imbalances, new growths. In most of these, exact allocation of the origin of the neurological, biochemical or psychological disorder often offers great difficulty, but there is no doubt of the metabolic causes or accompaniments or effects. One hypothesis as described, 1953, by James W. Papez (state laboratory for biological research, Columbus State Hospital) envisaged the possibility, in schizophrenia, of a causal character for a toxic waste product (an amine $NH_2$, possibly histamine) of an infectious living organism of a lower order of life of extracerebral origin. This organism was reported to cause degenerative cytochemical changes visible under the microscope in the cytoplasm of cells, especially cells in the region of the cerebral cortex and thalamus.

In studies between 1938 and 1941 in the Cornell anatomy department at Ithaca Papez noted that certain inclusion bodies observed in thalamic and cortical cells were especially numerous in material from some cases of schizophrenia. The finding of these inclusion bodies in more extensive work in well-fixed brain material from schizophrenics led to studies (with Calvin Baker) in which inclusion bodies were also observed in the cytoplasm of nerve cells taken from biopsies of seventy lobotomized schizophrenics.

The viral or rickettsial nature suggested by their appearance could not be conclusively confirmed by inoculation into chick embryos, mice, guinea pigs. Although inclusion bodies were subsequently found in several of the tissues of the inoculated animals, they did not appear in the brain. Certain consistent metabolic changes in nerve cells from schizophrenic subjects were associated with the presence of the inclusion bodies. The cytochemical changes and the cytoplasmic presence of inclusion bodies were reported, 1951, to be associated with living new organisms observed in preparation of human cortex (from biopsies taken during lobotomy) suspended in saline. Papez emphasized the need of work in other laboratories to confirm or disprove his observations, and others have made the same recommendation. Robert W. White (psychology, Harvard) observed 1953, "If these findings are confirmed they must be included somehow in our thinking of schizophrenia."

ILLUSTRATIVE STUDIES OF CERTAIN DRUGS AS A POSSIBLE SOURCE OF LIGHT ON SCHIZOPHRENIC PROCESSES

The present intensified interest in the effects of drugs in schizophrenia or other forms of mental illness is due, in part, to immediate therapeutic hope, and, in greater part, to the promise which some of these drugs seem to offer of shedding light on the biochemical mechanisms involved in mental disorder. There is nothing new, certainly, in the use of drugs in mental illness for sedation. In more recent years studies have been concerned also with drugs which, aside from sedative effect, have seemed to suggest more specific capacity to inhibit — or to produce — the psychological reactions of schizophrenia. A diminishing empiricism characterizes at least the outlook of certain of these drug studies. To discover a chemical convulsant that would act selectively on the brain, and thus avoid the potentially hazardous effects of current shock therapies on other body structures, has been, for instance, one objective in several laboratories of psychiatry, neurology, pharmacology and physiology. Recognition of the relation of oxygen consumption and therefore of cerebral blood flow to mental illness, including schizophrenia, partly explains the background of recently revived investigative interest (University of Iowa psychiatry department, McLean Hospital, Allen Memorial Institute, Montreal, and other centers) in the similarity between effects produced on behavior by drugs that modify cerebral blood flow (aminophylline and amphetamine) and schizophrenic hallucinations.

Among drugs of especial current interest because they induce psychological reactions resembling some of the symptoms of schizophrenia are two unrelated alkaloids, lysergic acid and mescaline, and adrenochrome (described as chemically intermediate between mescaline and adrenaline). Drugs creating great interest because they seem to promise therapeutic value in schizophrenia and also because of hope that the central complex of effects may lead to localization of the cerebral mechanisms of schizophrenia include serotonin, the alkaloids of *Rauwolfia serpentina* including reserpine, and the synthetic phenothiazine, chlorpromazine. While detailed knowledge of all the mechanisms and sites of action of these and other drugs upon the brain awaits advances in neurochemistry, the particular sensitivity of the reticular formation to narcotics has been recognized. Mescaline and like agents are reported to cause spiking in the hypothalamus. Chlorpromazine is reported to inhibit phosphorylations specifically in the basal ganglia-thalamus region of the brain, while having little or no effect upon the cortex.

Both lysergic acid and mescaline have been the subject of reports in recent years from the New York Psychiatric Institute (Hoch, Pennes and Cattell), the Boston Psychopathic Hospital (Solomon and associates) and laboratories at Ohio State and the University of Western Ontario. The schizogenic effect of lysergic acid was first suggested when a Swiss chemist working on it (1943) in other connections noticed peculiar reactions following mere inhalation of it. The actual madness of a number of citizens in a French village not long ago was attributed to lysergic acid in bread made from infected rye flour. The drug (synthesized, 1954, by Robert B. Woodward, chemistry, Harvard) has been found to produce in man a schizophrenic-like state (lasting for some hours). To studies of its effects in man have been added studies, reported in 1954, of its effects on Siamese fighting fish by Harold A. Abramson and Llewellyn T. Evans of the biological laboratory, Cold Spring Harbor. "Although recovery usually occurs within a week, exposure to the drug has in many cases actually altered the social behavior."

As a blocking agent against psychosis produced by lysergic acid, Howard D. Fabing tested meratran, alpha (2 piperidyl) benzhydrol hydrochloride. The Fabing group's clinical study of meratran led to the conclusion, 1955, that it appeared to have therapeutic value (though not consistently in the dosage used) in certain dissociation syndromes, including acute schizophrenia. Administration (in various forms) of meratran to students rendered psychotic by lysergic acid seemed to the investigators to bear out the blocking capacity of meratran, and thus to confirm its therapeutic possibility in mental illness.

Mescaline is essentially the ancient Indian peyote which has been used for its psychological effects by the Mexican Indians for hundreds of years and from which mescaline has been isolated. One hypothesis, based on both experimental work and work with students, would attribute its effects to its capacity to inhibit oxygen consumption of the brain. It was found that the inhibited oxygen consumption could be at least partly restored by succinate or succinic acid (an intermediary compound in the tricarboxylic acid or citric acid cycle of oxidative metabolism). This finding seemed not only to contribute to knowledge of the mechanism of mescaline but also to offer a therapeutic hope in succinate, a hope not sustained, 1952, by Hoch's trials of it at the New York State Psychiatric Institute. Solomon's group thought, 1952, that neither their own work nor the work of Hoch and his group had as yet provided any scientific explanation for the psychotic effect of mescaline.

The fact that normal persons can experience the effects of mescaline has stimulated public — and especially journalistic — imagination. Reports of trial of it by two normal volunteers point, however, in quite different directions. One of the volunteers, a Canadian journalist, considered that the drug had revealed to him, for the space of a few hours, the very hell in which the schizophrenic lives constantly. His report was designed to shock a negligent public into bestirring itself to rescue schizophrenics from their bondage of horror. In the other direction, Aldous Huxley imaginatively presented mescaline not as a demon walling the individual within an isolated chamber of horrors but rather as a liberator, opening to him the "doors of perception". More effectively than drink or tobacco, Huxley speculated, mescaline might show the rest of us who are nonschizophrenic (or only half schizophrenic) "for a few timeless hours the outer and inner worlds, not as they appear to an animal obsessed with survival or a human being obsessed with words and notions, but as they are apprehended directly by Mind at Large". However, the question has been raised whether most people are ready for such a dose of Mind at Large.

"Might not the universe manifest itself to some not very tough guinea pigs in a guise too overwhelming for them to face?"

From clinical trial of adrenochrome, Saskatchewan Hospital workers (Hoffer, Osmond and Smythies) reported, 1954, effects similar to those of mescaline, with especial emphasis on the loss of insight and the inability of treated subjects (for the twenty-four or more hours of the drug's effect) to see any connection between their experiences and the injection.

Serotonin, a "hormone-like" compound, occurring naturally in many tissues (including nerve) in many species has been under investigation chiefly in relation to hypertension since 1948. Some of the studies have been oriented by the hypothesis that serotonin may have a primary neural function; others by the possibility that interference with the function of serotonin by its antimetabolites may result in such mental illness as schizophrenia. Serotonin was synthesized in 1951 and work in several laboratories here and abroad has established the existence of naturally occurring and synthetic antimetabolites that specifically inhibit its action. The fact that all examples of three classes of alkaloid drugs employed as antimetabolites inhibit the action of serotonin on smooth muscle (including arterial muscle) suggested that serotonin may have a primary neural function in reflex regulation of normal blood pressure. In this view, the site of action of serotonin in the brain would be akin to "receptor" spots in arterial tissues on which the blood-borne serotonin acts in regulating blood pressure; mental aberrations, when they occur in connection with serotonin, would in that case be attributable to a deficiency of serotonin, indirectly resulting from diminished cerebral blood flow.

A more direct role for serotonin "in the maintenance of normal mental processes" through cerebral metabolic mechanisms was envisaged, however, in biochemical studies reported by D. W. Woolley and E. Shaw from the Rockefeller Institute. The work was based on the action of a few (not all) of the alkaloid antimetabolites that produce mental aberrations, as lysergic acid. The Rockefeller Institute investigators suggested that these antimetabolites exert their effects by penetration to the brain where they interfere with the function of serotonin. "If this view is correct, then naturally occurring psychiatric states such as schizophrenia might well be pictured as resulting from a deficiency in the brain brought about . . . by failure of the metabolic processes which normally synthesize or destroy this hormone there."

Further research has followed the line that enzymes involved in normal destruction of serotonin may be inhibited, leading to an excess, rather than to a deficiency of serotonin, in mental aberrations. Demonstration that excess serotonin produces mental aberrations in man cannot be tested because of the dangers of direct injection into the brain; the peripherally administered serotonin that has proved harmless to man fails to penetrate the brain where the accumulation is crucial, in this hypothesis. Woolley and Shaw suggested the need of further research to establish whether metabolic processes involved in the synthesis and destruction of serotonin in the brain are involved in normal mental processes and their disturbance. If this should prove to be the case, "one might picture the naturally occurring diseases as arising from an excess of serotonin brought about by increased production or diminished rate of destruction".

While objection to all of these hypotheses — "that the pharmacological and biochemical evidence is insufficient to justify any connection of serotonin with the neurological effects" — cannot, as Woolley and Shaw pointed out, 1954, be excluded, they considered the combined biochemical and pharmacological evidence "sufficient to encourage pursuit of the working hypothesis that this hormonelike compound plays an important part in the functioning of the nervous system". If this hypothesis should prove correct, antimetabolites might, in their view, be so constructed that they could penetrate the brain for action on specific enzymatic reactions affecting the serotonin level. They reported, 1954, the preparation of one such antimetabolite (medmain).

Seymour S. Kety, referring, 1954, to serotonin as an "hormonal agent", noted exhaustive research on it by radioactive techniques which had already delineated the pathways and rates of formation and destruction in the body. I. H. Page (who favored the view that one of the functions of serotonin is concerned with nerve metabolism), after citing, 1954, various speculative hypotheses as to its function — as a clotting factor, as an influence in gastrointestinal activity or in intrarenal hemodynamics — thought it clear that serotonin "is going to have many functions, real or fancied, before its true part in biological function is told".

Study in mental conditions, including schizophrenia, of alkaloids of *Rauwolfia serpentina*, the ancient "insanity herb" of India (named for a German botanist, Rauwolf, who published in 1582 his studies of medicinal plants used by early Greek and Arab physicians), began in 1953. Interest in extracts and alkaloids of the root had been active since 1951 in trials of the drug for clinical hypertension. Its sedative and hypnotic effects (noted since 1942) and the first report from Baroda, India, 1953, of apparent cures in schizophrenia coincided with isolation of the active alkaloid, reserpine (one of the trade names of which is serpasil), by H. J. Bein and associates at the Ciba laboratories at Basle. At about the same time, chlorpromazine, a synthetic drug with chemical structure and pharmacologic actions differing widely from those of reserpine, was introduced in France as an inhibitor of psychomotor excitement and manic states. At the Manteno State Hospital, serving the Chicago metropolitan district (8,200 patients), only eleven of more than 221 chronic schizophrenics that had responded temporarily to electroshock were unimproved on reserpine; of 139 shock-resistant patients, nineteen were discharged after thirteen years' hospitalization and fifty-two were given passes — all without psychotherapy. Results "more dramatic" than those produced by reserpine were announced, 1954, from the Rochester (New York) State Hospital on the basis of trial of chlorpromazine (a trade name of which is thorazine). According to the Rochester report, the drug was effective in eighty-eight per cent of approximately 300 patients. The effects of chlorpromazine on 500 mental patients at the Longview State Hospital were described, 1955, by Douglas Goldman (director) as more marked in chronic than in acute psychoses.

Reports of trials have frequently included both reserpine and chlorpromazine without clear distinction. At a 1955 symposium of the American Psychiatric Association held at the meeting of the American Association for the Advancement of Science, the two drugs were described as "remarkable new sedatives" especially useful in clarifying the minds of patients so that they become accessible to psychotherapy. In more than a thousand cases a high percentage of successes was reported in patients including chronic schizophrenics who had failed to respond to other therapy. It was emphasized, however, that the drugs are not a hundred per cent effective, that they do not in any sense "cure" mental diseases and that their long term value is yet to be established. Reports were made by E. F. Hollister, Palo Alto Veterans Administration Hospital, Lester H. Margolis of the University of California medical school, by A. A. Sainz, Iowa City Veterans Administration Hospital, and N. S. Kline of the Rockland State Hospital. Choice between reserpine and chlorpromazine appears to be on an individual basis. Without adequate criteria for administration and knowledge of the dangers, Bleuler and Stoll found the side effects to balance: reserpine caused less pain after injection and probably less liver damage and jaundice; chlorpromazine less frequently led to Parkinsonian symptoms (reversible).

These and other manifestations of the "reserpine syndrome" are of practical as well as theoretical interest in relation to schizophrenia. If the neurological and pharmacological effects of the drug could be elucidated with demonstration of the sites and mechanism of its action, the result, it was hoped, might be clues to the sites and mechanisms of the fundamental reactions of schizophrenia. Bein, 1953, had attributed the general effects to reduction of activity of the sympathetic regulatory centers of the brain. Later work at the Ciba laboratories indicated, 1955, that central sympathetic depression was not direct but rather was caused by inhibition of afferent impulses that activate these centers. Bein concluded, 1955, from animal studies, that reserpine apparently acts "upon central regulatory mechanisms which integrate autonomic and somatic functions". That functions not directly related to the autonomic system are affected by reserpine was suggested by the occurrence of signs of Parkinson's disease after prolonged and large doses, and by the "tranquilizing effect" which differs distinctly from the action of barbiturates upon the arousal mechanism in the brainstem with a definite pattern of sleep. In a series of rabbit studies, Himwich and coworkers found, 1955, that reserpine stimulates the reticular formation of the brainstem (arousal center) whereas drugs that are useful in Parkinson's disease inhibit the center. "This effect on the activating system is probably the reason why reserpine may produce a Parkinsonlike symptomology as a side effect." Having demonstrated that the cerebral cortex is necessary (in cats) to produce the full effects of reserpine, Schneider and co-workers proposed, as a working hypothesis, that a general pharmacodynamic effect of reserpine is augmentation of synaptic transmission "and possibly other functions of nerve transmission", one possibility being an effect on synapses in the cerebral cortex.

Certain forms of altered behavior "apparently can be understood only by assuming that conditions in the extracerebral environment exert an influence on the brain although the manner in which such an influence is exerted remains obscure". This 1951 statement of a more generalized biochemical hypothesis is Heinrich Klüver's, who speculated on the possibility that substances circulating in the blood may be able to produce profound behavioral changes, although they cannot be identified in the brain and apparently do not reach the central nervous system. Injections of gold compounds, "although no gold or gold compound could be demonstrated in the central nervous system", produced "not only neurological symptoms, such as ataxia, loss of orientation, and blindness, but also changes in the nerve cells . . ." The metabolic disturbance in the brain could then be viewed, according to Querido (as cited by Klüver), as the result of a collateral or "parallel" poisoning. The meaning is that the injected gold compound causes dysfunction of some other organ (as liver or kidney) which in turn produces a change affecting the cells in the central nervous system.

On the whole, expanding work on drugs and chemicals while not greatly increasing knowledge of the cause and cure of schizophrenia, has had an over-all effect in tending, as one psychologist expressed it, 1954, to "place mental illness again in the realm of diseases of disturbed metabolism".

## ONLY A REMOTE AND SPECULATIVE PRESENT ROLE FOR VITAMINS IN RELATION TO SCHIZOPHRENIA

The inadequacy of present knowledge of intermediary metabolism limits speculation on the possible role of the B vitamins in schizophrenia. That "lack of one or another of the B vitamins" may be concerned in functional disturbances of the peripheral or the central nervous system is a logical inference from the known facts that the B vitamins are instrumental in the catabolic reactions of the cell which break down carbohydrate, and that carbohydrate is the main source of energy for functioning of the nervous system.

That members of the B group of vitamins may be found to be of peculiar importance in the metabolism of nerve tissue is suggested by findings, in addition to present knowledge of the functions of thiamine, riboflavin, niacin, pyridoxine and pantothenic acid as parts of enzyme systems, outside the carbohydrate cycles. For example, biotin appears to have a part in a number of enzymes involved in amino acid and fatty acid metabolism (Herman C. Lichstein, bacteriology and immunology, Minnesota, 1951). In the biosynthesis and oxidation of purines and pyrimidines (components of nucleic acids and thus of nucleoproteins), some evidence exists that folic acid, riboflavin and biotin function in these metabolic sequences (William Shive, chemistry, Texas, 1951). Such information may eventually make possible study of the role of vitamins in areas of nerve metabolism not concerned with energy production. Sebrell and associates suggested that the B vitamins may be involved in other and less explored areas of metabolism in nerve cells, "for example growth, maintenance, nervous function, coordination and regeneration".

In man, deficiencies of only three of ten of the B vitamins have, as yet, been connected with well-recognized clinical disturbance of the nervous system, including pathological changes in parts of the central nervous system. The three are: thiamin deficiency, which results in the polyneuritis of beriberi (with some degenerative changes reported in spinal ganglion cells and nuclei of the medulla now generally accepted as inflammatory) and Wernicke's encephalopathy; niacin deficiency, which results in pellagra, with dementia and spinal cord damage as part of the classical picture (Eric K. Cruickshank, University College of the West Indies, 1952); vitamin $B_{12}$ deficiency, which results in pernicious anemia with involvement of sensory, motor disturbances and, if not compensated, destructive lesions in the spinal cord (Thomas H. Jukes and E. L. R. Stokstad, Lederle Laboratories, 1951).

## Endocrine Influences in Biochemical
### Phenomena in Schizophrenia

Great caution has been urged in interpreting abnormalities of the endocrine system in mental illness, notably schizophrenia. The abnormalities "may be secondary to a primary disturbance of brain or to a central process responsible for the mental as well as the physical picture, or may themselves be the factor that determines the abnormal mentation" (Hemphill and Reiss, 1950).

Of endocrine influences involved in mental illness, investigation has centered chiefly on the hormones of the adrenal medulla and the adrenal cortex. Hemphill and Reiss pointed out that in spite of the recognized importance of the adrenal medulla in the physiological regulation of the body and in spite of the important pharmacological properties of the hormone of the adrenal medulla, adrenaline, "no satisfactory studies of this field have been made in mental illness . . ." Need for such studies has been described as imperative in view of renewed interest everywhere in reactivity to stress.

### Hormones of the Adrenal Medulla and the Adrenal
### Cortex in Relation to Schizophrenia

The "recognized importance" of the adrenal medulla dates back to Cannon's emergency theory, which preceded much of the work on adrenal influence on cerebral activity and which was based on the functions of the autonomic nervous system and adrenaline in providing for rapid adjustment and in maintaining homeostasis in the internal environment of the body. While the Cannon emergency theory offered "what seemed to be a physiological foundation for understanding emotion", modern workers admit that it is inadequate to explain the whole psychological picture. Basic to understanding the whole picture of endocrine influences on behavior is understanding of the relative functions and connections of the adrenal medulla (under direct nerve control) and the adrenal cortex (stimulated by corticotropin, ACTH, discharged from the pituitary). Putting the relation very simply, Cobb said, 1950: "One can postulate that the adrenal cortex takes over where the medulla leaves off. The physiological reaction of the medulla is an emergency response, lasting for minutes only. It is brief, wasteful and maintained only by a sacrifice of normal functions . . ." The needs of continued stress are met by substances secreted by the adrenal cortex.

It is true that until recently the action of adrenaline as an emergency mechanism was believed to be only short and direct. In direct response to low blood sugar, adrenaline makes available glucose from stored glycogen in liver or from glycogen transported from muscles to the liver, thus restoring the blood glucose which is essential to the brain and to life. Over and beyond this emergency response, however, a function is now predicated for the medullary hormone, in stimulating release of corticotropin from the anterior pituitary (H. Gershberg, E. G. Fry, J. R. Brobeck, C. N. H. Long, 1950). Corticotropin then rapidly stimulates secretion of the adrenal cortical hormones which (as an example of the effects of the interrelation of the adrenal medulla and cortex) bring about sustained increase of blood sugar through conversion of tissue proteins to liver glycogen (Long, 1952). The pituitary-adrenal system is conceived as the means for meeting long-continued, rather than brief emergencies or stress. The consequences of cortical hormone action were described by Dwight J. Ingle, 1950, as spreading "through the organism in a manner reminiscent of the waves caused by the impact of a stone in a pool of water, but the point of impact of the hormone remains unknown for the present".

In England, G. W. Harris, in a series of experimental studies seeking neural factors that may control the pituitary, has suggested that release of the anterior pituitary hormones is controlled by the hypothalamus, through a hypothalamic secretion carried to the gland by the portal circulation. In this country, David M. Hume (surgical research, Harvard), 1952, proposed an emergency mechanism "under the control of the nervous system and mediated by a humoral substance" secreted by a hypothalamic center and liberated into the bloodstream.

Current hypotheses bearing on the influence of adrenocortical functioning on behavior, derived from concepts of the role of the adrenal cortex in adapting the organism to stress, naturally deal chiefly with cortisone (E) or hydrocortisone (F) and with corticotropin which stimulates their secretion. Although other steroids are apparently involved in the adrenal secretion, the question is unanswered whether these other steroids are true hormones or are intermediates or artefacts of extraction procedures. Only six of the twenty-eight steroid substances found in the adrenal cortex had (as of 1952) been positively identified as hormones for which more or less specific functions could be described. By 1955, methods of study of the content of the adrenal venous blood carrying secretions from the cortex (in animals and man) had revealed some fifty compounds, some "physiologically rational" and others with apparently no physiological role. The array of possible adrenocortical products is "staggering" (Pincus, 1955).

Especial stimulus to studies of the adrenal cortex was given by the 1949 report from the Worcester Foundation for Experimental Biology that adrenocortical response to stress was considerably lower or absent in approximately two thirds of a group of 200 hospitalized schizophrenics, as compared with the response of normal subjects. That this abnormal adrenal response was not due to lack of pituitary secretion of the adrenocorticotrophic hormone was suggested by failure of these patients to respond, as the normal subjects responded, by enhanced cortical secretion to administration of ACTH. These conclusions emerged in the course of a study of the adrenal cortex (its structure, secretions, metabolism and the function of its hormones) pursued at the foundation since 1941 (by Gregory Pincus, Hudson Hoagland and their associates). The work with the schizophrenics involved cooperation at the Worcester State Hospital with psychologists, psychiatrists and biochemists. As a result of earlier reports, a collaborative project, undertaken with federal funds, was set up for five years or more at the hospital, which is a cooperative research station of the National Institute of Mental Health. The National Institute of Mental Health has also financed studies of adrenocortical function in psychoses in several psychiatry departments, as those in the medical schools of the University of Utah and the University of Washington, Seattle.

Investigators in other institutions (Cleghorn in Montreal, Altschule at the McLean Hospital, Gildea in Washington University's psychiatry department) have reported findings in small series not altogether in agreement with the Worcester findings on 200 schizophrenics. No etiological significance was attached by the Worcester group to their findings on disturbed steroid metabolism in psychotics. The disturbance may, as Hoagland put it, in a communication to the American Foundation, 1953, "quite well be a result of the disease and may have nothing to do causally with the matter at all". He suggested that it may play a coincidental role or, through the influence attributed to various adrenocortical steroids on metabolism, influence oxygen consumption or glucose metabolism of the brain, either directly or indirectly.

Referring also to "successful treatment" reported, 1945, by British physicians (Allen and Broster) of paranoid psychosis in which hyperactive adrenal function was decreased by removal of one adrenal, Hoagland referred, 1953, to his own studies of bilateral adrenalectomy of schizophrenic patients "as a possible therapeutic procedure". In the first (press) reports, 1952, of an adrenalectomy project, representing collaboration between University of Chicago workers (C. B. Huggins performing the surgery, Nathaniel Apter the psychiatric evaluations) and the Worcester group (for the biochemical work), Hoagland was cited as considering that the results of adrenalectomy on six patients warranted continued study but did not provide evidence that cures had been accomplished.

A general clinical impression (Frederick Bernheim, 1952) has stressed the euphoric effect of cortisone and ACTH in such non-psychotic conditions as rheumatoid arthritis but also the danger of exacerbation of the psychoses of those already psychotic. A study at the Mayo Clinic of 100 patients (of whom only six were psychotic, three of them schizophrenic) indicated that latent schizophrenia appeared to be precipitated by cortisone and to subside with cessation of treatment. Psychiatric observations on another Mayo Clinic study of twenty-six patients receiving cortisone or ACTH for various medical conditions led Rome and Braceland to emphasize, 1950, the view expressed by many that psychic disorders developing during treatment with the hormones represent, in most instances, intensification of pre-existing personality disorders. To precisely what degree a pre-existing psychic state is responsible for untoward effects on behavior would naturally be a difficult question to answer. Gildea, 1952, summarizing the findings on his own series, had an "impression" that in patients to whom sufficiently large doses of either cortisone or ACTH are given, "these hormones usually produce a feeling of increased mental activity and well being and thus increase motor behavior", the speeding up in some cases being sufficient to produce anxiety and ultimately even manic excitement. This last statement has a degree of confirmation in Altschule's reference, 1953, to recent evidence indicating that "some persons, previously mentally normal, became manic or depressed even to the point of suicide when given ACTH or cortisone in large amounts".

Since, in the 200 schizophrenics studied by the Worcester group, some of those that still showed some adrenocortical reactivity to ACTH administration were found to benefit from electroshock treatment, test injections of ACTH were suggested as having prognostic value for cases of schizophrenia likely to benefit from electroshock therapy. Pincus, Hoagland and associates, suggested that electroshock as a form of violent stress activates the under-productive pituitary-adrenal system. The effects of all shock treatments on adrenocortical re-activity have been under study in several laboratories. Altschule observed, 1953, that the first insulin or electroshock treatments stimulate the adrenal cortex but that with additional treatments adrenal response decreases.

In work relating adrenal cortical functioning to mental illness few certainties are offered as to the mechanisms involved. Reiss, 1953, described causal relationships between brain function and the adrenal cortex as still largely unknown. In his view, "it appears probable that in some cases disturbed adrenal cortex reactivity can be a primary cause of disturbed mentation, while in others . . . it might be only a secondary consequence of exhaustion of the adrenal cortex".

### THYROID AND PARATHYROID INFLUENCE IN SCHIZOPHRENIA

Various workers have stressed the need of further studies, for instance through tracer techniques, to explain anomalies of thyroid activity (over- or under-production) and response to thyroid extract that have sometimes been observed in schizophrenia. Hemphill and Reiss commented on the value of radioactive iodine in distinguishing between primary hypothyroidism and hypothyroidism secondary to under-production of thyrotrophic hormone by the pituitary, which accounted for the majority of hypothyroid states found among mental patients. Using radioactive iodine (in addition to measurements of serum protein-bound iodine, basal metabolic rate, plasma cholesterol) Karl M. Bowman and associates (Langley Porter Clinic, University of California), 1950, found thyroid function significantly different in mental patients from that in normal controls, although the results of the tests fell within the normal range.

Altschule considered, 1953, that there is "no specific abnormality in thyroid function" in schizophrenia (or in involutional and manic-depressive psychoses). Lowering of the metabolic rate in these conditions could, in his view, be due to starvation or could be related to adrenal cortical hyperactivity. Cleghorn, 1952, pointed out that in advanced cases of hypothyroidism "delusions and hallucinations occur in nearly half the cases". Hemphill and Reiss suggested that the hyperthyroidism found in seventy-five per cent of their female schizophrenic patients was "apparently caused by increased production of thyrotrophic hormone, perhaps owing to primary nervous stimulation". With reference to psychosis in hyperthyroid patients, Cleghorn cited Means's view (1948) that the form of psychosis depends upon the premorbid condition of the patients. Among recent research projects concerned with thyroid functioning in schizophrenia is to be noted a study by E. H. Cranswick (Rockland Hospital research facility) of thyrotropic response in schizophrenia, under a grant from the National Institute of Mental Health.

With regard to parathyroid influence, Cleghorn, 1952, cited Richter and associates (1940) as having described, in monkeys and in human beings, cyclical changes in behavior and in mood, related to parathyroid deficiency.

## THE SEX HORMONES IN PSYCHOSES

The logic of a possible relation between the sex hormones and behavior has been suggested by the tendency of mental disturbances to occur during the puerperium, at adolescence, and at the climacteric. It has still not been possible, however, to determine whether what is involved is a primary derangement of the gonads or a result of abnormal pituitary function. Cleghorn did not, 1952, attribute to the sex hormones any determining role in psychoses. Of the few studies attempting to discover whether steroid hormones play a part in the metabolism of brain tissue, Gordon and Elliott reported, 1947, that several (progesterone, testosterone and stilbestrol as well as the synthetic adrenocortical hormone, desoxycorticosterone) inhibited oxygen uptake by brain suspensions. In 1949 and 1950 they noted that brain suspensions from castrated rats which appeared to show thirty-two per cent above normal consumption of oxygen could be reduced to normal by treatment with the above-named hormonal inhibitors of oxygen consumption.

## DOMINANTLY PSYCHOLOGICAL EMPHASIS IN THE STUDY OF MENTAL ILLNESS, INCLUDING SCHIZOPHRENIA

Many of the investigators engaged in work directed toward bringing neurophysiological and biochemical phenomena into at least tangential relation to thought processes have freely admitted that, as yet, something escapes them. What is the norm of the thought processes that are distorted and of the consciousness that is changed in schizophrenia? Consciousness, as pointed out by Robert B. MacLeod (psychology, Cornell), 1953, in reviewing the fourth Macy conference, is not a neat, clearly identifiable problem like the functions of the adrenal cortex, the conditions of blood clotting, or the nature of the nerve impulse. Kety suggested the immediate wisdom of acknowledging that at present neither the physiologist nor the psychologist ("the honest psychologist") can *explain* consciousness. "We can describe it, and correlate the various phenomena in our disciplines with it, but let us confess that we cannot explain it. . . . We can resolve consciousness into components: namely, sensations, but I defy anybody to describe a sensation." The cooperative work needed for filling the present gaps in knowledge would, Hebb once suggested, be furthered if some psychologists were to become thoroughly trained in neurophysiology and if some physiologists were to reciprocate by taking into account psychological factors in attacking their common problem — *i.e.*, to find out what connects the functional organization of the nervous system with behavior.

There are still many neurophysiologists and biochemists who, while realizing that something beyond their present orbit is concerned, sorely distrust a dominant psychological or psychiatric approach. And there are still many psychiatrists, who are not only ignorant of physiology and biochemistry but who also do not believe that either of these is likely to contribute fundamentally to explanation of schizophrenia. Some have fled to the psychiatric field because they have been disillusioned by neurophysiological or biochemical dead ends, citing the example of Freud when in 1890 he forsook neurology and devoted the remainder of his life to developing psychoanalysis.

## Influences that Somewhat Explain the Present Academic and Public Status of Psychiatry

One factor in the development, some would say the over-development, of psychiatry in the early part of this century was the revelation, in the first world war, of disabling psychological symptoms in a large proportion of the drafted men. Another factor was financial support and interest from outside the medical schools, notably the foundations, increasing facilities for teaching psychiatry as a clinical discipline (out of all proportion to the research funds available for testing its content and application), raising its status in the medical school curriculum and promoting governmental interest in mental health. Many states under the influence of the National Committee for Mental Hygiene established divisions or bureaus of mental health in state health departments.

"Psychosomatic" became almost a by-word in both medical and lay circles. There was a healthful aspect in this reinforcing of the ancient truth that all illness, mental or physical, organic or functional, has psychological concomitants, often so emphatic that they almost submerge the physiological factors involved. The psychological components of the most obviously "organic" illness, as heart disease or tuberculosis, may, even to (sensitive) patients themselves, seem dominant; as they seemed to Kafka when in the devastating grip of progressive tuberculosis he said: "I am mentally ill. The disease of the lungs is nothing but an overflowing of my mental disease." A realization quite so poignant as this is out of balance; but any situation is certainly more hopeful when patient and physician alike have some capacity to evaluate the inevitable association of psychic and somatic components.

A less healthful consequence of wide preoccupation with psychic influences lay in attempts to define them in formal but inexact and not uniformly accepted terms. In such attempts lay the danger of over-extending the discipline of psychiatry, of transforming its psychological hypotheses into determining principles. The formulation of psychiatric principles for teaching purposes (as pointed out, 1951, at the conference on psychiatric education organized by the American Psychiatric Association and the Association of American Medical Colleges) tended to "outrun the validation process" and accounted in part for the shortcomings of psychiatry as a medical discipline. Significant difference has been pointed out between a collection of good hunches deriving from the psychodynamists and a systematic body of experimentally demonstrable knowledge which characterizes a scientific discipline. Present day psychiatry was defined by Nolan Lewis a few years ago as "an odd mixture of internal medicine, neurology, psychology, clinical testing, 'psychosurgery' and various drug assaults on the personality, mental hygiene, philosophical speculation and the pseudoscientific diagnoses applied by those who operate on the margins of the specialty . . ."

One apprehension has been lest concentration on "genetic dynamic philosophy, for it is hardly more than that," as Walter Freeman once put it, may discourage exploration of the mind by other channels. There has been, for instance, especial comment on psychiatry's lack of concern with such characteristic resources of scientific research as animal experimentation. The contention that, since animals do not become spontaneously psychotic, animal experimentation is not a hopeful resource in study of schizophrenia has been characterized as unsound. J. Elkes (experimental psychiatry, University of Birmingham) at the 1952 Oxford conference attempted to demonstrate how animal experimentation could serve psychiatry even in lines so remote as psychoanalysis. He described as promising the whole attempt to "weave a thread between psychoanalytic theory and behavior studies in animal and man", and, with others, urged extending to mammals recent work on behavior patterns in birds and fishes. At the same conference, J. Bowlby (Tavistok Clinic, London) pointed out that since it may well be that the simplest human responses, those most charged with feeling, *i.e.* the responses of childhood, depend on centers in older parts of the brain (as the rhinencephalon), "not very different from those with which the older mammals are provided", it would be "sensible" to consider the nature of perceptions and responses in animals, as observed by animal psychologists and zoologists.

While some deplore lack of the chastening influence of concrete experiment in psychiatry, and criticize assumptions arrived at by imprecise methods, others, contrariwise, fear too literal application, at this stage, of the precision methods of other sciences. Preoccupation with quantitative variables and statistical evaluation of them has been described by one psychologist (S. J. Beck), 1954, as "one of the seductive fallacies to which all psychological theorizing is prone". The concept of quantitative variables drawn from other sciences does not, it is argued, play an equally determining role in psychology: "We cannot depend solely on quantity variables to make a system of psychological theory 'dynamic'."

Some critics would ask of psychiatry simply better use of traditional scientific methods, on the ground that, after all, "what exists exists in some quantity and can be measured". This group stresses the need, whether in large or in small scale experiments, of adequate controls (*i.e.*, groups of mental patients that have and that have not been subjected to a given procedure) and also adequate normal controls, repeated testing of results, consistent recognition of variables, in the patient, in the therapist, in the conditions of the experiment, in the environment outside the therapy. In sum, three outstanding needs are urged upon psychiatry: basic study of the normal; the use of numerous tests on numerous subjects; the constant checking of hypotheses by progressively acquired criteria.

Alienating to the general scientific student is the insularity of the current terminology used in psychiatric research and practice. It has, in the view of its critics, little relation either to simple literary clarity or to conventional scientific exactness. Many of its terms have been adopted by laymen, have been debauched by inexact and somewhat humorous use and have added nothing to public understanding of psychiatric concepts. In a comparatively brief time, psychiatry has added to the language terms which, because of their over-extended connotations, dictionaries now take care to label "psychol.": *e.g.*, id ("the primitive preformed psychic force in the unconscious"), ego, superego, libido, autism, anxiety, frustrations, cathexis, stress, regression, defenses, empathy, rationalization, oedipus complex, transference. Most of these terms define too little and connote too much. Ego, id and superego, Hebb once observed, are conceptions which, while they help one to see and state important factors of behavior, are also dangerously easy to treat as ghostly realities, as anthropomorphic agents. It may be that psychiatric concepts with reference to schizophrenia and mental illness may be more generally persuasive when they are less word-bound and are conveyed with more classic reference to original Greek and Latin derivations — and perhaps with more interest in Anglo-Saxon equivalents. The tax on the uninitiated reader is at present too great. Burnet remarked a few years ago that he found it "impossible to digest what of the psychological literature there is time to read". The reader can navigate only if he can bring into play the same degree of semantic skill as that displayed by the writer; the present reviewers felt unequal to translating "existential psychotherapy", by which term one neuropsychiatrist defined the field of his immediate interest.

Confidence in psychiatry will be advanced when it connotes the whole body of knowledge about biological and social forces that influence personal behavior, or when, to speak over-simply, it is merged in psychology, loosening its purely therapeutic slant and approaching mental illness on the firm ground of work on normal behavior, emotion, personality. In its present isolated psychodynamic trend, it is regarded by some medical educators as not a scientific or teachable discipline and as thus having no proper place in the medical school curriculum. They would give it only probationary academic status, pending its reincarnation as a discipline integrally related to the basic sciences dealing with normal physiology, biochemistry, psychology.

## CURRENT THERAPIES FOR SCHIZOPHRENIA AS VIEWED BY PSYCHIATRISTS

### THERAPIES HAVING OR ASSUMING A PHYSIOLOGIC RATIONALE

Therapies currently used in psychiatry range from those claiming physiological concepts (shock, psychosurgery, the new drugs) to psychoanalysis and many psychologic variants of it.  Some psychiatrists, notably among those in the psychoanalytic school, totally reject shock and psychosurgery in schizophrenia.  Other psychiatrists in various centers use or accept all types of therapy, physiological and psychological — lobotomy, insulin and electroshock, hypnosis, drugs, psychotherapy including psychoanalysis, and variants of it, and unassorted forms of group therapy.  When shock and psychosurgery are totally rejected, the ground is usually that neither of them has a rational basis or a proved record of greater efficacy than psychotherapy or than no therapy.  Nor, it is maintained, do they expand knowledge of the condition, as compared with psychotherapy.  This last contention is especially challenged, as indicated in foregoing sections of this chapter — in the section on neurophysiological work in which various forms of psychosurgery were cited as attempts at therapeutic application of present neurophysiological knowledge; in the section on work showing dominantly biochemical emphasis, in which the shock therapies were reviewed in connection with the biochemical processes assumed to be involved.  The brief review in the biochemical section of the new drugs that seem to shed a degree of light on schizophrenic processes by either favorably influencing symptoms or producing schizophrenialike reactions suggests that, whatever their present promise, these drugs are still in an experimental stage that makes present evaluation impossible.

Concern here is not with evaluation of any therapy.  In spite of the wide use of various forms of shock therapy, in spite of its prestige and of thousands of favorable reports on its use in small and large series, over many years, it is still to be said that its psychological results have not been comprehensively or fundamentally evaluated either as to schizophrenia or as to its more general use in manic depression.  In contrast to the few over-all conclusions, the range of opinion and clinical observation is wide — and sometimes illuminating.  Generally favorable reports are to a degree offset by such observations as that of Gjessing (Oslo City Mental Hospital), 1950, warning against a facile tendency to rate as "improved" the patient whom shock has made euphoric, uncritical, incapable of judging his own mental disability.  The physician is not to fall into the major error of considering the treatment satisfactory because the patient does.  Frieda

Fromm-Reichmann (Chestnut Lodge Sanitarium, Rockville, Maryland) joined the majority in ratifying the effectiveness of shock therapy in depressive states, yet she does not recommend it for the reasons mentioned below. She considered, 1953, that, in schizophrenia, it accomplishes, "according to most psychiatrists who have done research on the subject, at best a certain degree of social adaptation", without giving the schizophrenic any therapeutically effective understanding of the dynamics of his illness. In reply to the argument that shock therapy may be a useful adjuvant to other therapies in establishing a workable psychotherapeutic contact between patient and psychiatrist, Fromm-Reichmann recorded the view of her group and her institution that the necessary relation can be established without it. "All types of shock treatment temporarily dull and slow down the patient's mental functions. In the case of electroshock, serious cerebral damage has been observed in several cases (Goldstein, Riese)."

On psychosurgery (the surgeons themselves have objected to the hybrid term, although they use it, as do the rest of us, in the interest of economy), there is also no widely accepted body of generalized conclusions as to its psychological results, its effect upon intellectual power, initiative and emotional capacity. The lack of such generalizations is not strange, since, as has often been pointed out, there has not been adequate study of the approximately twenty thousand patients operated in this country since this expedient was first tried. There have been comprehensive detailed studies of limited groups, as two previously mentioned reports (covering under fifty operated patients) of the Columbia Greystone associates, consisting of medical scientists and clinicians from Columbia's College of Physicians and Surgeons and the New Jersey State Hospital and two reports of studies of lobotomized patients at the Boston Psychopathic Hospital (the second covering 116 operated patients). These reports of 1952 and 1953 contain detailed information and illustrate the kind of studies that must be made much more extensively.

The Greystone studies had the avowed purpose of defining factors needing study rather than evaluating over-all psychological results. Mettler and Landis in the concluding chapter of the second Greystone report observed: "Neither this nor our previous study made much progress in developing reliable objective methods for evaluating psychosurgical results. Indeed . . . it has become increasingly apparent that new objective methods are greatly needed for estimating the efficiency of any form of psychiatric therapy."

The Greenblatt and Solomon volume contains some quite definite conclusions based on study of the 116 cases. The editors divide schizophrenics into two groups as to recovery potential. In the schizophrenic that "maintains integration and abstraction during the illness" and is capable of tension, they state that lobotomy may have dramatic results. It is ineffective, however, with the schizophrenic patient that has "little potentiality for change", the "washed-out undemanding fragment case who so often receives the clinical label of hebephrenic schizophrenia and remains in the back wards of the hospital to the end of his days". Favorable reports of the more hopeful group included the finding that operated patients are "emotionally more integrated, more responsive to social demands and opportunities, and intellectually more free from anxiety-induced disruptions."

Even those most wary of substituting opinion for tests and validated study would with difficulty refrain from being influenced not only by such reports as the above, but also by the reserved attitude of various workers in mental illness toward psychosurgery. The question most frequently raised concerns the real nature of the release of tension and diminution of drive secured in the lobotomized patient. Adrian was disposed, 1954, to agree that there are certainly people who now lead "more placid, if perhaps less useful lives, because their anxieties have been diminished by leucotomy". And, as many others have pointed out, institutions charged with the custody of turbulent psychotics can certainly exist more placidly — and more economically — when their charges have been reduced to placidity. Remains the problem — it is the challenge recognized by many who would like to make a fair evaluation of psychosurgery — as to how far the placidity is to be honestly rated as improvement *so far as the patient's final recovery is concerned*. That, at present, psychiatrists, in order to evaluate psychosurgery, need vastly more knowledge of it was implied by Whitehorn, when, in consenting to open one of the sessions of the 1951 research conference on psychosurgery, he disclaimed direct knowledge of the subject, since he himself had invoked psychosurgical procedures in the case of only two patients. The very calling of the conference was described as indicating recognition of the need of evaluation.

In the discussions of the research conference, a wide range of opinion was expressed as to the effect of psychosurgery on initiative, drive, intelligence, personality. Some participants — a number — felt that, whatever the benefits, it must always be admitted that the net result for the patient is always "a minus"; some would refer grave personality changes only to drastic psychosurgery, some to any form of it. Most frequently mentioned at the research conference and in other discussions of psychological effects have been loss of important ego functions, replacement by new defenses, reduction in deliberative faculty, alterations in patterns of thought, feeling and judgment in relation to time, energy, money, avocations, religion, work performance, domestic and sexual habits, interpersonal relations; coarsening of esthetic, intellectual and moral judgment.

At an international meeting in Vienna, 1953, Nikolai I. Oserezki (psychiatric clinic, Pavlov Institute, Leningrad) attributed to Freeman, "one of the strongest advocates of the operation in the United States", a 1945 statement that lobotomy leads to "a disturbance in the activity of personality, the loss of interest by the patient in himself and his surroundings, emotional dullness, infantilism in behavior, loss of previously acquired training and difficulty in acquiring new learning". Oserezki himself characterized lobotomy as a means of making a patient sufficiently apathetic to be sent home, thus freeing a hospital bed. Rejecting lobotomy as an antiphysiological method that makes the patient an intellectual invalid, he announced, according to the *New York Times*, that lobotomy "widely performed in the United States has been outlawed in the Soviet Union as inhumane". Fromm-Reichmann, in expressing (1953) her view that psychosurgery deprives the patient of incentive and initiative, of ability to feel joy and grief, stressed the tragedy inherent in a situation in which, while the damage done to brain and to personality is great, it is also "not great enough for the patient not to be sadly aware of his loss".

In summing up a lengthy discussion of the effect of psychosurgery on the pain threshold (there was a good deal of agreement among members of the research conference on the effectiveness of psychosurgery in this regard), Kety, "perhaps naively and maybe heretically", raised this question: "What evidence do we have that lobotomy induces whatever effect it has on pain by virtue of specific cerebral trauma and not because of its psychological effects?" Hebb somewhat challenged distinguishing between perception of pain and the reaction to it as two quite different things. He stressed the need of knowing, in this connection, "what central processes there are". Grant expressed the view that those that have observed frontal lobe incisions know that appreciation of pain is not changed by the operation. What disappears is the dread of pain. "But what price do these patients pay for relief of their pain? Every observer agrees that no matter how little frontal lobe is removed, there is slight but definite personality change . . ."

On the moot question whether frontal lobe surgery necessarily leads to intellectual damage or deficit, Landis observed, 1954, that "it has been regularly found by every psychologist who has had the opportunity of applying intelligence tests before and after psychosurgery that there is no permanent damage to intellect, learning, or memory so long as the more posterior portions of the frontal lobe were not involved by the surgery". He added: "The myth that the frontal lobe tissue mediates higher intellectual processes dies hard." While a minority assumed that there is always some reduction in creativeness, many members of the 1951 research conference felt that creativeness is affected only if the operative procedure is very extensive.

The more or less agreed upon lack of concern and reduction of drive in lobotomized patients are very generally discussed in two quite opposed ways: one group deplores the reduction of a human being, through psychosurgery, to a "vegetable" (a word referred to at the 1951 conference as "loaded"); the other group commends the patient's "loss of aggression", greater friendliness, lessened susceptibility to frustration. The lobotomized patient, according to W. C. Halstead (experimental psychology, University of Chicago), manages to survive through progressive de-conditioning of aggressivity, "but always in terms of a highly stereotyped mode of living". What has been lost is "a biological heritage which attains its zenith in *homo sapiens*, the capacity for ego growth and differentiation". Freeman regarded Halstead's conclusions as "more sweeping than are justified by the material in the tests he used".

Mettler observed at the 1951 conference that, while lobotomized patients apparently go through an apathetic postoperative period, "it is not clear whether the ultimate condition of such patients is one of increased or decreased drive". This question came into high focus when, a few years ago, a young man, lobotomized in a mental hospital in New England, returned, as cured, to his college. Devastated at finding himself intellectually incapable of going on with college work, he sought out and killed a psychiatrist who had had no connection with his case, but with whose profession he somehow connected his tragedy. What this patient seems to have lost was not his drive but rather his power to think and to study, in whatever degree, large or small, he had once possessed it. One suggested explanation of the fact that this young man retained sufficient drive to go forth to kill was the hypothesis that lobotomized patients lose their drive so far as their internal but not so far as their external world is concerned. There persists the question whether the loss of internal drive, if it is to be expected from psychosurgery, impairs the patient's chance of final recovery. If our competitive culture requires drive "for a person to be effective" (Beck, 1951), it would appear to be essential also in achieving the social adjustment regarded as a major criterion of "cure" of mental illness.

To the leading question — "does psychosurgery materially influence the long-range outlook for large samples of psychiatric cases?" — the conference's answer was simply "it is the majority opinion that such an influence has not yet been demonstrated". However, on the associated question, as to whether any form of psychiatric therapy materially influences the long-range outlook for large samples of psychiatric cases, the conference had also no clear affirmation.

### Psychotherapy in its Various Forms

This is an uncharted field in which roam many schools of thought, deploying within uncertain boundaries. *Psychotherapy* includes not only psychoanalysis but many modifications and variants of it, indebted to classical psychoanalysis but often vastly broadened in their application and practiced by many outside the field of analysts — general practitioners, pastors, laymen, etc. Outside these again there are psychotherapeutic procedures, which make no conscious use of the rules of psychoanalysis but which are widely and freely used. Lack of canons governing their use by all and sundry perhaps accounts for such protests as Jung's against the assumption that "psychotherapy can be used 'technically' like a recipe or an operational method or a dyeing process".

The variety of current psychiatric treatments led S. Bernard Wortis (when chairmen of the certifying board in psychiatry) to recommend that every therapist should be humble in claiming the exclusive effectiveness of any one treatment. He counseled evaluating all therapies with due recognition of the fact that treatment fails, in any case, with approximately one third of patients, succeeds with one third, may benefit the remaining third in varying degrees.

### PSYCHOANALYTIC THEORY AND THERAPY AND PSYCHOANALYTICALLY-ORIENTED THERAPY

There is obvious difficulty in drawing a hard and fast line between psychoanalysis and psychoanalytically-oriented psychotherapy. Franz Alexander, director, Chicago Institute for Psychoanalysis (in the *Proceedings of the Association for Research in Nervous and Mental Diseases*, 1953), regarded the heated controversy on this question as purely a matter of words. On the other hand, in the same discussion, Oskar Diethelm (chairman, psychiatry department, Cornell) denied that the differences were purely "semantic". He wondered, indeed, whether brief psychoanalysis which foregoes the couch, which is directed primarily at amelioration of symptoms rather than at profound restructuring of the personality, which allows the therapist to be much more than the interpreter of classical psychoanalytic procedure should be called analysis at all.

"Psychoanalysis" was first used by Freud about 1895 to designate both a method and the theory of psychology upon which the method is based. Freud, as reported by his biographer, Ernest Jones, defined psychoanalysis as "simply the study of processes of which we are unaware, of what for the sake of brevity we call the unconscious, by the free association technique of analyzing observable phenomena of transference and resistance". Originally concerned in therapy primarily with neuroses, the method, with an increasing number of modifications since 1940, is being applied currently, on the one hand (to a limited degree) to psychoses, including schizophrenia, and, on the other, to a wide range of neuroses. These applications are made not only by physicians but also by lay practitioners, psychologists, anthropologists, social workers attached to clinics, hospitals, courts, correctional institutions, churches, schools, colleges and various social agencies.

## Development of the psychoanalytic school in the United States

The question is often asked — indeed, has become the subject of satire on the British and French stage — why psychoanalysis has gained firmer medical and popular support in the United States than in other countries, influencing not only the direction of psychological treatment in medicine, but also aspects of literature, psychology, sociology, anthropology, religion. Apart from the intellectual and scientific interest naturally aroused in the United States by Freud's discoveries with regard to the unconscious, and the formulation of a unified conceptual system (of interest to psychology, philosophy, as well as to medicine), psychoanalysis benefited by other influences: it offered in medicine the attraction of a coherent working theory and a methodistic therapy at a time when American psychiatry was largely descriptive and when, as previously mentioned, neurophysiological and biochemical approaches seemed to be stymied; it offered general practitioners of medicine a possibility of "doing something" about conditions increasingly recognized to be "psychosomatic"; it exercised close control through small societies which were for a number of years the sole sources of systematic education and certification in psychoanalysis. These societies were almost exclusively composed of medical men. The New York Psychoanalytic Society, founded in 1911 and by 1925 in possession of an endowment used for subsequent establishment of an institute for education and training, began and "still remains" a medical organization which regards psychoanalytic therapy "strictly as a branch of the practice of medicine" (Oberndorf, 1953).

Both world wars gave further impetus to expansion of psychoanalysis and of the membership of the American Psychoanalytic Association. The association's functioning as practically a closed corporation for education and training was due in part to the originally nonreceptive attitude of the medical schools and also to the "great reluctance of the societies to entrust the teaching program to any but their own members" (Oberndorf, 1953). The American Psychoanalytic Association by 1952 numbered fifteen city and regional societies with their respective training institutes. Although it was not until 1941 that the first graduate department of psychoanalytic training was established in a medical school (Columbia), Johns Hopkins had an elective course in psychoanalysis so early as 1918–1925 and cases were demonstrated to students in various medical schools and hospitals by psychoanalysts so early as 1910.

A recent survey of the activities of the American Psychoanalytic Association showed that approximately sixty per cent of its members were engaged in teaching psychiatry in the medical schools, university hospitals, psychoanalytic training centers, often in key positions. That the number of psychoanalytically-trained candidates for such positions is increasing is suggested by a statement made at the annual meeting of the association, 1951, that the seven hundred students currently training to become analysts exceeded the number of existing practicing analysts in the nation at that time. The institutes for education and training established by the local, later the national, psychoanalytic societies, have been described as "possibly without precedent in the American scholastic scheme". Beginning, as other scientific societies begin, with discussions by qualified members, they have undertaken the conduct and control of teaching institutions from which students graduate to a certification for membership. Such certification involves a medical degree, a year of interneship in a mental hospital, three years of graduate training at one of the approved institutes, along with a personal analysis.

A characteristic of psychoanalysis in the United States, especially since 1940, is the development of various substitutes for Freudian concepts offered by later students, both European and American. In the process of this development, some of the traditional psychoanalytic hypotheses have corrected themselves out of existence, as for instance Freud's pansexual hypothesis. Comprehensive and accurate enumeration of centers in this country in which psychodynamic approaches to therapy are now practiced is not possible because of the many variations in traditional psychoanalytic Freudian methods and because a number of psychoanalysts practice in psychiatric centers that use other therapeutic approaches besides analysis. Affiliated societies and training institutes, some of which also provide treatment, approved by the American Psychoanalytic Association include the societies in New York, Washington, Chicago, Boston, Philadelphia, Topeka, Detroit, San Francisco, Los Angeles, Baltimore, and the Southern California and Western New England societies. Columbia's psychoanalytic clinic and the psychoanalytic institute attached to the state university medical center at New York are also approved by the national society. The Institute for Psychoanalysis (Alexander), through variations in traditional methods employing shorter periods of treatment and emphasizing psychosomatic aspects, is not affiliated with the national society. Psychoanalytically oriented groups are centered in Yale's psychiatry department (Knight, Kubie, Lidz). While St. Elizabeth's Hospital in Washington has never been primarily a center of psychoanalysis, its former director, William Alanson White, has been described as "entirely psychoanalytically oriented" and this was also true of one of his early assistants, Sullivan, whose modifications of orthodox Freudian theory have influenced current practices in the United States. Other centers of psychoanalytic therapy include the Menninger Clinic in Topeka, Chestnut Lodge (Fromm-Reichmann and associates), the New York Institute of Psychoanalysis (Eissler, Kubie, others).

One outstanding research development owes its current vigor at least in part to the idea, long associated with psychoanalytic theory, that, in assaying the role of the unconscious, great importance attaches to the "unconscious hostilities, inadequacies and immaturities shaped in childhood by grievously unsatisfactory child-mother and child-father relationships". The familiar psychological doctrine that the "rejected" child is forced by later traumatic experiences to regress to earlier fixations is a briskly debated subject which cannot be disposed of here. Ralph Linton (anthropology, Yale), in a 1953 Salmon lecture, observed that "recent research seems to indicate that the predominant role assigned to infantile experience by certain schools of psychoanalysis is not supported by the evidence". It is, therefore, an important development that psychological speculation is in process of being documented by definite studies of various kinds. These include anthropological studies of infancy, childhood, adolescence, in connection with the formation of personality (normal and abnormal). They also include recent neurophysiological work — as Hebb's — providing a basis for the psychological concept. Studies of the significance of early years include work in such centers as Western Reserve, the Illinois Neuropsychiatric Institute, the New York Psychiatric Institute, the Pennsylvania Hospital, the Rockland State Hospital, the Roxbury Children's Center, the Orthogenic School in Chicago, the psychiatry department in Bellevue. Work at the University of Chicago includes therapeutic approaches to schizophrenia in children. In this connection, data accumulated in long-term studies of normal infants and children is particularly pertinent. Illustrative are comprehensive studies conducted since 1930 under the Child Research Council, University of Colorado, by A. H. Washburn (pediatrician); Arnold Gesell's studies (begun in 1911) in Yale University's Clinic of Child Development of the behavior of children from two to ten years; studies of childhood growth at Western Reserve involving interdepartmental collaboration (pediatrics, anatomy, other departments).

There should be no implication that interest in the importance of early years is confined to psychoanalysis. From whatever source has come the present emphasis on the signal importance of childhood years in mental illness, its influence has progressively permeated research. The World Health Organization, in projecting, 1954, "the first international program in the field of mental health", mentioned reports from consultants on such subjects as the relation of maternal care to mental health in early and later life, juvenile delinquency, the mental health side of adoption, etc. It is now widely accepted, some would say a little belatedly, the *London Times* recently observed, that the child is the father of the man.

Divergences from original Freudian procedures on the part of many analysts have been described as increasingly wide and strong. Illustrative of the departures is that of one of Freud's pupils, Ferenszi, who favored substituting for the classical objective role of the analyst "a more lenient and assisting approach to the patient", an active display of love on the part of the therapist toward the patient as a strong force in relief of anxiety and in recovery. In noting that classical psychoanalysts are inclined to scoff at such innovations, Oberndorf, 1953, observed: "However, so far as I know, no study has been published by any 'classical' or other psychoanalyst of results obtained in a series of consecutive cases followed for a reasonable period of time, let us say five years, after he has discharged the patients; hence there is no basis for comparison. . . ."

Quite apart from evaluation of current modifications of orthodox psychoanalysis, there appears to be difficulty in defining the psychological content of the therapeutic process even in orthodox analysis. After four years of deliberation (1947 to 1951), a committee of the American Psychoanalytic Association, 1952, found it "impossible to find a definition of psychoanalysis that is acceptable to even a large group of the members of the Association". They reported that "this four-year study has shown that a very strong resistance exists among the members of the American Psychoanalytic Association to any investigation on the problem of evaluating results, even on the basis of their own definitions".

### Applicability of psychoanalytic therapy to schizophrenia

Freud had doubts whether classical methods of analysis through lifting of repression, transference, etc., would be adequate in schizophrenia. Bleuler's (University of Zurich) testing of the validity of Freud's theories with psychotic patients in the mental hospital at Burgholzli was especially concerned with schizophrenics. Jung, in the *Psychology of Dementia Praecox*, corroborated Bleuler's view that Freud's psychoanalytic mechanisms could be demonstrated even more obviously in schizophrenia than in the neuroses.

Opinions vary greatly, however. As they would, since competent reports do not exist of psychoanalytic treatment of any considerable number of schizophrenics. Some of the reports of success in breaking through the schizophrenic's barrier to interpersonal relations by way of current modifications of classical analysis have been described as superficial processes, merely allaying symptoms; for any real curing of the basic personality disorder, "deep" and prolonged psychoanalysis is considered necessary. Some psychiatrists would definitely reserve psychoanalysis for the neuroses; others, however (as Otto Fenichel, 1945), consider that the therapeutic aim in schizophrenia and in neurosis is the same — to confront the patient with the anxieties from which he is trying to escape and to refuse to participate in his attempts to escape. One reason why, in Fenichel's view, an analytic effect on schizophrenics is possible is that the schizophrenic's "regression to narcissism is never a complete one".

As a complicating factor in psychoanalysis with schizophrenics, Eissler, 1952, cited the schizophrenic's faculty for learning to conceal "the psychic scar within the framework of the ego". Fromm-Reichmann, 1952, while not ruling out psychoanalysis in schizophrenia, mentioned as two of the factors that account for the reluctance of many psychotherapists to use it: first, the schizophrenic's bizarre language, difficult for the analyst to understand; secondly, his infantile self-engulfment which is an obstacle to the type of doctor-patient relation required for psychoanalysis. It has been suggested that with "basic schizophrenics" use of psychoanalysis may be often tragic in that removal of the repressive mechanism in potentially schizophrenic neurotics may precipitate psychosis.

The whole subject of the applicability of psychoanalytic techniques to schizophrenia is under review. Psychoanalytic concepts and principles were a focus in the discussions of a 1950 conference at Yale on psychotherapy with schizophrenics, participated in by workers from the Psychoanalytic Clinic for training and research, Columbia University, and the New York Psychoanalytic Institute (Arlow, Bak, Eidelberg, Eissler, Kubie); from the Johns Hopkins department of psychiatry (Frank); from Chestnut Lodge, Maryland (Fromm-Reichmann); from the Austen Riggs Foundation, Stockbridge, (Knight); from the Boston State Hospital (Semrad); from the Rhode Island Hospital (Wright); from the Yale psychiatry department (Lidz). With the exception of Wexler (then at the Menninger Foundation), a psychologist (Ph.D.), all were doctors of medicine with psychiatric, chiefly psychoanalytic, supplementary training.

### PSYCHOTHERAPY IN THE MORE GENERAL CONNOTATION — INDIVIDUAL, GROUP, MULTIPLE

Psychotherapy, with or without regard to traditional psychoanalytic practices, is widely used, whether alone or as a necessary adjuvant to other forms of therapy including lobotomies. Its necessity after

psychosurgery has been especially stressed. At the 1951 research conference, Kathleen Litten observed that any improvement following operation should be regarded as "only the beginning", to be
followed by psychotherapy ("to prevent psychiatric relapse" and
to re-educate the patient) for years rather than months and perhaps
permanently. Unless the lobotomized schizophrenic is re-adjusted to
his family and to his community, he is "left rootless or alone". Those
widely experienced in shock therapy have, as elsewhere suggested,
stressed the need of accompanying psychotherapy, particularly in its
social forms. That some workers have no difficulty in deciding which
is the more important of the two therapeutic expedients is illustrated
by Whitehorn's comparison, 1950, of improvement produced by
insulin treatment in from twenty-one to twenty-two per cent of schizophrenic cases in state hospitals, and improvement produced by intensive individualized psychotherapy in private mental hospitals: forty-
two per cent in a series of 500 (New York Hospital at Westchester)
recovered or sufficiently improved to justify discharge; fifty-two per
cent of 134 patients found to be "socially useful" nine years after
initial hospitalization (Phipps Psychiatric Institute).

Of psychotherapy, in the more generalized sense, outstanding current methods are intensive individual psychotherapy, including, but
not limited to, psychoanalysis; multiple psychotherapy (several
therapists and one patient); group therapy (a group of patients and
one therapist, with the role of the therapist ranging from that of the
traditional analyst to that of "participator"). Fromm-Reichmann
pointed out, 1953 (with especial reference to intensive individual
therapy as practiced by herself, by Sullivan, Rosen, Bychowski,
Eissler, Wexler, Knight, Federn), that therapeutic advances during
the past two decades are especially referable to these three forms of
therapy.

Intensive individual psychotherapy obviously covers factors so
numerous and so complex that they defy even illustration. Because
getting into any kind of *rapport* with the schizophrenic in individual
psychotherapy (and also in other forms of it) involves some method of
communication, study of the language of schizophrenics has been of
especial interest to several workers (Kasanin, University of California;
Sullivan; others). The schizophrenic is particularly apt to develop

"codification systems of his own — new words, mathematical systems" (Ruesch, 1953, in an observation to the American Foundation) and to use language revealing archaic and primitive symbolism. The problem of communication for schizophrenics was regarded as involving research on the network of communication in which the schizophrenic operates — his family and relatives and also study of communication in childhood (since the schizophrenic is believed to have failed to learn in his early childhood the necessary means of communicating efficiently with others). Ruesch emphasized the present need of "basic" work on communication, without thought of application in psychiatry. Students of communication have been swift to recognize that communication is not always dependent on language. Establishment of nonverbal communication between patient and therapist has been a subject of especial study in Emory's psychiatry department (Carl A. Whitaker) and in California under a five-year grant, 1948–1953, to Ruesch from the National Institute of Mental Health.

Intensive — and intense — individual psychotherapy can consume the energy of both patient and therapist to a degree intolerable to both. It is not only the cynics that have tended to regard some of the "cures" purporting to result from long-continued intensive treatment of this kind as more or less a discharge dictated by mutual exhaustion. There are also economic considerations: treatment that requires hundreds of hours, extending over many months and often years, is, as Knight put it, 1952, "bound to be quite expensive for somebody".

Multiple therapy is new and few data on the techniques used or the results achieved are as yet available. One of the advantages claimed for a system using more than one therapist (Malcolm L. Hayward, Joseph J. Peters and J. Edward Taylor, 1952) is that it offers to the schizophrenic patient opportunity to focus unfriendly emotions on one of the therapists and friendly emotions on another. In other words, by offering "more targets for expression of ambivalence, therapy can be greatly speeded and made more dynamic". Centers of research on multiple therapy include, besides the Institute of the Pennsylvania Hospital (the workers cited above), the psychiatry department at Emory University (Carl Whitaker), Chestnut Lodge (Rioch).

As for the third expedient, group therapy, the philosophy behind it (aside from its practical economic advantage) assumes that cooperation with a group aids the patient to "intellectualize" his problem (Brody, 1952). First tried in the army during the recent war as an expedient for dealing with large numbers suffering with various psychological reactions to battle strain and war stress, it is now being experimentally tested in centers for schizophrenia. Along with many other psychotherapeutic techniques, group therapy has been presented as owing a debt to Freud. Testimony offered in this direction includes one of Freud's observations in his *Group Psychology and the Analysis of the Ego:* "In the individual's mental life someone else is invariably involved, as a model, as an object, as a helper, as an opponent, and so, from the very first, individual psychology is at the same time social psychology as well."

Trigant Burrow has been mentioned as among the first in this country to call attention to psychoanalytic mechanisms operating in the group. The vigor of his interest, and that of others, in the group principle accounts for establishment of the American Group Psychotherapy Association which held its twelfth annual conference in January, 1955. Within the last decade, almost every "school" of individual psychotherapy has applied some of the group theories and methods (Saul Scheidlinger, 1953). Among the members of the group, the reasoning goes, a feeling of identity is gradually built up; the group becomes a unit in which emotional release in one patient can be achieved to some degree by expression through another patient. In the group discussions, utilized in group therapy, Ezriel, 1952, recommended that the therapist do nothing to "structure" the situation, offer no direct support or stimulus to the discussion; in Ezriel's view, the emotional relationships operating at the moment in the group are much more important than the content of the discussion. Group therapy is considered to offer schizophrenics experience in interpersonal relations, the breakdown of which is considered a major schizophrenic reaction. Since the group approximates "the atmosphere of the family and society as a whole" (Joseph Abrahams, 1947), it could be extended to a whole ward, and thus made a practical form of therapy in public as well as private institutions.

## QUALIFICATIONS OF THE THERAPIST IN ALL FORMS
### OF PSYCHOTHERAPY

Of the various schools of psychotherapy, the classic psychoanalytic school has shown most formal concern with the qualification of its practitioners. The requirement (maintained in all centers of psychoanalysis in this country) that the practitioner shall himself undergo analysis before engaging in psychotherapeutic work was aimed at ridding the therapist of his own psychological blind spots, enabling him to regard the patient with less bias and prejudice. Since, however, the therapist is envisaged in such different ways by psychotherapists generally, even those in various schools deriving from psychoanalytic theory, a neat catalogue of the qualities and policies desirable in the psychotherapist would obviously not be valid. One of the distinct cleavages divides the classical psychoanalytic view that the psychotherapist should be merely a recorder, an interpreter, an analyst, from the view that the psychotherapist should offer, as previously quoted, "a more lenient and helpful approach" to the patient, fulfilling a role which, in its extreme form, means "participating in the psychosis".

In John N. Rosen's method, described by him as "direct analysis" (in its "direct" concern with the patient's current reactions as contrasted with disregard of present "symptoms" by classic psychoanalysis), the psychotherapist's ability to "participate in the psychosis" is a *sine qua non*. "The therapist, like the good parent, must identify with the unhappy child and be so disturbed by the unhappiness of the child that he himself cannot rest until the child is again at peace." Participating, as contrasted with dispensing, requires a much greater expenditure of time, energy, interest, love on the part of the therapist. If time, energy, interest, love can be counted upon almost without limit, perhaps any technique would be productive. One of Rosen's colleagues expressed the view that many of his interpretations are "arbitrary if not incorrect", but that they are also notably "effective, irrespective of their truth or faultiness". This comment may be a recognition of the inevitable usefulness of the vast amount of time, energy and concern that "direct analysis" exacts of the therapist, or it may merely reflect current interest in anything that "works", an interest that is enlarging classical psychoanalytic concepts and methods in the United States.

The role of "participant-observer" for the therapist seemed (Sullivan) the "operational approach" to dealing with the anxiety in neurosis — and in schizophrenia. Wexler has been described (by Sanford, 1953) as having gone far in developing the technique by which the therapist aligns himself with the schizophrenic's archaic superego, speaking to the patient in the language of the superego (e.g., agreeing with aggressive, moral, self-accusations) and so gaining contact with him, and participating in the schizophrenic's reality.

There is a considerable amount of current interest in thinking through this matter of what the psychotherapist's qualities should be. For instance, recent interest, described in *Science*, 1954, in putting the management of interviews, as a cardinal technique in psychotherapy, upon a more scientific basis by devising a high fidelity recorder (Yale workers, Mahl, Dollard, Redlich, with advice from the Bell Telephone Company, the Psycho-Acoustic Laboratory and Department of Social Relations of Harvard, the Clark School for the Deaf and the Haskins Laboratory) was not entirely directed toward the patient. The declared hope was also to analyze more accurately the qualities of the interviewer that may determine the success or the failure of interview therapy.

The most usual common denominator in varying definitions of the therapist's qualifications bears on the degree of understanding, compassion and love which the therapist is able to feel for his patient (although the word love is usually avoided, probably as not sufficiently objective). The compassion and love are under constant strain. The therapist is under constant fire from the patient's perception which, although disturbed, may be abnormally keen. The schizophrenic, according to reports from some therapists, is often curiously sensitive to unverbalized feelings in the therapist of which the therapist himself is sometimes only partly conscious. The schizophrenic shows an uncanny faculty for "getting at the therapist's actual weaknesses". Ultimately the therapist must, as Knight put it, after weathering the patient's "emotional storms, insatiable demands, provocative testing maneuvers, primitive outbursts of hatred, and confusing communications", be able to convince the patient of the therapist's understanding, freedom from alarm, basic belief in human beings and, above all, affection for them. Knight admits that this relatively uncharted and tempestuous therapeutic voyage is taxing on the therapist's energies, though highly rewarding for those that can hold to their course.

Stressing the therapist's need of dedicated interest, Brody observed, 1952, that there would be no therapeutic response "if the therapist derives any conscious or unconscious gain in the sense of satisfying his own frustrated needs". He must be tough, built "to take whatever comes, for no matter how long, being recurrently hurt but not ever being destroyed in his role as the patient's physician" (Wright, psychiatry, Rhode Island Hospital, 1952). Always he must *care:* "The patient's recovery must be of high emotional importance to him . . . time spent on the patient must not count . . . the higher the stakes which the therapist places on the patient the greater will be his response" (Eissler, 1952).

In the view of some, these prescriptions seem to require of the psychotherapist, for success in his task, a practically extra-human capacity. On the one hand he is to *care* — intensely. On the other hand, he must guard, as Fromm-Riechmann put it, 1952, against "offering nonprofessional warmth to a schizophrenic patient". Her wise counsel never to go beyond the realistic professional relationship suggests at once the need of both a guide and a brake in maintaining the professional relationship and guarding against the patient's mistaking love of mankind for love of himself. Those whose lives are built around the need to be loved fall easily into this (temporarily) comforting error.

It becomes very clear that the ideal "intensive individualized psychotherapy" comes very close to religion. It may be on this ground that nonpsychodynamists resist the idea of deliberately procured "transference". It is certainly on this ground, among others, that some medical educators feel that much of the present psychiatry "belongs to the priesthood", as a function that can neither be taught in medical schools nor purchased in office hours. This could also be one of the reasons for the skepticism toward psychoanalysis attributed to some divisions of the church on the ground that psychoanalysis invades the province of the soul. The psychodynamic school generally noted with approbation Pope Pius XII's recent explicit approval of psychoanalysis as a healing device — to be used, however, "only in accordance with the truths established by reason and by faith, and the obligatory precepts of ethics".

## EMPHASIS ON SOCIAL AND CULTURAL FACTORS IN THE STUDY OF MENTAL ILLNESS, INCLUDING SCHIZOPHRENIA

### INTRODUCTORY: PERSONALITY AS A SOCIAL PRODUCT

Man's greater ability to communicate with his kind was attributed by H. J. Muller, 1955, only in part to the "moderate difference" between man's native intelligence and that of some other animals. It is attributable also to man's social disposition and his "queer proclivities for vocalizing and symbolizing". Every human individual embodies the "distilled experience of a vast ever-increasing body of his ancestors and associates". It is by virtue of this social evolution that man has become more potent than other forms of life on the earth "without any perceptible improvement having taken place in his genes even before civilization began".

The social approach to behavior, according to Clyde K. Kluckhohn (anthropology, Harvard) and Henry A. Murray (psychology, Harvard), 1953, does not deny the biological basis of human nature or the physiochemical basis of biology; it merely holds that human behavior is on a different level from physiological phenomena and hence should be studied in its own right "without waiting for more 'basic' sciences to provide the complete foundations". The psychiatrist has, therefore, "become an essential member of the social science fraternity". In mental illness, "the organism is ill in its relation to other organisms" (Denis Hill, Institute of Psychiatry, Maudsley Hospital, 1950). Freud conceived the individual as always part of a group, usually the family group. Jung thought that the psychology of the individual could be fully explained only by recognizing it as not merely a physiological, biological and personal problem, but also a question of contemporary history. Personality, as Kluckhohn summarized it, "is preeminently a social product".

The basic personality of the individual ("except in societies whose cultures are undergoing rapid change") will, according to Linton

(Salmon lecture, 1953), be congruous with his culture — *i.e.*, the ideas, habits and knowledge shared and transmitted by a society's members — and will permit him to participate in that culture "with a minimum of frustrations and a maximum of awards". The test of relative normalcy is "the extent to which the individual's experience has given him a personality conforming to the basic personality of his society". In our culture, when the individual's private world deviates too far from the official culture, we speak of mental disorders (Laurence Frank, 1953).

Social factors are fundamentally implied in many of the leading concepts and practices of psychiatry, in the concepts stressing "interpersonal relations", in the therapies addressed to adjusting morbid interpersonal relations. Different workers envisage social factors in different perspectives: Sullivan stressed the importance of interpersonal relations "in a broad extension of Freud's original analysis of the familial interpersonal relationship between parents and children"; Whitehorn referred, 1953, to the "school of thought in psychiatry which views the disturbance of social function not just as a symptomatic expression of psychiatric illness, but rather as the reverse", the cause of it. Ruesch attributed abolition of the ancient practice of jailing the mentally ill under unbearable social conditions to steadily increasing recognition of the importance of social relations in the complex picture of mental illness. "Investigators began to study the patients, their families, and ultimately the communities in which the patients lived." This development, in Ruesch's view, has led to virtual abandonment of the "individual-environment dichotomy". Especially since World War I, there has developed a branch of psychiatry which regards the mentally ill individual as a unit in "a network of human relations".

National and international gatherings, whether of psychiatrists, psychologists, or sociologists, regularly stress the importance of social factors and of interaction between the individual and his culture: various symposia of the fourteenth International Congress of Psychology, 1954, were devoted to social variables in personality determination and to many other social aspects of mental illness. At the 1951 research conference on psychosurgery, Hebb expressed the view that in mental illness "the decisive factor is often social", and

Mettler, in somewhat reverse form, conveyed the same truth: "The patient does not get into the mental institution because he is crazy but because of the environment in which he is no longer tolerated." At the 1951 Conference on Psychiatric Education the schizophrenic's outstanding failure was defined as inability to adapt to the other human beings in a "highly organized and enormously complex habitat". Great Britain's Mental Health Research Fund, 1954, among recommended studies included "research on the forms of social structure most likely to lead to the improvement of the mental quality and stamina of the community and most likely to reduce the incidence of addiction, delinquency and crime". As therapeutic essentials in mental illness, the World Federation for Mental Health, 1953, stressed the need of social measures "directed toward improving conditions, not only material but also psychological, in the home, in the school, in industry and in the community in general". The National Institute of Mental Health in a 1954 report described the field of mental health, in its full meaning, as "synonymous with human relations and as broad as life itself".

If we accept the premise that many people with the complete genetical equipment required for the development of a particular psychosis nevertheless do not develop it (Slater, 1952) because they are protected by environmental factors, and the further premise that other individuals apparently sound constitutionally do become psychotic under environmental stress, we are bound to investigate the real nature of these protecting, or precipitating, social factors. This will take us far afield — far beyond current studies of the family and the community, reaching back not only into anthropology but into all the economic and physical influences that account for any given civilization. The importance of the subjects concerned (A. Lewis, psychiatry, University of London, at the Oxford conference, 1952) "is in inverse proportion to our mastery of any means of studying them". Speculations in this field become, therefore, "rather like divination. The contrast with established fields of scientific inquiry is altogether too sharp."

More hopeful was Thomas Francis's view, 1953, cited in the second chapter of the first volume. He expressed to the first world conference on medical education in London his conviction that social factors, however large and complex, can be studied and evaluated in all types of illness. If social influences contribute to a complex etiology, they are pathogenic influences "which can be disclosed and integrated just as other factors can". Even if the social factors are not primary, study of them can provide effective information. Whether primary or secondary, they do not belong "in the rosy field of speculation".

## THE SOCIAL SCIENCES IN RESEARCH ON MENTAL ILLNESS

The pertinence of the social sciences in study of personality was attributed, at the 1951 conference on psychiatric education, to the fact that it is in the field of social functioning that the outstanding disturbances of psychiatric patients are perceived and must be controlled. The whole range of the social sciences (sociology, history, economics, psychology, anthropology) has certainly not yet been widely invoked in research on schizophrenia. Much of the work of various sociologists and social psychologists, as Cottrell, Burgess, Hollingshead, Parsons, Hawley and Dunham, including research on the family, research on the community (especially by ecological methods), the position of sociological theory, ethnic research, research in social psychology, has, according to Lewis, 1952, "played only a small part in the social research with which psychiatrists are familiar".

Social studies of this nature have been concerned with the ethnic, economic and cultural characteristics of patients admitted to mental hospitals; the situation in which the mental disorder developed; the social context of the illness; the degree of deviation from socially accepted behavior; the degree to which the social structure of the mental hospital reproduces in miniature the relations of the larger world; the effect of changing degrees of social contact on the individual's sense of his own personal and social worth at different ages (the aggravated mental failings of the elderly when they are isolated and unwanted); the social situation of patients returned to the community after discharge from a mental hospital. From another and more external point of view, social scientists have been concerned with popular criteria of "normal" behavior and popular concepts of mental illness; the nature of the institutions which communities and governments develop to meet the needs of the mentally sick; the attitude of society toward them; the changing attitudes in different classes of society and in different countries and cultures at different periods toward mental abnormality; the requirements for certification. On these and many other points, according to Lewis, "obvious though they seem, we have very little information". While in his view there would be no insurmountable difficulty in collecting it, the ground to be covered is "fantastically vast", the methods "hardly yet discernible".

How greatly modern techniques for fact-finding and new statistical methods may facilitate gathering comprehensive knowledge on social factors in human behavior was pointed out by Adrian, at the 1954 meeting of the British Association for the Advancement of Science. "The stage seems to be set for the new development and it might well be the most important scientific development of this century." Cybernetics, the mathematical system permitting computation of unpredictable as well as predictable factors, has been described as applicable to the social sciences in spite of the vagueness of some of the factors involved.

Serious reservations, however, are still entertained as to the functioning of the social sciences in the field of mental illness, on the ground that the kind of observations the social scientist can make will not "be sufficiently objective and sufficiently precise". Social scientists are urged to distinguish, as do workers in the physical and biological sciences, between concepts deduced from scattered individual observations and principles arrived at by the scientific method. Adrian does not despair of the possibility of conducting social research "on reasonably scientific lines". It is admitted that great difficulty is involved in making observations in a world where the units are men and women rather than in a laboratory where the units are cells or molecules. Nevertheless, social research is "too important a plant to be left in the hot-house atmosphere of research institutes and Unesco teams". Adrian would have more social scientists in the university "so that the rising generation can see what they are like".

Discussing "applied anthropology" in medicine generally, William Caudill, 1953, mentioned, among "some unusual things" which "social anthropologists" and social scientists have recently been doing, participating with physicians in conferences on social factors in medicine, teaching in medical schools, studying the social structure of hospitals and the flow of life on the wards, employing psychotherapy with Plains Indians and working with public health services in Peru. Caudill mentioned as one urgent practical reason for fostering application of social sciences in medicine, the need in the Point 4 program of interpreting our medical techniques and ideas to people of other cultures.

Sociological and psychological studies have been directed to the family, to the hospital ward, to the community. The *family* has been the particular focus of studies of neurotic behavior by Jules Henry and associates in Washington University's sociology department. Conceiving the family "as a field of forces made up of a complex of interactional systems", Henry developed a coding system to facilitate "a quick and relatively precise evaluation of fundamental behavior patterns and attitudes of an interactional system within the family". Some workers have even suggested making the family rather than the patient the unit of illness and regarding the patient as merely a station in which the disturbance is localized.

A Yale study (Lidz), supported in part by the National Institute of Mental Health, was concerned with the "interpersonal family environment of schizophrenia". The number of subjects with which family studies could be concerned is legion. At the Oxford conference, T. S. Simey (social science, University of Liverpool), who did not feel at all pessimistic about the possible results of field inquiries in this connection, suggested that family studies should be concerned with the kind of families that contain schizophrenics; their positions in the class structure; their occupations; their characteristic ways of life. Another speaker at this conference, J. M. Tanner, stressed the point that the family studies aimed at defining genetical and cultural background should certainly include studies on normal families; and if normal families are to be studied "for goodness' sake, let us study related normals and not accidentally chosen ones".

Since the hospital ward rather than the family is the "society" of so many of the mentally ill, social scientists have lately directed their attention to the wards in general hospitals and in mental institutions. Work especially concerned with this type of study includes that of Dunham, Barrabee, Stanton and Schwartz, Szurek, Fromm-Reichmann and a number of others, and still unpublished work by Grey and by Brody on the relationships between social class and ethnic factors and the behavior and treatment of psychiatric patients in mental hospitals. Other work (some of it as yet unpublished) concerned with the influence of the social setting in hospital therapy includes that of Milton Greenblatt, R. W. Hyde, and associates (based on observations on the men's acute wards), Boston Psychopathic Hospital; of Henry, McMillan Hospital in St. Louis; of Hobson, concerned with comparative study in four mental hospitals in the Boston area. A two-year study by the Russell Sage Foundation comprehended ward patient care in mental hospitals throughout the United States. A program motivated by the thesis that the unprofessional people "who perform the simple ward duties in mental hospitals and who have close daily contact with the patients play an important part in the job of helping them recover" was described, 1953, in a report of the National Institute of Mental Health. The program covered 360 federal, state and private mental hospitals.

The significance of interpersonal relationships among patients, and between patients and staff was touched upon in earlier references to group therapy. "The activities of the group form a describable pattern, the understanding of which is necessary for any complete understanding of particular members . . ." (Stanton and Schwartz). Understanding the ward group is not, however, a simple matter of applying to the ward the conventional criteria of social behavior in the world outside; Caudill once suggested that behavior which might be considered by the outer world primitive, instinctual and antisocial might, in the hospital, become social behavior, owing to a wider range of tolerance and suspension of judgment among patients. An important consideration is how far the rigid and custodial character of many overcrowded institutions can foster concern with the social interaction of its patients. In the general review of the present place of the mental hospital, the question has been raised whether patients that are able to function socially to any degree in any area of life should be hospitalized at all, other than for diagnostic study. Mention is made of belated but increasing interest in this country in having state mental hospital systems take more into account the possibilities of family and colony care, and of outpatient clinics for ambulatory patients. Such proposals recall Overholser's hopeful prediction, 1955, that the mental hospital in the year 2055 may occupy a far less important role in the care and treatment of the mentally ill than it does today, and, conversely, a much larger role in teaching, research and preventive psychiatry.

In the field of *community* studies, Caudill referred, 1953, to a number of "extremely promising projects . . . begun in recent years".  Under the direction of Alexander Leighton (Cornell), a large group of workers headed by Robert Rapoport (anthropologist), James S. Tyhurst (psychiatrist) and Allister MacMillan (psychologist) have been studying for several years a county in a Canadian province with a population of 20,000, equally divided into English- and French-speaking segments and occupationally separated into fishing, lumbering, farming and town groups.  The study aimed at: clarifying what constitutes mental health aside from the mere absence of pathology; illuminating the relationship between personality formation and social environment; indicating which types of stress in the social environment are most important in production of psychiatric disorders; and uncovering leads for further research.

Interrelations between social structure and mental illness were the subject of a Yale study (Redlich and Hollingshead) aided by a research grant from the National Institute of Mental Health.  The study aimed at correlating social variables in the community (New Haven) with the frequency and types of mental illness.  Included also was study of the attitudes of various local groups toward mental illness and psychiatry, types of psychiatric treatment used and comparative clinical response to them.

Psychiatrists at the 1951 conference on psychiatric education expressed the hopeful view that out of the "empirical, experimental and field studies in anthropology, psychology and sociology" there is gradually emerging a steadily increasing systematized body of immediately useful knowledge.  Anthropologists (Paul Fejos, anthropology, Yale, 1953) are concerning themselves more and more with the relation between culture and personality.  A. Irving Hallowell (anthropology, Pennsylvania) in the 1953 international symposium on anthropology cited this trend as "a twentieth-century development", especially among American anthropologists although in the twenties the major contributors were British. "Today many reciprocal lines of interest have developed between anthropologists and those working in the psychological disciplines." The net result of this is greatly to broaden the base of study of mental illness — to transfer stress from failure in perception to the normal processes of perception; from break-down in communication to the fundamental principles of all social communication; from childhood trauma to all the responses and cultural changes of the formative years.

Broad investigation of the childhood period was, as previously mentioned, recommended by Bowlby as a focus of research into the interaction between the individual and his culture. Bowlby pointed out that, in children, social relationships, clearly very relevant to mental illness, are restricted, intense, and at a higher pitch than they are in adults. Since, as pointed out earlier, the simplest and most highly motivated responses, those most charged with feeling, are learned in early childhood and depend on centers in the older parts of the brain, very similar to those with which other mammals are provided, Bowlby suggested the wisdom of systematic study of social influences and responses in animals as a source of light on man. He pointed out (citing the work of Scott, Fredericson and Fuller, 1951) that a lamb removed from the rest of the flock for the first ten days after birth does not follow the flock and never becomes strongly associated with it. There is, in other words, a fundamental change in the development of its social relationship. The needed studies of other mammals and of infants and very young children, Bowlby described as "not really even begun".

It would be a hardy soul that would cross in one broad jump the stream which at present separates zoological, physiological and psychological facts from psychiatric hypotheses. The hypotheses vary in their emphasis, according to schools of psychiatric thought. Discussing social origins of neurosis, Erich Fromm (social psychologist, Bennington), 1953, described, as the elementary root of neurosis, conflict between the child and parental authority. Since "man is not born to be broken", the child fights against the authority which his parents represent. The scars left from defeat in the child's fight against irrational authority are, Fromm reasoned, to be found at the bottom of every neurosis. The psychoanalytic method was lauded by

Elkes at the Oxford conference as "one of the few methods which has attempted to provide data on the formative role in man of objects in his very early natural environment", and the schizophrenic is described as having "lost his objects" or his "object relations". Culture changes during the formative years were described by Ruesch, 1953, as the experience which gives the future therapist the right psychological tool for understanding others. Fixation upon a quite definite period in the formative years, favored by some psychiatrists, has been challenged, as by Linton's view that "the period of maximum influence is undetermined".

In spite of especial concern of psychiatry with individuals and the abnormal, in evaluating childhood experience in relation to adult personality, and the concern of anthropology with societies and the normal (Francis L. K. Hsu, 1952), there is, among some psychiatrists, advancing recognition that child-rearing practices in different cultures suggest the need of much broader understanding of normal infant behavior before there can be a real understanding of personality development.

## ILLUSTRATIVE CULTURAL STUDIES

Indicative of the trend toward consideration of cultural factors in studies of personality development was the Rockefeller Foundation's grant (1948) to Harvard's anthropology department (Kluckhohn) for a field study of a homogeneous Indian culture in the west to determine the degree to which individual physiological and behavioral reactions are interwoven with community reactions and cultural standards. A study of 8,700 Hutterites, an ethnically Swiss sect of Anabaptist Christians, living in ninety-three separate farming colonies in North and South Dakota, Montana, Manitoba and Alberta, was made by Joseph W. Eaton (sociology and anthropology, Wayne University) with Robert J. Weil and Bert Kaplan as consultants in psychiatry and psychology. The Hutterites, considered to represent an extreme in resistance to the disorganizing effects of acculturation, "have for centuries lived in a slowly changing social system, including a religious communal system of property ownership, and a family system stripped of nearly all but the procreative and affection-giving functions" (Caudill, 1953). Among the Hutterites, "the incidence of most mental illnesses was found to be lower than that of other epidemiological surveys but higher than had been expected on the basis of cases known to hospitals, doctors, and previous students of the sect. There were four times as many cases of manic-depression as of schizophrenia."

Another cultural study, reported (1952) by B. J. F. Laubscher (Mental Hospital, Queenstown, Cape Province, South Africa) led to the conclusion that mental disorders, especially schizophrenia, are more frequent among the Bantu tribes of South Africa than is generally believed. Several African studies, described by Linton, 1953, as furnishing the best information in the very limited amount now available, indicated that all types of insanity found in Europe appear to be present in Africa also. Citing Geoffrey Tooth's studies of mental illness in the Gold Coast, Linton referred to the conclusion that Europeanization and the resulting cultural stresses are not a significant factor in psychosis. Outside Africa, the most interesting results were described by Linton as those reported by Stainbrook from Bahia in northern Brazil. Stainbrook found individuals (among the predominantly Negro subjects) in whom physical catatonia had "advanced to the point of waxy posture" but who manifested only very superficial social withdrawal.

There is much interest in the incidence of psychoses in different social classes, but studies and conclusions are limited. Reviews by Faris (1944) and by Dunham (1947) of ecological research in mental disorder seemed to indicate "major agreement" that high schizophrenic rates occur in areas of low economic status "while manic-depressive rates show much more scatter" through various economic levels. In the above-mentioned Yale study of incidence of psychoses in various social classes in New Haven the frequency of schizophrenia in the lowest class was shown (as cited by Linton) to be "twelve and one half as high a percentage as in the highest". Linton's comment was, however, "Numerous factors other than social and economic stress are involved in this picture and further study is needed."

There are warnings against attaching too much importance to cultural relativity. One school of thought holds to the concept that insanity everywhere will, after all, show the same basic pathological processes. The late Ruth Benedict often stressed the point that no one of the "particular cultural bridges should be regarded as the 'natural' path to maturity". Hallowell thought that regarding culture as determining or conditioning behavior was "to conceive the problem much too narrowly, if not inadequately". The contribution from anthropology of major interest to psychologists was, in his view, "the demonstrable relations between cultural variability and the motivational systems of human individuals, that is, the differential organization of drives, needs, emotions, attitudes, and so on, which lie at the core of relatively enduring *dispositions* to act in a predictable manner . . ." In all societies, Linton pointed out, "many individuals undergo the experiences which make some persons neurotic without becoming neurotic". The constitutional factor cannot be socialized out of existence.

In psychiatrically oriented comment, 1953, on the significance of various cultural studies, Henry Wegrocki (psychiatry, California Hospital, Los Angeles) pointed out that "human behavior has so long been seen in terms of the categories of Western civilization that a critical evaluation of cultures other than our own could not help exercising a salutary effect" on the tendency to keep to western criteria. The achievement of a "realization that one culture cannot be interpreted in terms of the cultures of another represents as tremendous an advance in the study of social behavior as did the brilliant insight of Freud into the field of depth psychology".

On the moot question whether abnormality is a relative or an absolute character, Ruth Benedict once implied that the canvas of research into mental illness must expand to take into account the existence of behavior considered abnormal in our culture but normal in other cultures; types of abnormality not occurring in western civilization; behavior considered normal in our society but abnormal in others. She defined the misfit as "one whose disposition is not capitalized in his culture". "When data are available in psychiatry, this minimum definition of abnormal human tendencies will be probably quite unlike our culturally conditioned, largely elaborated psychoses such as those described, *e.g.*, under the terms 'schizophrenic' and 'manic depressive'." The practicing psychiatrist "is so close to problems of his patients, which are within the same culture as his own" (Lewis, 1953) that he forgets that some of these problems "might cease to be problems if the culture changed".

# MAJOR SOURCES

The publications in the following highly selective list were chosen primarily to illustrate trends — since 1940 — in fundamental investigative work pertinent to the clinical problems discussed in all of the chapters of the second volume. A particular aim was to indicate those publications dealing with concepts that enlarge biological horizons and bring the specific medical problems into perspective with investigative work on life processes. The titles listed illustrate, in varying degrees, a marked trend in basic research, in the course of penetrating to progressively deeper levels, to cut across boundaries of specialization. That the list of "major sources" noted below is clearly not a list of sources cited in the text will be evident from comparison of the citations in any section of the text with the list. Less than one-sixth of the references that appear in the virus chapter, for instance, are specifically enumerated; similarly, the listed fifty publications dealing with cancer research were selected from some 700 publications referred to directly or indirectly in the cancer chapter and from hundreds of others antedating the period to which this list is restricted.

W. W. ACKERMANN: The relation of the Krebs cycle to viral synthesis, *J. Exper. Med.*, June, 1951.

E. D. ADRIAN: General principles of nervous activity, *Brain*, March, 1947.

————: The Physical Background of Perception, Clarendon Press, Oxford, 1947.

————: Science and human nature, *Science*, October 29, 1954.

FRANZ ALEXANDER: Development of the fundamental concepts of psychoanalysis, Dynamic Psychiatry, Franz Alexander and Helen Ross, eds., University of Chicago Press, 1952.

PETER ALEXANDER: The reactions of carcinogens with macromolecules, *Advances in Cancer Research*, 1954.

EDGAR ALLEN: Estrogenic hormones in the genesis of tumors and cancers, *Endocrinology*, June, 1942.

————: Physiology of the ovaries, Glandular Physiology and Therapy, Symposium prepared by Council on Pharmacy and Chemistry of the American Medical Association, 1942.

RUDOLF ALTSCHUL: Selected Studies of Arteriosclerosis, Thomas, Springfield, Illinois, 1950.

M. D. ALTSCHULE: Bodily Physiology in Mental and Emotional Disorders, Grune and Stratton, New York, 1953.

E. C. AMOROSO: Placentation, Marshall's Physiology of Reproduction, A. S. Parkes, ed., Longmans, Green, New York, 1952.

EVELYN ANDERSON and J. A. LONG: The hormonal influences on the secretion of insulin, *Recent Progress in Hormone Research*, Volume 2, 1948.

T. F. ANDERSON: The morphology and osmotic properties of bacteriophage systems, Viruses, *Cold Spring Harbor Symp. Quant. Biol.*, 1953.

H. B. ANDERVONT: Biological studies on the mammary tumor incitor in mice, Conference on viruses as causative agents in cancer, *Ann. New York Acad. Sc.*, July 10, 1952.

C. H. ANDREWES: Virulence of viruses in animals, *J. Gen. Microbiol.*, Volume 1, Suppl., January, 1947.

————: Viruses as organisms; Viruses as chemical agents, Poliomyelitis, Second International Poliomyelitis Conference, Lippincott, Philadelphia, 1952.

D. M. ANGEVINE: Structure and function of normal connective tissue, Conference (1st) on connective tissues, Charles Ragan, ed., Josiah Macy, Jr. Foundation, New York, 1951.

ITALO ARCHETTI and F. L. HORSFALL, JR.: Persistent antigenic variation of influenza A viruses after incomplete neutralization *in ovo* with heterologous immune serum, *J. Exper. Med.*, November, 1950.

CHARLES ARMSTRONG: Studies on choriomeningitis and poliomyelitis, *Harvey Lect.*, 1940–1941.

CAMILLO ARTOM: Formation of phospholipids in animal tissue, Phosphorus Metabolism, Volume 2, W. D. McElroy and Bentley Glass, eds., Johns Hopkins Press, Baltimore, 1952.

S. A. ASDELL: Reproduction, *Ann. Rev. Physiol.*, 1950.

W. R. ASHBY: Homeostasis, Conference (9th) on cybernetics, Heinz von Foerster, ed., Josiah Macy, Jr. Foundation, New York, 1953.

WINIFRED ASHBY: A report on the current status of an attempt to correlate abnormality of distribution of one brain enzyme with mental dysfunction, *J. Nerv. and Ment. Dis.*, November, 1950.

W. T. ASTBURY: The forms of biological molecules, Essays on Growth and Form, W. E. Clark and P. B. Medawar, eds., Clarendon Press, Oxford, 1945.

————: X-ray studies of muscle, A discussion on muscular contraction and relaxation: their physical and chemical basis, A. V. Hill, leader, *Proc. Roy. Soc. London*, April 13, 1950.

————: Adventures in molecular biology, *Harvey Lect.*, 1950–1951.

E. B. ASTWOOD, M. S. RABEN and R. W. PAYNE: Chemistry of corticotrophin, *Recent Progress in Hormone Research*, Volume 7, 1952.

W. B. ATKINSON: Studies on the effects of steroid sex hormones on alkaline phosphatase in the endometrium, Menstruation and Its Disorders, E. T. Engle, ed., Thomas, Springfield, Illinois, 1950.

O. T. AVERY, C. M. MACLEOD and Maclyn McCARTY: Studies on the chemical nature of the substance inducing transformation in pneumococcal types, *J. Exper. Med.*, February, 1944.

Z. M. BACQ: Metabolism of adrenalin, *J. Pharmacol. and Exper. Therap.*, April, Part 2, 1949.

C. C. BAILEY: Alloxan diabetes, *Vitamins and Hormones*, 1949.

PERCIVAL BAILEY: Relation of structure to function in the cerebral cortex, Biology of Mental Health and Disease, Milbank Memorial Fund, Hoeber, New York, 1952.

ERNEST BALDWIN: Dynamic Aspects of Biochemistry, University Press, Cambridge, 1953.

E. G. BALL: Oxidative mechanisms in animal tissues, A Symposium on Respiratory Enzymes, University of Wisconsin Press, Madison, 1942.

F. B. BANG: Cellular pathology of virus infections as seen with the electron microscope,

Conference on viruses as causative agents in cancer, *Ann. New York Acad. Sc.*, July 10, 1952.

JOSEPH BARCROFT: The respiratory function of the blood: III, The transition from placental to pulmonary respiration, *J. Roy. Inst. Pub. Health and Hyg.*, March, 1946.

————: Researches on Prenatal Life, Thomas, Springfield, Illinois, 1947.

PHILIP BARD: Neurophysiology: status, trends and needs, Survey of Neurobiology, Committee on Neurobiology of the National Research Council, Publication 237, National Academy of Sciences-National Research Council, Washington, 1952.

H. A. BARKER: Recent investigations on the formation and utilization of active acetate, Phosphorus Metabolism, Volume 1, W. D. McElroy and Bentley Glass, eds., Johns Hopkins Press, Baltimore, 1951.

D. P. BARR, E. M. RUSS and H. A. EDER: Protein-lipid relationships in plasma, Blood Cells and Plasma Proteins, J. L. Tullis, ed., Academic Press, New York, 1953.

D. H. BARRON: The changes in the fetal circulation at birth, *Physiol. Rev.*, April, 1944.

E. S. GUZMAN BARRON: Cellular metabolism and growth, The Chemistry and Physiology of Growth, A. K. Parpart, ed., Princeton University Press, 1949.

————: The effect of ionizing radiations on some systems of biological importance, Symposium on Radiobiology (National Research Council), J. J. Nickson, ed., Wiley, New York, 1952.

G. W. BARTELMEZ: Variability in menstrual cycles, *Science*, April 27, 1951.

G. R. BARTLETT and H. N. BARNET: Some observations on alcohol metabolism with radioactive ethyl alcohol, *Quart. J. Stud. on Alcohol*, December, 1949.

J. A. V. BATES: Ignorances in the physiological field, Prospects in Psychiatric Research, Oxford Conference of the Mental Health Research Fund, J. M. Tanner, ed., Blackwell Scientific Publications, Oxford, 1953.

D. J. BAUER: Metabolic aspects of virus multiplication, The Nature of Virus Multiplication, Symposium (2nd) Society for General Microbiology, University Press, Cambridge, 1953.

WALTER BAUER, J. E. GIANSIRACUSA and J. P. KULKA: The protean nature of the connective tissue diseases, Rheumatic Diseases, Proceedings (7th) International Congress on Rheumatic Diseases, Saunders, Philadelphia, 1952.

—————— and W. S. CLARK: The relationship of the adaptation concept to the connective tissue diseases, *Recent Progress in Hormone Research*, Volume 8, 1953.

F. C. BAWDEN: Virus and its interaction with the host cell; biochemical aspects, Poliomyelitis, International (2nd) Poliomyelitis Conference, Lippincott, Philadelphia, 1952.

—————— and N. W. PIRIE: Virus multiplication considered as a form of protein synthesis, The Nature of Virus Multiplication, University Press, Cambridge, 1953.

G. W. BEADLE: Biochemical genetics, *Chem. Rev.*, August, 1945.

J. W. BEARD: The chemical, physical and morphological properties of animal viruses, *Physiol. Rev.*, July, 1948.

S. J. BECK: The Six Schizophrenias (reaction patterns in children and adults), Research Monographs, No. 6, American Orthopsychiatric Association, New York, 1954.

E. T. BELL: The pathological anatomy in primary hypertension, Hypertension, E. T. Bell, ed., University of Minnesota Press, Minneapolis, 1951.

LEOPOLD BELLAK: Dementia Praecox, Grune and Stratton, New York, 1948.

RUTH BENEDICT: Continuities and discontinuities in cultural conditioning, Personality in Nature, Society, and Culture, Clyde Kluckhohn and H. A. Murray, eds., Knopf, New York, 1953.

C. W. BENNETT: Interference phenomena between plant viruses, *Ann. Rev. Microbiol.*, 1951.

L. L. BENNETT, RUTH E. KREISS, C. H. LI and H. M. EVANS: Production of ketosis by the growth and adrenocorticotropic hormones, *Am. J. Physiol.*, January, 1948.

R. R. BENSLEY: Chemical structure of cytoplasm, *Science*, October 30, 1942.

SYLVIA H. BENSLEY and A. W. HAM: The histophysiology of the connective tissues, Rheumatic Diseases, Proceedings (7th) International Congress on Rheumatic Diseases, Saunders, Philadelphia, 1952.

A. A. BENSON and M. CALVIN: The path of carbon in photosynthesis, Biological Applications of Tracer Elements, *Cold Spring Harbor Symp. Quant. Biol.*, 1948.

I. BERENBLUM: Carcinogenesis and tumor pathogenesis, *Advances in Cancer Research*, 1954.

MAX BERGMANN: A classification of proteolytic enzymes, *Advances in Enzymol.*, 1942.

────── and J. S. FRUTON: The significance of coupled reactions for the enzymatic hydrolysis and synthesis of proteins, Conference on energy relationships in enzyme reactions, *Ann. New York Acad. Sc.*, November 10, 1944.

FREDERICK BERNHEIM: The Interaction of Drugs and Cell Catalysts, Burgess, Minneapolis, 1942.

N. J. BERRILL: Malignancy in relation to organization and differentiation, *Physiol. Rev.*, April, 1943.

MORGAN BERTHRONG, A. R. RICH and P. C. GRIFFITH: A study of the effect of adrenocorticotropic hormone (ACTH) upon the experimental cardiovascular lesions produced by anaphylactic hypersensitivity, *Bull. Johns Hopkins Hosp.*, March, 1950.

C. H. BEST, W. S. HARTROFT, C. C. LUCAS and J. H. RIDOUT: Liver damage produced by feeding alcohol or sugar and its prevention by choline, *Brit. M. J.*, November 5, 1949.

──────, C. C. LUCAS and JESSIE H. RIDOUT: The lipotropic factors, Conference on nutritional factors and liver diseases, *Ann. New York Acad. Sc.*, May 10, 1954.

W. I. B. BEVERIDGE and F. M. BURNET: The cultivation of viruses and rickettsiae in the chick embryo, Medical Research Council, Special Report Series No. 256, Great Britain, 1946.

J. J. BIESELE and J. A. JACQUEZ: Mitotic effects of certain amino acid analogs in tissue culture, Conference on tissue culture techniques in pharmacology, *Ann. New York Acad. Sc.*, November 17, 1954.

G. H. BISHOP: Nerve and synaptic conduction, *Ann. Rev. Physiol.*, 1946.

──────: Neurophysiology and behavior, The Biology of Mental Health and Disease, Milbank Memorial Fund, Hoeber, New York, 1952.

J. J. BITTNER: The causes of mammary cancer in mice, Proceedings, International (4th) Cancer Research Congress, St. Louis, 1947.

J. BJORKSTEN: Cross-linkages in protein chemistry, *Advances in Protein Chem.*, 1951.

R. J. BLANDAU: Embryo-endometrial interrelationship in the rat and guinea pig, *Anat. Rec.*, July, 1949.

──────: The effects on development when eggs and sperm are aged before fertilization, Conference on parental age and characteristics of the offspring, *Ann. New York Acad. Sc.*, January 15, 1954.

EUGEN BLEULER: Dementia Praecox or the Group of Schizophrenias, 1911 (translated into English by Joseph Zinkin), International Universities Press, New York, 1950.

HUBERT BLOCH: The relationship between phagocytic cells and human tubercle bacilli, *Am. Rev. Tuberc.*, December, 1948.

KONRAD BLOCH: The metabolism of acetic acid in animal tissues, *Physiol. Rev.*, October, 1947.

————: Biological synthesis of cholesterol, *Harvey Lect.*, 1952–1953.

————, J. E. SNOKE and S. YANARI: Enzymatic synthesis of glutathione, Phosphorus Metabolism, Volume 2, W. D. McElroy and Bentley Glass, eds., Johns Hopkins Press, Baltimore, 1952.

WILLIAM BLOOM: Histological changes following radiation exposures, *Radiology*, September, 1947.

DAVID BODIAN: A reconsideration of the pathogenesis of poliomyelitis, *Am. J. Hyg.*, May, 1952.

HENRY BORSOOK: Protein turnover and incorporation of labeled amino acids into tissue proteins *in vivo* and *in vitro*, *Physiol. Rev.*, April, 1950.

————: Peptide bond formation, *Advances in Protein Chem.*, 1953.

J. P. BOUCKAERT and CHR. DEDUVE: The action of insulin, *Physiol. Rev.*, January, 1947.

J. BOWLBY: The contribution of studies of animal behavior, Prospects in Psychiatric Research, Oxford Conference of the Mental Health Research Fund, J. M. Tanner, ed., Blackwell Scientific Publications, Oxford, 1953.

J. D. BOYD and W. J. HAMILTON: Cleavage, early development and implantation of the egg, Marshall's Physiology of Reproduction, A. S. Parkes, ed., Longmans, Green, New York, 1952.

JEAN BRACHET: The localization and the role of ribonucleic acid in the cell, Conference on structure in relation to cellular function, *Ann. New York Acad. Sc.*, February 24, 1950.

R. O. BRADY, F. D. W. LUKENS and SAMUEL GURIN: Hormonal influences upon the *in vitro* synthesis of radioactive fatty acids, *Science*, April 13, 1951.

W. R. BRAIN: Mind, Perception and Science, Blackwell, Oxford, New York, 1951.

EDUARDO BRAUN-MENÉNDEZ, J. C. FASCIOLO, L. F. LELOIR, J. M. MUNOZ and A. C. TAQUINI: Renal Hypertension, Thomas, Springfield, Illinois, 1946.

MARY A. B. BRAZIER: The Electrical Activity of the Nervous System, Macmillan, New York, 1951.

E. S. BREED and C. F. BAXTER: Renal function in surgery, Symposium on basic sciences in surgical practice, *Surg. Clin. North America*, April, 1952.

FRANK BRINK, JR., D. W. BRONK, F. D. CARLSON and C. M. CONNELLY: The oxygen uptake of active axons, The Neuron, *Cold Spring Harbor Symp. Quant. Biol.*, 1952.

E. B. BRODY: The treatment of schizophrenia, Psychotherapy with Schizophrenics, E. B. Brody and F. C. Redlich, eds., International Universities Press, New York, 1952.

S. C. BROOKS: Permeability and enzymic reactions, *Advances in Enzymol.*, 1947.

H. W. BROSIN: Contributions of psychoanalysis to the study of organic cerebral disorders, Dynamic Psychiatry, Franz Alexander and Helen Ross, eds., University of Chicago Press, 1952.

G. B. BROWN: Biosynthesis of nucleic acids as a basis for an approach to chemotherapy, Conference on 6-mercaptopurine, *Ann. New York Acad. Sc.*, December 6, 1954.

A. M. BRUES and G. A. SACHER: Analysis of mammalian radiation injury and lethality, Symposium on Radiobiology (The National Research Council), J. J. Nickson, ed., Wiley, New York, 1952.

————: Ionizing radiations and cancer, *Advances in Cancer Research*, 1954.

W. L. BRUETSCH: Mental disorders arising from organic disease, The Biology of Mental Health and Disease, Milbank Memorial Fund, Hoeber, New York, 1952.

J. M. BUCHANAN and A. B. HASTINGS: The use of isotopically marked carbon in the study of intermediary metabolism, *Physiol. Rev.*, January, 1946.

R. C. BUCK and R. J. ROSSITER: Minerals in normal and atherosclerotic aortas, *Fed. Proc.*, March, 1951.

G. J. BUDDINGH: Dermatropic viruses, *Ann. Rev. Microbiol.*, 1949.

H. B. BULL: The enzyme-substrate complex as an intermediate in enzyme-catalyzed reactions, A Symposium on the Mechanism of Enzyme Action, W. D. McElroy and Bentley Glass, eds., Johns Hopkins Press, Baltimore, 1954.

J. J. BUNIM, LEON SOKOLOFF, E. J. BIEN, S. L. WILENS, MORRIS ZIFF and CURRIER McEWEN: Histological and chemical changes in skeletal muscle of patients with rheumatic and nonrheumatic diseases, Rheumatic Diseases, Proceedings (7th) International Congress on Rheumatic Diseases, Saunders, Philadelphia, 1952.

HENRY BUNTING: The distribution of acid mucopolysaccharides in mammalian tissues as revealed by histochemical methods, Conference on the ground substance of the mesenchyme and hyaluronidase, *Ann. New York Acad. Sc.*, May 31, 1950.

B. R. BURMESTER: Studies on fowl lymphomatosis, Conference on viruses as causative agents in cancer, *Ann. New York Acad. Sc.*, July 10, 1952.

F. M. BURNET: Virus as Organism, Harvard University Press, 1945.

———— and FRANK FENNER: The Production of Antibodies, Macmillan, Melbourne, Australia, 1949.

———— and P. E. LIND: A genetic approach to variation in influenza viruses, *J. Gen. Microbiol.*, February, 1951.

TRIGANT BURROW: Science and Man's Behavior, W. E. Galt, ed., Philosophical Library, New York, 1953.

MILTON BURTON: Elementary chemical processes in radiobiological reactions, Symposium on Radiobiology (National Research Council), J. J. Nickson, ed., Wiley, New York, 1952.

MELVIN CALVIN: The path of carbon in photosynthesis, *Harvey Lect.*, 1950–1951.

D. H. CAMPBELL: The nature of antibodies, *Ann. Rev. Microbiol.*, 1948.

P. R. CANNON, L. E. FRAZIER and R. H. HUGHES: Influence of potassium on tissue protein synthesis, *Metabolism*, January, 1952.

JORDI CASALS: Immunological relationships among central nervous system viruses, *J. Exper. Med.*, April, 1944.

T. O. CASPERSSON: Cell Growth and Cell Function, Norton, New York, 1950.

WILLIAM CAUDILL: Applied anthropology in medicine, Anthropology Today, International symposium on anthropology, A. L. Kroeber, chairman, University of Chicago Press, Chicago, 1953.

I. L. CHAIKOFF and C. ENTENMAN: Antifatty liver factor of the pancreas — present status, *Advances in Enzymol.*, 1948.

————: Metabolic blocks in carbohydrate metabolism in diabetes, *Harvey Lect.*, 1951–1952.

ROBERT CHAMBERS and B. W. ZWEIFACH: Intercellular cement and capillary permeability, *Physiol. Rev.*, July, 1947.

———: The cell as an integrated functional body, Conference on structure in relation to cellular function, *Ann. New York Acad. Sc.*, February 24, 1950.

BRITTON CHANCE: On the reaction of catalase peroxides with acceptors, *J. Biol. Chem.*, February, 1950.

———: Enzyme mechanisms in living cells, A Symposium on the Mechanism of Enzyme Action, W. D. McElroy and Bentley Glass, eds., Johns Hopkins Press, Baltimore, 1954.

H. T. CHANG: Electrical activity of dendrites, The Biology of Mental Health and Disease, Milbank Memorial Fund, Hoeber, New York, 1952.

M. C. CHANG: The effect of seminal plasma on fertilized rabbit ova, *Proc. Nat. Acad. Sc.*, March, 1950.

——— and G. PINCUS: Physiology of fertilization in mammals, *Physiol. Rev.*, January, 1951.

ERWIN CHARGAFF: Structure and function of nucleic acids as cell constituents, *Fed. Proc.*, September, 1951.

M. W. CHASE: Cellular transfer of cutaneous hypersensitivity to tuberculin, *Proc. Soc. Exper. Biol. and Med.*, June, 1945.

———: Immunological reactions mediated through cells, The Nature and Significance of the Antibody Response, A. M. Pappenheimer, ed., Columbia University Press, New York, 1953.

S. CHERNICK, P. A. SRERE and I. L. CHAIKOFF: The metabolism of arterial tissue, *J. Biol. Chem.*, May, 1949.

C. M. CHILD: Patterns and Problems of Development, University of Chicago Press, 1941.

K. L. CHOW, J. S. BLUM and R. A. BLUM: Effects of combined destruction of frontal and posterior "associative areas" in monkeys, *J. Neurophysiol.*, January, 1951.

H. N. CHRISTENSEN: Mode of transport of amino acids into cells, A Symposium on Amino Acid Metabolism, W. D. McElroy and Bentley Glass, eds., Johns Hopkins Press, 1955.

A. A. CHRISTMAN: Purine and pyrimidine metabolism, *Physiol. Rev.*, April, 1952.

S. L. CLARK: Trends and needs in neuroanatomy, Survey in Neurobiology, Committee on Neurobiology of the National Research Council, Publication 237, National Academy of Sciences-National Research Council, Washington, 1952.

W. E. L. CLARK: Ignorances in the anatomical field, Prospects in Psychiatric Research, Oxford Conference of the Mental Health Research Fund, J. M. Tanner, ed., Blackwell Scientific Publications, Oxford, 1953.

ALBERT CLAUDE: Studies on cells: Morphology, chemical constitution and distribution of biochemical functions, *Harvey Lect.*, 1947–1948.

———: Proteins, lipids, and nucleic acids in cell structures and functions, *Advances in Protein Chem.*, 1949.

STANLEY COBB: Foundations of Neuropsychiatry, Williams and Wilkins, Baltimore, 1952.

P. P. COHEN: The synthesis of peptide bonds, Phosphorus Metabolism, Volume 1, W. D. McElroy and Bentley Glass, eds., Johns Hopkins Press, Baltimore, 1951.

S. S. COHEN: Studies on controlling mechanisms in the metabolism of virus-infected bacteria, Viruses, *Cold Spring Harbor Symp. Quant. Biol.*, 1953.

E. J. COHN, J. L. ONCLEY, L. E. STRONG, W. L. HUGHES, JR. and S. H. ARMSTRONG, JR.: The characterization of the protein fractions of human plasma, *J. Clin. Invest.*, July, 1944.

————: Chemical specificity in biological interactions, Chemical Specificity in Biological Interactions, Harvard Memoirs, No. 3, F. R. N. Gurd, ed., Academic Press, New York, 1954.

W. E. COHN, D. G. DOHERTY and ELLIOT VOLKIN: The products of ribonucleic acid hydrolysis and their relationship to its structure, Phosphorus Metabolism, Volume 2, W. D. McElroy and Bentley Glass, eds., Johns Hopkins Press, Baltimore, 1952.

————: The influence of ion-exchange chromatography upon our concept of the structure of ribonucleic acid, Chemical Specificity in Biological Interactions, Harvard Memoirs, No. 3, F. R. N. Gurd, ed., Academic Press, New York, 1954.

L. J. COLE, V. P. BOND and M. C. FISHLER: Preprotection of mice against x-irradiation mortality by sodium nitrite, *Science*, June 13, 1952.

S. P. COLOWICK, GERTY T. CORI and M. W. SLEIN: Effect of adrenal cortex and anterior pituitary extracts and insulin on the hexokinase reaction, *J. Biol. Chem.*, May, 1947.

COLUMBIA GREYSTONE ASSOCIATES (second group): Psychosurgical Problems, F. A. Mettler, ed., Blakiston, Philadelphia, 1952.

J. L. CONEL: Histologic development of the cerebral cortex, The Biology of Mental Health and Disease, Milbank Memorial Fund, Hoeber, New York, 1952.

E. G. CONKLIN: Cleavage and differentiation in marine eggs, Conference on the mechanisms of cell division, *Ann. New York Acad. Sc.*, March 23, 1951.

J. W. CONN: Effects of adrenal cortical steroids on carbohydrate metabolism in man, Experimental Diabetes and its Relation to the Clinical Disease, Symposium (Council for International Organizations of Medical Sciences), Blackwell, Oxford, 1954.

A. H. COONS: The penetration of antigens into connective tissue, Rheumatic Fever, A Symposium, Lewis Thomas, ed., University of Minnesota Press, Minneapolis, 1952.

A. C. CORCORAN: The renal pressor system and experimental and clinical hypertension, *Recent Progress in Hormone Research*, Volume 3, 1948.

C. F. CORI: Enzymatic reactions in carbohydrate metabolism, *Harvey Lect.*, 1945–1946.

————: The enzymic synthesis and molecular configuration of glycogen, Symposium on Carbohydrate Metabolism, V. A. Najjar, ed., Johns Hopkins Press, Baltimore, 1952.

GERTY T. CORI: Glycogen structure and enzyme deficiencies in glycogen storage disease, *Harvey Lect.*, 1952–1953.

G. W. CORNER: Ourselves Unborn, Yale University Press, New Haven, 1945.

———— and B. W. BARTELMEZ: Early abnormal embryos of the rhesus monkey, Pregnancy Wastage, Proceedings, Conference sponsored by Committee on Human Reproduction, National Research Council, E. T. Engle, ed., Thomas, Springfield, Illinois, 1953.

H. J. CORPER: Fundamental information on the mechanism of specific tuberculo-immunity, *J. Lab. and Clin. Med.*, March, 1946.

C. A. COULSON: Electronic configuration and carcinogenesis, *Advances in Cancer Research*, 1953.

COUNCIL FOR INTERNATIONAL ORGANIZATIONS OF MEDICAL SCIENCES OF THE WORLD HEALTH ORGANIZATION: Anoxia of the New-Born Infant, K. W. Gross, Marcel Lelong and C. A. Smith, eds., Blackwell, Oxford, 1953.

E. V. COWDRY: Epidermal carcinogenesis, *Advances in Cancer Research*, 1953.

H. R. COX: Growth of viruses and rickettsiae in the developing chick embryo, Conference on the chick embryo in biological research, *Ann. New York Acad. Sc.*, August 8, 1952.

————: Living modified viruses as immunizing agents: *Brit. M. J.*, July 31, 1954.

L. A. CRANDALL, JR., ALYS LIPSCOMB and S. B. BARKER: Sources for hepatic glucose production in fasting normal and diabetic dogs, *Fed. Proc.*, March, 1947.

A. CSAPÓ: Actomyosin of uterus, *Am. J. Physiol.*, January, 1950.

D. H. CURNOW and E. C. DODDS: The metabolism and excretion of synthetic estrogens, with special reference to the formation of the glycuronides, Steroid hormones and enzymes, *Ciba Foundation Colloquia on Endocrinology*, Volume 1, 1952.

H. J. CURTIS: The biological effects of radiations, *Advances in Biological and Medical Physics*, Volume 2, 1951.

W. M. DALE: Some aspects of the biochemical effects of ionizing radiations, Symposium on Radiobiology (National Research Council), J. J. Nickson, ed., Wiley, New York, 1952.

GILBERT DALLDORF and G. M. SICKLES: An unidentified filtrable agent isolated from the feces of children with paralysis, *Science*, July 16, 1948.

————: The relationships of viruses and cells, with particular reference to the interference phenomenon, The Pathogenesis and Pathology of Viral Diseases, J. G. Kidd, ed., Columbia University Press, New York, 1950.

C. H. DANFORTH: Physiological aspects of genetics, *Ann. Rev. Physiol.*, 1946.

C. D. DARLINGTON: Heredity, development, and infection, *Nature*, August 5, 1944.

D. V. DAUBER and L. N. KATZ: Experimental atherosclerosis in the chick, *Arch. Path.*, November, 1943.

G. S. DAWES and J. H. COMROE, JR.: Chemoreflexes from the heart and lungs, *Physiol. Rev.*, April, 1954.

INÉS L. C. DE ALLENDE and OSCAR ORÍAS: Cytology of the Human Vagina, Hoeber-Harper, New York, 1950.

HELEN W. DEANE and A. M. SELIGMAN: Evaluation of procedures for the cytological localization of ketosteroids, *Vitamins and Hormones*, 1953.

R. C. DEBODO and M. W. SINKOFF: Anterior pituitary and adrenal hormones in the regulation of carbohydrate metabolism, *Recent Progress in Hormone Research*, Volume 8, 1953.

E. D. DELAMATER, M. E. HUNTER and STUART MUDD: Current status of the bacterial nucleus, Symposium on the chemistry and physiology of the nucleus, *Exper. Cell Res.*, Suppl. 2, 1952.

MAX DELBRÜCK: Bacterial viruses or bacteriophages, *Biol. Rev.*, January, 1946.

MILISLAV DEMEREC: Origin of bacterial resistance to antibiotics, *J. Bact.*, July, 1948.

E. W. DEMPSEY and R. S. MORISON: The electrical activity of a thalamocortical relay system, *Am. J. Physiol.*, January, 1943.

———— and G. B. WISLOCKI: Histochemical contributions to physiology, *Physiol. Rev.*, January, 1946.

E. deRobertis and F. O. Schmitt: Effect of nerve degeneration on the structure of neurotubules, *J. Cell. Comp. Physiol.*, August, 1948.

K. W. Deutsch: Communication theory and social science, *J. Orthopsychiat.*, July, 1952.

J. G. Dewan: Chemical steps in the metabolism of alcohol by brain *in vitro, Quart. J. Stud. on Alcohol*, December, 1943.

Louis Dienes, M. W. Ropes, W. E. Smith, S. Madoff and W. Bauer: The role of pleuropneumonia-like organisms in genitourinary and joint diseases, *New England J. Med.*, April, 1948.

Konrad Dobriner: Steroid hormones and cancer, *Ciba Foundation Colloquia on Endocrinology*, Volume 1, 1952.

William Dock: The predilection of atherosclerosis for the coronary arteries, *JAMA*, July 13, 1946.

E. C. Dodds: Possibilities in the realm of synthetic estrogens, *Vitamins and Hormones*, 1945.

A. H. Doermann: The vegetative state in the life cycle of bacteriophage: evidence for its occurrence, and its genetic characterization, Viruses, *Cold Spring Harbor Symp. Quant. Biol.*, 1953.

E. A. Doisy: Estrogens, *Endocrinology*, June, 1942.

Albert Dorfman: The biochemistry of connective tissue and rheumatic fever, Rheumatic Fever, A Symposium, Lewis Thomas, ed., University of Minnesota Press, Minneapolis, 1952.

R. I. Dorfman: Steroids and tissue oxidation, *Vitamins and Hormones*, 1952.

T. F. Dougherty: Effect of hormones on lymphatic tissue, *Physiol. Rev.*, October, 1952.

A. L. Dounce: The enzymes of isolated nuclei, Symposium on the chemistry and physiology of the nucleus, *Exper. Cell Res.*, Suppl. 2, 1952.

Henry Dowling: The effect of the emergence of resistant strains on the future of antibiotic therapy, Antibiotics Annual, 1953–1954, Symposium on antibiotics (Food and Drug Administration, Department of Health, Education and Welfare), Henry Welch, chairman, Medical Encyclopedia, Inc., New York, 1953.

A. W. Downie: Infection and immunity in smallpox, *Lancet*, February 24, 1951.

D. R. Drury and A. N. Wick: Effect of b-hydroxy-butyric acid on glucose oxidation in insulinized animals, *J. Biol. Chem.*, May, 1952.

R. J. Dubos: The Bacterial Cell, Harvard University Press, Cambridge, 1945.

————: Biologic and immunologic properties of tubercle bacilli, *Am. J. Med.*, November, 1950.

————: Biochemical Determinants of Microbial Diseases, Harvard University Press, Cambridge, Massachusetts, 1954.

Renato Dulbecco and Marguerite Vogt: Some problems of animal virology as studied by the plaque technique, Viruses, *Cold Spring Harbor Symp. Quant. Biol.*, 1953.

C. L. Dunham, E. P. Cronkite, G. V. Le Roy and Shields Warren: Atomic bomb injury: radiation, *JAMA*, September 1, 1951.

H. L. Dunn: Frequency of Abortion, Special reports — vital statistics, Bureau of the Census, July, 1942.

L. C. Dunn: Genetically determined variations in male fertility in the house mouse,

Studies on Testis and Ovary, Eggs and Sperm, E. T. Engle, ed., Thomas, Springfield, Illinois, 1952.

FRANCISCO DURAN-REYNALS: Tissue permeability and the spreading factors in infection, *Bact. Rev.*, December, 1942.

———: Virus-induced tumors and the virus theory of cancer, The Physiopathology of Cancer, Freddy Homburger and W. H. Fishman, eds., Hoeber-Harper, New York, 1953.

W. R. DURYEE and J. K. DOHERTY: Nuclear and cytoplasmic organoids in the living cell, Conference on tissue culture techniques in pharmacology, *Ann. New York Acad. Sc.*, November 17, 1954.

VINCENT DU VIGNEAUD: Migration of the methyl group in the body, *Proc., Am. Philosophical Soc.*, July 19, 1948.

———: Some studies on the active principles of the posterior gland, Chemical Specificity in Biological Interactions, Harvard Memoirs, No. 3, F. R. N. Gurd, ed., Academic Press, New York, 1954.

HARRY EAGLE: Drug resistance, Conference, Paul Ehrlich Centennial, *Ann. New York Acad. Sc.*, September 23, 1954.

W. R. EARLE: A summary of certain data on the production of malignancy *in vitro*, A.A.A.S. Research Conference on Cancer, F. R. Moulton, ed., A.A.A.S., Washington, 1945.

———, J. C. BRYANT and E. L. SCHILLING: Certain factors limiting the size of tissue culture and the development of massive cultures, Conference on tissue culture techniques in pharmacology, *Ann. New York Acad. Sc.*, November 17, 1954.

J. C. ECCLES: The Neurophysiological Basis of Mind, Clarendon Press, Oxford, 1953.

J. T. EDSALL: Some correlations between physicochemical data and the amino acid composition of the simple proteins, Conference on amino acid analysis of proteins, *Ann. New York Acad. Sc.*, August 29, 1946.

M. GRACE EGGLETON and ISABEL G. SMITH: The effect of ethyl alcohol and some other diuretics on chloride excretion in man, *J. Physiol.*, April, 1946.

W. E. EHRICH and T. N. HARRIS: The site of antibody formation, *Science*, January 12, 1945.

——— and JOSEPH SEIFTER: The effect of corticosteroids on lymphoid tissue, The Effect of ACTH and Cortisone upon Infection and Resistance, Gregory Shwartzman, ed., Columbia University Press, New York, 1953.

HERBERT ELFTMAN: Cytochemistry of human spermatogenesis, Studies on Testis and Ovary, Eggs and Sperm, E. T. Engle, ed., Thomas, Springfield, Illinois, 1952.

K. A. C. ELLIOTT: Brain tissue respiration and glycolysis, The Biology of Mental Health and Disease, Milbank Memorial Fund, Hoeber, New York, 1952.

L. A. ELSON: The growth inhibiting action of cancer producing substances in relation to hormonal control of protein and carbohydrate metabolism, Steroid hormones and enzymes, *Ciba Foundation Colloquia on Endocrinology*, Volume 1, 1952.

C. A. ELVEHJEM: The biological action of the vitamins, Biological Action of Vitamins, E. A. Evans, Jr., ed., University of Chicago Press, Chicago, 1942.

J. F. ENDERS, T. H. WELLER and F. C. ROBBINS: Cultivation of the Lansing strain of poliomyelitis virus in cultures of various human embryonic tissues, *Science*, January 28, 1949.

———: Propagation of viruses and rickettsiae in tissue cultures, Viral and Rickettsial Infections of Man, T. M. Rivers, ed., Lippincott, Philadelphia, 1952.

F. L. ENGEL: Adrenal cortex and stress in protein metabolism, *Recent Progress in Hormone Research*, Volume 6, 1951.

————: The significance of the metabolic changes during shock, Conference on shock syndrome, *Ann. New York Acad. Sc.*, September 3, 1952.

V. A. ENGELHARDT: Adenosinetriphosphatase properties of myosin, *Advances in Enzymol.*, 1946.

E. T. ENGLE: Introduction, The Problem of Fertility, E. T. Engle, ed., Princeton University Press, 1946.

E. A. EVANS, JR.: The fixation of $CO_2$ by animal tissues, *Harvey Lect.*, 1943–1944.

————: Biochemical relationship of viruses with cells, Conference on viruses as causative agents in cancer, *Ann. New York Acad. Sc.*, July 10, 1952.

H. M. EVANS and MIRIAM E. SIMPSON: Physiology of the gonadotrophins, The Hormones, Volume 2, Gregory Pincus and K. V. Thimann, eds., Academic Press, New York, 1950.

T. C. EVANS: The influence of quantity and quality of radiation on the biologic effect, Symposium on Radiobiology (National Research Council), J. J. Nickson, ed., Wiley, New York, 1952.

N. B. EVERETT: The present status of the germ-cell problems in vertebrates, *Biol. Rev.*, April, 1945.

HENRY EYRING, RUFUS LUMRY and J. D. SPIKES: Kinetic and thermodynamic aspects of enzymecatalyzed reactions, Symposium on the Mechanism of Enzyme Action, W. D. McElroy and Bentley Glass, eds., Johns Hopkins Press, Baltimore, 1954.

H. K. FABER: The question of extraneural growth *in vivo* of poliomyelitis virus, *Science*, November 30, 1951.

OTTO FENICHEL: The Psychoanalytic Theory of Neurosis, Norton, New York, 1945.

L. F. FIESER: Hydrocarbon carcinogenesis, A.A.A.S., Research Conference on Cancer, F. R. Moulton, ed., Washington, 1945.

———— and MARY FIESER: Natural Products Related to Phenanthrene, Reinhold, New York, 1949.

————: Some aspects of the chemistry and biochemistry of cholesterol, *Science*, May 21, 1954.

JACOB FINE, HOWARD FRANK, FRITZ SCHWEINBURG, STANLEY JACOB and THEODORE GORDON: The bacterial factor in traumatic shock, Conference on shock syndrome, *Ann. New York Acad. Sc.*, September 3, 1952.

E. E. FISCHEL: Adrenal hormones and the development of antibody and hypersensitivity, The Effect of ACTH and Cortisone upon Infection and Resistance, Symposium, Gregory Shwartzman, ed., Columbia University Press, 1953.

W. H. FISHMAN: B-glucuronidase and the action of steroid hormones, Conference on the influence of hormones on enzymes, *Ann. New York Acad. Sc.*, December 28, 1951.

————: Enzymes and cancer, The Physiopathology of Cancer, Freddy Homburger and W. H. Fishman, eds., Hoeber-Harper, New York, 1953.

L. B. FLEXNER and ALFRED GELLHORN: The comparative physiology of placental transfer, *Am. J. Obst. and Gynec.*, June, 1942.

————: Physiologic development of the cortex of the brain and its relationship to its morphology, chemical constitution and enzyme systems, The Biology of Mental Health and Disease, Milbank Memorial Fund, Hoeber, New York, 1952.

HOWARD FLOREY: Some problems in the chemotherapy of tuberculosis, *Proc. Roy. Soc. Med.*, February, 1952.

JORDI FOLCH: Biochemical problems related to psychiatry, Psychiatric Research, Harvard University Press, Cambridge, Massachusetts, 1946.

H. H. FOX: The chemical approach to the control of tuberculosis, *Science*, August 8, 1952.

C. M. FRANCHI and E. DE ROBERTIS: Electron microscope observations on elastic fibers, *Proc. Soc. Exper. Biol. and Med.*, March, 1951.

THOMAS FRANCIS, JR.: Influenza: methods of study and control, *Bull. New York Acad. Med.*, July, 1945.

————: Mechanisms of infection and immunity in virus diseases of man, *Bact. Rev.*, September, 1947.

————: Distribution of poliomyelitis virus in the epidemic community, *Trans. A. Am. Physicians*, 1952.

WALTER FREEMAN and J. W. WATTS: Psychosurgery: Intelligence, Emotion and Social Behavior Following Lobotomy for Mental Disorders, Thomas, Springfield, Illinois, 1942.

JULES FREUND: The response of immunized animals to specific and nonspecific stimuli, The Nature and Significance of the Antibody Response, A. M. Pappenheimer, Jr., ed., Columbia University Press, New York, 1953.

E. H. FRIEDEN and F. L. HISAW: The biochemistry of relaxin, *Recent Progress in Hormone Research*, Volume 8, 1953.

J. S. FRIEDENWALD: The action of nitrogen mustards and related substances on cell division, Conference on the mechanisms of cell division, *Ann. New York Acad. Sc.*, March 23, 1951.

———— and GERTRUDE D. MAENGWYN-DAVIES: Elementary kinetic theory of enzymatic activity, The Mechanism of Enzyme Action, W. D. McElroy and Bentley Glass, eds., Johns Hopkins Press, Baltimore, 1954.

W. F. FRIEDEWALD and PEYTON ROUS: The pathogenesis of deferred cancer. A study of the after-effects of methylcholanthrene upon rabbit skin, *J. Exper. Med.*, May, 1950.

S. M. FRIEDMAN, J. R. POLLEY and C. L. FRIEDMAN: The effect of desoxycorticosterone acetate on blood pressure, renal function, and electrolyte pattern in the intact rat, *J. Exper. Med.*, April, 1948.

CLAUDE FROMAGEOT: The quantitative analysis of amino acids in proteins: insulin and lysozyme, Amino Acids and Proteins, *Cold Spring Harbor Symp. Quant. Biol.*, 1950.

ERICH FROMM: Individual and social origins of neurosis, Personality in Nature, Society and Culture, Clyde Kluckhohn and H. A. Murray, eds., Knopf, New York, 1953.

FRIEDA FROMM-REICHMANN: Some aspects of psychoanalytic psychotherapy with schizophrenics, Psychotherapy with Schizophrenics, E. B. Brody and F. C. Redlich, eds., International Universities Press, New York, 1952.

J. S. FRUTON: The synthesis of peptides, *Advances in Protein Chem.*, 1949.

J. F. FULTON: Physiology of the Nervous System, 3rd ed., Oxford University Press, New York, 1949.

————: Frontal Lobotomy and Affective Behavior; a Neurophysiological Analysis, Norton, New York, 1951.

JACOB FURTH: Facility of induction of ovarian tumors by X rays; character and histogenesis of these growths, Proceedings, International (4th) Cancer Research Conference, St. Louis, 1947.

J. C. GALE: Electron microscope studies of collagen from normal and diseased tissues, *Am. J. Path.*, May-June, 1951.

T. F. GALLAGHER: Biochemical problems of the steroid hormones, Chemical Specificity in Biological Interactions, Harvard Memoirs, No. 3, F. R. N. Gurd, ed., Academic Press, New York, 1954.

ERNEST GARDNER: Physiology of movable joints, *Physiol. Rev.*, April, 1950.

W. U. GARDNER: Hormonal aspects of experimental tumorigenesis, *Advances in Cancer Research*, 1953.

ROBERT GAUNT, J. H. BIRNIE and W. J. EVERSOLE: Adrenal cortex and water metabolism, *Physiol. Rev.*, October, 1949.

P. G. H. GELL: Antigens and antibodies in hypersensitivity, Immunochemistry, Biochemical Society Symposia, Number 10, 1953.

ERNST GELLHORN: Physiological Foundations of Neurology and Psychiatry, University of Minnesota Press, 1953.

C. L. GEMMILL: Glycolysis in pharmacology, Metabolism and Function, David Nachmansohn, ed., Elsevier, Amsterdam, 1950.

R. W. GERARD: The acetylcholine system in neural function, *Recent Progress in Hormone Research*, Volume 5, 1950.

ISIDORE GERSH and H. R. CATCHPOLE: The organization of ground substance and basement membrane and its significance in tissue injury, disease and growth, *Am. J. Anat.*, November, 1949.

G. O. GEY and F. B. BANG: Viruses and cells — A study in tissue culture applications, *Trans. New York Acad. Sc.*, November, 1951.

——, —— and MARGARET K. BANG: Responses of a variety of normal and malignant cells to continuous cultivation, and some practical applications of these responses to problems in the biology of disease, Conference on tissue culture techniques in pharmacology, *Ann. New York Acad. Sc.*, November 17, 1954.

F. A. GIBBS: Electrical activity of the brain, *Ann. Rev. Physiol.*, 1945.

N. H. GILES, JR.: Recent evidence on the mechanism of chromosome abberration production by ionizing radiations, Symposium on Radiobiology (National Research Council), J. J. Nickson, ed., Wiley, New York, 1952.

H. S. GINSBERG: Modification of the course of a viral pneumonia in mice, *Bull. New York Acad. Med.*, August, 1950.

BENTLEY GLASS and H. L. PLAINE: Genetic control of tryptophan metabolism in Drosophila, Symposium on Amino Acid Metabolism, W. D. McElroy and H. B. Glass, eds., Johns Hopkins Press, Baltimore, 1955.

DAVID GLICK: Principles of enzymic histo- and cytochemistry, *Advances in Enzymol.*, 1949.

ALFRED GLUCKSMANN: Quantitative histological analysis of radiation-effects in human carcinomata, *Brit. Med. Bull.*, Volume 4, Number 1, 1946.

J. W. GOFMAN: Biophysical approaches to atherosclerosis, *Advances in Biological and Medical Physics*, Volume 2, 1951.

HARRY GOLDBLATT: The Renal Origin of Hypertension, Thomas, Springfield, Illinois, 1948.

WILLIAM GOLDRING and HERBERT CHASIS: Hypertension and Hypertensive Disease, Commonwealth Fund, New York, 1944.

A. S. GORDON and GRACE F. KATSH: The relation of the adrenal cortex to the structure and phagocytic activity of the macrophagic system, *Ann. New York Acad. Sc.*, July 27, 1949.

J. E. GORDON and T. H. INGALLS: Death, defect, and disability in prenatal life, *Am. J. Pub. Health*, January, 1948.

J. W. GOWEN: Inheritance of immunity in animals, *Ann. Rev. Microbiol.*, 1948.

SAMUEL GRAFF, MICHAEL HEIDELBERGER and C. D. HAAGENSEN: Observations on the mouse mammary carcinoma virus, Conference on viruses as causative agents in cancer, *Ann. New York Acad. Sc.*, July 10, 1952.

SAM GRANICK: The structural and functional relationships between heme and chlorophyll, *Harvey Lect.*, 1948–1949.

D. E. GREEN: Biochemistry from the standpoint of enzymes, Currents in Biochemical Research, D. E. Green, ed., Interscience, New York, 1946.

————: Integrated enzyme activity in soluble extracts of heart muscle, *Science*, June 20, 1952.

R. G. GREEN: The species character of cancer cells, *Science*, January 24, 1947.

D. M. GREENBERG, FELIX FRIEDBERG, M. P. SCHULMAN and THEODORE WINNICK: Studies on the mechanism of protein synthesis with radioactive carbon-labeled compounds, Biological Applications of Tracer Elements, *Cold Spring Harbor Symp. Quant. Biol.*, 1948.

MILTON GREENBLATT and H. C. SOLOMON: Frontal Lobes and Schizophrenia, Second lobotomy project of the Boston Psychopathic Hospital, Milton Greenblatt and H. C. Solomon, eds., Springer, New York, 1953.

H. S. N. GREENE: A conception of tumor autonomy based on transplantation studies: a review, *Cancer Res.*, December, 1951.

J. P. GREENSTEIN: Enzymes in normal and neoplastic animal tissues, A.A.A.S. Research Conference on Cancer, A.A.A.S., Washington, 1945.

————: Biochemistry of Cancer, Academic Press, New York, 1947.

R. O. GREEP and HELEN W. DEANE: The cytology and cytochemistry of the adrenal cortex, Conference on the adrenal cortex, *Ann. New York Acad. Sc.*, June 27, 1949.

M. I. GREGERSEN: Experimental studies on traumatic and hemorrhagic shock, Conference on hemorrhage, *Ann. New York Acad. Sc.*, May 11, 1948.

R. R. GRINKER: Problems of consciousness, Conference (4th) on problems of consciousness, H. A. Abramson, ed., Josiah Macy, Jr. Foundation, New York, 1954.

ARTHUR GROLLMAN: The role of the kidney in the pathogenesis of hypertension as determined by a study of the effect of nephrectomy on the blood pressure of normal and hypertensive animals, Conference (2nd) on Factors Regulating Blood Pressure, B. W. Zweifach and Ephraim Shorr, eds., Josiah Macy, Jr. Foundation, New York, 1948.

JEROME GROSS: Evaluation of structural and chemical changes in connective tissue, Conference on mechanism of corticosteroid action in disease processes, *Ann. New York Acad. Sc.*, July 17, 1953.

R. E. GROSS: Surgical Treatment for Abnormalities of the Heart and Great Vessels, Thomas, Springfield, Illinois, 1947.

HARRY GRUNDFEST: Mechanism and properties of bioelectric-potentials, Modern

Trends in Physiology and Biochemistry, E. S. Guzman Barron, ed., Academic Press, New York, 1952.

F. R. N. GURD, J. L. ONCLEY, J. T. EDSALL and E. J. COHN: The lipo-proteins of human plasma, Discussions of the Faraday Society, No. 6, Lipo-Proteins, Aberdeen University Press, 1949.

SAMUEL GURIN and R. O. BRADY: The *in vitro* synthesis of lipids and its hormonal control, *Recent Progress in Hormone Research*, Volume 8, 1953.

ALEXANDER HADDOW: Transformation of cells and viruses, *Nature*, August 12, 1944.

————: The chemical and genetic mechanisms of carcinogenesis, II.   Biological alkylating agents, The Physiopathology of Cancer, Freddy Homburger and W. H. Fishman, eds., Hoeber-Harper, New York, 1953.

H. W. HAGGARD, L. A. GREENBERG, L. H. COHEN and N. J. RAKIETEN: Studies on the absorption, distribution and elimination of alcohol, *J. Pharmacol. and Exper. Therap.*, April, 1941.

R. E. HAIST: Factors affecting the insulin content of the pancreas, *Physiol. Rev.*, October, 1944.

J. B. S. HALDANE: The Biochemistry of Genetics, Macmillan, New York, 1954.

A. I. HALLOWELL: Culture, personality and society, Anthropology Today, International symposium on anthropology, University of Chicago Press, Chicago, 1953.

W. C. HALSTEAD: Brain and intelligence, Cerebral Mechanisms in Behavior, L. C. Jeffress, ed., Wiley, New York, 1951.

W. M. HAMMON and W. C. REEVES: Recent advances in the epidemiology of the arthropod-borne virus encephalitides, including certain exotic types, *Am. J. Pub. Health*, October, 1945.

JOHN HAMMOND: Fertility, Marshall's Physiology of Reproduction, A. S. Parkes, ed., Longmans, Green, New York, 1952.

H. F. HARLOW: Functional organization of the brain in relation to mentation and behavior, The Biology of Mental Health and Disease, Milbank Memorial Fund, Hoeber, New York, 1952.

G. W. HARRIS: Neural control of the pituitary gland, *Physiol. Rev.*, April, 1948.

R. J. C. HARRIS: Properties of the agent of Rous No. 1 sarcoma, *Advances in Cancer Research*, 1953.

C. V. HARRISON: Experimental pulmonary arteriosclerosis, *J. Path. and Bact.*, April, 1948.

E. J. HART: Radioactive chemistry, *Ann. Rev. Physical Chem.*, 1954.

C. G. HARTMAN: Reproduction, *Ann. Rev. Physiol.*, 1952.

F. A. HARTMAN and KATHARINE A. BROWNELL: The Adrenal Gland, Lea and Febiger, Philadelphia, 1949.

E. N. HARVEY: Enzymes in luminescence, The Enzymes: Chemistry and Mechanism of Action, J. B. Sumner and Karl Myrbäck, eds., Volume 2, Part 1, Academic Press, New York, 1951.

A. B. HASTINGS: Factors affecting the metabolism of glucose and pyruvate, *in vitro*, Symposium on carbohydrate metabolism, Johns Hopkins Press, Baltimore, 1952.

FELIX HAUROWITZ: Chemistry and Biology of Proteins, Academic Press, New York, 1950.

———— and C. F. CRAMPTON: The role of the nucleus in protein synthesis, Symposium on the chemistry and physiology of the nucleus, *Exper. Cell Res.*, Suppl. 2, 1952.

F. W. HAYNES and L. DEXTER: Renin, hypertensinogen, and hypertensinase concentration of blood of dogs during the development of hypertension by constriction of the renal artery, *Am. J. Physiol.*, July, 1947.

R. G. HEATH: Studies in Schizophrenia, by the Tulane department of psychiatry and neurology, reported by R. G. Heath, chairman, Commonwealth Fund, Harvard University Press, Cambridge, 1954.

D. O. HEBB: The Organization of Behavior, Wiley, New York, 1949.

OSCAR HECHTER: Mechanisms of spreading factor action, Conference on the ground substance of the mesenchyme and hyaluronidase, *Ann. New York Acad. Sc.*, May 31, 1950.

—— and GREGORY PINCUS: Genesis of adrenocortical secretion, *Physiol. Rev.*, July, 1954.

CHARLES HEIDELBERGER and S. M. WEISS: The distribution of radioactivity in mice following administration of 3,4-benzpyrene-5-$C^{14}$ and 1,2,5,6-dibenzanthracene-9,10-$C^{14}$, *Cancer Res.*, November, 1951.

MICHAEL HEIDELBERGER: Immunochemistry of antigen and antibodies, Allergy in Theory and Practice, R. A. Cooke, ed., Saunders, Philadelphia, 1947.

——: Persistence of antibodies in man after immunization, The Nature and Significance of the Antibody Response, A. M. Pappenheimer, Jr., ed., Columbia University Press, New York, 1953.

L. V. HEILBRUNN: The physiology of cell division, Modern Trends in Physiology and Biochemistry, E. S. Guzman Barron, ed., Academic Press, New York, 1952.

——: An Outline of General Physiology, Saunders, Philadelphia, 1952.

D. H. HEILMAN, W. H. FELDMAN and F. C. MANN: Specific cytotoxic action of tuberculin, *Am. Rev. Tuberc.*, July, 1945.

R. E. HEMPHILL and M. REISS: Perspectives in the endocrinology and pathophysiology of mental disturbances, Perspectives in Neuropsychiatry, Derek Richter, ed., Lewis, London, 1950.

P. S. HENCH, E. C. KENDALL, C. H. SLOCUMB and H. F. POLLEY: The effect of a hormone of the adrenal cortex (17 hydroxy-11-dehydrocorticosterone; compound E) and of the pituitary adrenocorticotropic hormone on rheumatoid arthritis, *Proc. Staff Meet., Mayo Clin.*, April, 1949.

WERNER HENLE: Interference phenomena between animal viruses, *J. Immunol.*, March, 1950.

——, SUSANNA HARRIS, GERTRUDE HENLE, T. N. HARRIS, M. E. DRAKE, FRANCOISE MANGOLD and JOSEPH STOKES, JR.: Studies of the agent of infectious hepatitis, *J. Exper. Med.*, September, 1950.

——: Developmental cycles in animal viruses, Viruses, *Cold Spring Harbor Symp. Quant. Biol.*, 1953.

P. S. HENSHAW, E. F. RILEY and G. E. STAPLETON: The carcinogenic effect of pile radiations, *Cancer Res.*, January, 1947.

R. M. HERRIOTT: Nucleic-acid-free T2 virus "ghosts" with specific biological action, *J. Bact.*, June, 1951.

A. D. HERSHEY: Functional differentiation within particles of bacteriophage $T^2$, Viruses, *Cold Spring Harbor Symp. Quant. Biol.*, 1953.

A. T. HERTIG and JOHN ROCK: Two human ova of the pre-villous stage, having an ovulation age of about eleven and twelve days respectively, *Contributions to Embryology*, Carnegie Institution of Washington, Volume 29, 1941.

718     UNSOLVED CLINICAL PROBLEMS

—— and ——: Abortive human ova and associated endometria, Menstruation and Its Disorders, E. T. Engle, ed., Thomas, Springfield, Illinois, 1950.

Roy Hertz: The role of dietary trace factors in hormone-induced tissue growth, *Ciba Foundation Colloquia on Endocrinology*, Volume 1, 1952.

W. E. Heston: Genetics of cancer, *Advances in Genetics*, 1948.

George Hevesy: Ionizing radiation and cellular metabolism, Symposium on Radiobiology (National Research Council), J. J. Nickson, ed., Wiley, New York, 1952.

Corneille Heymans: Introduction to the Regulation of Blood Pressure and Heart Rate, Thomas, Springfield, Illinois, 1950.

I. Hieger: Carcinogenic activity of sterols, Steroid hormones and tumor growth, *Ciba Foundation Colloquia on Endocrinology*, Volume 1, 1952.

E. R. Hilgard: Theories of Learning, Appleton-Century-Crofts, New York, 1948.

H. E. Himwich: Brain Metabolism and Cerebral Disorders, Williams and Wilkins, Baltimore, 1951.

E. F. Hirsch and Sidney Weinhouse: The role of lipids in atherosclerosis, *Physiol. Rev.*, July, 1943.

G. K. Hirst: The agglutination of red cells by allantoic fluid of chick embryos infected with influenza virus, *Science*, July 4, 1941.

F. L. Hisaw: Development of the graafian follicle and ovulation, *Physiol. Rev.*, January, 1947.

—— and R. D. Owen: Physiological aspects of genetics, *Ann. Rev. Physiol.*, 1954.

G. H. Hitchings and Gertrude B. Elion: The chemistry and biochemistry of purine analogues, Conference on 6-mercaptopurine, *Ann. New York Acad. Sc.*, December 6, 1954.

Hudson Hoagland: Metabolic and physiologic disturbances in psychoses, The Biology of Mental Health and Disease, Milbank Memorial Fund, Hoeber, New York, 1952.

P. H. Hoch: Experimental induction of psychoses, The Biology of Mental Health and Disease, Milbank Memorial Fund, Hoeber, New York, 1952.

E. C. Hoff, J. F. Kell, Jr., N. Hastings, D. M. Sholes and E. H. Gray: Vasomotor, cellular and functional changes produced in kidney by brain stimulation, *J. Neurophysiol.*, July, 1951.

G. H. Hogeboom, W. C. Schneider and Mary Jo Striebich: Localization and integration of cellular function, *Cancer Res.*, September, 1953.

C. W. Hooker: The biology of the interstitial cells of the testis, *Recent Progress in Hormone Research*, Volume 3, 1948.

Davenport Hooker: Human fetal activity, The Biology of Mental Health and Disease, Milbank Memorial Fund, Hoeber, New York, 1952.

N. H. Horowitz and H. K. Mitchell: Biochemical genetics, *Ann. Rev. Biochem.*, 1951.

F. L. Horsfall, Jr.: Experiments on chemical alteration of virus infections, *Harvey Lect.*, 1952–1953.

Dorothy M. Horstmann: The epidemiology and pathogenesis of poliomyelitis, *Bull. New York Acad. Med.*, December, 1953.

R. D. Hotchkiss: The genetic chemistry of the pneumococcal transformations, *Harvey Lect.*, 1953–1954.

B. A. Houssay: The history of hypophyseal diabetes, Essays in Biology, University of California Press, Berkeley, 1943.

J. W. Howland and S. L. Warren: The effects of the atomic bomb irradiation on the Japanese, *Advances in Biological and Medical Physics*, Volume 1, 1948.

L. Hoyle: The multiplication of the influenza virus considered in relation to the general problem of biological multiplication, The Nature of Virus Multiplication, Symposium (2nd) Society for General Microbiology, University Press, Cambridge, 1953.

W. C. Hueper: Arteriosclerosis, *Arch. Path.*, January, March, 1945.

———: Environmental cancer, The Physiopathology of Cancer, Freddy Homburger and W. H. Fishman, eds., Hoeber-Harper, New York, 1953.

A. St. G. Huggett and John Hammond: Physiology cf the placenta, Marshall's Physiology of Reproduction, A. S. Parkes, ed., Longmans, Green, New York, 1952.

Charles Huggins: The physiology of the prostate gland, *Physiol. Rev.*, April, 1945.

———: The anti-androgenic control of human cancer, Steroids in cancer therapy, *Ciba Foundation Colloquia on Endocrinology*, Volume 1, 1952.

D. M. Hume: Role of the hypothalamus in release of ACTH, The Biology of Mental Health and Disease, Milbank Memorial Fund, Hoeber, New York, 1952.

G. H. Humphreys: General principles in cardiovascular surgery, Symposium on basic sciences in surgical practice, *Surg. Clin. North America*, April, 1952.

T. H. Ingalls: Principles underlying experimentally induced anomalies, Conference on prematurity, congenital malformation and birth injury, Association for the Aid of Crippled Children, New York, 1953.

D. J. Ingle: Parameters of metabolic problems, *Recent Progress in Hormone Research*, Volume 6, 1951.

——— and B. L. Baker: A consideration of the relationship of experimentally produced and naturally occurring pathologic changes in the rat to the adaptation diseases, *Recent Progress in Hormone Research*, Volume 8, 1953.

M. H. Jacobs: The measurement of cell permeability with particular reference to the erythrocyte, Modern Trends in Physiology and Biochemistry, E. S. Guzman Barron, ed., Academic Press, New York, 1952.

E. Jacobsen: The metabolism of ethyl alcohol, *Nature*, April 19, 1952.

H. H. Jasper: Electrical activity and mechanisms of cerebral integration, The Biology of Mental Health and Disease, Milbank Memorial Fund, Hoeber, New York, 1952.

Hans Jensen and J. L. Gray: The influence of hormones on the amino acid dehydrogenase systems of the liver and kidney, Conference on the influence of hormones on enzymes, *Ann. New York Acad. Sc.*, December 28, 1951.

K. E. Jensen and Thomas Francis, Jr.: The antigenic composition of influenza virus measured by antibody-absorption, *J. Exper. Med.*, December, 1953.

F. H. Johnson, Henry Eyring and M. J. Polissar: The Kinetic Basis of Molecular Biology, Wiley, New York, 1954.

G. E. S. Jones, G. O. Gey and M. K. Gey: Hormone production by placental cells maintained in continuous culture, *Bull. Johns Hopkins Hosp.*, January, 1943.

K. L. Jones: Variation in *Streptomyces*, Conference on speciation in asexual fungi, *Ann. New York Acad. Sc.*, October 29, 1954.

C. G. Jung: Psychological reflections, translated and selected by Jolande Jacobi, Pantheon Books, New York, 1953.

E. A. KABAT: Immunochemistry of the proteins, *J. Immunol.*, December, 1943.

————: The unity and diversity of antibodies, The Nature and Significance of the Antibody Response, A. M. Pappenheimer, Jr., ed., Columbia University Press, New York, 1953.

HERBERT KAHLER and B. J. LLOYD, JR.: Electron microscopic study of the Shope papilloma virus, *J. Nat. Cancer Inst.*, June, 1952.

H. M. KALCKAR: The biological incorporation of purines and pyrimidines into nucleosides and nucleic acid, Metabolism and Function, David Nachmansohn, ed., Elsevier, Amsterdam, 1950.

F. J. KALLMANN: The genetics of psychotic behavior patterns, Genetics and the Inheritance of Integrated Neurological and Psychiatric Patterns, Williams and Wilkins, Baltimore, 1954.

N. O. KAPLAN: Pyridine nucleotides and coupled phosphorylation, Phosphorus Metabolism, Volume 1, W. D. McElroy and Bentley Glass, eds., Johns Hopkins Press, Baltimore, 1951.

E. H. KASS, MARY J. KENDRICK and MAXWELL FINLAND: Effects of certain corticosteroids and of growth hormone on nucleoproteins of lymph nodes, Conference on mechanism of corticosteroid action, *Ann. New York Acad. Sc.*, July 17, 1953.

B. P. KAUFMANN, HELEN GAY and MARGARET R. McDONALD: Localization of cellular proteins by enzymatic hydrolysis, Amino Acids and Proteins, *Cold Spring Harbor Symp. Quant. Biol.*, 1950.

D. KEILIN and E. F. HARTREE: Properties of catalase, catalysis of coupled oxidation of alcohols, *Biochem. J.*, Volume 39, No. 4, 1945.

AARON KELLNER: Lipid metabolism and atherosclerosis, *Bull. New York Acad. Med.*, January, 1952.

E. C. KENDALL: The chemistry and partial synthesis of adrenal steroids, Conference on the adrenal cortex, *Ann. New York Acad. Sc.*, June 27, 1949.

————: Hormones of the adrenal cortex, *Bull. New York Acad. Med.*, February, 1953.

E. L. KENNAWAY: The chemists' contribution, Ten Years' Progress in Cancer Research, Symposium, The International Cancer Research Foundation, Lord Baltimore Press, Baltimore, June 8, 1942.

E. P. KENNEDY and A. L. LEHNINGER: The enzymatic oxidation of fatty acids, Phosphorus Metabolism, Volume 2, W. D. McElroy and Bentley Glass, eds., Johns Hopkins Press, Baltimore, 1952.

C. J. KENSLER: Dietary factors that influence the carcinogenic activity of azo dyes and related compounds, Conference on nutrition in relation to cancer, *Ann. New York Acad. Sc.*, September 7, 1947.

W. J. KERR and P. A. CAVELTI: New immunologic aspects of the pathogenesis of glomerulonephritis and rheumatic fever, *Tr. A. Am. Physicians*, 1947.

S. S. KETY and C. F. SCHMIDT: The effects of altered arterial tensions of carbon dioxide and oxygen on cerebral blood flow and cerebral oxygen consumption of normal young men, *J. Clin. Investigation*, July, 1948.

————: Blood flow and metabolism of the human brain in health and disease, *Tr. and Stud. Coll. Physicians, Philadelphia*, December, 1950.

ANCEL KEYS, OLAF MICKELSEN, E. v. O. MILLER, E. R. HAYES and R. L. TODD: The concentration of cholesterol in the blood serum of normal man and its relation to age, *J. Clin. Investigation*, October, 1950.

J. G. KIDD: Distinctive constituents of tumor cells and their possible relations to the phenomena of autonomy, anaplasia, and cancer causation, Heredity and Variation in Microorganisms, *Cold Spring Harbor Symp. Quant. Biol.*, 1946.

———: Effects of an antibiotic from *Aspergillus fumigatus* Fresenius on tumor cells *in vitro*, and its possible identity with gliotoxin, *Science*, May 16, 1947.

———: Proliferative lesions caused by viruses and virus-like agents, The Pathogenesis and Pathology of Viral Diseases, J. G. Kidd, ed., Columbia University Press, New York, 1950.

J. E. KIRK: Metabolism of arterial tissues, Symposium on studies on arteriosclerosis, Gerontological Society, *J. Gerontol.*, April, 1951.

J. G. KIRKWOOD: The nature of the forces between protein molecules in solution, A Symposium on the Mechanism of Enzyme Action, W. D. McElroy and Bentley Glass, eds., Johns Hopkins Press, Baltimore, 1954.

GERALD KLATSKIN, H. M. GEWIN and W. A. KREHL: Effects of prolonged alcohol ingestion on the liver of the rat under conditions of controlled adequate dietary intake, *Yale J. Biol. and Med.*, February, 1951.

PAUL KLEMPERER: The concept of collagen diseases, *Am. J. Path.*, July, 1950.

———: The significance of the intermediate substances of the connective tissue in human disease, *Harvey Lect.*, 1953–1954.

N. S. KLINE and A. M. STANLEY: Use of reserpine in a neuropsychiatric hospital, Conference on reserpine in the treatment of neuropsychiatric, neurological and related clinical problems, *Ann. New York Acad. Sc.*, April 15, 1955.

I. M. KLOTZ: Thermodynamic and molecular properties of some metal-protein complexes, Symposium on the Mechanism of Enzyme Action, W. D. McElroy and Bentley Glass, eds., Johns Hopkins Press, Baltimore, 1954.

CLYDE KLUCKHOHN and H. A. MURRAY: Outline of a conception of personality; Personality formation: the determinants, Personality in Nature, Society and Culture, Clyde Kluckhohn and H. A. Murray, eds., Knopf, New York, 1953.

HEINRICH KLÜVER: Functional differences between the occipital and temporal lobes, with special reference to the interrelations of behavior and extracerebral mechanisms, Cerebral Mechanisms in Behavior, Hixon Symposium, L. A. Jeffress, ed., Wiley, New York, 1951.

B. C. J. G. KNIGHT: Growth factors in microbiology, *Vitamins and Hormones*, 1945.

C. A. KNIGHT: Amino acid composition of highly purified viral particles of influenza A and B, *J. Exper. Med.*, August, 1947.

R. P. KNIGHT: Introduction, Psychotherapy with Schizophrenics, E. B. Brody and F. C. Redlich, eds., International Universities Press, New York, 1952.

M. H. KNISELY: Methods for direct investigation of factors leading to thrombosis, Conference (4th) on blood clotting and allied problems, J. E. Flynn, ed., Josiah Macy, Jr. Foundation, New York, 1951.

C. D. KOCHAKIAN: The effects on enzymes of androgens and growth hormone, Steroid hormones and enzymes, *Ciba Foundation Colloquia on Endocrinology*, Volume 1, 1952.

M. J. KOPAK: Probable ultrastructures involved in cell division, Conference on the mechanisms of cell division, *Ann. New York Acad. Sc.*, March 23, 1951.

ARTHUR KORNBERG: The metabolism of phosphorus-containing coenzymes, Phosphorus Metabolism, Volume 1, W. D. McElroy and Bentley Glass, eds., Johns Hopkins Press, Baltimore, 1951.

D. E. KOSHLAND, JR.: Group transfer as an enzymatic substitution mechanism, A

Symposium on the Mechanism of Enzyme Action, W. D. McElroy and Bentley Glass, eds., Johns Hopkins Press, Baltimore, 1954.

L. M. KOZLOFF: Origin and fate of bacteriophage material, Viruses, *Cold Spring Harbor Symp. Quant. Biol.*, 1953.

M. E. KRAHL: The effect of insulin and pituitary hormones on glucose uptake in muscle, Conference on the influence of hormones on enzymes, *Ann. New York Acad. Sc.*, December 28, 1954.

H. A. KREBS: The tricarboxylic acid cycle, *Harvey Lect.*, 1948–1949.

L. O. KUNKEL: Variation in phytopathogenic viruses, *Ann. Rev. Microbiol.*, 1947.

A. LACASSAGNE: Carcinogenic activity of some polycyclic nitrogen compounds, *International (4th) Cancer Research Congress*, St. Louis, 1947.

REBECCA C. LANCEFIELD: Specific relationship of cell composition to biological activity of hemolytic streptococci, *Harvey Lect.*, 1940–1941.

KARL LANDSTEINER: The Specificity of Serological Reactions, Harvard University Press, Cambridge, 1945.

A. I. LANSING: Chemical morphology of elastic fibers, Transactions, Conference (2nd) on connective tissues, Charles Ragan, ed., Josiah Macy, Jr. Foundation, New York, 1951.

H. A. LARDY and P. H. PHILLIPS: The interrelation of oxidative and glycolytic processes as sources of energy for bull spermatozoa, *Am. J. Physiol.*, July, 1941.

———: The metabolic regulator in mammalian spermatozoa, Studies on Testis and Ovary, Eggs and Sperm, E. T. Engle, ed., Thomas, Springfield, Illinois, 1952.

K. S. LASHLEY: The problem of serial order in behavior, Cerebral Mechanisms in Behavior, Hixon Symposium, L. A. Jeffress, ed., Wiley, New York, 1951.

———: Functional interpretation of anatomic patterns, Patterns of Organization in the Central Nervous System, Proceedings, Association for Research in Nervous and Mental Diseases, Williams and Wilkins, Baltimore, 1952.

———: Neuropsychology, Survey of Neurobiology, Committee on Neurobiology of the National Research Council, Publication 237, National Academy of Sciences-National Research Council, Washington, 1952.

M. A. LAUFFER, W. C. PRICE and A. W. PETRE: The nature of viruses, *Advances in Enzymol.*, 1949.

J. H. LAURENCE and N. L. BERLIN: Relative polycythemia; polycythemia of stress, *Yale J. Biol. and Med.*, June, 1952.

L. W. LAW: Genetic studies in experimental cancer, *Advances in Cancer Research*, 1954.

ARNOLD LAZAROW: Factors controlling the development and progression of diabetes, *Physiol. Rev.*, January, 1949.

A. L. LEHNINGER: Oxidative phosphorylation, *Harvey Lect.*, 1953–1954.

L. M. LEONARD and D. D. RUTSTEIN: Interaction of steroid compounds and single cells, Conference on mechanisms of corticosteroid action in disease processes, *Ann. New York Acad. Sc.*, July 17, 1953.

PIERRE LÉPINE: On the nomenclature and classification of arthropod-borne encephalitides, Conference on virus and rickettsial classification and nomenclature, *Ann. New York Acad. Sc.*, March 31, 1953.

MICHAEL LEVINE: The action of colchicine on cell division in human cancer, animal, and plant tissues, Conference on the mechanisms of cell division, *Ann. New York Acad. Sc.*, March 23, 1951.

MILTON LEVY and EVELYN SLOBODIANSKY: The application of the isotopic derivative technic to the study of protein structure, Amino Acids and Proteins, *Cold Spring Harbor Symp. Quant. Biol.*, 1950.

A. LEWIS: Points of research into the interaction between the individual and the culture, Prospects in Psychiatric Research, Oxford Conference of the Mental Health Research Fund, J. M. Tanner, ed., Blackwell Scientific Publications, Oxford, 1953.

W. H. LEWIS: Cell division with special reference to cells in tissue cultures, Conference on the mechanisms of cell division, *Ann. New York Acad. Sc.*, March 23, 1951.

C. H. LI, MIRIAM E. SIMPSON and H. M. EVANS: Isolation of adrenocorticotropic hormone from sheep pituitaries, *Science*, November 13, 1942.

―――― and H. M. EVANS: The isolation of pituitary growth hormone, *Science*, March 3, 1944.

――――: Growth and adrenocorticotropic hormones of anterior pituitary, *Harvey Lect.*, 1950–1951.

J. C. LILLY: Forms and figures in the electrical activity seen in the surface of the cerebral cortex, The Biology of Mental Health and Disease, Milbank Memorial Fund, Hoeber, New York, 1952.

STUART LINDSAY, I. L. CHAIKOFF and J. W. GILMORE: Arteriosclerosis in the dog, *A.M.A. Arch. Path.*, April, 1952.

K. P. LINK: The anticoagulant dicumarol, *Proc. Inst. Med. of Chicago*, October 15, 1945.

RALPH LINTON: Culture and Mental Disorders, Salmon Lecture Series, 1953 (in press).

FRITZ LIPMANN: Acetylphosphate, *Advances in Enzymol.*, 1946.

――――: Biosynthetic mechanisms, *Harvey Lect.*, 1948–1949.

――――: Development of the acetylation problem, a personal account (Nobel prize address, 1953), *Science*, November 26, 1954.

――――: On the mechanism of some ATP-linked reactions and certain aspects of protein synthesis, A Symposium on the Mechanism of Enzyme Action, W. D. McElroy and Bentley Glass, eds., Johns Hopkins Press, Baltimore, 1954.

C. C. LITTLE: The genetics of spontaneous tumor formation, Biology of the Laboratory Mouse by the Staff of the Roscoe B. Jackson Memorial Laboratory, G. D. Snell, ed., Blakiston, Philadelphia, 1941.

ROBERT LIVINGSTON: General statements about chemical reactions induced by ionizing radiation, Symposium on Radiobiology (National Research Council), J. J. Nickson, ed., Wiley, New York, 1952.

LEO LOEB: Tumors and organismal differentials, The Biological Basis of Individuality, Part 4, Thomas, New York, 1945.

R. F. LOEB: The adrenal cortex and electrolyte behavior, *Harvey Lect.*, 1941–1942.

OTTO LOEWI: Aspects of the transmission of the nervous impulse: II, Theoretical and clinical implications, *J. Mt. Sinai Hosp.*, September–October, 1945.

――――: On the mechanism of drug action, Modern Trends in Physiology and Biochemistry, E. S. Guzman Barron, ed., Academic Press, New York, 1952.

C. N. H. LONG: The endocrine control of the blood sugar, *Lancet*, February 16, 1952.

――――: Regulation of ACTH secretion, *Recent Progress in Hormone Research*, Volume 7, 1952.

E. R. LONG: Constitution and related factors in resistance to tuberculosis, *Arch. Path.*, July–August, 1941.

RAFAEL LORENTE DE NÓ: A Study of Nerve Physiology, Studies from the Rockefeller Institute for Medical Research, Volumes 131 and 132, New York, 1947.

EGON LORENZ: Effects of long-continued total-body gamma irradiation on mice, guinea pigs, and rabbits; Biological Effects of External X and Gamma Radiations (National Nuclear Energy Series, Volume 22 B, Part 1), R. E. Zirkle, ed., McGraw-Hill, New York, 1954.

O. H. LOWRY: The quantitative histochemistry of the brain, *Science*, November 14, 1952.

J. M. LUCK: The liver proteins, Amino Acids and Proteins, *Cold Spring Harbor Symp. Quant. Biol.*, 1950.

BALDUIN LUCKÉ: Kidney carcinoma in the leopard frog: A virus tumor, Conference on viruses as causative agents in cancer, *Ann. New York Acad. Sc.*, July 10, 1952.

R. J. LUDFORD: Can somatic cell mutations explain the properties of malignant cells?, Proceedings International (7th) Genetical Congress, P. C. Punnett, ed., University Press, Cambridge, 1941.

F. D. W. LUKENS: Alloxan diabetes, *Physiol. Rev.*, July, 1948.

E. LUNDSGAARD: The ATP content of resting and active muscle, A discussion on muscular contraction and relaxation: their physical and chemical basis, A. V. Hill, leader, *Proc. Roy. Soc. London*, April 13, 1950.

M. B. LURIE: Heredity, constitution, and tuberculosis, *Am. Rev. Tuberc.*, Supp., September, 1941.

———, PETER ZAPPOSODI and A. M. DANNENBERG, JR.: Constitutional factors in resistance to infection, The Effect of ACTH and Cortisone Upon Infection and Resistance, Gregory Shwartzman, ed., Columbia University Press, New York, 1953.

FEODOR LYNEN: Acetyl coenzyme A and the "fatty acid cycle," *Harvey Lect.*, 1952–1953.

JOHN MACLEOD: Metabolism and motility of human spermatozoa; The Problem of Fertility, E. T. Engle, ed., Princeton University Press, 1946.

L. D. MACLEOD: Biochemistry and alcoholism, *Brit. J. Addiction*, July, 1950.

H. W. MAGOUN: Caudal and cephalic influences of the brain stem reticular formation, *Physiol. Rev.*, October, 1950.

THADDEUS MANN: Metabolism of semen, *Advances in Enzymol.*, 1949.

R. J. MARDONES: On the relationships between deficiency of B vitamins and alcohol intake in rats, *Quart. J. Stud. on Alcohol*, December, 1951.

J. E. MARKEE: The relation of blood flow to endometrial growth and the inception of menstruation, Menstruation and its Disorders, E. T. Engle, ed., Thomas, Springfield, Illinois, 1950.

ROY MARKHAM: Nucleic acids in virus multiplication, The Nature of Virus Multiplication, Symposium (2nd) Society for General Microbiology, University Press, Cambridge, 1953.

J. R. MARRACK: Enzymes and immunology, The Enzymes: Chemistry and Mechanism of Action, J. B. Sumner and Karl Myrbäck, eds., Volume 1, Part 1, Academic Press, New York, 1950.

G. F. MARRIAN: Some aspects of progesterone metabolism, *Recent Progress in Hormone Research*, Volume 4, 1949.

S. P. MARTIN, C. H. PIERCE, G. MIDDLEBROOK and R. J. DUBOS: The effect of tubercle bacilli on the polymorphonuclear leucocytes of normal animals, *J. Exper. Med.*, April, 1950.

K. E. MASON: Physiological action of vitamin E and its homologues, *Vitamins and Hormones*, 1944.

J. H. MASSERMAN: Experimental approaches to psychodynamic problems, *J. Mt. Sinai Hosp.*, January–February, 1953.

DANIEL MAZIA: Physiology of the cell nucleus, Modern Trends in Physiology and Biochemistry, E. S. Guzman Barron, ed., Academic Press, New York, 1952.

MACLYN McCARTY: The biology of group A hemolytic streptococci, Rheumatic Diseases, Proceedings (7th) International Congress on Rheumatic Diseases, Saunders, Philadelphia, 1952.

W. S. McCULLOCH, J. Y. LETTVIN, W. H. PITTS and P. C. DELL: An electrical hypothesis of central inhibition and facilitation, Patterns of Organization in the Central Nervous System, Proceedings, Association for Research in Nervous and Mental Disease, Williams and Wilkins, Baltimore, 1952.

W. D. McELROY: Phosphate bond energy and bioluminescence, Phosphorus Metabolism, Volume 1, W. D. McElroy and Bentley Glass, eds., Johns Hopkins Press, Baltimore, 1951.

H. McILWAIN: Glutamic acid and glucose as substrates for mammalian brain, *J. of Ment. Sc.*, October, 1951.

P. B. McMASTER and R. J. PARSONS: The movement of substances and the state of fluid in the intradermal tissue, Conference on the ground substance of the mesenchyme and hyaluronidase, *Ann. New York Acad. Sc.*, May 31, 1950.

———: Sites of antibody formation, The Nature and Significance of Antibody Response, Columbia University Press, New York, 1953.

J. H. MEANS: The Thyroid and its Diseases, Lippincott, Philadelphia, 1948.

P. B. MEDAWAR: Cellular inheritance and transformation, *Biol. Rev.*, October, 1947.

L. J. MEDUNA: Oneirophrenia, University of Illinois Press, Urbana, 1950.

J. L. MELNICK: Poliomyelitis and poliomyelitis-like viruses of man and animals, *Ann. Rev. Microbiol.*, 1951.

F. A. METTLER: Anatomy and physiology, Selective Partial Ablation of the Frontal Cortex, F. A. Mettler, ed., Hoeber, New York, 1949.

KARL MEYER: The biological significance of hyaluronic acid and hyaluronidase, *Physiol. Rev.*, July, 1947.

R. K. MEYER: Relation of glucuronidase to action of gonadal hormones, Steroid hormones and enzymes, *Ciba Foundation Colloquia on Endocrinology*, Volume 1, 1952.

OTTO MEYERHOF: Intermediate carbohydrate metabolism, Symposium on Respiratory Enzymes, University of Wisconsin Press, Madison, 1942.

———: The main chemical phases of the recovery of muscle, Conference on muscular contraction, *Ann. New York Acad. Sc.*, May 30, 1947.

GARDNER MIDDLEBROOK, R. J. DUBOS and C. PIERCE: Virulence and morphological characteristics of mammalian tubercle bacilli, *J. Exper. Med.*, August, 1947.

——— and JULES FREUND: The mycobacteria, Bacterial and Mycotic Infections of Man, R. J. Dubos, ed., Lippincott, Philadelphia, 1952.

E. C. MILLER and J. A. MILLER: *In vivo* combinations between carcinogens and tissue constituents and their possible role in carcinogenesis, Symposium on immunogenetics and carcinogenesis, *Cancer Res.*, August, 1952.

J. G. MILLER: Future trends in clinical psychology, Conference on current trends in clinical psychology, *Ann. New York Acad. Sc.*, October 8, 1948.

J. M. MILLER and C. B. FAVOUR: The lymphocytic origin of a plasma factor responsible for hypersensitivity *in vitro* of tuberculin type, *J. Exper. Med.*, January, 1951.

A. E. MIRSKY: The chemical composition of chromosomes, *Harvey Lect.*, 1950–1951.

I. A. MIRSKY, BEN SIMKIN and R. H. BROH-KAHN: The inactivation of insulin by tissue extracts, *Arch. Biochem.*, October, 1950.

E. A. MOELWYN-HUGHES: Physical chemistry and chemical kinetics of enzymes, The Enzymes: Chemistry and Mechanism of Action, J. B. Sumner and Karl Myrbäck, eds., Volume I, Part 1, 1950.

W. F. H. M. MOMMAERTS: Phosphate metabolism in the activity of skeletal and cardiac muscle, Phosphorus Metabolism, Volume 1, W. D. McElroy and Bentley Glass, eds., Johns Hopkins Press, Baltimore, 1951.

————: Studies on the contractile protein system of muscle, Modern Trends in Physiology and Biochemistry, E. S. Guzman Barron, ed., Academic Press, New York, 1952.

LUDWIK MONNÉ: Functioning of the cytoplasm, *Advances in Enzymol.*, 1948.

H. D. MOON, M. E. SIMPSON and H. M. EVANS: Inhibition of methylcholanthrene carcinogenesis by hypophysectomy, *Science*, September 26, 1952.

C. R. MOORE: Comparative biology of testicular and ovarian hormones, *Biol. Symposia*, Volume 9, 1942.

————: Gonad hormones and sex differentiation, *Am. Naturalist*, March–April, 1944.

ISABEL M. MORGAN and DAVID BODIAN: The role of antibody in experimental poliomyelitis, *Am. J. Hygiene*, May, 1947.

PHILIP MORRISON: Radiation in living matter: The physical processes, Symposium on Radiobiology (National Research Council), J. J. Nickson, ed., Wiley, New York, 1952.

H. W. MOSSMAN: The embryonic nature of the adult ovary, Studies on Testis and Ovary, Eggs and Sperm, E. T. Engle, ed., Thomas, Springfield, Illinois, 1952.

STUART MUDD: Cytology of bacteria, Part 1, The bacterial cell, *Ann. Rev. Microbiol.*, 1954.

H. J. MULLER: The development of the gene theory, Genetics in the 20th Century, L. C. Dunn, ed., Macmillan, New York, 1951.

————: Gene mutations caused by radiation, Symposium on Radiobiology (National Research Council), J. J. Nickson, ed., Wiley, New York, 1952.

————: Life, *Science*, January 7, 1955.

G. E. MURPHY and H. F. SWIFT: The induction of rheumatic-like cardiac lesions in rabbits by repeated focal infections with group A streptococci, *J. Exper. Med.*, May, 1950.

————: The histopathology of rheumatic fever: a critical review, Rheumatic Fever, A Symposium, Lewis Thomas, ed., University of Minnesota Press, Minneapolis, 1952.

J. P. MURPHY and E. GELLHORN: The influence of hypothalamic stimulation on cortically induced movements and on action potentials of the cortex, *J. Neurophysiol.*, November, 1945.

DAVID NACHMANSOHN: Metabolism and function of the nerve cell, *Harvey Lect.*, 1953–1954.

————: Generation of bioelectric potentials, *Science*, November 12, 1954.

DOROTHY M. NEEDHAM: Myosin and adenosinetriphosphate in relation to muscle contraction, Metabolism and Function, David Nachmansohn, ed., Elsevier, Amsterdam, 1950.

JOSEPH NEEDHAM: Biochemistry and Morphogenesis, University Press, Cambridge, 1942.

HANS NEURATH: Some consideration of the chemical structure and biological activity of chymotrypsin, Modern Trends in Physiology and Biochemistry, E. S. Guzman Barron, ed., Academic Press, New York, 1952.

H. W. NEWMAN: Some factors influencing the rate of metabolism of ethyl alcohol, *Quart. J. Stud. on Alcohol*, December, 1947.

MARK NICKERSON: Sympathoadrenal factors in hypertension, Hypertension, E. T. Bell, ed., University of Minnesota Press, Minneapolis, 1951.

W. J. NICKERSON: Experimental control of morphogenesis in microorganisms, Conference on speciation and variation in asexual fungi, *Ann. New York Acad. Sc.*, October 29, 1954.

J. H. NORTHROP: Enzymes and the synthesis of proteins, Chemistry and Physiology of Growth, A. K. Parpart, ed., Princeton University Press, New Jersey, 1949.

G. D. NOVELLI and FRITZ LIPMANN: The catalytic function of coenzyme A in citric acid synthesis, *J. Biol. Chem.*, January, 1950.

—— and MORRIS SOODAK: Coenzymes, Biochemistry and Physiology of Nutrition, Volume 2, G. H. Bourne and G. W. Kidder, eds., Academic Press, New York, 1953.

W. J. NUNGESTER: Nonspecific factors in immunity, *Ann. Rev. Microbiol.*, 1954.

CHARLES OBERLING: The Riddle of Cancer, translated by W. H. Woglom, Yale University Press, New Haven, 1944.

—— and M. GUÉRIN: The role of viruses in the production of cancer, *Advances in Cancer Research*, 1954.

C. P. OBERNDORF: A History of Psychoanalysis in America, Grune and Stratton, New York, 1953.

SEVERO OCHOA: Enzyme studies in biological oxidations and synthesis, *Harvey Lect.*, 1950–1951.

——: Pyruvate oxidation in brain, The Biology of Mental Health and Disease, Milbank Memorial Fund, Hoeber, New York, 1952.

——: Tricarboxylic acid cycle: enzymatic mechanisms, The National Institutes of Health Annual Lectures — 1953, United States Public Health Service, Washington, 1954.

ERIC OGDEN: The physiological significance of the renal pressor mechanism, *Tex. Reps. Biol. and Med.*, Volume 2, 1944.

P. K. OLITSKY and JORDI CASALS: Viral encephalitides, Viral and Rickettsial Infections of Man, T. M. Rivers, ed., Lippincott, Philadelphia, 1952.

E. L. OPIE and MARY B. ROTHBARD: Water exchange of collagenous tissues and of gelatin, *J. Exper. Med.*, April, 1953.

I. H. PAGE: The renin-angiotonin pressor system, Hypertension, E. T. Bell, ed., University of Minnesota Press, Minneapolis, 1951.

——: Serotonin (5-Hydroxytryptamine), *Physiol. Rev.*, July, 1954.

G. N. PAPANICOLAOU and H. F. TRAUT: Diagnosis of Uterine Cancer by the Vaginal Smear, Commonwealth Fund, New York, 1943.

J. W. PAPEZ and J. F. BATEMAN: Changes in nervous tissues and study of living organisms in mental disease, *J. Nerv. and Ment. Dis.*, November, 1951.

A. M. PAPPENHEIMER, JR.: Valence of antibodies, The Nature and Significance of the Antibody Response, A. M. Pappenheimer, Jr., ed., Columbia University Press, New York, 1953.

A. S. Parkes: The adrenal-gonad relationship, *Physiol. Rev.*, April, 1945.

H. M. Patt: Protective mechanisms in ionizing radiation injury, *Physiol. Rev.*, January, 1953.

————: Radiation effects on mammalian systems, *Ann. Rev. Physiol.*, 1954.

Linus Pauling, D. H. Campbell and David Pressman: The nature of the forces between antigen and antibody and of the precipitation reaction, *Physiol. Rev.*, July, 1943.

————, R. B. Corey and H. B. Branson: The structure of proteins: two hydrogen-bonded helical configurations of the polypeptide chain, *Proc. Nat. Acad. Sc.*, April, 1951.

———— and ————: A proposed structure for the nucleic acids, *Proc. Nat. Acad. Sc.*, February, 1953.

————: Abnormality of hemoglobin molecules in hereditary hemolytic anemias, *Harvey Lect.*, 1953–1954.

Wilder Penfield and Theodore Rasmussen: The Cerebral Cortex of Man, Macmillan, New York, 1950.

————: Some observations on the functional organization of the human brain, *Proc., Am. Philosophical Society*, October 15, 1954.

———— and H. H. Jasper: Epilepsy and the Functional Anatomy of the Human Brain, Little Brown, Boston, 1954.

G. A. Perera: The adrenal cortex and hypertensive vascular disease, Hypertension, E. T. Bell, ed., University of Minnesota Press, Minneapolis, 1951.

I. Perlman and J. M. Hollander: Radioactivity and nuclear structure, *Ann. Rev. Physical Chem.*, 1954.

J. P. Peters: The interrelations of foodstuffs in metabolism, *Yale J. Biol. and Med.*, September, 1951.

Carroll A. Pfeiffer: Endocrinology of reproduction, *Ann. Rev. Physiol.*, 1943.

G. W. Pickering: The vascular physiology of hypertension, *Advances in Internal Med.*, 1950.

Gregory Pincus: Factors controlling the growth of rabbit blastocysts, *Am. J. Physiol.*, June, 1941.

————: The chemistry and metabolism of the steroid hormones, *Ann. Rev. Biochem.*, 1950.

R. L. Platzman: On the primary processes in radiation chemistry and biology, Symposium on Radiobiology (National Research Council), J. J. Nickson, ed., Wiley, New York, 1952.

————: Influences of details of electronic binding on penetration phenomena, and the penetration of energetic charged particles through liquid water, Symposium on Radiobiology (National Research Council), J. J. Nickson, ed., Wiley, New York, 1952.

A. W. Pollister: Nucleoproteins of the nucleus, Symposium on the chemistry and physiology of the nucleus, *Exper. Cell Res.*, Suppl. 2, 1952.

W. T. Pommerenke and M. A. Breckenridge: Biochemical studies of the female genital tract, Conference on world population problems in birth control, *Ann. New York Acad. Sc.*, May 2, 1952.

K. R. Porter and F. L. Kallman: Significance of cell particulates as seen by electron microscopy, Conference on viruses as causative agents in cancer, *Ann. New York Acad. Sc.*, July 10, 1952.

R. W. PORTER: Alterations in electrical activity of the hypothalamus induced by stress stimuli, *Am. J. Physiol.*, June, 1952.

EDITH L. POTTER and F. L. ADAIR: Fetal and Neonatal Death, University of Chicago Press, Chicago, 1950.

V. R. POTTER: Enzymes, Growth and Cancer, Thomas, Springfield, Illinois, 1950.

—— and CHARLES HEIDELBERGER: Alternative metabolic pathways, *Physiol. Rev.*, October, 1950.

DOROTHY PRICE: Analysis of factors influencing growth and development of mammalian reproductive tract, *Physiol. Zöl.*, July, 1947.

W. H. PRICE and C. F. CORI: The separation of adenosinetriphosphatase from myosin and its activation by creatine, *J. Biol. Chem.*, February, 1946.

C. L. PROSSER: Problems in the comparative physiology of nervous systems, Modern Trends in Physiology and Biochemistry, E. S. Guzman Barron, ed., Academic Press, New York, 1952.

M. G. M. PRYOR: The molecular mechanism of contraction, A discussion on muscular contraction and relaxation: their physical and chemical basis, A. V. Hill, leader, *Proc. Roy. Soc. London*, April 13, 1950.

PUBLIC HEALTH SERVICE (NATIONAL INSTITUTE OF MENTAL HEALTH): Evaluation of Psychosurgery, Proceedings, Research Conference (3rd, 1951) on Psychosurgery, Public Health Service publication No. 221, U.S. Government Printing Office, Washington, 1954.

F. W. PUTNAM: Bacteriophages: nature and reproduction, *Advances in Protein Chem.*, 1953.

HENRY QUASTLER: Feedback mechanism in cellular biology, Conference (9th) on cybernetics, Heinz von Foerster, Margaret Mead and H. L. Teuber, eds., Josiah Macy, Jr. Foundation, New York, 1953.

A. J. QUICK: Is the action of calcium in the coagulation of blood stoichiometric or catalytic?, *Science*, December 12, 1947.

W. RAAB: Specific sympathomimetic substances in brain, *Am. J. Physiol.*, February, 1948.

E. I. RABINOWITCH: Photosynthesis and Related Processes, Interscience, New York, 1945.

SIDNEY RAFFEL: The relationship of acquired resistance, allergy, antibodies and tissue reactivities to the components of the tubercle bacillus, *Am. Rev. Tuberc.*, December, 1946.

——: Immunity, Hypersensitivity, Serology; Appleton-Century-Crofts, New York, 1953.

CHARLES RAGAN and KARL MEYER: Hyaluronic acid — hyaluronidase and the rheumatic diseases, Conference on the ground substance of the mesenchyme and hyaluronidase, *Ann. New York Acad. Sc.*, May, 1950.

——: The physiology of the connective tissue (loose areolar), *Ann. Rev. Physiol.*, 1952.

GEOFFREY RAKE: The lymphogranuloma-psittacosis group, Conference on virus and rickettsial classification and nomenclature, *Ann. New York Acad. Sc.*, March 31, 1953.

ELAINE P. RALLI and MARY E. DUMM: Relation of pantothenic acid to adrenal cortical function, *Vitamins and Hormones*, 1953.

J. T. Randall and M. H. G. Friedlaender: The microstructure of ram spermatozoa, *Exper. Cell Res.*, January, 1950.

S. W. Ranson: The Anatomy of the Nervous System; Its Development and Function, 9th ed., revised by S. L. Clark, Saunders, Philadelphia, 1953.

I. S. Ravdin: The direction of surgical effort, Research in Medical Science, D. E. Green and W. E. Knox, eds., Macmillan, New York, 1950.

F. C. Redlich: The concept of schizophrenia and its implications for therapy, Psychotherapy with Schizophrenics, E. B. Brody and F. C. Redlich, eds., International Universities Press, New York, 1952.

C. I. Reed, Herman Joffe and N. R. Joseph: Autonomic control of the synovial-fluid reaction, *J. Bone and Joint Surg.*, April, 1947.

Tadeus Reichstein and C. W. Shoppee: Hormones of the adrenal cortex, *Vitamins and Hormones*, 1943.

E. Reid: Growth hormone and adrenocortical hormones in relation to experimental tumors, *Cancer Res.*, May, 1954.

W. O. Reinhardt and C. H. Li: Experimental production of arthritis in rats by hypophyseal growth hormone, *Science*, March 20, 1953.

S. R. M. Reynolds: Determinants of uterine growth and activity, *Physiol. Rev.*, July, 1951.

C. P. Rhoads: Neoplastic abnormal growth, The Chemistry and Physiology of Growth, A. K. Parpart, ed., Princeton University Press, New Jersey, 1949.

————: Rational cancer chemotherapy, *Science*, January 15, 1954.

A. R. Rich: The significance of hypersensitivity in infections, *Physiol. Rev.*, January, 1941.

————: Hypersensitivity in disease with especial reference to periarteritis nodosa, rheumatic fever, disseminated lupus erythematosus and rheumatoid arthritis, *Harvey Lect.*, 1946–1947.

————: The Pathogenesis of Tuberculosis, Thomas, Springfield, Illinois, 1951.

D. W. Richards, Jr.: Pulmonary physiology, Research in Medical Science, D. E. Green and W. E. Knox, eds., Macmillan, New York, 1950.

Derek Richter: The biochemistry of cerebral function, Perspectives in Neuropsychiatry, Oxford Conference of the Mental Health Research Fund, Derek Richter, ed., Lewis, London, 1950.

R. L. Riley and A. F. Cournand: Pulmonary function studies in relation to chest surgery, *Advances in Surg.*, 1949.

J. F. Rinehart and L. D. Greenberg: Pathogenesis of experimental arteriosclerosis in pyridoxine deficiency, with notes on similarities to human arteriosclerosis, *A.M.A. Arch. Path.*, January, 1951.

David Rittenberg and Konrad Bloch: The utilization of acetic acid for the synthesis of fatty acids, *J. Biol. Chem.*, October, 1945.

————: The application of the isotope technique to the study of the metabolism of glycine, Biological Applications of Tracer Elements, *Cold Spring Harbor Symp. Quant. Biol.*, 1948.

————: Dynamic aspects of the metabolism of amino acids, *Harvey Lect.*, 1948–1949.

T. M. Rivers: General aspects of viral and rickettsial infections, Viral and Rickettsial Infections of Man, T. M. Rivers, ed., Lippincott, Philadelphia, 1948.

A. H. T. Robb-Smith: The nature of reticulin, Transactions, Conference (3rd) on connective tissues, Charles Ragan, ed., Josiah Macy, Jr. Foundation, New York, 1952.

ELI ROBINS and D. E. SMITH: A quantitative histochemical study of eight enzymes of the cerebellar cortex and subjacent white matter in the monkey, Metabolic and Toxic Diseases of the Nervous System, Proceedings, Association for Research in Nervous and Mental Disease, Williams and Wilkins, Baltimore, 1953.

JOHN ROCK and M. F. MENKIN: In vitro fertilization and cleavage of human ovarian eggs, *Science*, August 4, 1944.

MARIAN W. ROPES and WALTER BAUER: Synovial Fluid Changes in Joint Disease, Commonwealth Fund, Harvard University Press, Cambridge, 1953.

W. C. J. ROSS: The chemistry of cytotoxic alkylating agents, *Advances in Cancer Research*, 1953.

SIDNEY ROTHBARD: Protective effect of hyaluronidase and type-specific anti-M serum on experimental group A streptococcus infections in mice, *J. Exper. Med.*, September, 1948.

PEYTON ROUS: Viruses and tumors, Virus Diseases, Members of the Rockefeller Institute for Medical Research, Cornell University Press, Ithaca, 1943.

———: Recent advances in cancer research, *Bull. New York Acad. Med.*, February, 1947.

JURGEN RUESCH and GREGORY BATESON: Communication: The Social Matrix of Psychiatry, Norton, New York, 1951.

JOHN RUNNSTRÖM: Fertilization in metazoa, *Advances in Enzymol.*, 1949.

———: The cytoplasm, its structure and role in metabolism, growth and differentiation, Modern Trends in Physiology and Biochemistry, E. S. Guzman Barron, ed., Academic Press, New York, 1952.

H. B. RUSCH: Extrinsic factors that influence carcinogenesis, *Physiol. Rev.*, April, 1944.

E. M. RUSS, H. A. EDER and D. P. BARR: Protein-lipid relationships in human plasma; in normal individuals, *Am. J. Med.*, October, 1951.

L. B. RUSSELL and W. L. RUSSELL: Radiation hazards to embryo and fetus, *Radiology*, March, 1952.

W. L. RUSSELL: Mammalian radiation genetics, Symposium on Radiobiology (National Research Council), J. J. Nickson, ed., Wiley, New York, 1952.

A. B. SABIN: The dengue group of viruses and its family relationships, Symposium on viral and rickettsial diseases, *Bact. Rev.*, September, 1950.

———: Genetic, hormonal and age factors in natural resistance to certain viruses, Conference on viruses as causative agents in cancer, *Ann. New York Acad. Sc.*, July 10, 1952.

———: Infection and immunity in poliomyelitis: avirulent viruses for immunization against poliomyelitis, International (3rd) Poliomyelitis Conference, September, 1954.

FLORENCE R. SABIN: Cellular reactions to fractions from tubercle bacilli, *Am. Rev. Tuberc.*, October, 1941.

JACOB SACKS: Mechanism of phosphate transfer across cell membranes, Biological Applications of Tracer Elements, *Cold Spring Harbor Symp. Quant. Biol.*, 1948.

MANFRED SAKEL: The classical Sakel shock treatment, *J. Clin. and Exper. Psychopath.*, July–September, 1954.

J. E. SALK: Immunization against poliomyelitis, Symposium on Poliomyelitis, National Foundation for Infantile Paralysis, *Pediatric Clinics of North America*, Volume 1, No. 1A, 1953.

BENNETT SALLMAN and J. M. BIRKELAND: The role of hyaluronidase in hemolytic streptococcal infection, Conference on the ground substance of the mesenchyme and hyaluronidase, *Ann. New York Acad. Sc.*, May 31, 1950.

K. F. SANDERS: Possible multiplication cycles in neurotropic viruses, The Nature of Virus Multiplication, Symposium (2nd) Society for General Microbiology, University Press, Cambridge, 1953.

NEVITT SANFORD: Clinical methods: psychotherapy, *Ann. Rev. Psychology*, 1953.

F. SANGER: Some chemical investigations on the structure of insulin, Amino Acids and Proteins, *Cold Spring Harbor Symp. Quant. Biol.*, 1950.

L. H. SARETT, G. E. ARTH, R. M. LUKES, R. E. BEYLER, G. I. POOS, W. F. JOHNS and J. M. CONSTANTIN: Stereospecific total synthesis of cortisone, *J. Am. Chem. Soc.*, October, 1952.

GEORGE SAYERS, ABRAHAM WHITE and C. N. H. LONG: Preparation of pituitary adrenotropic hormone, *Proc. Soc. Exper. Biol. Med.*, March, 1943.

————: The adrenal cortex and homeostasis, *Physiol. Rev.*, July, 1950.

GEORGE SCATCHARD, W. L. HUGHES, JR., F. R. N. GURD and P. E. WILCOX: The interaction of proteins with small molecules and ions, Chemical Specificity in Biological Interactions, Harvard Memoirs, No. 3, F. R. N. Gurd, ed., Academic Press, New York, 1954.

FRITZ SCHLENK: Pyrimidine nucleosidases, Phosphorus Metabolism, Volume 1, W. D. McElroy and Bentley Glass, eds., Johns Hopkins Press, Baltimore, 1951.

R. W. SCHLESINGER: Immunological barriers to viral growth, Conference on viruses as causative agents in cancer, *Ann. New York Acad. Sc.*, July 10, 1952.

————: Developmental stages of viruses, *Ann. Rev. Microbiol.*, 1953.

J. G. SCHLICTER: Vascularization of the aorta in different species in health and disease, *Am. Heart J.*, May, 1948.

C. F. SCHMIDT: Recent studies of the cerebral circulation, *Harvey Lect.*, 1948–1949.

GERHARD SCHMIDT: Nucleoproteins and cancer, The Physiopathology of Cancer, Freddy Homburger and W. H. Fishman, eds., Hoeber-Harper, New York, 1953.

F. O. SCHMITT: Ultrastructure and the problem of cellular organization, *Harvey Lect.*, 1944–1945.

————: Molecular morphology and growth, The Chemistry and Physiology of Growth, A. K. Parpart, ed., Princeton University Press, New Jersey, 1949.

————: Morphology in muscle and nerve physiology, Metabolism and Function, David Nachmansohn, ed., Elsevier, Amsterdam, 1950.

RUDOLF SCHOENHEIMER: The Dynamic State of Body Constituents, Harvard University Press, Cambridge, 1942.

GEORGE SCHOLES and JOSEPH WEISS: Chemical action of x-rays on nucleic acids and related substances in aqueous systems, *Exper. Cell Res.*, Suppl. No. 2, 1952.

JACK SCHUBERT: Interactions of metals with small molecules in relation to metal protein complexes, Chemical Specificity in Biological Interactions, Harvard Memoirs, No. 3, F. R. N. Gurd, ed., Academic Press, New York, 1954.

PAULA SCHWERIN, S. P. BESSMAN, HEINRICH WAELSCH: The uptake of glutamic acid and glutamine by brain and other tissues of the rat and mouse, *J. Biol. Chem.*, May, 1950.

T. F. M. Scott: Diseases caused by the virus of herpes simplex, Viral and Rickettsial Infections of Man, T. M. Rivers, ed., Lippincott, Philadelphia, 1952.

W. H. Sebrell, Jr. and Klaus Schwarz: The role of B vitamins in the metabolism of the nervous system, Metabolic and Toxic Diseases of the Nervous System, Proceedings, Association for Research in Nervous and Mental Disease, Williams and Wilkins, Baltimore, 1953.

W. H. Seegers: Coagulation of the blood, *Harvey Lect.*, 1951–1952.

Florence B. Seibert: Constituents of mycobacteria, *Ann. Rev. Microbiol.*, 1950.

————: The chemistry of the proteins of the acid-fast bacilli, *Bact. Rev.*, March, 1951.

William Seifriz: The properties of protoplasm with special reference to the influence of enzymic reactions, *Advances in Enzymol.*, 1947.

————: Pathogenicity and isosterism, *Science*, January 2, 1948.

Joseph Seifter, W. E. Ehrich, D. H. Baeder, A. J. Butt and E. A. Hauser: Evidence for the direct effect of steroids on the ground substance, Conference on mechanism of corticosteroid action in disease processes, *Ann. New York Acad. Sc.*, July17, 1953.

Hans Selye: The Physiology and Pathology of Exposure to Stress, ACTA, Montreal, 1950.

M. C. Sevag, J. S. Gots and E. Steers: Enzymes in relation to genes, viruses, hormones, vitamins, and chemotherapeutic drug action, The Enzymes: Chemistry and Mechanism of Action, J. B. Sumner and Karl Myrbäck, eds., Volume 1, Part 1, Academic Press, N.Y., 1950.

M. J. Shear and J. Leiter: Studies in carcinogenesis; production of subcutaneous tumors in mice by miscellaneous polycyclic compounds, *J. Nat. Cancer Inst.*, December, 1941.

David Shemin and David Rittenberg: Some interrelations in general nitrogen metabolism, *J. Biol. Chem.*, May, 1944.

————: Some aspects of the biosynthesis of amino acids, Amino Acids and Proteins, *Cold Spring Harbor Symp. Quant. Biol.*, 1950.

C. S. Sherrington: Integrative Action of the Nervous System, University Press, Cambridge, 1947.

Sol Sherry: Current concepts of diabetes, *Bull. New York Acad. Med.*, March, 1953.

William Shive: The functions of B-vitamins in the biosynthesis of purines and pyrimidines, *Vitamins and Hormones*, 1951.

N. W. Shock: Ageing of homeostatic mechanisms, Cowdry's Problems of Ageing, A. I. Lansing, ed., Williams and Wilkins, Baltimore, 1952.

R. E. Shope: "Masking", transformation, and interepidemic survival of animal viruses, Conference on the similarities and dissimilarities between viruses attacking animals, plants, and bacteria, respectively, Viruses, Max Delbrück, ed., California Institute of Technology, Pasadena, 1950.

C. W. Shoppee: Steroids in relation to cancer from the chemical aspect, Steroid hormones and tumor growth, *Ciba Foundation Colloquia on Endocrinology*, Volume 1, 1952.

Ephraim Shorr, B. W. Zweifach and R. F. Furchgott: Hepato-renal factors in circulatory homeostasis, Conference on hemorrage, *Ann. New York Acad. Sc.*, May 11, 1948.

Gregory Shwartzman and S. M. Aronson: Alteration of experimental poliomyelitis by means of cortisone with reference to other viruses, The Effect of ACTH and Cortisone Upon Infection and Resistance, Gregory Shwartzman, ed., Columbia University Press, New York, 1953.

MARTIN SILBERBERG and RUTH SILBERBERG: The effects of endocrine secretions on articular tissues and their relation to ageing processes, Rheumatic Diseases, Proceedings (7th) International Congress on Rheumatic Diseases, Saunders, Philadelphia, 1952.

E. L. SIMMONS, L. O. JACOBSON, NORMAN PEARLMAN and C. L. PROSSER: The effectiveness of drugs in preventing or alleviating x-ray damage, Biological Effects of External X and Gamma Radiation (National Nuclear Energy Series, Volume B, Part 1), R. E. Zirkle, ed., McGraw-Hill, New York, 1954.

H. S. SIMMS: A review of research on lipfanogens and antilipfanogen, Symposium: studies on arteriosclerosis, J. Gerontol., April, 1951.

M. D. SIPERSTEIN, I. L. CHAIKOFF and S. S. CHERNICK: Significance of endogenous cholesterol in arteriosclerosis, Science, June 29, 1951.

E. T. O. SLATER: Perspectives in psychiatric genetics, Perspectives in Neuropsychiatry, Oxford Conference of the Mental Health Research Fund, Derek Richter, ed., Lewis, London, 1950.

S. R. SLAVSON: An Introduction to Group Therapy, Commonwealth Fund, New York, 1943.

M. W. SLEIN: Some studies of fructose metabolism, Phosphorus Metabolism, Volume 1, W. D. McElroy and Bentley Glass, eds., Johns Hopkins Press, Baltimore, 1951.

J. E. SMADEL: Serologic reactions in viral and rickettsial infections, Viral and Rickettsial Infections of Man, T. M. Rivers, ed., Lippincott, Philadelphia, 1952.

————: Smallpox and Vaccinia, Viral and Rickettsial Infections of Man, T. M. Rivers, ed., Lippincott, Philadelphia, 1952.

E. L. SMITH: Aspects of the specificity and mode of action of some peptidases, Enzymes and Enzyme Systems, J. T. Edsall, ed., Harvard University Press, Cambridge, 1951.

H. W. SMITH: The Kidney: Structure and Function in Health and Disease, Oxford University Press, New York, 1951.

K. U. SMITH: Learning and the associative pathways of the human cerebral cortex, Science, August 3, 1951.

W. E. SMITH, J. G. KIDD and PEYTON ROUS: Experiments on cause of rabbit carcinomas derived from virus-induced papillomas; propagation of several cancers in sucklings, with etiological tests, J. Exper. Med., March, 1952.

E. E. SNELL and G. M. BROWN: Pantethine and related forms of the Lactobacillus bulgaricus factor, Advances in Enzymol., 1953.

G. D. SNELL: Semi-sterility in the mouse caused by radiation-induced chromosome changes, Studies on Testis and Ovary, Eggs and Sperm, E. T. Engle, ed., Thomas, Springfield, Illinois, 1952.

T. M. SONNEBORN: Experimental control of the concentration of cytoplasmic genetic factors in paramecium, Heredity and Variation in Microorganisms, Cold Spring Harbor Symp. Quant. Biol., 1946.

A. H. SPARROW, M. J. MOSES and R. J. DUBOW: Relationships between ionizing radiation, chromosome breakage and certain other nuclear disturbances, Exper. Cell Res., Suppl. No. 2, 1952.

F. G. SPEAR: The biological effects of penetrating radiations, Brit. M. Bull., Volume 4, 1946.

SOL SPIEGELMAN and M. D. KAMEN: Genes and nucleoproteins in the synthesis of enzymes, Science, December 20, 1946.

————: Modern aspects of enzymatic adaptation, The Enzymes: Chemistry and

Mechanism of Action, J. B. Sumner and Karl Myrbäck, eds., Volume 1, Part 1, Academic Press, New York, 1950.

O. L. Sponsler and J. D. Bath: Molecular structure in protoplasm, A Symposium on The Structure of Protoplasm, William Seifriz, ed., Iowa College Press, 1942.

D. B. Sprinson: Studies on the metabolism of proteins, A Symposium on the Use of Isotopes in Biology and Medicine, University of Wisconsin Press, Madison, 1948.

D. H. Sprunt: The ground substance in infection, Conference on the ground substance of the mesenchyme and hyaluronidase, Ann. New York Acad. Sc., May 31, 1950.

W. C. Stadie: Current concepts of the action of insulin, Physiol. Rev., January, 1954.

E. R. Stadtman: On the energy-rich nature of acetyl imidazole, an enzymatically active compound, A Symposium on the Mechanism of Enzyme Action, W. D. McElroy and Bentley Glass, eds, Johns Hopkins Press, Baltimore, 1954.

W. M. Stanley: Chemical structure and the mutation of viruses, Virus Diseases, by Members of the Rockefeller Institute for Medical Research, Cornell University Press, Ithaca, 1943.

———: Viruses as chemical agents, Poliomyelitis, International (2nd) Poliomyelitis Conference, Lippincott, Philadelphia, 1952.

———, H. L. Bachrach and C. E. Schwerdt: Biochemical and physicochemical identification of Type II human poliomyelitis viruses, Science, November 13, 1953.

J. F. Stauffer and M. P. Backus: Spontaneous and induced variation in selected stocks of the Penicillium chrysogenum series, Conference on speciation and variation in asexual fungi, Ann. New York Acad. Sc., October 29, 1954.

W. H. Stein and Stanford Moore: Chromatographic determination of the amino acid composition of proteins, Amino Acids and Proteins, Cold Spring Harbor Symp. Quant. Biol., 1950.

H. B. Steinbach: The sodium and potassium balance of muscle and nerve, Modern Trends in Physiology and Biochemistry, E. S. Guzman Barron, ed., Academic Press, New York, 1952.

Curt Stern: Genetic aspects of sterility, Fertil. and Steril., September, 1950.

J. R. Stern and Severo Ochoa: Enzymatic synthesis of citric acid by condensation of acetate and oxalacetate, J. Biol. Chem., May, 1949.

K. G. Stern: Growth as a problem of chemical catalysis, Growth, Volume 6, Suppl., 1942.

———: Problems in nuclear chemistry and biology, Symposium on the chemistry and physiology of the nucleus, Exper. Cell Res., Suppl. 2, 1952.

DeWitt Stetten, Jr.: The endocrine regulation of carbohydrate metabolism, JAMA, October 19, 1946.

———: The alterations in metabolism incident to administration of insulin, adrenaline, and thyroid substances, studied with the aid of isotopes, Recent Progress in Hormone Research, Volume 4, 1949.

———: Biochemical explorations of certain disturbances of carbohydrate metabolism, Tr. and Stud. Coll. Physicians, Philadelphia, February, 1955.

H. C. Stoerk: Depression by cortisone of inherited and acquired resistance to infection and to tumor grafting, The Effect of ACTH and Cortisone upon Infection and Resistance, Gregory Shwartzman, ed., Columbia University Press, New York, 1953.

L. C. Strong: A new theory of mutation and origin of cancer, Yale J. Biol. and Med., March, 1949.

A. H. STURTEVANT: Social implications of the genetics of man, *Science*, September 10, 1954.

H. S. SULLIVAN: The Interpersonal Theory of Psychiatry, Helen S. Perry and Mary L. Gawel, eds., Norton, New York, 1953.

J. B. SUMNER: The chemical nature of enzymes, Nobel Laureate Lecture, *J. Wash. Acad. Sc.*, April 15, 1948.

—— and KARL MYRBÄCK: Introduction, The Enzymes: Chemistry and Mechanism of Action, J. B. Sumner and Karl Myrbäck, eds., Volume 1, Part 1, Academic Press, New York, 1950.

E. W. SUTHERLAND: The effect of the hyperglycemic factor and epinephrine on enzyme systems of liver and muscle, Conference on the influence of hormones on enzymes, *Ann. New York Acad. Sc.*, December 28, 1951.

H. F. SWIFT: The streptococcal etiology of rheumatic fever, Rheumatic Diseases, Proceedings (7th) International Congress on Rheumatic Diseases, Saunders, Philadelphia, 1952.

W. W. SWINGLE and J. W. REMINGTON: The role of the adrenal cortex in physiological processes, *Physiol. Rev.*, January, 1944.

J. T. SYVERTON and W. F. SCHERER: Applications of strains of mammalian cells to the study of animal viruses, Viruses, *Cold Spring Harbor Symp. Quant. Biol.*, 1953.

ALBERT SZENT-GYÖRGYI: Thermodynamics and muscle, Modern Trends in Physiology and Biochemistry, E. S. Guzman Barron, ed., Academic Press, New York, 1952.

——: Chemistry and Physiology of Contraction in Body and Heart Muscle, Academic Press, New York, 1953.

M. L. TAINTER and F. P. LUDUENA: Sympathetic hormonal transmission, *Recent Progress in Hormone Research*, Volume 5, 1950.

W. H. TALIAFERRO: The cellular basis of immunity, *Ann. Rev. Microbiol.*, 1949.

ALBERT TANNENBAUM and HERBERT SILVERSTONE: Nutrition in relation to cancer, *Advances in Cancer Research*, 1953.

E. L. TATUM: Induced biochemical mutations in bacteria, Heredity and Variation in Microorganisms, *Cold Spring Harbor Symp. Quant. Biol.*, 1946.

C. B. TAYLOR and R. G. GOULD: Effect of dietary cholesterol on rate of cholesterol synthesis in the intact animal measured by means of radioactive carbon, *Circulation*, September, 1950.

TORSTEN TEORELL: Permeability, *Ann. Rev. Physiol.*, 1949.

MAX THEILER: Yellow fever, Viral and Rickettsial Infections of Man, T. M. Rivers, ed., Lippincott, Philadelphia, 1952.

HUGO THEORELL: Heme-linked groups and mode of action of some hemoproteins, *Advances in Enzymol.*, 1947.

K. V. THIMANN: Plant hormones and the analysis of growth, Currents in Biochemical Research, D. E. Green, ed., Interscience, New York, 1946.

LEWIS THOMAS: The generalized Shwartzman reaction in rabbits infected with group A hemolytic streptococci, Rheumatic Fever, A Symposium, Lewis Thomas, ed., University of Minnesota Press, Minneapolis, 1952.

——: The effects of cortisone on bacterial infection and intoxication, The Effect of ACTH and Cortisone upon Infection and Resistance, Gregory Shwartzman, ed., Columbia University Press, New York, 1953.

D. W. THOMPSON: On Growth and Form, University Press, Cambridge, 1942.

W. S. TILLETT: Infectious diseases, *Ann. Rev. Med.*, 1953.

A. R. TODD: The nucleotides: Some recent chemical research and its biological implications, *Harvey Lect.*, 1951–1952.

————: Chemical structure of the nucleic acids, *Proc. Nat. Acad. Sc.*, August, 1954.

G. M. TOMKINS, H. SHEPPARD and I. L. CHAIKOFF: Cholesterol synthesis by liver, *J. Biol. Chem.*, August, 1953.

H. P. TREFFERS: Serology and immunochemistry, Bacterial and Mycotic Infections of Man, R. J. Dubos, ed., Lippincott, Philadelphia, 1952.

G. R. TRISTRAM: Amino acid composition of purified proteins, *Advances in Protein Chem.*, 1949.

R. B. TURNER: Physical and chemical properties of the steroids related to protein binding, Chemical Specificity in Biological Interactions, Harvard Memoirs, No. 3, F. R. N. Gurd, ed., Academic Press, New York, 1954.

R. H. TURNER, J. R. SNAVELY, W. H. GOLDWATER and M. L. RANDOLPH: The study of serum proteins and lipids with the aid of the quantity ultracentrifuge, *Yale J. Biol. and Med.*, June, 1952.

T. B. TURNER and D. H. HOLLANDER: Studies on the mechanism of action of cortisone in experimental syphilis, The Effect of ACTH and Cortisone upon Infection and Resistance, Gregory Shwartzman, ed., Columbia University Press, New York, 1953.

ALBERT TYLER: Fertilization and immunity, *Physiol. Rev.*, April, 1948.

H. C. UREY: Methods and objectives in the separation of isotopes, *Proc., Am. Philosophical Soc.*, January 29, 1946.

H. B. VAN DYKE: The regulation of water excretion by the neurohyphysis, Hormones in Health and Disease, R. L. Craig, ed., Macmillan, New York, 1954.

C. B. VAN NIEL: The bacterial photosyntheses and their importance to the general problem of photosynthesis, *Advances in Enzymol.*, 1941.

————: The kinetics of growth of microorganisms, The Chemistry and Physiology of Growth, A. K. Parpart, ed., Princeton University Press, Princeton, 1949.

GERTRUDE VAN WAGENEN: Reproduction, *Ann. Rev. Physiol.*, 1947.

H. B. VICKERY: The contribution of the analytical chemist to protein chemistry, Conference on amino acid analysis of proteins, *Ann. New York Acad. Sc.*, August 29, 1946.

CARL VOEGTLIN: Trends in cancer research, *J. Nat. Cancer Inst.*, February, 1942.

MARTHE VOGT: Biological assays of cortical hormones and estimation of the rate of secretion of the mammalian suprarenal cortex, *J. Endocrinol.*, November, 1947.

H. VON EULER: Adaptation of microorganisms to antibacterial substances, International (4th) Congress for Microbiology, 1947, Rosenkilde and Bagger, Copenhagen, 1949.

U. S. V. EULER: Sympathin E and nor-adrenalin, *Science*, April 23, 1948.

HEINZ VON FOERSTER, MARGARET MEAD and H. L. TEUBER: A note by the editors, Transactions, Conferences (8th and 9th) on cybernetics, Josiah Macy, Jr. Foundation, New York, 1952, 1953.

ALEXANDER VON MURALT: The development of muscle-chemistry, a lesson in neurophysiology, Metabolism and Function, David Nachmansohn, ed., Elsevier, Amsterdam, 1950.

HEINRICH WAELSCH: Certain aspects of intermediary metabolism of glutamine, asparagine, and glutathione, *Advances in Enzymol.*, 1952.

S. A. WAKSMAN: Microbial Antagonisms and Antibiotic Substances, The Commonwealth Fund, New York, 1945.

GEORGE WALD: The interconversion of the retinenes and vitamins A *in vitro*, Metabolism and Function, David Nachmansohn, ed., Elsevier, Amsterdam, 1950.

A. E. WALKER and R. G. FISHER: Recent advances in the treatment of craniocerebral injuries, *Advances in Surg.*, Volume 2, 1949.

MERRILL WALLENSTEIN, A. L. WAHRHAFTIG, HENRY ROSENSTOCK and HENRY EYRING: Chemical reactions in the gas phase connected with ionization, Symposium on Radiobiology (National Research Council), J. J. Nickson, ed., Wiley, New York, 1952.

OTTO WARBURG: Heavy Metal Prosthetic Groups, Clarendon Press, Oxford, 1949.

SHIELDS WARREN: The effects of X ray and other radiations on proteins and living tissues, Chemical Specificity in Biological Interactions, Harvard Memoirs, No. 3, F. R. N. Gurd, ed., Academic Press, New York, 1954.

J. D. WATSON and F. H. C. CRICK: The structure of DNA, Viruses, *Cold Spring Harbor Symp. Quant. Biol.*, 1953.

H. H. WEBER: Adenosine triphosphate and motility of living systems, *Harvey Lect.*, 1953–1954.

L. T. WEBSTER: Rabies, Macmillan, New York, 1942.

H. J. WEGROCKI: A critique of cultural and statistical concepts of abnormality, Personality in Nature, Society, and Culture, Clyde Kluckhohn and H. A. Murray, eds., Knopf, New York, 1953.

SIDNEY WEINHOUSE: Isotope studies on two-carbon acids, Phosphorus Metabolism, Volume 1, W. D. McElroy and Bentley Glass, eds., Johns Hopkins Press, Baltimore, 1951.

PAUL WEISS: Problem of specificity in growth and development, *Yale J. Biol. and Med.*, January, 1947.

———: The biological basis of adaptation, Adaptation, John Romano, ed., Cornell University Press, Ithaca, New York, 1949.

———: Differential growth, The Chemistry and Physiology of Growth, A. K. Parpart, ed., Princeton University Press, Princeton, 1949.

———: Medicine and society: The biological foundations, *J. Mt. Sinai Hosp.*, March–April, 1953.

I. D. WELT and A. E. WILHELMI: The effect of adrenalectomy and of the adrenocorticotrophic and growth hormones on the synthesis of fatty acids, *Yale J. Biol. and Med.*, November, 1950.

N. T. WERTHESSEN, ERWIN SCHWENK and CYRIL BAKER: Biosynthesis of estrone and β-estradiol in the perfused ovary, *Science*, April 10, 1953.

ABRAHAM WHITE: Preparation and chemistry of anterior pituitary hormones, *Physiol. Rev.*, October, 1946.

R. W. WHITE: Abnormalities of behavior, *Ann. Rev. Psychol.*, 1953.

J. C. WHITEHORN: Psychodynamic approach to the study of psychoses, Dynamic Psychiatry, Franz Alexander and Helen Ross, eds., University of Chicago Press, Chicago, 1952.

A. N. WICK, D. R. DRURY and E. M. MACKAY: The disposition of glucose by the extrahepatic tissues, Conference on the influence of hormones on enzymes, *Ann. New York Acad. Sc.*, December 28, 1951.

NORBERT WIENER: Cybernetics or Control and Communication in the Animal and the Machine, Technology Press, Wiley, New York, 1949.

R. C. WILLIAMS: The shapes and sizes of purified viruses as determined by electron microscopy, Viruses, *Cold Spring Harbor Symp. Quant. Biol.*, 1953.

R. J. WILLIAMS: B vitamins and cancer, A.A.A.S. Research Conference on Cancer, F. R. Moulton, ed., A.A.A.S., Washington, 1945.

———, L. J. BERRY and ERNEST BEERSTECHER, JR.: Individual metabolic patterns, alcoholism, genetotrophic diseases, *Science*, June, 1949.

B. H. WILLIER: Phases in embryonic development, *J. Cell. and Comp. Physiol.*, Volume 43, Suppl. 1, 1954.

I. B. WILSON: Biochemical similarities and differences between synaptic transmission and axonal conduction, Conference (3rd) on nerve impulse, H. H. Merritt, ed., Josiah Macy, Jr. Foundation, New York, 1952.

J. G. WILSON and JOSEF WARKANY: Cardiac and aortic anomalies in the offspring of vitamin A deficient rats correlated with similar human anomalies, *Pediatrics*, April, 1950.

P. W. WILSON and R. H. BURRIS: Biological nitrogen fixation — a reappraisal, *Ann. Rev. Microbiol.*, 1953.

R. R. WILSON: Beams of high-energy particles, Symposium on Radiobiology (National Research Council), J. J. Nickson, ed., Wiley, New York, 1952.

R. J. WINZLER: The chemistry of cancer tissue, The Physiopathology of Cancer, Freddy Homburger and W. H. Fishman, eds., Hoeber-Harper, New York, 1953.

G. B. WISLOCKI and E. W. DEMPSEY: Histochemical reactions in the endometrium in pregnancy, *Am. J. Anat.*, November, 1945.

EMIL WITSCHI: Developmental physiology, *Ann. Rev. Physiol.*, 1941.

C. A. WOERNER: Microscopic anatomy of the arterial wall, Symposium: studies on arteriosclerosis, *J. Gerontol.*, April, 1951.

H. G. WOLFF: Changes in the vulnerability of tissue: an aspect of man's response to threat, The National Institutes of Health Annual Lectures — 1953, United States Public Health Service, Washington, 1954.

H. G. WOOD: The fixation of carbon dioxide and the inter-relationships of the tricarboxylic acid cycle, *Physiol. Rev.*, April, 1946.

W. B. WOOD, JR.: Studies on the cellular immunology of acute bacterial infections, *Harvey Lect.*, 1952–1953.

M. W. WOODS and H. G. DUBUY: Cytoplasmic diseases and cancer, *Science*, December 7, 1945.

R. B. WOODWARD, FRANZ SONDHEIMER, DAVID TAUB, KARL HEUSLER and W. M. McLAMORE: The total synthesis of steroids, *J. Am. Chem. Soc.*, September 6, 1952.

D. W. WOOLLEY: A Study of Antimetabolites, Wiley, New York, 1952.

——— and E. SHAW: Some neurophysiological aspects of serotonin, *Brit. M. J.*, July 17, 1954.

C. N. WOOLSEY: Patterns of localization in sensory and motor areas of the cerebral cortex, The Biology of Mental Health and Disease, Milbank Memorial Fund, Hoeber, New York, 1952.

SEWALL WRIGHT: Discussion on population genetics and radiation, *J. Cell. and Comp. Physiol.*, Volume 35, Suppl. 1, 1950.

R. W. G. WYCKOFF: The fine structure of connective tissues, Conference (3rd) on connective tissues, Charles Ragan, ed., Josiah Macy, Jr. Foundation, New York, 1952.

J. B. YOUMANS: Nutritional Deficiencies, 2nd edition, Lippincott, Philadelphia, 1942.

F. G. YOUNG: The growth hormone and diabetes, *Recent Progress in Hormone Research*, Volume 8, 1953.

W. C. YOUNG: Gamete-age at the time of fertilization and the course of gestation in mammals, Pregnancy Wastage, Proceedings, Conference sponsored by Committee on Human Reproduction (National Research Council), E. T. Engle, ed., Thomas, Springfield, Illinois, 1953.

R. E. ZIRKLE: Speculations on cellular actions of radiations, Symposium on Radiobiology (National Research Council), J. J. Nickson, ed., Wiley, New York, 1952.

—— and WILLIAM BLOOM: Irradiation of parts of individual cells, *Science*, May 8, 1953.

BERNHARD ZONDEK and FELIX SULMAN: The mechanism of action and metabolism of gonadotropic hormones in the organism, *Vitamins and Hormones*, 1945.

B. W. ZWEIFACH and ROBERT CHAMBERS: The action of hyaluronidase extracts on the capillary wall, Conference on the ground substance of the mesenchyme and hyaluronidase, *Ann. New York Acad. Sc.*, May 31, 1950.

——: Functional deterioration of the terminal vascular bed in irreversible hemorrhagic shock, Conference on shock syndrome, *Ann. New York Acad. Sc.*, September 3, 1952.